Atlas of Intestinal Stomas

Victor W. Fazio • James M. Church • James S. Wu
Editors

Atlas of Intestinal Stomas

Springer

Editors
Victor W. Fazio, A.O., M.B., B.S., M.S., F.R.A.C.S., F.R.A.C.S. (Hon), F.A.C.S., F.R.C.S (E. Hon), F.R.C.S (Ed. Hon), M.D. (Pol. Hon), F.R.C.S.I. (Hon)
Department of Colorectal Surgery
Digestive Diseases Institute
Cleveland Clinic Lerner College of Medicine of Case Western Reserve University
Cleveland Clinic Foundation
Cleveland, OH
USA
faziov@ccf.org

James M. Church, B.Sc. (Hum Bio), M.B. Ch.B., M.Med. Sci. (Anatomy), F.R.A.C.S.
Department of Colorectal Surgery
Digestive Disease Institute
Cleveland Clinic Foundation
Cleveland, OH
USA
churchj@ccf.org

James S. Wu, Ph.D., M.D.
Department of Colorectal Surgery
Digestive Disease Institute
Cleveland Clinic Foundation
Cleveland, OH
USA
wuj@ccf.org

ISBN 978-0-387-78850-0 ISBN 978-0-387-78851-7 (eBook)
DOI 10.1007/978-0-387-78851-7
Springer New York Dordrecht Heidelberg London

Library of Congress Control Number: 2011933843

Printed on acid-free paper

Springer is part of Springer Science+Business Media (www.springer.com)

This book is dedicated first and foremost to our late mentors, Dr. Rupert B. Turnbull, Jr., M.D. and Frank L. Weakley, M.D. And to Dr. Fazio's grandchildren, Halle, Kisandra, Griffin, James Hunter and Talon, to Dr. Church's grandchildren, James and Olivia; and to Dr. Wu's family, Margaret and Michelle.

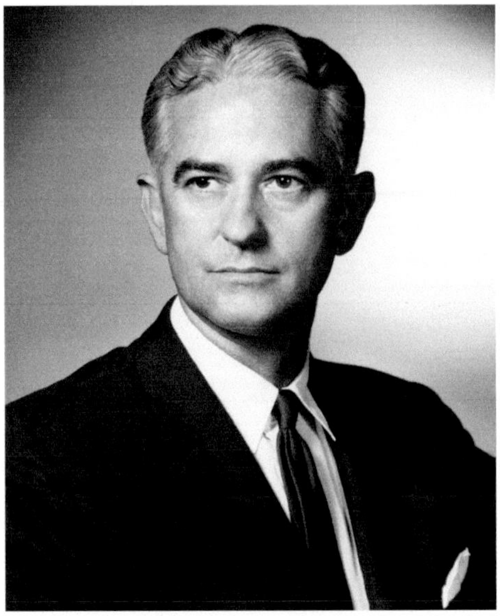

Fig. 1 Rupert B. Turnbull, Jr.

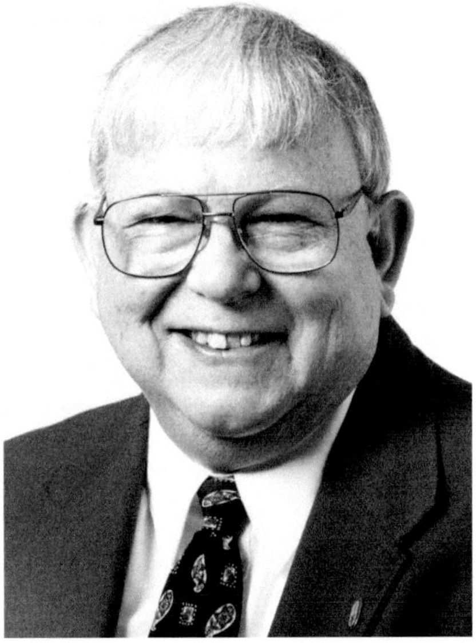

Fig. 2 Frank L. Weakley

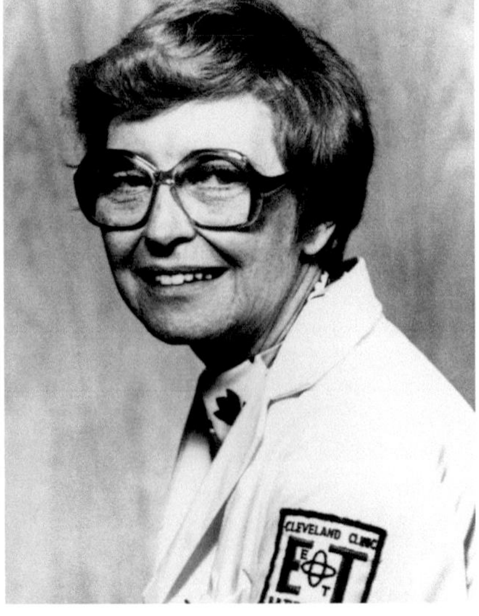

Fig. 3 Norma N. Gill, the first director of the Cleveland Clinic Foundation School of Enterostomal Therapy

Preface

The first edition of the *Atlas of Intestinal Stomas* by Rupert B. Turnbull (Fig. 1) and Frank L. Weakley (Fig. 2) was published in 1967 specifically to provide the practicing intestinal surgeon access to the techniques of ostomy construction. The principles leading to methods that worked were products of centuries-old experiences of surgeons around the world. Many of the techniques selected for illustration by Turnbull and Weakley are still standard in clinical practice. However, in the 43 years since the publication of the first edition, new procedures and new techniques have emerged. These advances stimulated us to update the Turnbull/Weakley Atlas with the *Atlas of Intestinal Stomas*. Additions include chapters on anatomy and physiology, biliary stomas, pediatric ostomies, the continent ileostomy, urostomy, laparoscopic stoma construction, stomas in trauma surgery, stomas for antegrade continence enema, percutaneous ostomies, and quality of life. There are also updated sections on ileostomy, colostomy, enterostomal therapy (Fig. 3), and on the management of complications of stomas such as management of the high output ostomy, enterocutaneous fistula, parastomal hernia, prolapse, and skin conditions. We also have included a chapter on particularly challenging stomas that we hope will be particularly helpful for surgeons faced with difficult circumstances.

This new edition differs from the first in that it is multi-authored. However, each chapter is written with a clarity and directness that is similar to the original.

The Turnbull/Weakley Atlas was illustrated by a single artist, Robert M. Reed, former head of the Cleveland Clinic Medical Illustration Department. *Atlas of Intestinal Stomas* is illustrated entirely by Joe Pangrace and his staff of the same department. Pangrace, mentored by Reed early in his career, has developed his own style of illustration that we describe as accurate, crisp, and beautiful.

Few of the contributing authors to the *Atlas of Intestinal Stomas* had the privilege of working closely with our "well diggers," Drs. Turnbull and Weakley. Those of us who did believe that they would be pleased with our work.

Victor W. Fazio, M.D.
James M. Church, M.D.
James S. Wu, M.D.

Acknowledgments

The editors acknowledge first the Cleveland Clinic Foundation for its enthusiastic support of this work. In particular, we acknowledge Ann Paladino, Director of the Cleveland Clinic Center for Medical Art and Photography and members of her team whose talent, skill, and efforts made this project possible. We thank Joe Pangrace, CMI; William Garriott; Elizabeth Halasz, CMI; and Wendy Knapp for their ability to clearly convey, through illustration, the surgical and medical concepts of this surgical atlas. We extend our appreciation to Kathleen Miller for digitalizing the quality of photographic slides and historical photos. We thank Jeffrey Loerch for processing licenses for hundreds of Cleveland Clinic illustrations and photographic works. We thank Joyce Balliet of the Department of Colorectal Surgery for her extensive photographic contributions to the book. We thank Marty Hodgson of the Department of Colorectal Surgery for her tireless support of this work over many years. We thank the Staff of the Cleveland Clinic Library for providing superlative access to the literature. We acknowledge each of the authors to this work who have selflessly given their knowledge, experience, and time. We thank Mr. Sreejith Viswanathan, Ms. Sajeni Ravindranathadas, and Ms. Vinitha Vipin our Project Managers at SPi Global for constructing the book. We gratefully thank our editors at Springer, Maureen Pierce, Paula Callaghan, Andy Kwan, Susan Westendorf, and Richard Hruska, who, with limitless patience and gentle nudging, guided us from drawing table to a completed work. Without the contributions of these individuals and their offices, this Atlas would not have been possible.

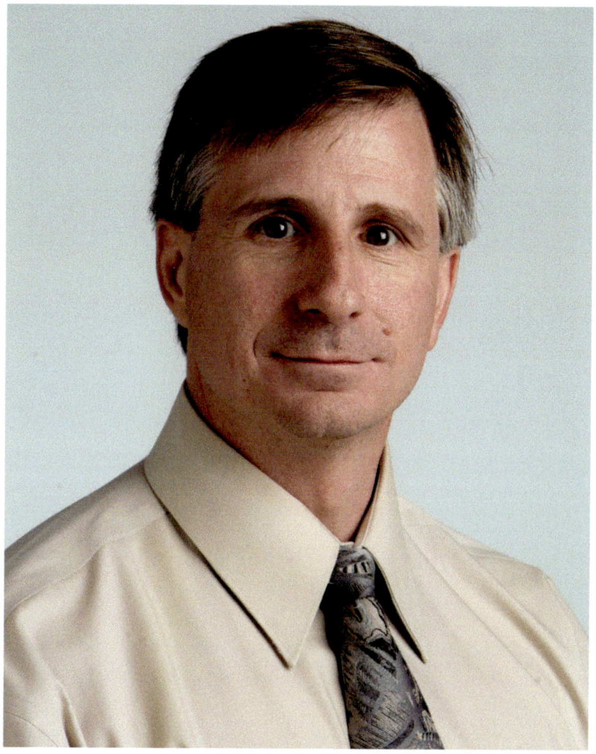

Fig. 4 Joseph A. Pangrace, CMI

For the past 28 years, Joseph Pangrace (Fig. 4) has applied his knowledge and skill as a medical illustrator for the Cleveland Clinic. Upon graduating in 1983 from the Cleveland Institute of Art's Medical Illustration program, he immediately began working at the Clinic, creating illustrations for use in publications, presentations, and videos. Over the course of his career, Pangrace's works have been published in major medical journals, textbooks, and atlases. In 2001, Pangrace assumed the responsibilities of Senior Medical Illustrator and Art Director for the *Cleveland Clinic Journal of Medicine*. In 2005, he was awarded the Association of Medical Illustrator's Max Bröedel award for continuous tone illustration. Pangrace currently acts as the Medical Illustration section leader for the Center for Medical Art and Photography. His artwork and that of his staff consistently reach the highest standards. We are indebted to Pangrace for his monumental contribution to the *Atlas of Intestinal Stomas*.

Victor W. Fazio, M.D.
James M. Church, M.D.
James S. Wu, M.D.

Contents

Contributors

Greg J. Beilman, M.D. Department of Surgery, University of Minnesota, Minneapolis, MN, USA

Ann E. Brannigan, M.Ch., F.R.C.S.I., F.R.C.S. Mater Misericordiae University Hospital, Dublin, Ireland

Matthew C. Byrnes, M.D. Department of Surgery, University of Minnesota, Minneapolis, MN, USA

James M. Church, B.Sc. (Hum Bio), M.B. Ch.B., M.Med. Sci. (Anatomy), F.R.A.C.S. Department of Colorectal Surgery, Digestive Diseases Institute, Cleveland Clinic Foundation, Cleveland, OH, USA

Eoghan Condon, M.B., B.Ch., B.A.O., F.R.C.S.I., M.D. Department of Surgery, Limerick University Hospital, Limerick, Ireland

Meagan M. Costedio, M.D. Department of Colorectal Surgery, Digestive Disease Institute, Cleveland Clinic Foundation, Cleveland, OH, USA

David Dietz, M.D., F.A.C.S., F.A.S.C.R.S. Department of Colorectal Surgery, Digestive Disease Institute, Cleveland Clinic Foundation, Cleveland, OH, USA

Richard L. Drake, Ph.D. Cleveland Clinic Lerner College of Medicine of Case Western Reserve University, Cleveland, OH, USA

Paula Erwin-Toth, M.S.N., R.N., E.T., C.W.O.C.N., C.N.S. The Rupert B. Turnbull School of WOC/ET, Cleveland Clinic/ET, Cleveland, OH, USA

Victor W. Fazio, A.O., M.B., B.S., M.S., F.R.A.C.S., F.R.A.C.S. (Hon), F.A.C.S., F.R.C.S (E. Hon), F.R.C.S (Ed. Hon), M.D. (Pol. Hon), F.R.C.S.I. (Hon) Department of Colorectal Surgery, Digestive Diseases Institute, Cleveland Clinic Lerner College of Medicine of Case Western Reserve University, Cleveland Clinic Foundation, Cleveland, OH, USA

Amr F. Fergany, M.D., Ph.D. Glickman Urological and Kidney Institute, Cleveland Clinic Foundation, Cleveland, OH, USA

Crina V. Floruta, M.S.N., C.N.P., C.W.O.C.N. Department of Colorectal Surgery, Digestive Disease Institute, Cleveland Clinic Foundation, Cleveland, OH, USA

John Fung, M.D., Ph.D. Digestive Disease Institute, Transplant Center, Cleveland Clinic Lerner College of Medicine, Cleveland Clinic Foundation, Cleveland, OH, USA

Thomas Garofalo, M.D., F.A.C.S. Department of Colorectal Surgery, Digestive Disease Institute, Cleveland Clinic Foundation, Cleveland, OH, USA

Daniel P. Geisler, M.D. West Penn Allegheny Health System, Pittsburgh, PA, USA

Brooke Gurland, M.D. Department of Colorectal Surgery, Digestive Disease Institute, Cleveland Clinic Foundation, Cleveland, OH, USA

Barbara Hocevar, B.S.N., R.N., C.W.O.C.N. Nursing Institute/Digestive Disease Institute, Cleveland Clinic/ET, Cleveland, OH, USA

Tracy A. Hull, M.D. Department of Colon and Rectal Surgery, Digestive Disease Institute, Cleveland Clinic Foundation, Cleveland, OH, USA

Michelle D. Inkster, M.D., Ph.D. Digestive Disease Institute, Cleveland Clinic Foundation, Cleveland, OH, USA

Michael D. Johnson, M.D. The Nebraska Medical Center, Surgical Services of the Great Plains, P.C., Omaha, NE, USA

Matthew F. Kalady, M.D., F.A.C.S., F.A.S.C.R.S. Department of Colorectal Surgery, Cleveland Clinic, Cleveland, OH, USA

Hermann Kessler, M.D., Ph.D. Department of Surgery, University of Erlangen, Erlangen, Germany

Ravi Pokala Kiran, M.B.B.S., M.S., F.R.C.S. (Eng), F.R.C.S. (Glas), F.A.C.S., F.A.S.C.R.S. Department of Colorectal Surgery, Digestive Disease Institute, Cleveland Clinic Foundation, Cleveland, OH, USA

Hasan T. Kirat, M.D. Department of Colorectal Surgery, Digestive Disease Institute, Cleveland Clinic Foundation, Cleveland, OH, USA

Ian C. Lavery, M.B.B.S., F.A.C.S. Department of Colorectal Surgery, Digestive Disease Institute, Cleveland Clinic Foundation, Cleveland, OH, USA

David K. Magnuson, M.D. Department of Pediatric Surgery, Cleveland Clinic Foundation, Cleveland, OH, USA

Jennifer M. McBride, Ph.D. Cleveland Clinic Lerner College of Medicine of Case Western Reserve University, Cleveland, OH, USA

James I. Merlino, M.D., F.A.C.S., F.A.S.C.R.S. Department of Colorectal Surgery, Digestive Disease Institute, Cleveland Clinic Foundation, Cleveland, OH, USA

Neha Parekh, M.S., R.D., L.D., C.N.S.D. Intestinal Rehabilitation and Transplant Nutrition, Digestive Disease Institute, Cleveland Clinic Foundation, Cleveland, OH, USA

Amit R. Patel, M.D. Urologic Oncology, University of Chicago Medical Center, Chicago, IL, USA

Feza H. Remzi, M.D., F.A.C.S., F.A.S.C.R.S. Department of Colorectal Surgery, Digestive Disease Institute, Cleveland Clinic Foundation, Cleveland, OH, USA

John Rombeau, M.D. Department of Veterans Affairs, Palo Alto Health Care System, Palo Alto, CA, USA

Douglas L. Seidner, M.D., F.A.C.G., C.N.S.P. Division of Gastroenterology, Hepatology and Nutrition, Vanderbilt Center for Human Nutrition, Vanderbilt University Medical Center, Nashville, TN, USA

Oliver S. Soldes, M.D., F.A.C.S., F.A.A.P. Department of Pediatric Surgery, Cleveland Clinic Foundation, Cleveland, OH, USA

Luca Stocchi, M.D., F.A.C.S., F.A.S.C.R.S. Department of Colorectal Surgery, Digestive Disease Institute, Cleveland Clinic Foundation, Cleveland, OH, USA

Linda J. Stricker, M.S.N/E.D., R.N., C.W.O.C.N., L.N.C. WOC Nursing Education, Cleveland Clinic/ET, Cleveland, OH, USA

Ursula M. Szmulowicz, M.D. Department of Colorectal Surgery, Cleveland Clinic Foundation, Cleveland, OH, USA

John J. Vargo II, M.D., M.P.H: A.G.A.F., F.A.C.P., F.A.C.G., F.A.S.G.E. Department of Gastroenterology and Hepatology, Digestive Disease Institute, Cleveland Clinic Foundation, Cleveland, OH, USA

Ryan S. Williams, M.D. Department of Colorectal Surgery, Digestive Diseases Institute, Cleveland Clinic Lerner College of Medicine of Case Western Reserve University, Cleveland Clinic Foundation, Cleveland, OH, USA

James S. Wu, Ph.D., M.D. Department of Colorectal Surgery, Digestive Disease Institute, Cleveland Clinic Foundation, Cleveland, OH, USA

Intestinal Stomas: Historical Overview 1

James S. Wu

Introduction

The word "stoma" is derived from the Greek, *stomat*, for mouth [1]. Gastrointestinal stomas are artificial connections of the gut to the skin. Reports of colostomies designed to relieve obstruction appear in the eighteenth century (Table 1.1) [1–21]. Small intestinal stomas are associated most closely with the twentieth century operations devised to treat inflammatory bowel, urologic, pediatric, and hepatobiliary conditions. Ostomies of the stomach were introduced to decompress the gut or to instill nutrition. This chapter recognizes contributions of pioneers from many disciplines whose work improved the lives of gastrointestinal stoma patients.

Anus Praeternaturalis, Künstlichen Afters, Anus Artificiel, Abdominal Anus [18]

Caelii Aureliani **Celerum Vel Acutarum Passionum** [19]	Caelius Aurelianus **On Swift or Acute Diseases** [21]
De Acuto Tormento, Quod Graeci Ileon Appellant [20]	*Acute Intestinal Obstruction (Greek ILEOS)* [22]
Tormentum dictum est quod existiment aegrotantes convolvi atque torqueri suorum intestinorum verticula, vel quod spiritus ob abstinentiam clausus sese involvens vinctiones atque tormenta efficiat, vel quod vehementia dolorum supra eas partes quae patiuntur aegrotantes arcuati convolutique plicentur.	Intestinal obstruction (*tormentum*, "ileus") gets its name either because the patient has a feeling that the folds of his intestines are tied up and twisted; or because the pneuma is blocked and shut off, the resulting involution of the flow producing cramps and twisting pains; or else because the violent pains over the parts affected cause the patient to be bent over, twisted, and doubled up.

The agony of intestinal obstruction has been recognized since antiquity. Treatments described by Caelius Aurelianus [23] were predominantly supportive and included: rest, fasting, wine, venesection, the application of mild heat to relieve the pain, clysters (enemas), hernia reduction, emetics, and the ingestion of a lead pill to drive out the obstructing matter [24]. Caelius attributes a surgical solution for intestinal obstruction to Praxagorus of Cos, a surgeon who reportedly lived in the fourth century BC [25].

Praxagoras tertio libro Curationum clysterem iubet adhiberi, dans medicamina purgativae virtutis, atque per vomitum corpora dissecari [26].	In Book III of his work *On Treatments*, Praxagorus prescribes a clyster, purgative drugs, and emetics to dry out the body [27].
Item confectis quibusdam supradictis adiutoriis dividendum probat pubetenus, dividendum etiam intestinum rectum atque detracto stercore consuendum dicit, in protervam veniens chirurgiam [28].	And in some cases, after the procedures already described have been carried out, Praxagorus recommends making an incision in the pubic region, then cutting open the rectum, removing the excrement, and sewing up [the rectum and the abdomen] [29].

J.S. Wu
Department of Colorectal Surgery, Digestive Disease Institute, Cleveland Clinic Foundation, Cleveland, OH, USA
e-mail: wuj@ccf.org

V.W. Fazio et al. (eds.), *Atlas of Intestinal Stomas*,
DOI 10.1007/978-0-387-78851-7_1,

Surgical ostomies to divert feces away from a point of intestinal blockage appear in the European literature in the eighteenth century [30]. Causes of intestinal obstruction included hernia and colorectal cancer in adults and congenital anorectal malformation in infants. The surgeon's impulse to intervene, however, would have been tempered by uncertainty with respect to outcome. Patients presenting with obstruction would have been dehydrated and malnourished. Coexisting medical illness would have been untreated. Operation would have been undertaken without the benefit of the anesthesia, mechanical ventilation, intravenous fluid resuscitation, blood transfusion, radiology, antibiotics, parenteral nutritional supplementation, or ostomy care-adjuncts that now are taken for granted (Table 1.1).

Table 1.1 Timeline of advances in intestinal stoma surgery and related areas

Surgical advances		Nonsurgical advances
	1700	
1710: Littre introduces the concept of ventral colostomy		
1757: Heister recommends suturing the wounded intestine to the abdominal wall		
1776: Pillore treats obstructing rectal cancer by cecostomy		
1783: Dubois performs the operation of Littre on an infant with imperforate anus		
1793: Duret reports iliac colostomy to treat an infant with imperforate anus.		
1797: Fine treats obstructing rectal cancer by transverse colostomy		
	1800	
1800 Callisen describes lumbar colostomy to treat imperforate anus		
1839 Amussat performs lumbar colostomy to treat obstructing rectal carcinoma		
		1842: Long performs surgery with ether inhalation anesthesia [2]
		1847-Simpson describes chloroform inhalation anesthesia [3]
		1880 Macewen introduces endotracheal intubation [4]
1876: Verneuil describes gastrostomy to treat esophageal stricture		
1879: Schede adds proximal diverting colostomy after transsacral rectal resection		
1884: Madelung recommends complete division of the colon during colostomy creation to achieve complete diversion		
1885: Knie emphasizes the importance of the spur to achieve diversion in colostomy creation		
1885: Davies-Colley suggests colon exteriorization followed by delayed resection to decrease the risk of suppuration after colotomy		
1887: Reclus performs colonic exteriorization with delayed opening of the colon to treat rectal cancer		
1888: Madyl describes loop colostomy		
1892: Smith recommends enterostomy to treat peritonitis		
1894: Bloch described staged extraperitoneal resection of the left colon for cancer		
1895: Keetley suggests appendicostomy as a treatment for ulcerative colitis		1895: Röntgen reports X-rays [5, 6]
1895: Paul performs exteriorization/resection for cancer with tube colostomy		
1893: Henrotin relieves distension caused by appendicitis by cecostomy		
		1899: Bier describes spinal anesthesia with cocaine [7]

Table 1.1 (continued)

Surgical advances		Nonsurgical advances
	1900	1901: Landsteiner reports on blood groups [8]
1902: Weir: Appendicostomy as a treatment for ulcerative colitis		
1903: Mikulicz – Three step treatment of colon cancer: exteriorization, resection, delayed reconstitution of bowel continuity		
		1909: Meltzer and Auer – Continuous respiration without respiratory movements [9]
1908: Mayo – left iliac colostomy following abdominoperineal resection for cancer		
1913: Brown – Ileostomy and cecostomy for colitis		
1921: Hartmann – Sigmoid resection with colostomy and rectal stump		
		1923: Fischer – Barium enema [10]
		1929: Fleming – Penicillin [11]
1931: Rankin – Ileostomy and total colectomy for polyposis coli and ulcerative colitis		
1935: Koenig–Rutzen ostomy appliance		
1941: Dragstedt – Skin grafted ileostomy		
		1942: Grifith and Johnson – Curare [12]
		1940s: World War II – Blood banking
1946: Butler-Primary colostomy maturation		
		1950: Thorn – ACTH treatment for ulcerative colitis [13]
1950: Bricker – Bladder substitution using segments of intestine		
1950: Mt Sinai Hospital – First organized support group for ostomates		
1951: Brooke – Primary maturation of the ileostomy		
1951: Waren and McKitrick – Ileostomy dysfunction		
1952: Turnbull – mucosal grafted ileostomy		
1954: Lemmer and Mehnert – Maintenance of alignment of all layers of the abdominal wall during colostomy creation		1954: Trulove and Witts – Cortisone in ulcerative colitis [14]
1950s: Elise Sorensen – Plastic disposable ostomy appliances		
1957: Bishop and Koop – Roux Y Ileostomy to treat meconium ileus		
1958: Sames and Golligher independently describe retroperitoneal colostomy		
1961: First School of Enterostomal Therapy		
		1966: Dudrick, Wilmore, Vars, and Rhoads – Total intravenous feeding and growth in puppies [15]
1969: Kock introduces the continent ileostomy		
1972: Seruga describes Hepaticojejunostomy with jejunostomy for biliary access		
		References: [16, 17]

In his text, *The Anatomy of the Human Body*, published in 1750, Cheselden [31] described the case of Margaret White of Newington in Surry who acquired a colostomy at the site of a ruptured umbilical hernia:

> In the fiftieth year of her age, she had a rupture at her navel, which continued till her seventy third year, when after a fit of cholic, it mortified, and she being presently after taken with a vomiting, it burst. I went to her and found her in this condition, with about six and twenty inches and a half of the gut hanging out mortified. I took away what was mortified, and left the end of the sound gut hanging out at the navel, to which it afterwards adhered; she recovered, and lived many years after, voiding the excrements through the intestine at the navel…

In 1839, Amussat [32] published a comprehensive treatise on the subject of the *anus artificiel.* He reviewed two major approaches that had emerged to achieve decompression of the obstructed large intestine: ventral and lumbar colostomy (Fig. 1.1a, b).

Fecal diversion by ventral colostomy had been proposed in 1710 by Littre [33].

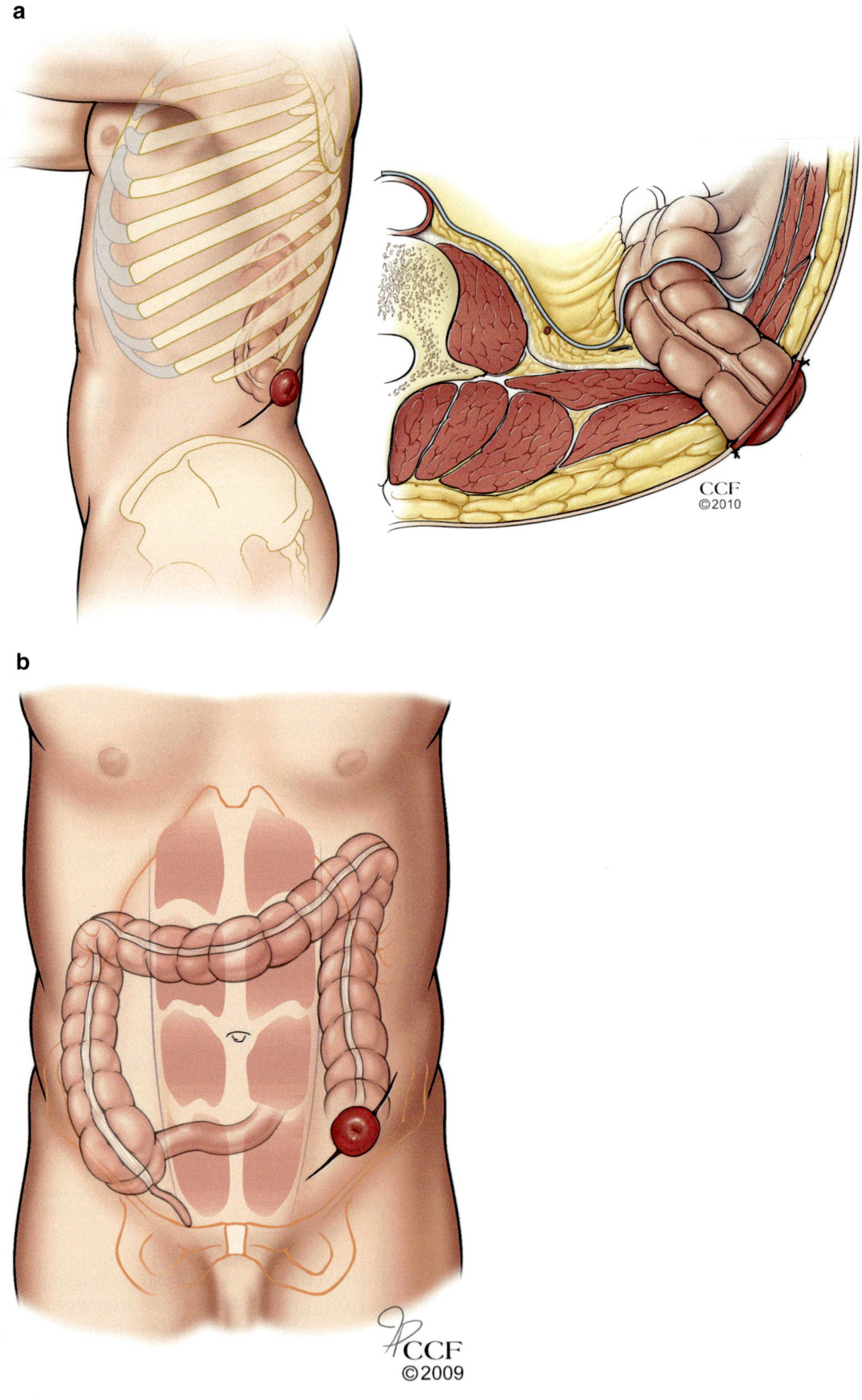

Fig. 1.1 Lumbar and ventral colostomy: (**a**) lumbar colostomy was made using a retroperitoneal approach; (**b**) ventral colostomy originally was created by an iliac or inguinal incision (Illustration © CCF)

Diverses Observations Anatomiques	**Diverse Anatomic Observations**
"Dans le cadavre d'un Enfant mort à 6. jours, M. Littre a vû le Rectum divisé en deux parties, qui ne tenoient l'une à l'autre que par quelches petits filets, longs environ d'un pouce. M. Littre qui a voulu rendre son observation utile, a imaginé & proposé une opération chirurgique fort délicate pour les cas où l'on auroit reconnu une semblable conformation. Il faudroit faire une incision au Ventre, & recoudre ensemble les deux parties d'Intestin après les avoir rouvertes, ou du moins faire venir la partie superieure de l'Intestin à la playe du Ventre, que l'on ne refermeroit jamais, & qui feroit la fonction d'anus."	"In the cadaver of an infant who died at the age of 6 days, M. Littre saw that the rectum was divided into two parts which did not touch each other except by several strands about an inch long. M. Littre, who wished to make his observation useful, imagined and proposed a very delicate surgical operation in case a similar situation should present itself again. It would be necessary to make a ventral incision and sew together the two parts of the intestine after they have been reopened or at least bring the superior part of the intestine to the ventral abdomen, which would never be closed and which would function as an anus." [34].

In 1776, Pillore of Rouen was the first to apply the ideas of Littre [35, 36]. His surgery, however, was not sufficiently brought to light in the contemporary literature of the time. In 1839, Pillore's achievement was documented by Amussat [37]. The patient, Monsieur Morel, presented with a totally obstructing scirrhous tumor of the rectum. Among the methods used to try to open bowel passage was the ingestion of mercury. None of the ingested metal was evacuated even after 1 month. Pillore recommended surgery to create an artificial anus to which M. Morel replied:

Opération d'anus artificiel, par la méthode de LITTRE [38]	**Operation to Create an Artificial Anus, by the method of LITTRE** [34]
"Eh, bien! leur répondit-il, il faut bien avoir recours à l'opération, puisqu'elle seule peut me sauver, vous en convenez, et qu'il est de fait que ma maladie est mortelle."	"Well then," he answered, "the operation will have to be performed, since it is the only thing that can save me, you'll agree, and the fact is that my illness is fatal."

Pillore continues his recollection of the procedure as follows:

Encouragé par des raisons aussi fortes, je fis l'opération en présence de messieurs mes confrères, et de six élèves pensionnaires que j'avais alors. J'avais choisi le coecum comme celui des intestins qui était le plus propre à remplir mes vues tant par sa situation que parce qu'il nous fournissait un réservoir… Je commençai par une incision transversale des tégumens un peu au-dessus du pli de l'aine; je la continuai obliquement de bas en haut; à la faveur du tissu cellulaire en sous-œuvre, j'arrivai à l'aponévrose du muscle grand oblique du bas-ventre; je l'incisai un peu au-dessus du ligament de Fallope dans la même proportion pour avoir au moins un bon pouce de canal depuis le réservoir jusqu'à l'ouverture des tégumens; je fis aux muscles et au péritoine une ouverture transversale à peu près de la même étendue; le fonds de cœcum, facile à reconnaître par son appendice, se présenta, je n'eus pas la peine de le chercher; je l'amenai sans effort le plus en avant possible; là, soutenu par un aide et par moi, je l'ouvris transversalement et l'assujettis aux deux lèvres de la plaie par le moyen d'un point de suture que je fis à l'une et à l'autre avec deux aiguilles enfilées du même fil; je les passai de dedans en dehors et je coupai le fil par le milieu pour obtenir deux anses que je nouai tant supérieurement qu'inférieurement sur deux compresses pour empêcher le froncement des lèvres. Les matières sortirent abondamment…	Encouraged by such strong reasons, I performed the operation in the presence of my colleagues and six resident students whom I had at that time. I had chosen the coecum as the intestine that was the most likely to serve my ideas, both because of its location and because it provided us with a reservoir… I began with a transverse incision of the teguments slightly above the fold of the groin; continuing it obliquely from bottom to top, with the help of the cellular tissue underpinning, I reached the aponeurosis of the large oblique muscle of the lower part of the abdomen; I made an incision slightly above the fallopian ligament in the same proportion, in order to have at least a good inch of channel from the reservoir to the opening of the teguments; I made a transverse opening in the muscles and the peritoneum of approximately the same extent; the coecum bottom, easily recognizable by its appendix, appeared, I did not have to look for it; effortlessly, I drew it as far forward as possible; there, with an assistant and I supporting it, I opened it transversely and fastened it to the two lips of the wound by means of a suture that I made in the lips with two needles threaded with the same thread; I passed them from inside to outside and cut the thread in the middle in order to obtain two loops that I knotted at top and bottom on two compresses to prevent the lips from puckering. An abundance of material came out…

Pillore successfully decompressed the obstructed large intestine by cecostomy created through a right lower quadrant incision. M. Morel survived 28 days. At autopsy, Pillore found a totally obstructed scirrhous tumor at the junction between the end of the colon and the beginning of the rectum. The mercury that the patient had been given was found in a gangrenous segment of jejunum.

Amussat quotes Allan who recorded that Dubois performed Littre's operation in a case of anal atresia in 1783 [39].

"Antoine Dubois a fait, en 1783 l'essai du procédé de Littre, sur un enfant né depuis trois jours sans apparence d'anus. Cet enfant est mort dix jours après l'opération. A l'ouverture du petit cadavre, en trouva les bords de l'intestin consolidés à la circonférence de la plaie de l'abdomen."	In 1783, Antoine Dubois, performed Littre's procedure on a child born 3 days earlier without any appearance of an anus. This child died 10 days after the operation. On opening the small corpse, the edges of the intestines were found to be circumferentially healed to the abdominal wound [34].

In 1793, Duret [40] of Brest successfully performed an iliac colostomy on an infant with imperforate anus.

Observation sur un enfant né sans anus, et auquel il a été fait une ouverture pour y suppléer; par le C. Duret, professeur d'anatomie et de chirurgie, à l'hôpital militaire de la marine à Brest

"J'ouvris le ventre du petit malade au-dessus de la région iliaque, dans l'endroit où l'S du colon formoit une tumeur, à la vérité peu apparente, et où le méconium sembloit imprimer une couleur plus foncée à la peau; je donnai à cette ouverture à-peu-près un pouce et demi d'étendue; elle servit à introduire mon doigt index dans l'abdomen, avec lequel j'attirai au dehors l'S du colon; et dans le crainte qu'il ne rentrât par la suite dans le ventre, je passai dans le mezo-colon deux fils cirés; ensuite j'incisai l'intestin en long; l'air et le méconium sortirent en abondance par cette ouverture…"

Observations on an infant born without an anus, for which an opening was made to provide one; by C. Duret, Professor of Anatomie and Surgery, the Military Hospital, Brest

"I opened the belly of the little sick child over the iliac region, in the place where the sigmoid colon formed a mass, visible from the skin, and where the meconium appeared to impart a dark color to the skin; I made an opening at that site that was extended a one and a half inches; it served to introduce my index finger into the abdomen, with which I pulled out the sigmoid colon; and out of fear that the colon would retreat back into the belly, I passed two waxed threads though the mesocolon; then I incised the intestine longitudinally; gas and meconium ran out in abundance through this opening…"

Dinnick records that this child survived and lived to the age of 45 years [41]. In praise, Verneuil and Reclus wrote that Duret developed his technique by experimentation on cadavers, practiced his technique many times with success, and passed his knowledge on to pupils [42]. A year later, in 1794, Desault reported another case of artificial anus by the method of Littre on an infant with imperforate anus [43]. The child lived for 4 days. In 1797, Dumas [44] described an infant with imperforate anus in whom surgery was suggested but not done.

Observations et réflexions sur une imperforation de l'anus.
C. L. Dumas, professeur de l'École de Santé de Montpellier

En examinant l'enfant, je trouvai l'anus absolument clos… Je fis appeller Estor, chirurgien, pour qu'il m'aidât de ses conseils et de son ministère…

Je proposai à Estor de pratiquer un anus artificiel vers l'extrêmité gauche du colon. Il approuva mon idée, mais il n'eut pas le courage de l'exécuter, parce que les parens sembloient y répugner: il craignait de compromettre sa réputation par les suites d'une opération aussi importante, dont le succès sembloit fort incertain. L'enfant mourut le troisième jour de sa naissance. Nous procédâmes à l'ouverture du cadavre. Après avoir fait une incision dans la région iliaque gauche, nous mîmes à découvert la partie inférieure du colon qui se présenta la première, et qui, par conséquent, étoit contigue à la lame interne du péritoine. Cet intestin étoit boursoufflé par l'air, et plein de matières liquides et gazeuses. Il occupoit un espace considérable, et faisoit saillie vers les muscles abdominaux. Il eût été dès-lors bien facile d'établir un anus artificiel, qui auroit au moins prolongé la vie du sujet, en même tems qu'il eût fourni à la science une observation intéressante et rare

Observations and reflexionson a case of imperforate anus.
C.L. Dumas, professor, School of Health, of Montpellier

On examination, I found that the anus was completely closed… I asked Estor, a surgeon, to aid me with his counsel and ministries…

I proposed to Estor to place an artificial anus toward the left end of the colon. He approved of my idea, but he did not have the courage to carry it out, because the parents seemed to be reluctant to have it done: he was afraid of compromising his reputation with the consequences of such an important surgery, whose success seemed quite uncertain. The child died 3 days after his birth. We undertook the opening up of the corpse. After having made an incision in the left iliac region, we uncovered the lower part of the colon, which came first, and which, consequently, was next to the internal strip of the peritoneum. This intestine was swollen by air, and full of liquid and gaseous matters. It was occupying considerable space and bulging towards the abdominal muscles. It would have been, therefore, easy to insert an artificial anus, which would at least have prolonged the life of the patient, and at the same time would have provided an interesting and rare observation to science [34].

In 1797, Fine, chief surgeon of the hospital of Geneva, published two papers on the subject of artificial anus in the *Annals of the Society of Medicine of Montpellier* [45]. Noting that Fine's work had been "complètement ignores," Amussat reproduced the papers in their entirety.

Mémoire et observation sur l'entérotomie, par M. Pierre Fine, chirurgien en chef de l'hôpital de Genève, et correspondant de la Société de médecine pratique de Montpellier.

Ad extremos morbos, extrema remedia exquisitè optima.

Hipp. APH. 6, sect. I

Opération d'anus artificiel, par la méthode de Littre, sur une femme âgée de 63 ans, qui a vécu trois mois et demi.

Depuis que j'exerce l'art de guérir, j'ai eu à soigner plusieurs cas de tympanite, soit essentielle, soit le plus souvent symptomatique; frappé depuis longtemps de l'insuffisance des moyens que la médecine prescrit contre cette terrible maladie, affligé de la perte que je venais de faire tout récemment d'un malade atteint de cet état morbide pour lequel j'avais inutilement conseillé l'entérotomie, je me promis bien qu'à l'avenir j'insisterais fortement sur l'emploi de ce moyen, lorsque le cas dont je vais présenter le journal s'offrit peu de temps après [46].

Memoir and observation on enterotomy, by M. Pierre Fine, surgeon in chief, Hospital of Geneva, and correspondent of the Society of practical medicine of Montpellier.

For extreme illness, extreme remedies.

Hipp. APH. 6, sect. I

Operation of artificial anus by the method of Littre on a woman aged 63 years who lived three and half months.

Since I began practicing the healing art, I have had to treat several cases of tympanites, sometimes idiopathic but more often symptomatic. I had long been struck by the inadequacy of the measures prescribed by medical science for this terrible illness, and was afflicted by my very recent loss of a patient suffering from this morbid condition, and for whom I had in vain advised enterotomy, I promised myself that in the future I would strongly insist on using this method, when the case on which I am going to report occurred a short time later [47].

Fine's patient suffered from an obstructed rectal cancer. Through an incision between the navel and the pubis, he created a decompressing ostomy. His patient lived three and a half months. Postmortem examination revealed that he had created a transverse colostomy [48].

A second method of colonic decompression using a retroperitoneal approach was introduced because of concern that peritonitis might occur from intra-abdominal intestinal injury using a ventral incision. In 1800, Callisen [49], professor of surgery at Copenhagen, recommended lumbar access to the descending colon in order to create an artificial anus.

Henrici Callisen. Systema Chirurgiae Hodiernae in usum publicum et privatum adornatum pars posterior editio nova auctior et emendatior	Henrich Callisen. A System of Contemporary Surgery Prepared for Public and Private Use. A new enlarged and corrected later edition
"MLXXII: *Chirurgia imperforationis ani*	"1072: Surgery on an imperforation of the anus.
Quae proposita sub hoc rerum statu fuit incisio intestini coeci vel coli descendentis, sectione in regione lumbari sinistra ad marginem musculi quadrati lumborum facta, ut anus paretur artificialis, remedium praebet omnino incertum, atque hac operatione vix vita miselli seruari poterit. Quanquam intestinum in hoc loco facilius attingatur, quam supra regionem inguinalem."	Under these circumstances an incision has been suggested in the cecum or the descending colon, with a section made in the left lumbar region near the edge of the quadratus lumborum muscle, so that an artificial anus may be made ready. This offers a very doubtful remedy, and it will only be possible with difficulty to save the life of the wretched sufferer by this operation. And yet the intestine may be more easily reached in this place than above the region of the groin." [50]

Callisen performed the operation on a cadaver [51]. The greatest advocate of the retroperitoneal approach to the colon was Amussat [52, 53]. Amussat developed his surgical technique studying the surgical and pathologic anatomy of the colon in the lumbar regions using cadavers [54] and, in 1839, reported the particulars of his first case to treat obstructing carcinoma of the rectum in a 48-year-old woman, Madame D., born in Nantes.

Mémoire sur la possibilité d'établir un anus artificiel dans la région lombaire sans pénétrer dans le péritoine.	Treatise on the possibility of establishing an artificial anus in the lumbar region without penetrating the peritoneum.
J. Z. Amussat	J.Z. Amussat
Introduction.	Introduction.
"L'idée d'ouvrir le colon lombaire gauche sans intéresser le péritoine est assez ancienne; mais elle avait paru inexécutable jusqu'à présent, comme je vais le prouver par quelques citations." [55]	"The idea of opening the left colon from a lumbar approach without concerning the peritoneum is rather old, but it has not been carried out until the present as I shall prove by several citations."
CHAPITRE IV.	**CHAPTER IV.**
FAITS PARTICULIERS.	**PARTICULAR FACTS**
1re OBSERVATION.	**1st OBSERVATION.**
Obstruction complète de la fin de l'S iliaque par des tumeurs, chez une femme âgée de quarante-huit ans; constipation datant de vingt-six jours; tympanite stercorale des plus violentes. Anus artificiel établi avec succès, en ouvrant le colon lombaire gauche *sans pénétrer dans le péritoine* [56].	Complete obstruction of the end of the sigmoid colon by tumor, in a 48-year-old woman; constipated for 26 days; a most violent distention of the bowels. Artificial anus created successfully by opening the lumbar aspect of the left colon *without opening the peritoneum* [34].

Modestly, he referred to his approach as the "Callisen modification." [57] In the follow-up, 4 months after surgery, Amussat records that Madame D's health was as satisfactory as possible [58]. In a passage preceding this case description, Amussat explained his motivation for undertaking this work. Affected by the painful death caused by stercoral obstruction, he acted.

j'etais bien préparé à ne plus rester spectateur passif de la mort par obstruction du rectum [56].	I was well prepared to no longer remain a passive spectator of death by obstruction of the rectum.

In 1841, Erichsen [59] introduced Amussat's work to the English medical public. Subsequently, in 1844, Amussat [54] published a memoir on "enterotomia," successfully performed without opening the peritoneum, in the *Medical Times*. Concerning the application of this operation to cases of obstruction, Amussat concluded:

> Finally, this case confirms all that I have asserted in the different memoirs, already published on the subject, and it emboldens me, and ought likewise to embolden other practitioners, to perform this operation, instead of, as is often the case, allowing their patients to die unrelieved.

Decompression proximal to the site of obstruction was not always achieved by lumbar colostomy. In 1850, Avery [60] at Charing-cross Hospital described a case of intestinal obstruction in which an operation for artificial anus in the left lumbar region was performed. Unfortunately, the patient succumbed; and autopsy revealed "twisting of the caecum and ascending colon, producing obstruction of the bowels." In 1873, Mason [61] in New York described 6 cases of lumbar colostomy and presented a summary of 80 cases.

In 1821, Pring reported [62] the case of Mrs. White who had an obstruction in the lower bowels detected by a rectal-bougie. The formation of an artificial anus was proposed. Pring recorded his course of action as follows:

> The patient was desirous of living upon any terms, and agreed to submit to the operation. Accordingly, having placed her on a table, I made an incision on the left side of the abdomen, beginning about two inches above, and one inch on the inside, of the anterior superior spinous process of the ilium. This incision was extended obliquely downwards and inwards to within three-quarters of an inch of the edge of Poupart's ligament: the fascia covering the abdominal muscles was thus exposed to the extent of between three and four inches. An opening was then made through the external and internal oblique, and the transversalis, muscles; which opening was enlarged, with a bistoury conducted by my finger, to the extent of the external incision. The peritoneum being now laid bare, a small opening was made in this membrane… The colon was thus freely exposed a little above its sigmoid flexure, at which place I made an incision into it… The contents of the bowels were immediately expelled with great force to a considerable distance: as the feces escaped, the gut collapsed, and began to subside from its place: a ligature was therefore passed through it at the lower part of the opening, the apposition of which to the external wound was then preserved until the bowels were copiously evacuated.

At follow-up between 5 and 6 months, Pring reported that his patient's general health was apparently good and that "the object of the operation has been completely attained." An account of "an analogous Operation" by Freer in the same article [62] described a case of artificial anus made through "the parietes of the abdomen, in the left iliac region, so as to expose the colon near its sigmoid flexure" on an infant born without an anus. Freer recalled:

> I accordingly performed the operation: a considerable quantity of meconium was evacuated; and during the three weeks that the child lived, the feces passed freely at the wound. The child sucked and slept well, and seemed free from suffering, but died apparently from marasmus.
>
> In this case, though ultimately unsuccessful, the operation had undoubtedly prolonged the life of the child, and seemed to justify us in recommending it in the present instance.

In 1851, Luke [63] in London reported a case of colonic obstruction situated about the "sigmoid flexure." The site of blockage was determined by the fact that insertion of an esophagus tube into the rectum met with obstruction about 12 in. distant from the anus and water injected into the tube also immediately returned. In pondering his surgical options, Luke wrote:

> Assuming the correctness of our conclusion, that operation which passes under the name of Amussat, appeared to recommend itself by the circumstance of its avoiding the necessity of peritoneal section… Yet, as I thought it not prudent to assume that our conclusion respecting the seat of obstruction was certainly correct, I determined to adopt that operation which would at least give me some opportunity of extending my search, provided I did not find the obstruction at the point where it was supposed to be, thinking that the increased probability thus afforded, of finding the obstruction, would be more than an adequate compensation for the little increased danger from peritoneal section. I therefore opened the abdominal parietes near the groin.

The colon proximal to a stricture was exteriorized and opened immediately. Luke recorded that: "Through the aperture thus made, half a chamber-utensil full of fluid faeculent matter made its escape, after which the patient expressed himself much relieved." This person recovered and was able to return to work.

In 1881, Richter reported the presentation of Schinzinger [64] in Salzburg who described two cases of inoperable sigmoid colon cancer treated by colostomy in which the colon is divided.

Redner theilt vor Allem 2 Fälle von inoperablem Krebs der Flex. sigm. mit, in welchen er zur Erleichterung der Kranken einen künstlichen After oberhalb der Leistenbeuge anlegte. Er empfiehlt, in solchen Fällen den Darm ganz zu durchtrennen, das obere Ende desselben in die Wunde einzunähen, das untere aber ganz zu schliessen und zu versenken.	The speaker reports in particular on 2 cases of inoperable cancer of the sigmoid flexure, in which he created an artificial anus above the groin to ease the discomfort of the patients. He recommends in such cases that the intestine should be cut through completely, the upper end sutured into the wound, and the lower end closed off completely and buried [34].

In a larger study, published in 1884, Madelung [65] in Rostock described totally diverting colostomy to treat rectal carcinoma in which the bowel is completely divided, the proximal end is secured in the abdominal wall, and the distal end is closed and returned to the abdominal cavity.

Madelung (Rostock). Über eine Modifikation der Colotomie wegen Carcinoma recti	**Madelung (Rostock). Concerning a modification for colostomy for rectal carcinoma**
"Es soll in das Colon nicht nur ein Fenster eingeschnitten, sondern der Darm vollständig durchschnitten werden. Sein centrales Ende wird zur Bildung des künstlichen Afters in die Bauchwandungen eingepflanzt, das periphere wird nach Verschluss seines Lumen in die Bauchhöhle versenkt. Diese Operation ist schwieriger als die gewöhnliche Colotomie. Vor Allem muss natürlich genau bestimmt werden, welches der zuführende, welches der abführende Darmtheil ist."	"Not only should a window be cut into the intestine, but also the colon should be completely divided. The proximal end used to create the artificial anus is implanted into the abdominal wall while the lumen of the distal end is closed and buried in the abdominal cavity. This operation is more difficult than the usual colostomy. Above all, of course, it is necessary to determine very precisely which is the incoming, which the outgoing part of the intestine." [34]

In 1885, Knie [66], in Moscow, looked for an alternative technique to create a two-sided colostomy that would be totally diverting. He proposed that the spur connecting the limbs of a two-sided colostomy should effectively make the distal end of the colostomy impassable (*undurchgängig*). He tested his ideas through animal experiments.

Zur Technik der Kolotomie
Von Dr. A Knie
(Aus dem Laboratorium für experimentelle Pathologie in Moskau)

"Ausgehend davon, dass bei spontan enstandenem Anus praeternaturalis der Darminhalt durch den Sporn nach außen geleitet wird, und in vielen Fällen von Spornbildung es gar nicht mehr zur Entleerung per Rectum kommt, unternahm ich eine Versuchsreihe, die die Bedingungen feststellen sollte, unter welchen es möglich wäre, bei noch nicht eröffnetem Darmrohr einen Sporn zu bilden."

On the Technique of the Colotomy
By Dr. A Knie
(Laboratory for Experimental Pathology, Moscow)

"Proceeding on the basis that, in cases of spontaneously formed anus praeternaturalis, the intestinal content is conducted to the outside through the spur and that, in many cases where a spur is formed, the content is no longer emptied via the rectum at all, I conducted a series of experiments to determine the conditions under which it would be possible to form a spur before the intestinal tube is opened." [34]

In 1887, Allingham [67] reported the results of six inguinal colostomies. He argued for inguinal colostomy over lumbar colostomy for artificial anus applied to obstruction in the rectum or sigmoid flexure.

> Now that surgery, through perfect cleanliness, has made such gigantic strides, and the peritoneum is no longer held in awe as in former days, the opening of that serous cavity, if due care be taken, does not to any great extent increase the dangers of the operation, and is certainly not more harmful to the patient than the disturbance of cellular tissue and parts around, so frequently incurred when there is difficulty in finding the bowel in lumbar colotomy.

In Allingham's technique, a loop of gut was exteriorized and stitched to the abdominal wall with thread passed through the mesentery close to the intestine and then through the abdominal wall on both sides. In the same year, Reclus [68] described a patient with a large cancer of the rectum treated by iliac artificial anus. He used a staged technique involving support of the exteriorized sigmoid colon by a wick of iodoform gauze and delayed intestinal decompression.

Anus artificiel iliaque
Par M. le Dr. Paul Reclus

J'ai pratiqué, il y a sept mois, un anus artificiel iliaque pour obvier aux accidents que provoquait, chez une femme de 59 ans, un cancer volumineux de la partie moyenne du rectum.

Et d'abord, un mot sur le manuel opératoire, car le mode d'intervention auquel j'ai eu recours, n'est pas usité en France, et c'est peut-être la première opération de ce genre qui ait été faite chez nous.

…nous retirons une anse bosselée, grisâtre, à bandes longitudinales visibles et hérissée d'appendices épiploiques; c'est bien la partie que nous cherchons, et nous nous apprêtons à la faire au dehors.

Au lieu de pratiquer des points de suture, temps long et délicat, nous avons maintenu l'anse en passant au-dessous d'elle et au travers du mésentère une mèche aseptique, une lanière de tarlatane iodoformée saisie par une pince à forcipressure.…Puis, avec du collodion, les deux extrémités libres de la lanière ont été collées sur la peau; l'anse se trouvait ainsi solidement fixée et ne pouvait plus rentrer dans le ventre.

Le sixième jour seulement, l'appareil a été levé et nous avons incisé au thermocautère la convexité de l'anus; le huitième jour, comptant sur des adhérences péritonéales suffisantes, nous avons enlevé la lanière de tarlatane iodoformée; l'intestin n'a pas bougé; le douzième jour, la malade est allée abondamment à la garderobe par son anus artificiel…

Iliac artificial anus
By Dr. Paul Reclus

Seven months ago, I created an iliac artificial anus in a 59-year-old woman to prevent problems caused by a voluminous cancer in the middle part of the rectum.

First of all, a word about the operating manual, because the surgical procedure I used is not in common use in France, and may be the first operation of this kind done in our country.

…we pulled out a lumpy, grayish loop with visible longitudinal bands and covered with appendices epiploica. It was in fact the part we were looking for, and we prepared to bring it out.

Rather than making sutures, a long and delicate procedure, we held the loop by passing aseptic packing, a strip of iodoform gauze, under it and through the mesentery grasped by forcipressure clamps… The two free ends of the strip were then adhered to the skin with collodion. Thus, the loop was solidly attached, so that it could not slip back into the abdomen.

Only on the sixth day was the device removed, and we made an incision in the convexity of the anus using thermocautery. On the eighth day, counting on the peritoneum being sufficiently healed, we removed the iodoform gauze strip. The intestine did not move. On the 12th day, the patient had a copious bowel movement through her artificial anus [34].

In 1888, Maydl [69, 70] in Vienna reported on diversion of the fecal stream in cases of malignancy. In his operation, a mobile loop of large or small intestine is exteriorized and then suspended outside the abdominal wall by a transmesenteric rubber (vulcanite) rod. In emergencies, he used a goose feather.

Zur Technik der Kolotomie
Von Dr. Karl Maydl

"Und nun will ich das Verfahren kurz schildern, wie ich es in der letzen Zeit zu üben pflege.

On the Technique of Colotomy
By Dr. Karl Maydl

"And now I want to describe briefly the procedure which I have been using recently.

Nach Eröffnung der Bauchhöhle ziehe ich einen beweglichen Darmabschnitt (Col. transv., Flexura rom. oder Ileum) so weit vor, dass der Mesenterialansatz der vorgezogenen Darmschlinge vor die Bauchwunde zu liegen kommt; durch einen Schlitz des Mesenteriums knapp am Darm stecke ich einen mit Jodoformgaze umwickelten Hartkautschukbolzen (im Nothfall Gänsefederkiel) durch…	After opening the abdominal cavity, I pull a movable section of the intestine (transverse colon, flexura rom. or ileum) so far forward that the mesenterial attachment of the pulled-out loop of intestine comes to rest in front of the abdominal wound; through a slit cut in the mesentery right at the intestine, I insert a hard rubber pin wrapped with iodoform gauze (in an emergency, a goosefeather quill)…
Soll der Anus praeternaturalis persistiren, so eröffnet man bei einzeitiger Operation gleich, bei zweizeitiger in 4–6 Tagen den Darm quer, auf ein Drittel seiner Peripherie…	If the artificial anus is intended to last, open the intestine transversely around one third of its periphery – this is done right away if this is a one-time operation, or after 4–6 days, if the operation is performed in two phases…
Für gewöhnlich genügt die Eröffnung allein, die den Gasen einen Ausweg schafft; die flüssigen oder festen Darminhaltsmassen können später entleert werden; die Möglichkeit der Gasentweichung bietet den Pat. eine genügende Linderung ihres bisherigen Zustandes. Die Eröffnung des Darmes mache ich, um alle Blutung zu vermeiden, mit dem Thermokauter. Hat der Kranke alle Operationsfolgen gut überstanden, so wird nach 14 Tagen bis 3 Wochen die übrige Darmperipherie auf dem Kautschukbolzen getrennt, wobei dieser sehr gut als Unterlage und Marke verwendet wird. Zum Überfluss kann man den Rand der Darmlumina mit einigen Nähten an die Haut befestigen, da sie stets eine Tendenz zur Retraktion haben;…"	The process of opening is usually enough in itself to create an escape route for the gases; the liquid or solid intestinal contents can be emptied out later; the ability of the gases to escape gives the patient sufficient relief from his current state. To avoid any bleeding, I open the intestine with a thermocauterizer. If the patient has survived all of the consequences of the operation in good shape, then after 14 days to 3 weeks, the rest of the periphery of the intestine is cut through on the rubber pin – the pin serves very effectively as a support surface and as a marker. It is not strictly necessary, but one can fasten the edge of the intestinal lumen to the skin with a few sutures, because it always has a tendency to retract…" [34]

In 1889, Kelsey [71] in New York described an "improvement in the technique of inguinal colostomy" that involved supporting the exteriorized colon by means of a hare-lip pin passed through the abdominal wall and through the intestinal mesentery.

> The incision is that of Crips—across a line from the anterior-superior spinous process to the umbilicus. After getting the sigmoid flexure outside the body, a hair-lip pin is passed under it in the following manner: It is entered through the skin on the side of the wound toward the median line, and at the junction of the lower with the middle third of the incision. It perforates first the skin, next the parietal peritoneum, next the mesentery of the gut close to the bowel, and at the junction of the lower and middle thirds of the exposed loop, next the parietal peritoneum on the other side of the incision, and finally the skin. By this means the gut is so firmly held in position that it cannot be dislodged by any vomiting, and a perfectly satisfactory spur is formed, which will prevent any passing of fecal matter beyond the opening.

In 1892, Reeves [72] described sigmoid loop colostomy suspended outside of the abdominal wall by means of a transmesenteric rod. At the end of a week, the bowel was opened longitudinally and the gut edges stitched to the skin (Fig. 1.2a). In 1900, Hartmann [73] illustrated the use of iodoform gauze to suspend the loop iliac colostomy (Fig. 1.2b).

Extraperitoneal Resection of Colon Cancer

In 1885, Davies-Colley [74] in London described three cases of colostomy with delayed opening of the intestine. He found that delayed opening is accompanied by less suppuration. By extension, he suggested exteriorization with delayed resection:

> …in the case of a tumour of the colon, it might be better to draw out the loop of intestine containing the growth with the investing peritoneum and wait for a few days before excising the loop by the knife, the cautery, or some caustic agent.

In 1894, Bloch [75, 76] of Copenhagen described extraperitoneal resection of the left colon for cancer in a 24-year-old woman. The freely movable tumor was exteriorized and incised above the tumor. This was followed by extraperitoneal resection and delayed closure of the artificial anus.

Extraabdominal Resektion af hele Colon descendens og et Stykke af Colon transversum for Cancer.	**Extra-abdominal Resection of the whole descending colon and a piece of the transverse colon for cancer.**
Af Oscar Bloch	**By Oscar Bloch**
Den 6/5 94 foretoges Laparotomi; den stærkt angrebne Colon descendens med det tilgrænsende Stykke af Flexura coli lienalis blev trukket frem, saa at det laa udenfor Abdominalsaarets Hudrande, frit ovenpaa Bugvæggen; det blev holdt i dette Leje ved Hjælp af tre med Jodoformgaze omviklede Glasstænger, der bleve stukne gennem Mesocolon…	On 6/5 94, laparotomy was performed. The heavily attached descending colon with an adjacent piece of the splenic flexure was pulled forward such that it lay beyond the abdominal incision, exposed on top of the abdominal wall. It was kept in position with the help of three glass rods wrapped in iodoform gauze, which were inserted through the mesocolon…
15de Dag efter Operationen reseceres det syge Tarmstykke i sundt Væv. Et Par Uger senere kom Patienten op, og lidt over to Maaneder efter Laparotomien med Fremlægningen var Saaret lægt; Anus præternaturalis fungerede godt.	On the 15th day after surgery the diseased piece of intestine is resected in healthy tissue. A couple of weeks later the patient is mobilized, and a little more than 2 months after the laparotomy, with the exposure the wound was healed. The anus praeternaturalis functioned well.
Som det vil ses af ovenstaaende Meddelelse er det muligt ved extraabdominal Fremlægning og senere Resektion at fjærne et meget stort Stykke Tarm, selv om dette ved Adhærencer er fast bundet til Bughulens bageste Væg; i det meddelte Tilfælde har Forløbet efter den store Operation været paafaldende roligt.	As it will be seen from the above message, it is possible to remove a rather large part of the intestine by extra-abdominal exposure and subsequent resection, even when this by adherence is firmly attached to the posterior abdominal wall. "In the case described, the course of events since the large operation has been strikingly uneventful." [34]

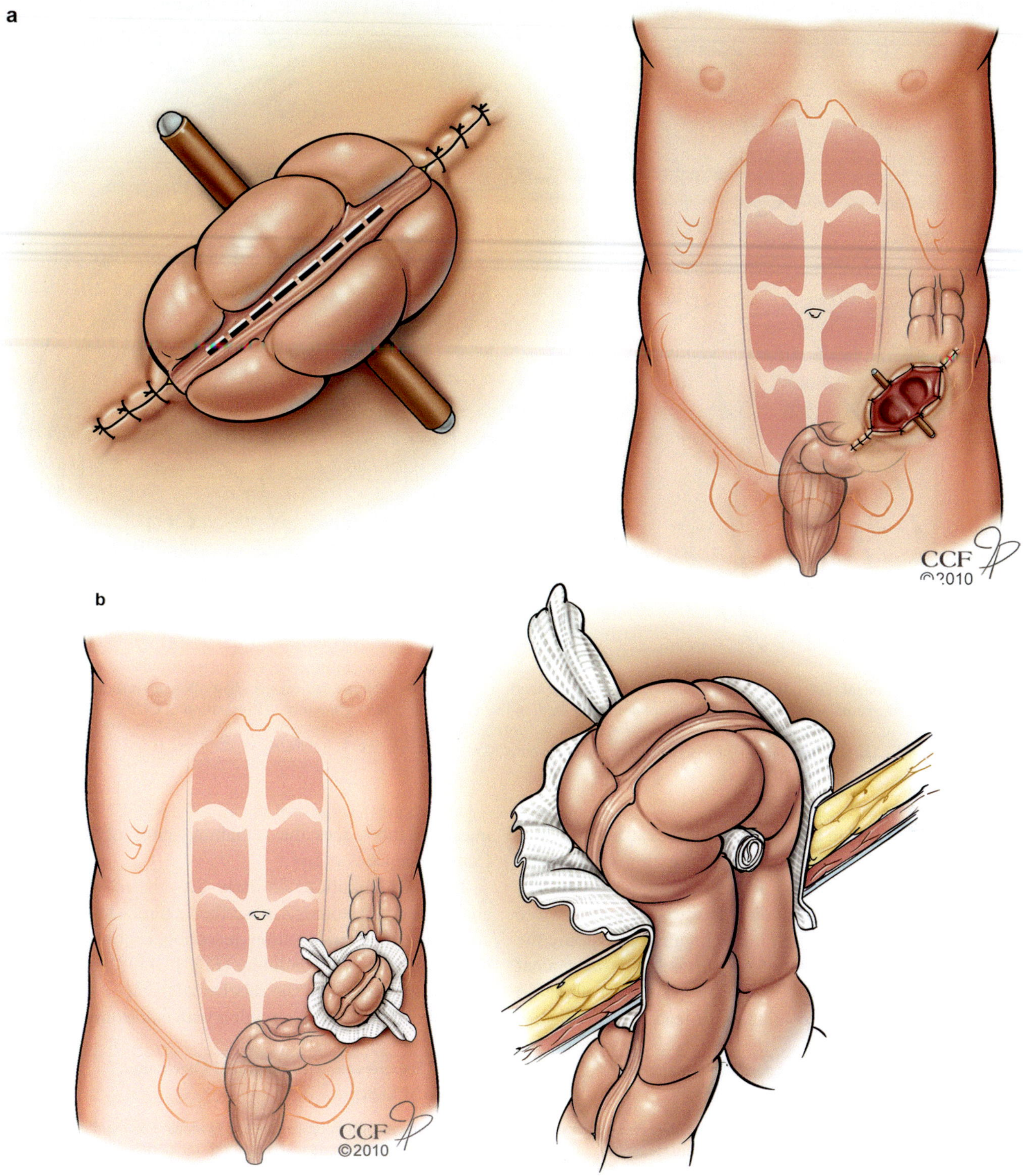

Fig. 1.2 Loop Colostomy: (**a**) Sigmoid loop colostomy (Reeves). The exteriorized sigmoid colon is secured above the skin by a transmesenteric rod; (**b**) Treatment of rectal cancer by proximal diversion as illustrated by Hartmann. The bowel is exteriorized through a left iliac incision, supported using iodoform gauze and then opened several days later (Illustration © CCF)

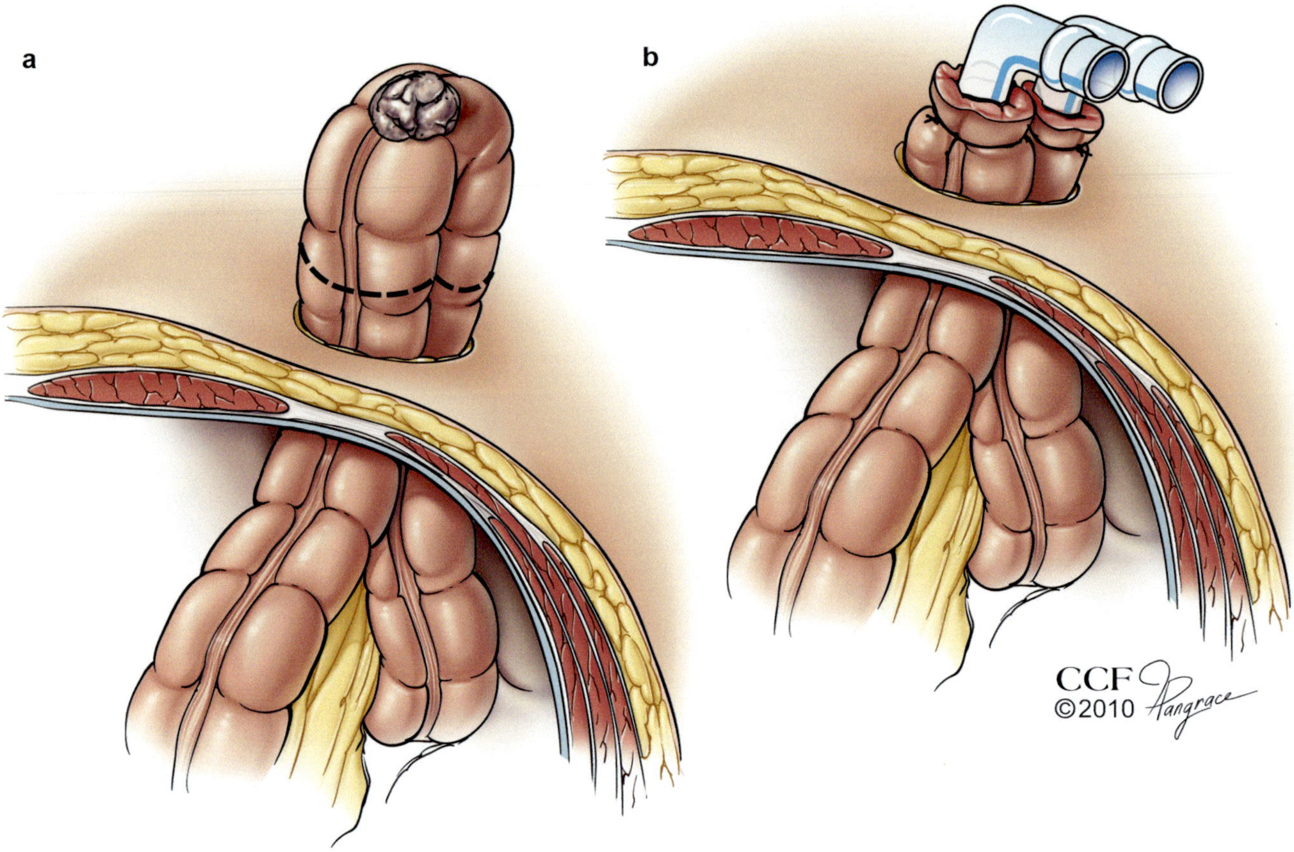

Fig. 1.3 Extraperitoneal resection of colon cancer. (**a**) The tumor bearing segment of colon is exteriorized. (**b**) Following resection of the tumor bearing segment, the remaining limbs of intestine are decompressed, in this case using Paul's glass tubes (Illustration © CCF)

In 1895, Paul [77] in Liverpool, wrote a treatise that began with a description of a patient with a malignant sigmoid stricture that was excised. A primary anastomosis unfortunately leaked, and the patient died. In retrospect, Paul wrote that had he been content with initial inguinal colostomy the patient "could scarcely have failed to survive." In a subsequent case, he excised a sigmoid malignancy, but then made no attempt to restore bowel continuity. Instead, he sewed glass intestinal tubes into the remaining ends of the intestine. Convalescence was rapid.

In 1903, Mikulicz, similarly dissatisfied with resection and primary anastomosis, described a three-step treatment of colon cancer: exteriorization, resection, followed by delayed restitution of bowel continuity (Fig. 1.3) [78].

Mikulicz discussed the relative advantages and disadvantages of extraperitoneal resection with colostomy as follows:

Chirurgische Erfahrungen über das Darmcarcinom
Von J. von Mikulicz

Die Vortheile dieses Verfahrens sind ersichtlich. Die Hauptoperation ist kürzer als bei der einzeitigen Methode, die Infection des Peritoneums während der Operation wird absolut vermieden, man kann sie daher einem durch das Leiden heruntergekommenen Kranken viel eher zumuten.

Die Methode ist also nicht nur ungefährlicher, sondern auch leistungsfähiger. Allerdings hat das Verfahren auch seine Schattenseiten. Die Behandlungsdauer ist eine viel längere und der Operirte muss eine Zeit lang die Unannehmlichkeiten eines widernatürlichen Afters über sich ergehen lassen. Aber das sind, denke ich, Nachtheile, die durch den Vortheil der grösseren Sicherheit und Leistungsfähigkeit reichlich aufgewogen werden.

Surgical Experiences with Intestinal Carcinoma
by J. von Mikulicz

The advantages of this procedure are evident. The main operation is shorter than by the single stage method, the peritoneal infection during the operation is absolutely avoided, and one can thus attempt it much earlier on a patient debilitated by the disease.

The method is not only less dangerous but also more easily performed. Of course the procedure also has its drawbacks. The duration of treatment is longer and the patient operated on must bear with the unpleasantness of an artificial anus for a long time. But I think these disadvantages are greatly outweighed by the advantages of greater safety and increased ease of performance [79].

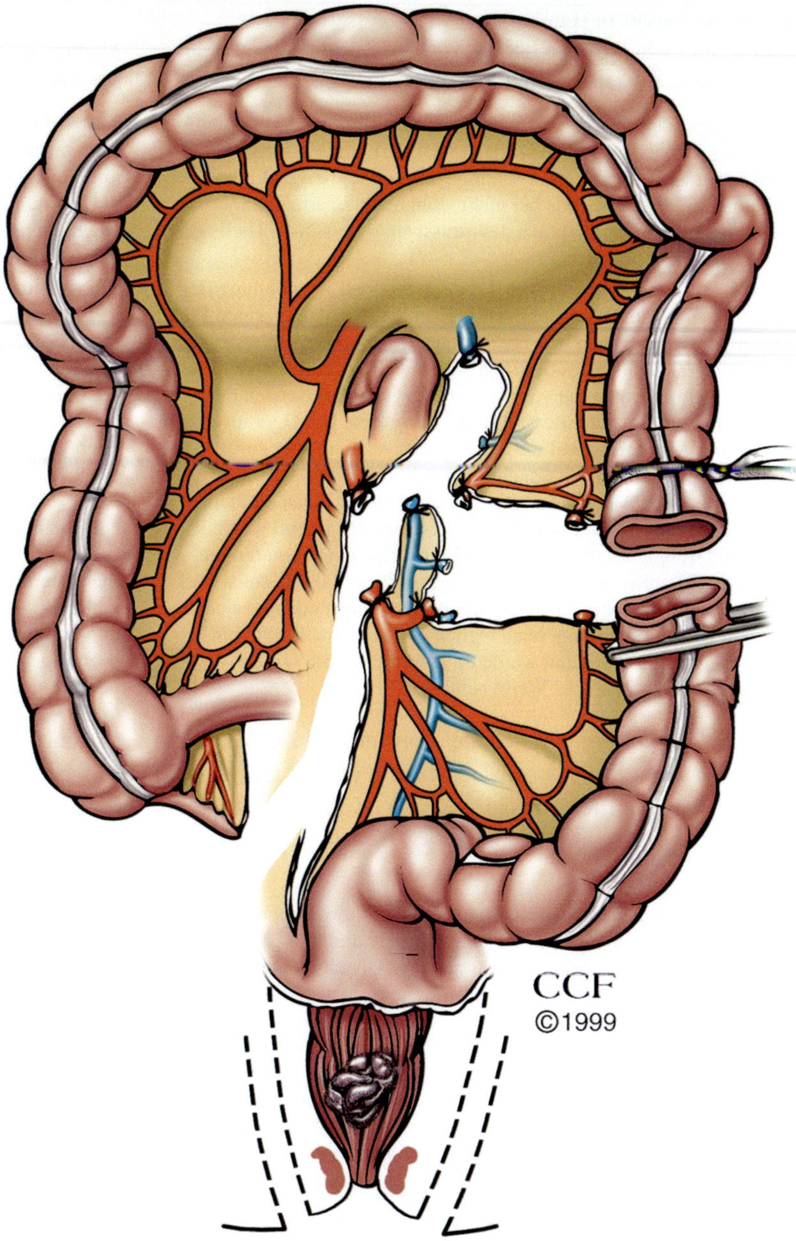

Fig. 1.4 Colostomy resulting from abdominoperineal resection of the rectum for cancer (Illustration © CCF)

In 1928, Sistrunk [80] in Rochester recommended proximal transverse colostomy as an initial step for Mikulicz resection of sigmoid cancers. Two and a half weeks later, a second operation was performed to remove the growth. This was followed by subsequent simultaneous closure of the two colostomies.

Rectal Cancer Resection with Proximal Diversion

In 1904, Mayo [81] described abdominoperineal resection of the rectum for carcinoma (Fig. 1.4) as follows:

> The block removal of the rectum and glands where possible from below and in high location of the cancer, the combined abdominal and perineal methods of removing rectum, glands, and all malignant tissue en masse, is the surgery for the cancer of this region. This method is merely the application of principles of the surgery of cancer, regardless of location, as exemplified by Halstead's operation for the removal of cancer of the breast.
>
> The combined abdominal and perineal method is now advocated for high rectal carcinoma by the pioneers in rectal surgery, Kocher, Kraske, Gaudier, Quenu, Trendelenberg, Abbe, Weir, and numerous others.

In Mayo's technique, "colostomy, as usually performed, has been the lifting of a loop of sigmoid through an abdominal iliac incision."

In 1887, Schede [82] described rectal cancer excision according to the method of Kraske [83]. In one case, he added an abdominal colostomy, effectively diverting the feces away from the operative field.

Aerztlicher Verein zu Hamburg.
Sitzung am 13. September 1887.
Herr Schede: Zur Operation des Mastdarmkrebses.

Der Vortragende knüpft an den wichtigen Fortschritt an, der in der operativen Behandlung hochsitzender Mastdarmkrebse durch den glücklichen Gedanken Kraske's...angebahnt ist, die Zugängigkeit der vom unteren Mastdarmende her nicht wohl mehr zu erreichenden Neubildung durch Wegnehmen des Steissbeines und eines Theils des Kreuzbeines zu erleichtern.

Deselbe betraf einen 35 jährigen Arbeiter. Sitz und Ausdehnung des Carcinoms unterschieden sich nicht wesentlich von dem vorigen Falle, doch war, trotzdem auch hier bereits die Drüsen und Lymphstränge des retrorectalen Gewebes ergriffen waren, die Operation wesentlich leichter, und brauchten die von Kraske angegebenen Grenzen der Kreuzbeinresection nicht überschritten zu werden. Die Operation wurde genau ebenso ausgeführt, wie die vorige, dann aber sofort am Colon descendens von der Bauchseite ein künstlicher After angelegt und von diesem aus das periphere Darmende durch einen einfachen, an einen Faden befestigen Wattetampon verschlossen. Irgend welche Reaction erfolgte auf den Eingriff nicht; überhaupt aber waren die Leiden des Kranken ganz unvergleichlich geringer, als sie sonst nach Mastdarmexstirpationen zu sein pflegen. Der Patient erfreute sich einer sehr geregelten Verdauung, hatte täglich des Morgens einmal einen reichlichen festen Stuhl und wurde im Uebrigen durch seinen künstlichen After in keiner Weise belästigt.

Meeting on September 13, 1887.
Mr. Schede: On the Surgery of the Rectal Carcinoma

The speaker took as his starting point the important advance in the surgical treatment of carcinomas positioned high in the rectum initiated by Kraske's fortunate idea of removing the coccyx and part of the sacrum to facilitate access to a tumor that can no longer be reached practicably from the lower end of the rectum.

This was the situation in the case of a 35-year-old worker. The location and size of the carcinoma did not differ significantly from the previous case, but here, in spite of the fact that the lymph nodes and vessels of the retrorectal tissue were already involved, the operation was much easier and the boundaries of the sacrum resection given by Kraske did not have to be exceeded. The operation was executed in exactly the same way as the previous one, but then an artificial anus was created immediately at the descending colon on the abdominal side and, proceeding from this, the peripheral end of the intestine was closed by a simple cotton tampon fastened by a thread. No reaction to the intervention occurred, but the suffering of the patient was quite significantly less than that which is otherwise the case after rectal extirpations. The patient enjoyed very regular digestion, produced a large, solid stool every morning, and was otherwise not discommoded in any way by his artificial anus [34].

In the discussion of Schede's presentation, Lauenstein recounted a case of his own in which a patient had died of sepsis 2 weeks after Kraske excision of rectal cancer. He attributed Schede's comparative success to the fact that stool had been prevented from passing over the fresh operative field.

Discussion

Herr Lauenstein hatte Gelegenheit, in einem Falle von hochsitzendem Mastdarmkrebs nach Kraske zu operiren... Die durch die Naht vereinigten Mastdarmenden wichen nach der Operation aus einander, und liess sich nicht verhindern, dass Koth in die Wundhöhle übertrat. Der Kranke starb gegen Ende der 2. Woche unter den Erscheinunen einer subacut verlaufenden Sepsis, deren Ursache wohl in jenem Kothaustritt zu suchen war. L. glaubt, dass das von Schede empfohlene und mit Erfolg geübte Verfahren, der Exstirpation des Mastdarmkrebses die Anlegung eines künstlichen Afters hinzuzufügen, der die Kothpassage über das frische Operationsfeld verhindere, geeignet sei, der Kraske'schen Operation erst ihren wahren Werth zu verleihen.

Discussion

Mr. Lauenstein had the opportunity to perform an operation by Kraske's method on a patient with cancer seated high in the rectum. The ends of the rectum which had been joined by the suture came apart after the operation and it was impossible to prevent feces from entering the wound cavity. The patient died toward the end of the second week in a condition characterized by subacute sepsis, the cause of which was apparently to be found in the escape of feces. L. believes that the procedure recommended and successfully performed by Schede, namely, adding to the extirpation of the rectal cancer the creation of an artificial anus which prevents the passage of feces over the fresh surgical field, shows the true value of Kraske's operation [34].

In 1921, Hartmann described an entirely abdominal operation for cancers of the distal sigmoid colon and rectum [84]. This brief report, two paragraphs in length, has had a far-reaching impact on intestinal surgery.

Nouveau procédé d'ablation des cancers de la partie terminale du colon pelvien,
Par M. Henri Hartmann, de Paris

Il est de règle, pour l'extirpation des cancers de la partie terminale du côlon pelvien, de faire une opération actuellement encore très grave, l'amputation abdomino-périnéale du rectum. Chez deux malades, colostomisés pour des accidents d'occlusion, je me suis, dans un deuxième temps, borné à extirper le segment de côlon intermédiaire à l'anus artificiel et au rectum avec le territoire ganglionnaire correspondant. Puis j'ai fermé le bout supérieur du rectum et l'ai péritonisé, ne touchant pas au plancher périnéal.

Les suites de l'opération ont dans les deux cas été aussi simples que celles d'une opération d'appendicite à froid. La conservation d'un petit cul-de-sac rectal sus-sphinctérien n'a pas présenté le moindre inconvénient, mes opérations datent de 9 et de 10 mois; les malades vont très bien.

New Ablation Procedure for Cancers of the Distal the Pelvic Colon
By Mr. Henri Hartmann, of Paris

An operation that is currently still very serious, abdominoperineal resection of the rectum, is the standard practice for removing cancers of the distal pelvic colon. In two patients who underwent colostomy for occlusions, I was forced to perform a second operation to remove the segment of the colon between the artificial anus and the rectum, together with the corresponding lymph node area. I then closed the upper part of the rectum and peritonealized it without affecting the perineal floor.

The consequences of the surgery in both cases have been as simple as those of an operation of appendicitis without anesthesia/preparation. The keeping of a small rectal cul-de-sac above the sphincter did not present the least inconvenience, my surgeries were done 9 and 10 months ago, and the patients are doing very well [34].

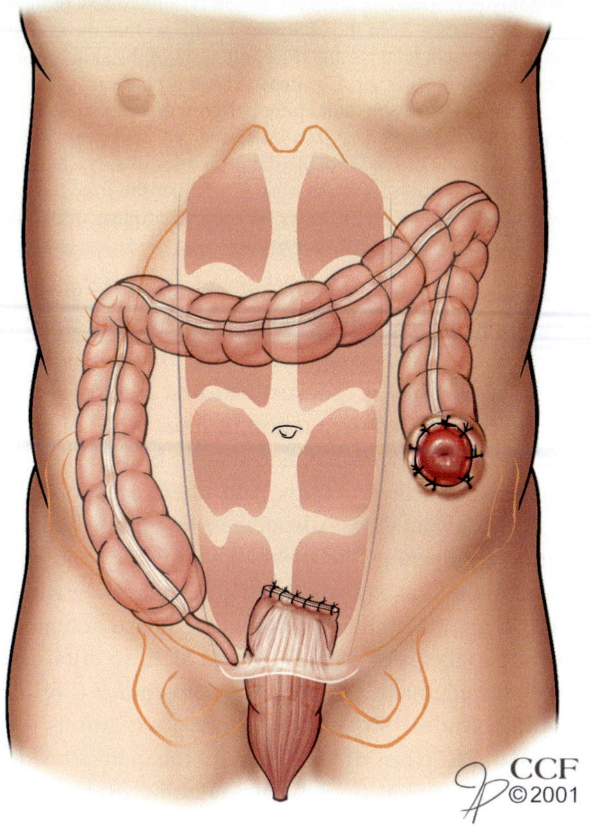

Fig. 1.5 Hartmann's resection. The pelvic colon and variable amounts of rectum are removed. The proximal colon is brought out of the abdomen as an end colostomy and the rectal stump is closed and returned to the abdomen (Illustration © CCF)

The tumor is resected, the rectal stump is left in place and the proximal colon is exteriorized as an end colostomy (Fig. 1.5).

Colon and Rectal Trauma

In the 6th edition of *A General System of Surgery*, published in 1757, Heister [85] recommended management of intestinal wounds by suturing the wounded part of the intestine to the abdominal wound:

> As the modern Surgeons have found by Experience, that scarce any are saved who have received Wounds in the Intestines, and that in those few who do recover, the wounded Parts, from the Fineness of the Coats of the Gut, do not properly unite, but rather adhere to the inner Part of the *Peritonæum*, or to the *Omentum*, or to some of the other Intestines; it is no wonder, therefore, that they intirely lay aside the Practice of stitching up the wounded Parts of the Intestine, especially with uninterrupted Stitches, like the *Glover's Suture:* which by the frequency of the Puncture brings on a violent Inflammation, the most acute Pains, Convulstions, nay sometimes Cancer or Mortification, and Death itself. But they rather chuse now to deal more tenderly with the Patient, and to substitute a gentler Method of Cure. In Consequence of which, the present Practice is to pass a waxed Thread through a fine Needle, and with this to fasten the wounded Part of the Intestine to the internal Orifice of the Wound of the Abdomen. The Thread that hangs out the Abdomen is to be so firmly fixed by the Application of sticking Plasters to the Wound, that the Intestine cannot recede from the Part to which it was fastened, nor can it evacuate any of its Contents into the Cavity of the Abdomen.

Dr. Dufresne recorded in the *Medical Times* of London in 1844 that in 1795, Daguescea treated a traumatic colonic injury by ventral colostomy [86].

> *Artificial Anus.* --In August, 1795, V—-, æt. 57, was, during harvest, occupied in loading his cart with wheat; during an effort to lift a sheaf, the band having broken, he lost his equilibrium, fell, and the left side of his abdomen struck one of the stakes forming the sides of the cart, with sufficient force to cause it to penetrate deeply. Taken home, M. Daguesceau, a surgeon residing at Chadurec, was called in immediately, and decided upon establishing an artificial anus, according to Littrés method. No consecutive accidents occurred; and the patient soon got well, and lived twenty-four years, for he died in 1819, aged eighty-one.

Routine abdominopelvic operation to treat colon and rectal injuries were described in World War I. In 1917, Captains J. Fraser and H. Drummond [87] reported on 300 perforating war wounds of the abdomen, 85 of which involved the colon and 10 of which involved the rectum (Table 1.2).

Table 1.2 Fraser and Drummond. Results of colon and rectum wounds, World War I

Colon Wounds	*Number*
Bullet wounds	34
Revolver bullet wounds	2
Shell wounds	42
Bomb and grenade wounds	7
Complicated wounds	64
Pure colon wounds	21
Treatment	
Simple suture	55
Suture with proximal colotomy	25
Colotomy at the site of injury	4
Resection	1
Results	
Recovered	37
Died	48
Wounds of Rectum	*Number*
Bullet wounds	4
Bomb and shell wounds	6
Complicated wounds	9
Treatment	
Suture	3
Simple drainage	2
Drainage and colotomy	5
Results	
Died	7
Recovered	3

High mortality associated with colon and rectal war wounds in the American and British armies persisted until 1943 [88]. From 1943 onward, however, a remarkable decline in death was seen.

The most significant change was mandatory exteriorization of colon injuries advocated by Major-General W.H. Ogilvie [89].

> *The exteriorization of colon injuries.* A step which I have repeatedly advocated since the outbreak of war, the exteriorization of colon injuries, is, perhaps the greatest single factor in the improved results we are able to record. The principle that all damaged parts of the large intestine must be excluded till the process of repair is complete applies to all injuries even suspected ones, and to all parts of the large bowel, particularly the extraperitoneal portion of the rectum.

For the United States Army, the policy was stated in Circular letter No. 178: [90]

"ARMY SERVICE FORCES
Office of the Surgeon General
Washington 25, D. C.
23 October 1943.
CIRCULAR LETTER NO. 178
Subject: Care of the wounded in theaters of operation.
(5) Abdomen
(e) In large bowel injuries, the damaged segment will be exteriorized by drawing it out through a separate incision, preferably in the flank. In order to facilitate subsequent closure the two limbs of the loop should be approximated by suture for a distance of about 2 1/2 inches and then returned to the abdomen leaving the apex exteriorized with a short length of rubber tubing or other suitable material beneath it. If the segment cannot be mobilized the injury should be repaired and a proximal colostomy done.
(f) Penetrating injuries of the rectum should have exploratory laparotomy and posterior drainage by excision of the coccyx and incision of the fascia propria.
For The Surgeon General:
ROBERT J. CARPENTER
Lieut. Colonel, Medical Corps
Executive Officer.
DISTRIBUTION:
All officers of the Medical Corps, U S Army"

The 1945 technique of colostomy closure used in the US Army was illustrated by Colcock [91] as shown in Fig. 1.6.

Indications for colostomy in trauma subsequently have changed significantly.

Primary Colostomy Maturation

In 1951, Patey [92] argued for primary epithelial apposition in colostomy creation:

> The question I wish to raise in dealing with my small series of cases in this paper is a point in the technique of colostomy… As commonly performed, in all types the gut is deliberately brought out some distance from the abdominal wall, so that the epithelium of the bowel mucosa and the epithelium of the skin are at a distance from each other. Eventually, after a phase of granulation, fibrous contraction, and epithelial growth, epithelial continuity is re-established… The securing of early epithelial apposition is one of the fundamental principles of surgical healing, and the question I wish to raise is whether the time has not now come when we ought to try to achieve primary epithelial apposition at the time of the colostomy.

Patey asserts that the traditional technique seems to have been developed to guard against sepsis from intestinal contents, retraction, and sloughing. Patey maintained that in most wounds healing is quickest and best if early epithelial apposition is instituted. In a report of three types of colostomies (in continuity, terminal, and double barreled) done for acute obstruction, diverticulitis, and after resections, Patey found no disadvantages. Advantages to primary epithelial apposition by opening the bowel immediately and sewing the bowel to the skin edge included quicker healing and "earlier functioning of the bowel without the phase of temporary obstruction to the passage of flatus and feces so often associated with the edematous granulating colostomy" (Fig. 1.7).

In 1952, Butler [93] presented his observations on the treatment of 267 cases of rectal carcinoma in his President's Address to the Royal Society of Medicine. Regarding the method of colostomy creation following abdominoperineal resection, Butler stated: "In 1946, at Mr. Hermon Taylor's suggestion, we began the practice of sewing the colon to the skin at the end of the operation…" The technique, depicted in Fig. 1.8, produced "a final effect like a sea-anemone…" The immediate benefit of primary maturation was "an immediate free vent for escape of gas and fæces." In addition, the authors found that stenosis and retraction were avoided and that infection was uncommon.

In 1954, Lemmer and Mehnert [94] further defined the technique of colostomy creation advising that "all layers of the abdominal wall be kept in their proper vertical perspective when making a colostomy incision." To accomplish this, they placed "traction forceps on the peritoneum, on the fascia, and in the subcutaneous tissues near the skin before making the colostomy incision."

Extraperitoneal Colostomy

In 1958, Sames [95] in Bath brought attention to "lateral-space obstruction," a complication of left iliac colostomy. To remedy this problem, he brought the descending colon out "extraperitoneally before passing through the other layers of the abdominal wall." In the same year, Goligher [96] at Leeds independently published on the technique of extraperitoneal colostomy or ileostomy (Fig. 1.9).

Goligher used the technique to establish a colostomy in 45 cases and an ileostomy in 14. With relatively short

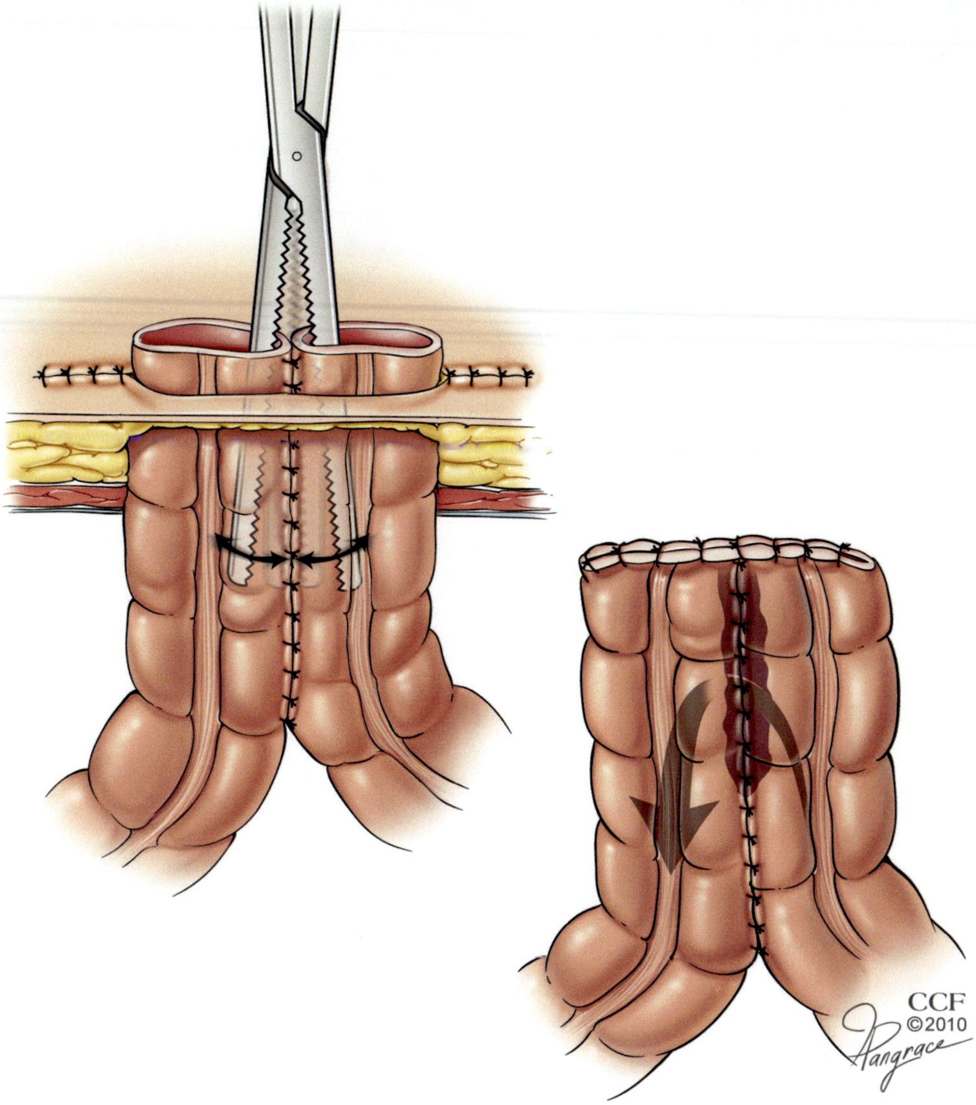

Fig. 1.6 Colostomy closure is facilitated by crushing the spur between two limbs of intestine fixed next to each other (Illustration © CCF)

follow-up, although no drawbacks were discovered in the method, two or three of the colostomy cases had shown "slight pericolostomic bulging" and one of the ileostomy cases had developed "some degree of recession of her ileostomy bud on recumbency…"

Hidden Colostomy

In 1967, Turnbull and Weakley [97] described an approach for patients with metastatic left-sided colorectal carcinoma with impending obstruction. The mobile transverse colon is secured above the fascia but beneath the skin. When obstruction occurs, decompression via the previously "hidden loop colostomy" is easily achieved by a local subcutaneous procedure instead of laparotomy. An India ink tattoo suggests the line of incision (Fig. 1.10).

Cecostomy

The cecum is a relatively accessible mobile structure that may be used to decompress the large intestine. In 1893, Henrotin [98] in Chicago recommended that in "*severe* general diffuse septic peritonitis with tympanities, from whatever cause, the chances of recovery will be enhanced if two openings are made, one to drain the peritoneal cavity and the other, an artificial anus, to relieve the distension." He reported a case of perforated appendicitis in a 15-year-old boy successfully treated by cecostomy and drainage.

> I opened the abdomen in the right semilunar line, and there welled out fully one pint of the most offensive greenish-black pus that can well be imagined. The appendix was matted down into an apparently inextricable exudate, and along its side were found two fecal concretions, evidently part of one body before being broken. The cecum on one side and the adjoining coils of

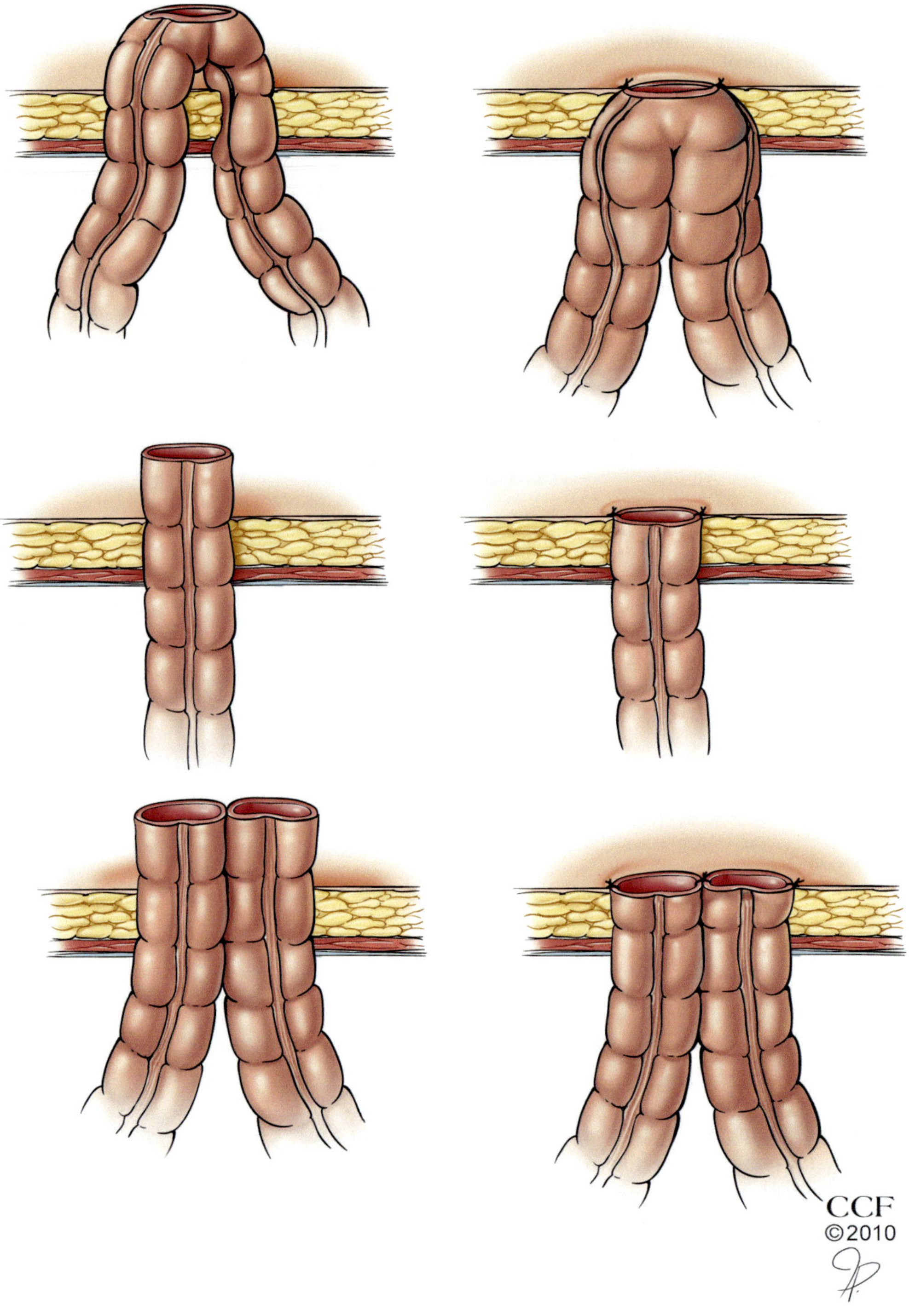

Fig. 1.7 Primary colostomy maturation (Patey). The illustrations on the *left* represent the three main colostomy types (in continuity, terminal, and double-barreled) as performed by the "traditional" technique; those on the *right*, by primary epithelial apposition (Illustration © CCF)

ileum were immensely distended, dark in color, and covered with more or less organized lymph. Pushing in a long glass tube, connected with a reservoir filled with hot sterilized physiological salt solution, to the upper abdomen, I turned my attention to the bowel. Making an incision into the abdominal wall at the side above the anterior superior spine of the ilium and parallel to the cecum, I pushed out a fold of that distended organ and made through its walls an incision about an inch and a quarter in length, the edges of which incision I stitched to the abdominal wall, thereby making a large artificial anus at that point. As soon as opened, the cecum began to discharge gas and fecal matter; and now, passing in a large rubber tube upward in the course of the ascending colon, I practised a thorough lavage of the colon. Meanwhile the abdomen from the more median incision had been constantly undergoing a flushing process. After ten or fifteen minutes more of this combined washing out the boy was put to bed, care meanwhile having been taken to introduce iodoform gauze strips to the left side, down into the pelvis, and particularly down into the region of the appendix and around the recently constructed artificial anus. The first twenty-four hours the meteorism was reduced to one-half, and in three days his belly was almost flat.

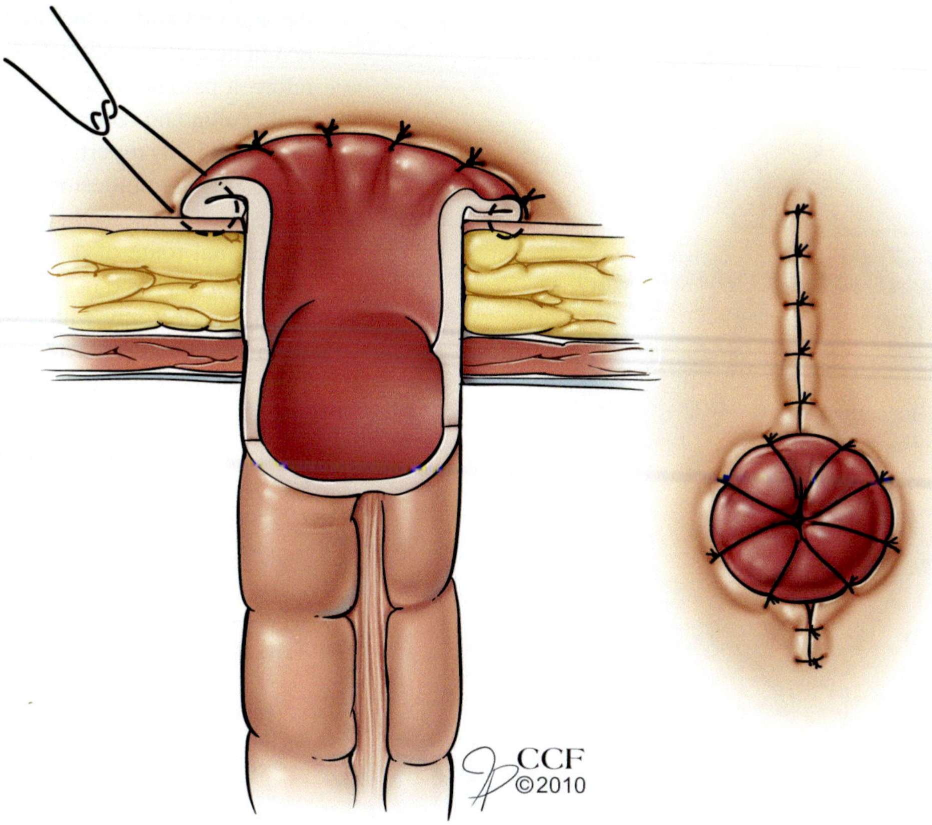

Fig. 1.8 Colostomy primary maturation following abdominoperineal resection according to Butler (1951): "Each stitch enters the skin half an inch from the wound and emerges at the skin edge itself. It then passes through the edge of the bowel wall from mucosa to serosa and pierces the colon again from serosal aspect an inch proximally, finally emerging from the depths of the lumen. As the suture is tied, the bowel wall is drawn out on to the surface of the skin while its edge is tucked under." [94] (Illustration © CCF)

Enterostomy

Similar to colostomy, the earliest small intestinal stomas were created to decompress the distended intestine. In 1888, Maydl noted that either colostomy or enterostomy could be used in the treatment of rectal carcinoma [99, 100]. In 1892, Smith [101] in Bristol read a paper advocating "operative evacuation and drainage of intestinal contents in cases of obstruction of the bowels where distension was a marked feature" by enterostomy. Surgical options included: "(1) simple evacuation of contents with immediate return of the gut; or (2) evacuation with drainage for several hours or days, and subsequent closure and return of the gut; or (3) evacuation with drainage that may be permanent."

Enterostomy to treat intestinal distension also was described by Lund [102] of Boston in 1903:

> Enterostomy is indicated for obstruction or paralytic distension of the intestine from whatever cause, after the ordinary means for relief of such distension have failed. It is especially applicable for distension after operations for acute appendicitis or general peritonitis. Under such circumstances it may restore to life cases in which death seems inevitable.

In his technique, the skin and subcutaneous tissue are anesthetized with cocaine. The abdomen is entered through a 1 in. subumbilical incision. The nearest distended coil of small intestine is sutured to the opening by a continuous suture, opened and a large glass tube inserted into the afferent coil. Lund noted that "the patient generally expresses relief even for the slight diminution of distension which is at once evident."

The development of small intestinal ostomy surgery is closely associated with operations directed at ulcerative colitis. Early reports of the treatment of ulcerative colitis did not involve colectomy because the majority of patients brought to surgery often were extremely ill and not considered good surgical candidates. In 1913, Brown [103] in St. Louis summarized current therapy as follows:

> While many of the ulcerative types of colitis respond to medical treatment and colonic lavage, the severer types are now recognized as surgical. In the operative treatment of such cases, three procedures have been resorted to: First, appendicostomy; second, cæcostomy; third, ileosigmoidostomy. All of these operations are objectionable. The first two simply permit of colonic irrigation and medication. As fast as the colon is flushed with solutions it refills with the fæcal contents from the small bowel; thus the area under treatment is constantly contaminated. A very serious objection to the short-circuiting operation is that the lower pelvic colon is almost invariably involved in the colitis, and it is impossible in the majority of cases to bring a loop of ileum to a part of the sigmoid distal to the disease; hence, when this is done, some degree of the symptoms, namely, that due to the sigmoid below anastomosis, will persist.

Brown described an operation that involved tube ileostomy and cecostomy to treat acute and chronic obstruction of

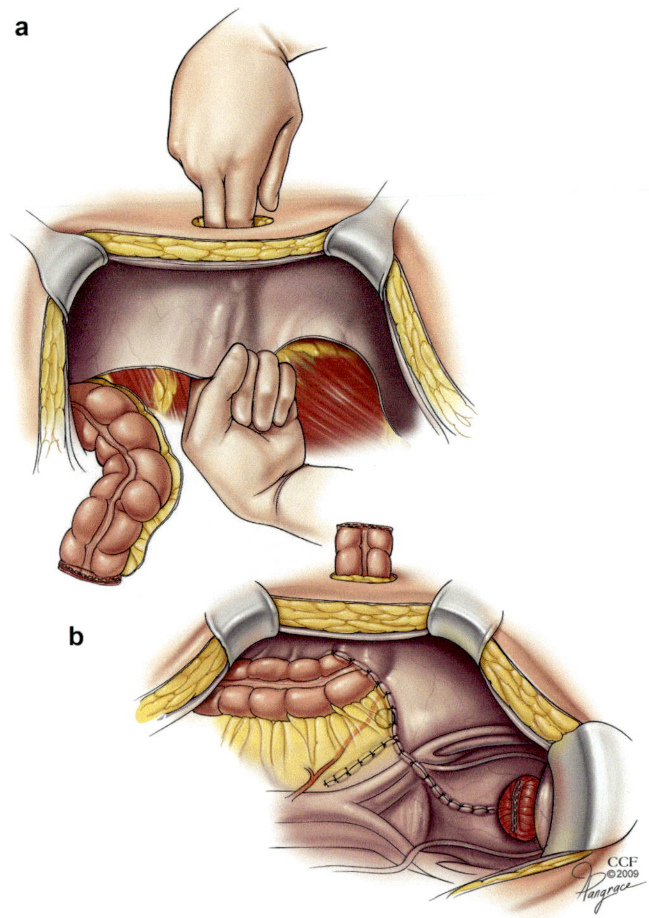

Fig. 1.9 Extraperitoneal colostomy: (**a**) an extraperitoneal tunnel is created; (**b**) the extraperitoneal colostomy in place (Illustration © CCF)

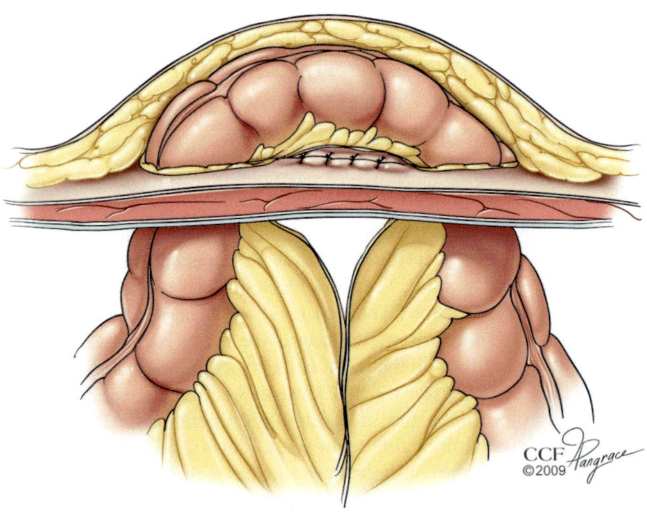

Fig. 1.10 Hidden loop colostomy. The mobile transverse colon is secured above the fascia in a subcutaneous position. In the event of a distal obstruction, decompression is accomplished by incising the skin overlying the transverse colon (Illustration © CCF)

the sigmoid and rectum and also to permit complete bowel rest in ulcerative colitis. Using this procedure, he was able to return a patient with extensive ulcerative colitis of the sigmoid colon and rectum to good health (Fig. 1.11).

Despite this report, ileostomy was not embraced immediately. Ileosigmoidostomy remained popular because it bypasses the diseased colon and at the same time preserves the normal route of defecation. An example of this type of operation, reported in 1931 by Arn [104] of Dayton involved ileosigmoidostomy with distal ileostomy (Fig. 1.12).

In his 1944 review of the surgical management of ulcerative colitis, Corbett [105] wrote: "There is no doubt that appendicostomy was the most popular form of surgical treatment in London only just 4 years ago." He attributed to Keetley the suggested use of the appendix for irrigation in 1895 and to Weir the performance of the first appendicostomy for ulcerative colits in 1902.

The Ascension of Ileostomy

The evolution of ileostomy as the foremost surgical procedure for the treatment of chronic ulcerative colitis of the thromboulcerative type has had a long and devious course. The long years during which it was being evaluated, as well as study of the cases in which it was done, brought to the fore sporadic attempts to substitute for it such maneuvers as appendicostomy, cecostomy, colostomy and ileosigmoidostomy. These operations were always eventually replaced by the seemingly inevitable ileostomy.

J. Arnold Bargen, Wallace W. Lindahl,
Frank S. Ashburn, John DeJ Pemberton
Rochester, 1943 [106]

Ileostomy.-This operation consists of draining the contents of the small gut through an opening in the terminal part of the ileum near the ileocæcal valve and so putting out of action completely, the whole of the colon. It is a drastic procedure and for this reason few physicians or surgeons are prepared to submit their patients to it, except after very careful consideration.

R. S. Corbett
President's Address
Section of Proctology
Royal Society of Medicine, 1944 [105]

Internists understandably and properly delayed sending patients with ulcerative colitis to surgeons for ileostomy until such was the serious state of the patient from advanced (toxic) stages of the disease that the internists, family physicians, all members of the family and the surgical consultants were unanimous in their opinion that ileostomy, however repulsive it might be, was the sole available measure by which the patient's life could possibly be saved.

Frank H. Lahey
Boston, 1951 [107]

An ileostomy must work perfectly if the surgical treatment of ulcerative colitis is not to fall into disrepute.

B. N. Brooke
The University of Birmingham, 1952 [108, 109]

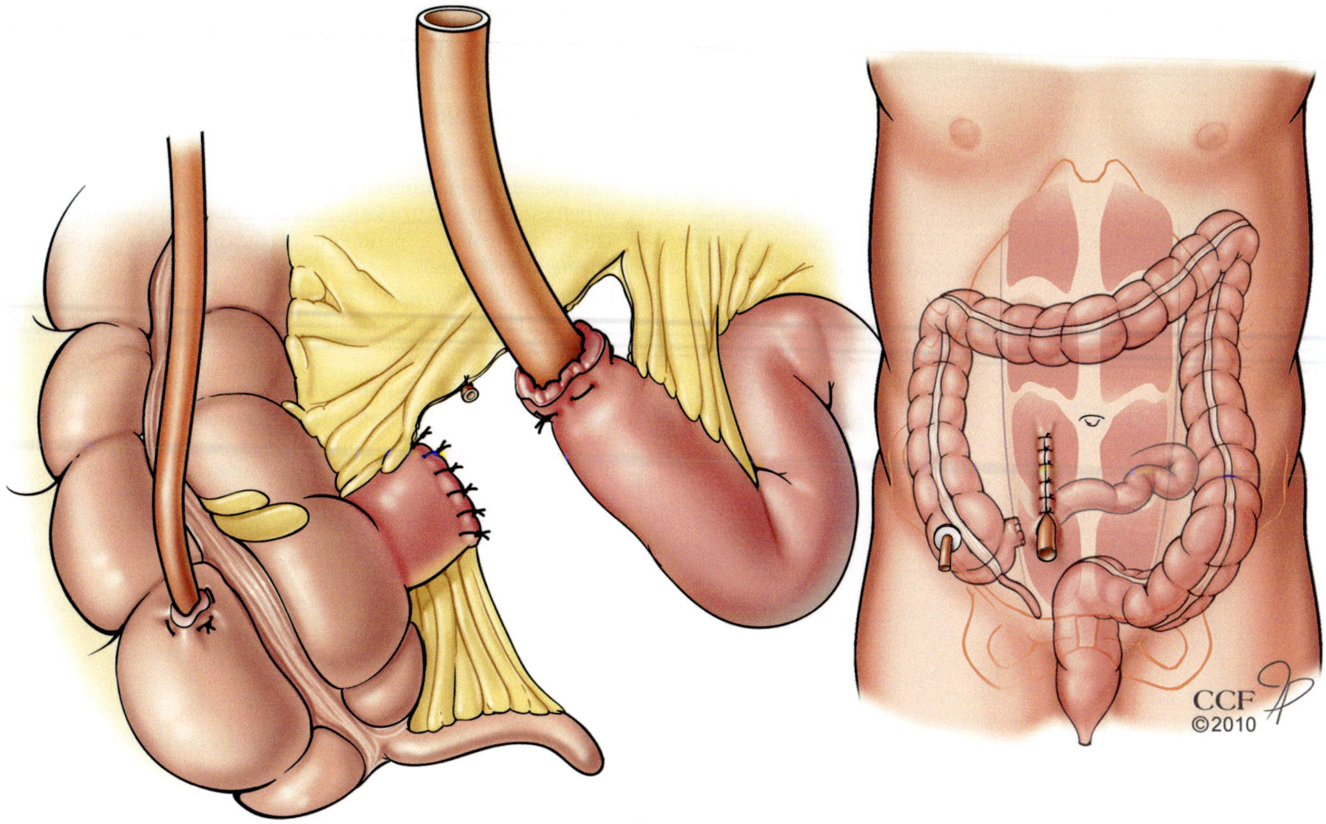

Fig. 1.11 Tube ileostomy and cecostomy to treat ulcerative colitis (Brown's operation). The ileum is divided. The distal ileum is tied off. The proximal end is exteriorized as an artificial anus with a stiff rubber tube inserted. A tube cecostomy is brought out through a separate incision (Illustration © CCF)

Although potentially a life-saving intervention, early ileostomy creation unfortunately was associated with significant morbidity and high mortality. Lahey noted that surgery frequently was performed as a last resort when patients were critically ill from toxicity, hepatitis, fistulas, and advanced malnutrition following failure of medical therapy. At that point, the performance of even the simplest type of ileostomy could be fatal. Once created, ileostomies were associated with numerous complications including: liquid discharge, bad odor, skin erosion, digestion of the abdominal wall, stomal retraction into the abdomen, appliance insecurity, depression, and in some cases, suicide [107]. In 1931, Rankin [110] described total colectomy with ileostomy for polyposis and ulcerative colitis. Initial diversion by ileostomy was followed by staged proctocolectomy. To create the ileostomy, the abdomen was accessed through a McBurney incision, without exploration. The ileum was divided close to the ileocecal valve. The proximal end was brought out, leaving a clamp on the end for 2 days. In a subsequent paper, in 1932, Bargen et al. [111] placed a small drainage catheter into the ileum after removal of the clamp; they also noted that the immediate convalescence after ileostomy was complicated by considerable loss of fluid and drastic efforts to maintain a satisfactory water balance were necessary. In 1935, Cattell [112] also reported that a large amount of fluid, substances of food value and chlorides were lost following ileostomy. In 1940, Cave and Nickel [113] reported 51 deaths in a group of 154 patients (33%) following ileostomy. They stated that: "In no small measure has the high mortality been due to a rapid and excessive loss of fluid and chlorides immediately after operation."

In 1951, Warren and McKittrick [114] of the Massachusetts General Hospital described the outcome of 210 ulcerative colitis patients treated by ileostomy between 1930 and 1949. The authors enunciated principles for stoma site selection and incision that are still in use: "Select a point in the right lower quadrant of the abdomen as far as possible from irregularities of surface such as the anterior superior iliac spine, the umbilicus and the symphysis pubis." Through a rectus muscle-splitting incision, approximately 3 cm of ileum were brought out beyond the skin, and a glass tube or catheter was placed in the stoma to lead the discharge away. Unfortunately, a syndrome with signs and symptoms of partial small bowel obstruction were seen in 130 (62%) of the patients. The authors coined the term

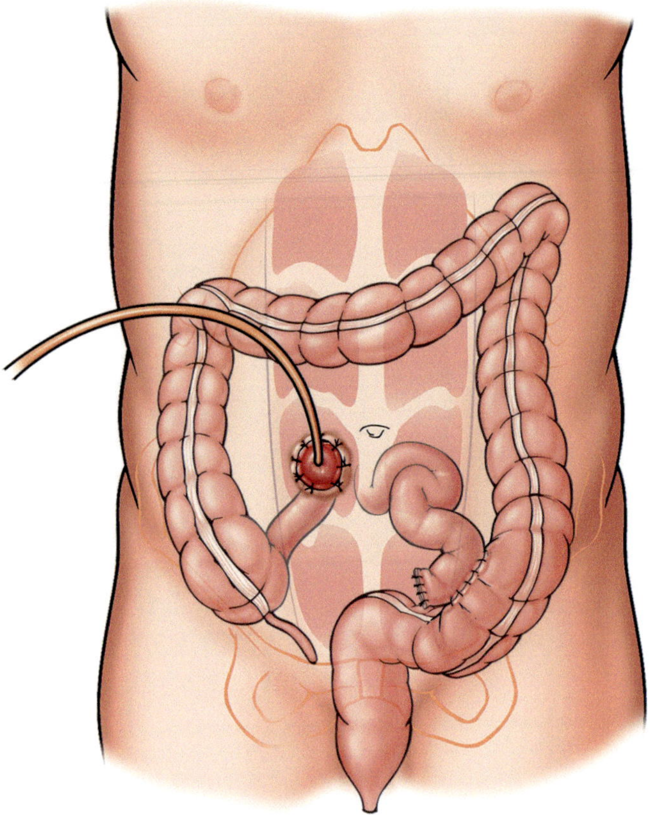

Fig. 1.12 Ileosigmoidostomy and end ileostomy (Arn). The ileostomy was used for colonic irrigation (Illustration © CCF)

"ileostomy dysfunction" to describe this condition. They described the clinical characteristics of the syndrome as follows:

> It is characterized by cramp-like pain and, paradoxically, an increase in the volume of ileostomy discharge. The discharge becomes watery. In the severe cases vomiting occurs and ileostomy diarrhea becomes so severe that serious water and electrolyte deficiencies may result. The first systemic manifestation may be sudden evidence of profound fluid and electrolyte imbalance as manifested by a shock-like state.

Concerning the cause of ileostomy dysfunction, the authors wrote:

> The cases which occur early are usually due to interference with the normal flexibility and peristaltic action of the ileum by the comparatively rigid abdominal wall, those which occur late, the result of a constricting band of scar tissue which replaces the granulation tissue on the serosa of the exposed ileum and draws the mucosal margin down toward the skin.

Symptomatic relief could be achieved by decompression using a catheter. Plastic operations were introduced that were intended to release the constricting effects of scar tissue at the exteriorized intestine (Fig. 1.13). In Warren and McKittrick's series, such procedures had to be done in more than a third of all ileostomy patients and in more than half of those developing dysfunction.

In 1954, Crile and Turnbull [115] summarized ileostomy dysfunction as follows:

> A naked, unprotected segment of ileum is suddenly brought into the septic environment of its own discharges. Serositis with fibrinopurulent exudate is noted by the third or fourth day. This is in reality a peritonitis of the protruding segment. Edema, rigidity, and loss of peristalsis of the exteriorized segment soon follow, just as they do in any peritonitis. Although a tube or finger can be passed easily, functional obstruction is present…
>
> The classic ileostomy must progress through certain phases before it begins to function normally. We have referred to this sequence of events as 'maturation of the ileostomy,' and until maturation is complete, varying degrees of dysfunction (obstruction) persist. In the course of maturation, the infected serosal surface slowly contracts and pulls the free mucosal border down toward the abdominal skin. This spontaneous eversion of the ileostomy takes place over a period of four to six weeks, and is nature's way of covering the exposed and infected serosal surface. (Fig. 1.14)

The Solution to Ileostomy Dysfunction

> Improvements in technics of establishing ileostomy to prevent serositis have resulted from contributions by Dragstedt and associates (skin grafting), Brooke, (full-thickness eversion), and Turnbull and Crile (mucosal grafting).
> Oliver H. Beahrs
> Rochester, 1971 [116]

In 1941, Dragstedt et al. [117] in Chicago described a method of ileostomy creation that involved skin grafting the serosal surface of the exposed ileum (Fig. 1.15). The resulting ileostomy prevented skin excoriation and was easily fitted with an appliance.

In 1949, Monroe and Olwin [118] found a tendency of both the bowel and a split thickness skin graft to contract over time, resulting in shortening of the ileostomy. To prevent this, the authors described a technique for constructing a skin-covered ileostomy by wrapping the terminal ileum in a flap of skin, subcutaneous tissue, and fascia nourished by the superficial epigastric vessels.

Primary Ileostomy Maturation

> A more simple device is to evaginate the ileal end at the time of operation and suture the mucosa to the skin.
> B. N. Brooke
> The University of Birmingham, 1952 [108]

In 1952, Brooke recommended primary complete eversion of the ileostomy. The ileal end is evaginated at the time of operation, and the mucosa is sutured to the skin (Fig. 1.16).

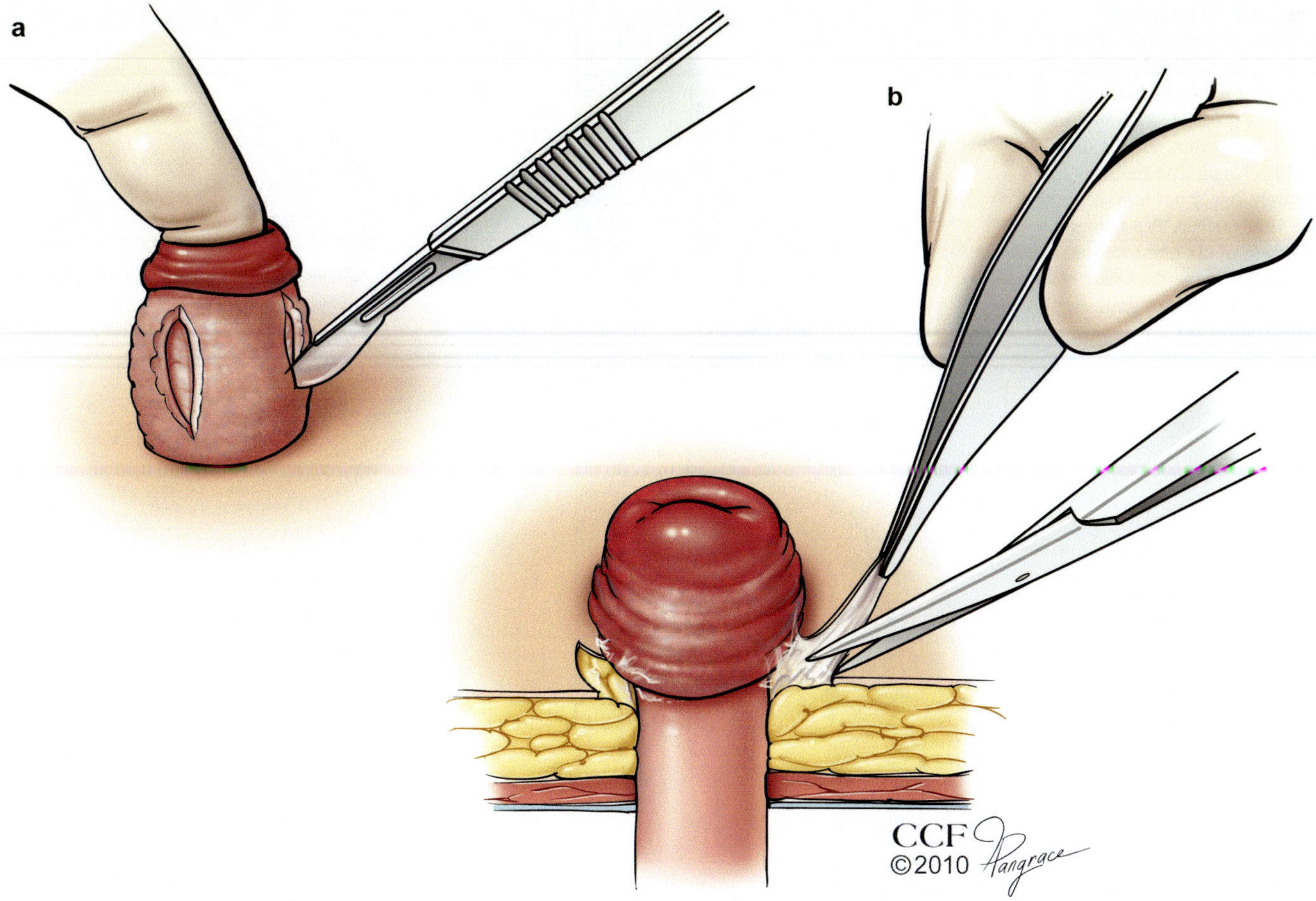

Fig. 1.13 Plastic operation designed to release constricting effect of scar tissue at the exteriorized stoma: (**a**) multiple longitudinal incisions to release the contracting collar of scar; (**b**) excision of stricturing scar at the stoma base

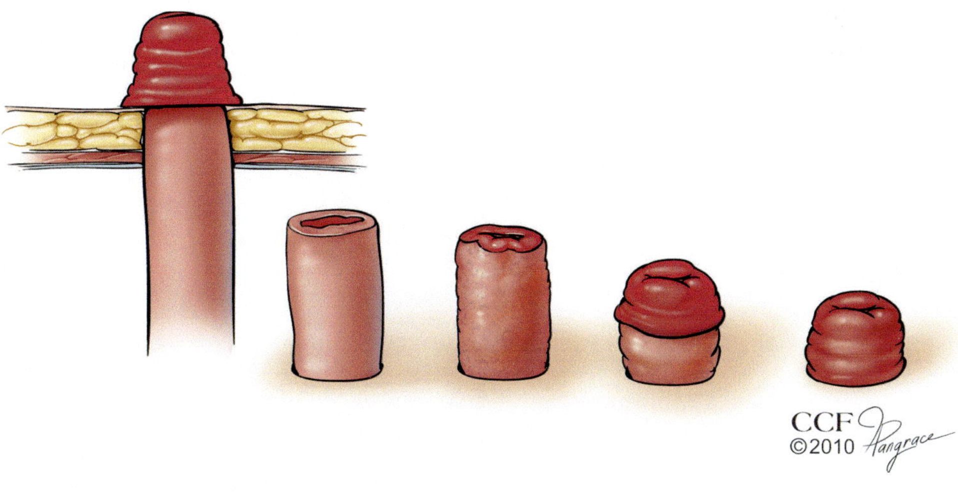

Fig. 1.14 Spontaneous maturation of the ileostomy. The cut end of the small intestine will spontaneously evert and seal with the skin. Spontaneous eversion takes weeks to complete and is accompanied by symptoms and signs of partial intestinal obstruction, a syndrome referred to as "ileostomy dysfunction." (Illustration © CCF)

His method helped to overcome complications such as stenosis and postoperative diarrhea associated with ileostomy dysfunction. Years later, Brooke modestly stated that it was "by chance" that the problem of ileostomy dysfunction was overcome by his eversion method [119]. The "Brooke ileostomy" remains to this day the standard technique for ileostomy creation.

In 1953, Turnbull [120, 121] described a technique for hastening stomal maturation developed in partnership with Dr. George Crile in which the seromuscular coats of the distal exteriorized ileostomy are removed and the residual mucosa-submucosal tube sewn down to the skin to produce a mucosal-grafted ileostomy (Fig. 1.17). The trimming procedure was done on the seventh day after initial surgery.

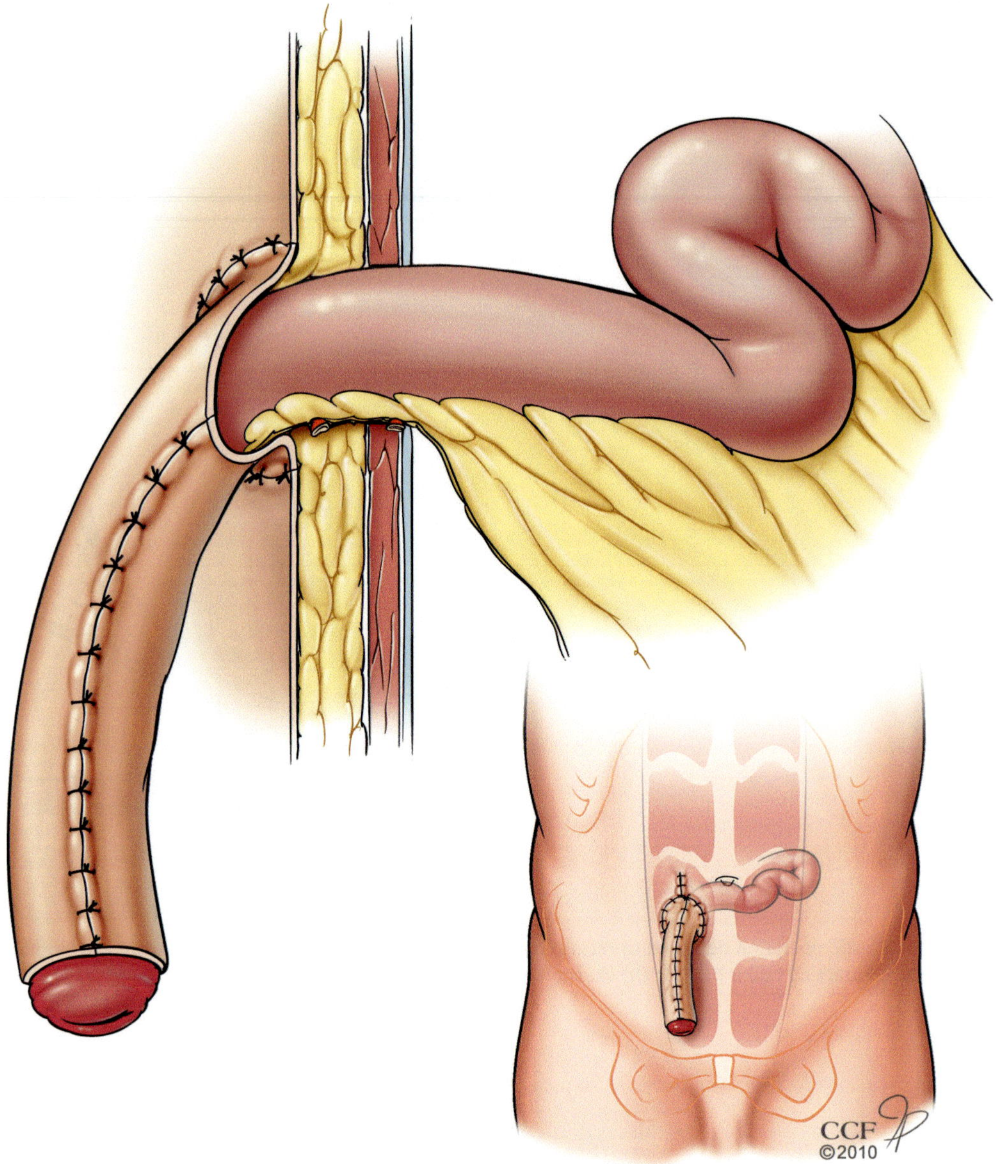

Fig. 1.15 Skin grafted ileostomy (Dragstedt). The abdomen is opened through a low right rectus incision. The ileum is transected about 4 in. from the cecum, and the distal end is closed. The ileum is brought out about 6 in. beyond the skin surface. A rectangular segment of six one-thousandths of an inch is the thickness of the split thickness skin graft. (Illustration © CCF)

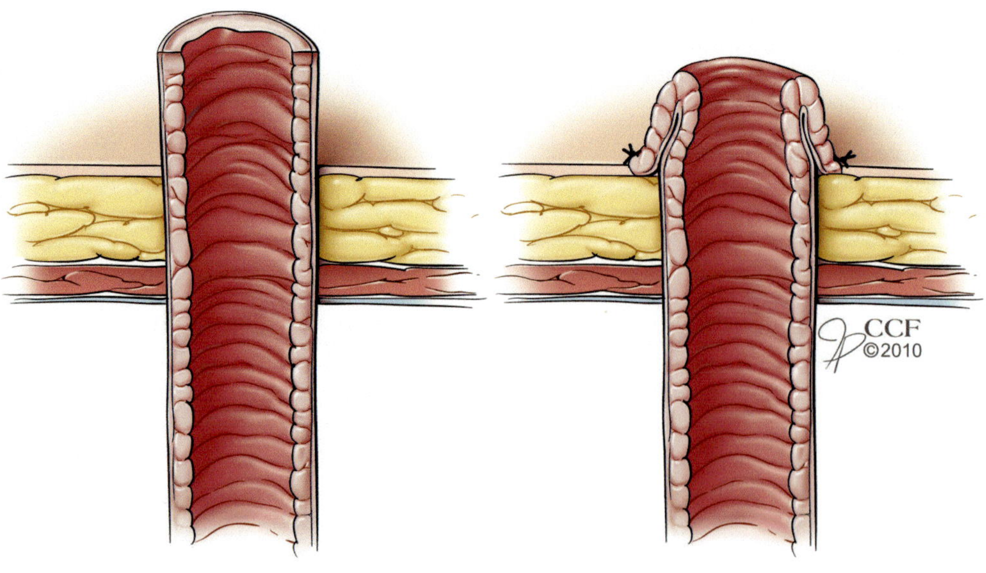

Fig. 1.16 Brooke's Ileostomy. The edges of the intestine are everted and sewn directly to the skin (Illustration © CCF)

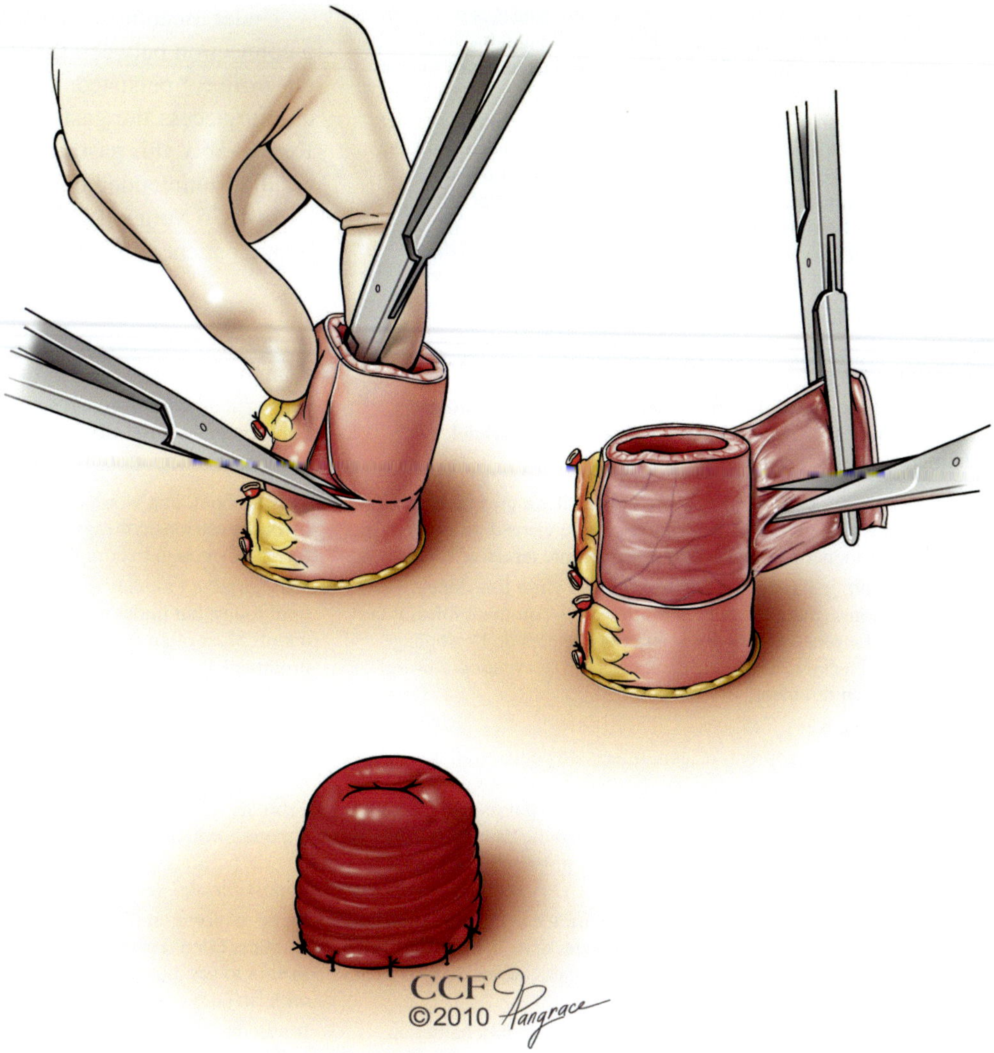

Fig. 1.17 Turnbull and Crile's Ileostomy. After seromuscular stripping, stomal maturation is achieved by bringing the mucosa-submucosal tube down to the abdominal skin and fixing it with sutures (Illustration © CCF)

Gastrostomy

In 1833, William Beaumont, Surgeon in the US Army, published a treatise on experiments and observations on gastric juice and the physiology of digestion. [122]

> Experiments and observations on the Gastric Juice and the Physiology of Digestion.
>
> William Beaumont,
> Surgeon in the US Army

Introduction

> The experiments which follow were commenced in 1825, and have been continued, with various interruptions, to the present time, (1833.) The opportunity for making them was afforded to me in the following way.
>
> Whilst stationed at Michillimackinic, Michigan Territory, in 1822, in the military service of the United States, the following case of surgery came under my care and treatment.
>
> Alexis St. Martin, who is the subject of these experiments, was a Canadian, of French descent, at the above mentioned time about eighteen years of age, of good constitution, robust and healthy. He had been engaged in the service of the American Fur Company, as a voyageur, and was accidentally wounded by the discharge of a musket, on the 6th of June, 1822.
>
> The charge, consisting of powder and duck shot, was received in the left side of the youth, he being at a distance of not more than one yard from the muzzle of the gun. The contents entered posteriorly, and in an oblique direction, forward and inward, literally blowing off integuments and muscles of the size of a man's hand, fracturing and carrying away the anterior half of the sixth rib, fracturing the fifth, lacerating the lower portion of the left lobe of the lungs, the diaphragm, and perforating the stomach.
>
> I saw him in twenty-five or thirty minutes after the accident occurred, and, on examination, found a portion of the lung, as large as a Turkey's egg, protruding through the external wound, lacerated and burnt; and immediately below this, another protrusion, which, on further examination, proved to be a portion of the stomach,…

> Frequent dressings with soft compresses and bandages were necessarily applied, to relieve his suffering and retain his food and drinks, until the winter of 1823-4. At that time, a small fold or doubling of the coats of the stomach appeared, forming at the superior margin of the orifice, slightly protruding, and increasing till it filled the aperture, so as to supersede the necessity for the compress and bandage for retaining the contents of the stomach. This valvular formation adapted itself to the accidental orifice, so as completely to prevent the efflux of the gastric contents when the stomach was full, but was easily depressed with the finger.

Under Beaumont's care, St. Martin recovered. However, a connection between the stomach and the abdominal wall, an "orifice, " persisted. Through this aperture Beaumont was able to access the gastric cavity for the purposes of study. Remarkably, this gastrocutaneous connection, created as the result of unintended trauma, achieved continence.

In 1876 Verneuil [123] described *gastro-stomie* to treat a young patient with an impassable esophagus.

Communications	Communications
M. Verneuil communique une Observation de gastro-stomie pratiquée avec succès pour un rétrécissement cicatriciel infranchissable de l'œsophage.	**M. Verneuil communicates an observation of gastrostomy performed successfully for an impassable scar narrowing of the esophagus.**
Il s'agit en un mot de la *gastro-stomie* conçue il y a près de trente ans par notre illustre collègue M. Sédillot, et que je viens d'être assez heureux pour mener à bonne fin dans une récente tentative.	This is about, in a word, a gastrotomy designed nearly 30 years ago by our illustrious colleague M. Sédillot, and that I've just been fortunate enough to complete successfully in a recent attempt.
Cette operation, je l'ai déjà dit, a été pratiquée vingt fois depuis 1849 jusqu'à nos jours, mais dans des conditions très-peu favorables, il faut en convenir. Le plus souvent il s'agissait de cancers de l'œsophage ayant amené un état cachectique dans lequel l'intervention chirurgicale réussit bien rarement;	This surgery, I already said, was performed twenty times since 1849 until today, but under not very favorable conditions, we have to admit. Most often it was about cancers of the esophagus having prompted a cachexia in which the surgery is seldom successful.
Voici, le fait (1):	Here, the fact (1):
R.M..., dix-sept ans, apprenti maçon, mince, de petite taille et d'apparence encore enfantine, s'était toujours bien porté, lorsque le 4 février 1876 il avala par mégarde une solution de potasse d'Amérique, qui provaqua dan la gorge une sensation immédiate de brûlure vive. La fièvre s'alluma et la déglutition resta pendant plusieurs jours presque impossible et très-douloureuse;	R.M..., 17 years old, an apprentice bricklayer, thin, small and with a still childish look, had always been in good health, when, on February 4, 1876, he accidentally swallowed a solution of potash of America, which brought in his throat an immediate sensation of intense burning. Fever started and swallowing remained almost impossible and very painful for several days
A l'exploration de l'œsophage la sonde est arrêtée à 7 centimètres de l'anneau cricoïdien, assez avant par conséquent dans la poitrine, J'essaye en vain d'arriver dans l'estomac avec des olives du plus petit numéro et avec des sondes de baleine.	In the exploration of the esophagus, the probe is stopped at 7 cm from the cricoid cartilage, therefore deep enough in the chest. I try in vain to get into the stomach with olives of the smallest size and with rib (stay) probes.
Il fallait donc ou assister les bras croisés à une mort prochaine, ou exécuter l'opération de Sédillot. Je consultai la famille qui me donna carte blanche, et j'allais procéder quand une lueur d'espoir brilla à mes yeux.	It was therefore necessary either to witness an early death without being able to do anything, or to execute Sédillot's operation. I consulted the family who gave me carte blanche, and I was going to proceed when a glimmer of hope shone in my eyes.
Je crus plus sûr d'agir purement et simplement comme dans l'entérotomie ordinaire, telle qu'on l'exécute quand on veut créer un anus artificiel à la paroi abdominale antérieure.	I thought it was safer to act simply as for an ordinary enterotomy, which is done when you want to create an artificial anus in the anterior abdominal wall.
Une incision de 5 centimètres fut pratiquée à la limite de l'épigastre... La peau, le tissu cellulaire sou-cutané et l'aponévrose furent successivement divisés; ... l'estomac fut facilement reconnu...Je me mis en devoir alors de fixer les parois stomacales et abdominales; je mis en usage, à cet effet, le procédé de Nélaton pour l'entérotomie, qui consiste, comme chacun le sait, à passer une série circulaire de sutures *avant d'ouvrir* la cavité intestinale.	A 5 cm incision was performed at the edge of the upper abdomen... The skin, the subcutaneous cellular tissue, and fascia were divided successively;... the stomach was easily recognized... I then decided to attach the stomach and abdominal walls, using for this purpose, Nélaton's [124] process for enterotomy, which is, as everyone knows, to pass a circular series of sutures *before opening* the gut cavity.
Je me servis du chasse-fil courbe et de fils d'argent, et plaçai ainsi successivement 14 points, distants l'un de l'autre de 5 à 6 millimètres environ...les fils furent serrés avec des boutons de chemise et un anneau de plomb écrasé avec un davier. Tous ces boutons rangés circulairement et régulièrement donnaient à la ligne de réunion une certaine élégance.	I used a curved needle and silver threads, and thus successively placed 14 points apart from each other of about 5–6 mm... the threads were tightened with shirt buttons and a lead ring crushed with a forceps. All these buttons circularly and regularly placed gave to the line of meeting some elegance.
Je fis cette ouverture sur le point culminant de la bosselure stomacale herniée avec des ciseaux, et dans l'étendue seulement d'un centimètre.	I made this opening to the climax of the herniated stomach small bump with scissors, and for only 1 cm.
Je crus bon, enfin, de placer à demeure dans l'ouverture un corps étranger creux qui permît d'introduire des aliments fluides dans l'estomac.	I thought it would be good, finally, to place in the opening a hollow foreign object which would permit the introduction of liquid food in the stomach [34].

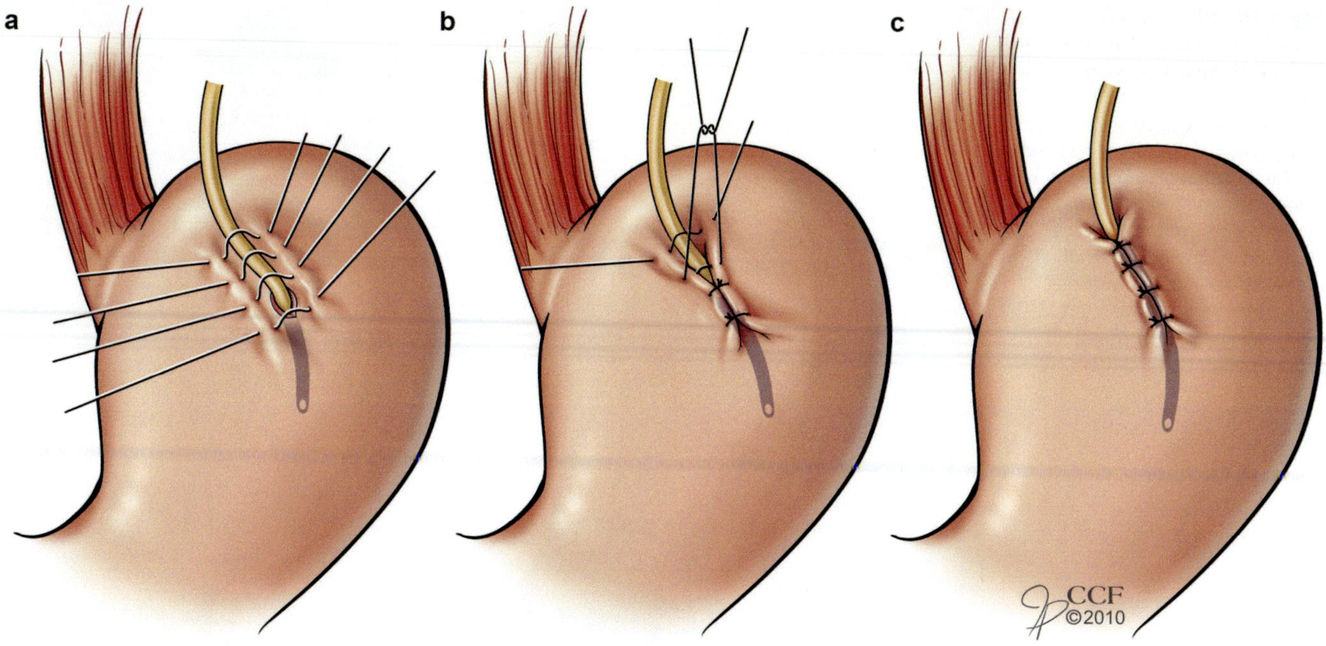

Fig. 1.18 Witzel's tunneled tube gastrostomy: (**a**) sutures are placed on either side of the tube after insertion into the stomach; (**b**) the sutures are sewn over the tube to make a tunnel (**c**) (Illustration © CCF)

In 1891, Witzel [125] described a technique for creating a fistula to the stomach using a tube that passes through a surgically created tunnel (Fig. 1.18). Witzel stated that the technique provides a route for the tube similar to that traveled by the ureter into the bladder.

Zur Technik der Magenfistelanlegung	On the Technique of Gastrostomy
Von Prof. Oscar Witzel, Bonn	**by Oscar Witzel, Bonn**
Nun würde es mir eine Freude sein, wenn das Vorgehen, welches im Folgenden geschildert wird, Beachtung bei den Fachgenossen fände, die Technik wurde von mir zunächst an der Leiche erprobt, sie hat sich in 2 Fällen am Lebenden als gut erwiesen.	I would be glad if the method described below would find favor with my colleagues. I tested the technique first on a cadaver, and it has also given good results in two live patients.
Das Verfahren geht darauf hinaus, durch Vernähung der freien Ränder zweier parallelen Längsfalten am vorgezogenen Theile der Magenwand einen schräg von oben rechts nach unten links hin ziehenden Kanal zu schaffen, der, unten auf die klein angelegte Magenöffnung führend, dem eingelegten Röhrchen einen Verlauf geben soll gleich dem des unteren Endstückes des Ureters in der Blasenwandung.	The procedure consists in pulling two parallel longitudinal folds out from the stomach wall and in suturing their free edges together to create a channel which slants downward from the top right to the bottom left, leading to the small opening made in the stomach. The channel is intended to provide a route for the inserted tube similar to that which the lower end of the ureter takes in the wall of the bladder [34].

In 1894, Stamm [126] of Fremont, Ohio, reported a new technique for tube gastrostomy in which the tube is secured to the stomach by means of a purse-string suture. This suture guards against leakage from the stomach.

Ostomy Appliances

With stoma creation came the problem of waste collection. As noted previously, in 1795, Daguescea successfully treated a man who had sustained a penetrating abdominal injury by establishing an artificial anus according to Littrés method. A small leather sac was used to collect feces discharged from the artificial anus [86]. During World War II, resourcefulness, ingenuity, and necessity led to the creation of receptacles made from canteens for soldiers with ileostomy or colostomy (Fig. 1.19 [127, 128]).

Rigid containers placed over a stoma and held in place with belts were cumbersome and often plagued by leakage and by injury either to the ostomy or to the adjacent skin.

From the mid twentieth century onward, indications for intestinal stomas expanded. In 1950, Bricker [129] reviewed bladder substitution after pelvic evisceration. Following bilateral ureteral anastomosis, segments of ileum, sigmoid colon, or ileocecum were drained to the abdominal surface as ileostomy, colostomy, or cecostomy. In 1957, Bishop and

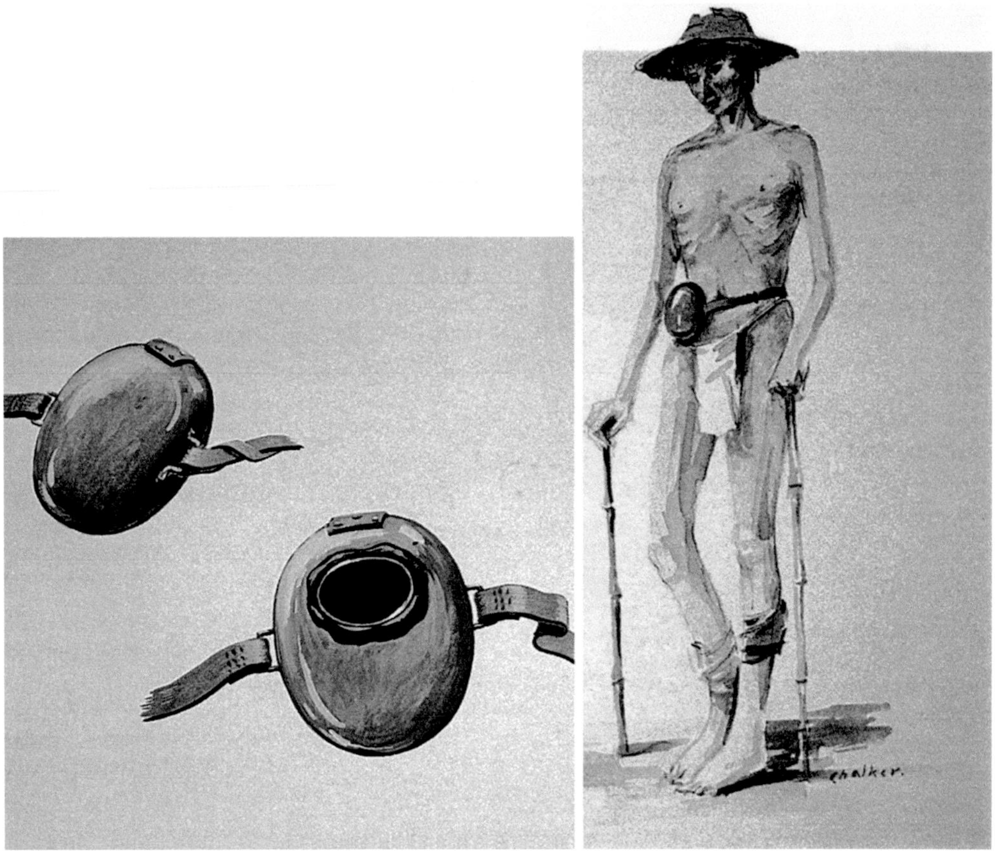

Fig. 1.19 *"Ileostomy and colostomy bottles, Chungkai and Nakorn Pathon, 1943–1945:* Made from Dutch army water bottles with the aperture faced with pieces of old motor tyre and held in position on the patient with army webbing. The water-bottle spouts have been removed and the hole sealed up." These resourceful innovations proved very successful (Reproduced with permission from Chalker [127, 128]

Koop [130] described the method of resection, Roux-en-Y anastomosis, ileostomy, and postoperative irrigation with pancreatic enzymes to treat meconium ileus associated with fibrocystic disease of the pancreas.

In 1969, Kock [131] introduced the continent intra-abdominal reservoir in patients with permanent ileostomy. In 1972, Suruga et al. [132] described treatment of biliary atresia by portojejunostomy in which additional cutaneous enterostomy of the draining loop was created in order to allow observation of bile flow. In 1976, Feustel et al. [133] reported a continent colostomy using a magnetic ring implanted into the abdominal wall around the stoma.

Ostomy to the Isolated Intestinal Segment

In 1864, Thiry [134, 135] described a method to isolate the small intestine in order to study intestinal physiology detached from the flow of the fecal stream. After restoring continuity of the intestinal canal, one end of the excluded loop was closed; the other was attached to the skin (Fig. 1.20).

The Thiry loop and related methods currently are used by intestinal surgeons to preserve segments of out-of-circuit small intestine for possible future reintegration into the main intestinal stream.

Intestinal Stomas and Industry

In a history of ostomy products manufacturers, Davidson and Fischer [136] note that improvements in stoma appliances often were created by forward-thinking visionaries who saw the need for something better either because they had an ostomy themselves or because they were close to someone with an ostomy.

The Koenig–Rutzen Appliance

In 1934 Koenig, of Chicago, submitted an application for a colostomy appliance (Fig. 1.21):

United States Patent Office, 2,048,392, COLOSTOMY APPLIANCE, Henry F. Koenig, Chicago, Ill. Application March 19, 1934, Serial No. 716, 235.

> The present invention relates to appliances in the form of receptacles or containers adapted to be associated with artificial orifices in abdominal walls, and has for its object to simplify and improve such appliances.
>
> Heretofore appliances of this type have been bulky and rather cumbersome and, viewed in one of its aspects, the present invention may be said to have for its object to produce an appliance which will be thin and flat and thus produce no considerable outward projection from the abdominal wall.

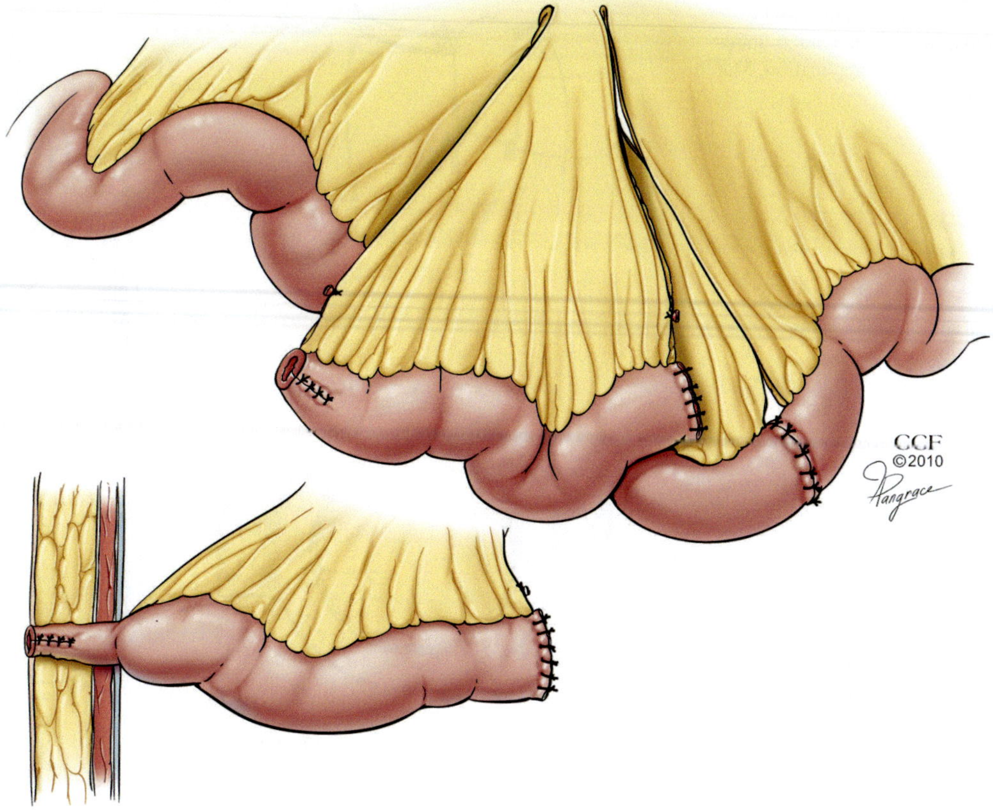

Fig. 1.20 Thiry fistula. A segment of small intestine is isolated. One end is closed; the other end is brought to the surface of the abdomen as a stoma (Illustration © CCF)

> Heretofore it has been practically impossible to secure a fluid-tight joint between the appliance and the abdominal wall and, viewed in another of its aspects, the present invention may be said to have for its object to provide a simple and novel means whereby, without undue pressure or other cause or act that may produce inconvenience or discomfort, all danger of outward leakage between the contacting surfaces of the appliance and the abdominal wall is prevented. [137]

The appliance was made of two thin sheets of flexible rubber lying flat upon each other. Consequently, the container was flat or very thin. A washer-like piece made of soft rubber, adapted to contact with the abdominal wall of the wearer around an orifice, produced a seal to prevent escape of fluid. In a 1944 review of surgery for ulcerative colitis, Strauss and Strauss [138] identified irritation of the skin produced by the intestinal contents as a major problem associated with ileostomy:

> We have completely solved this with a bag devised by one of us (A.A.S) and Mr. Koenig, a chemical student on whom we corrected an ileostomy done elsewhere, and on whom we eventually performed a colectomy. At our suggestion he developed a bag which covers the ileostomy and does not permit secretions to come in contact with the skin. The bag is held to the skin with a latex preparation which we will describe later, and completely prevents the irritation of the skin, as well as the possible escape of secretions, collecting them in light, soft, rubber container.

Koenig teamed up with Herman W. Rutzen to manufacture the appliance in Chicago. In a conversation on 10 Septemper 2009, Mr. Earl Rutzen, 81 years old, recalled:

> My father had received an ileostomy to treat amoebic dysentery. His surgeons were Dr. Herman Sondel in Chicago and Dr. Clarence Dennis in Minneapolis [139]. Dad owned a rubber mill. Unfortunately, it wouldn't run because he didn't have a motor. Henry Koenig brought in an old Chevy engine and together they got the mill going to make the stoma bags. Henry Koenig was a genius; he designed the bag. My father, however, ran production. I joined the company, H. W. Rutzen & Son, in 1946. Soft rubber bales from the West Indies were fashioned into bags, treated with zinc oxide, stearic acid and mercaptobenzothiazol, and then Vulcanized to make the rubber firm. The Vulcanization process initially was done using a kitchen pressure cooker. We had to watch the pressure really closely to make sure it wouldn't explode. The face-plate was made separately and glued to the bag. We would go to the hospitals when called and measure patients individually before making their appliance. The Rutzen bag, as it came to be called, effectively protected the skin around the stoma by fixing the bag to the skin using rubber cement. The seal would last between 12 and 24 hours. I worked for the company for 60 years. We supplied appliances to patients around the world. We closed our doors in April 2007. It was plastics and disposables that subsequently replaced us.

The Koenig–Rutzen appliance has received accolades from the highest places:

> About seven days after surgery the patient is fitted with one of a supply of Koenig-Rutzen bags kept on hand for the purpose, and may be up and about the ward. As soon as the patient masters the management of the bag, usually in another two to three days, he goes home.
>
> Clarence Dennis
> Minneapolis, 1945 [139]

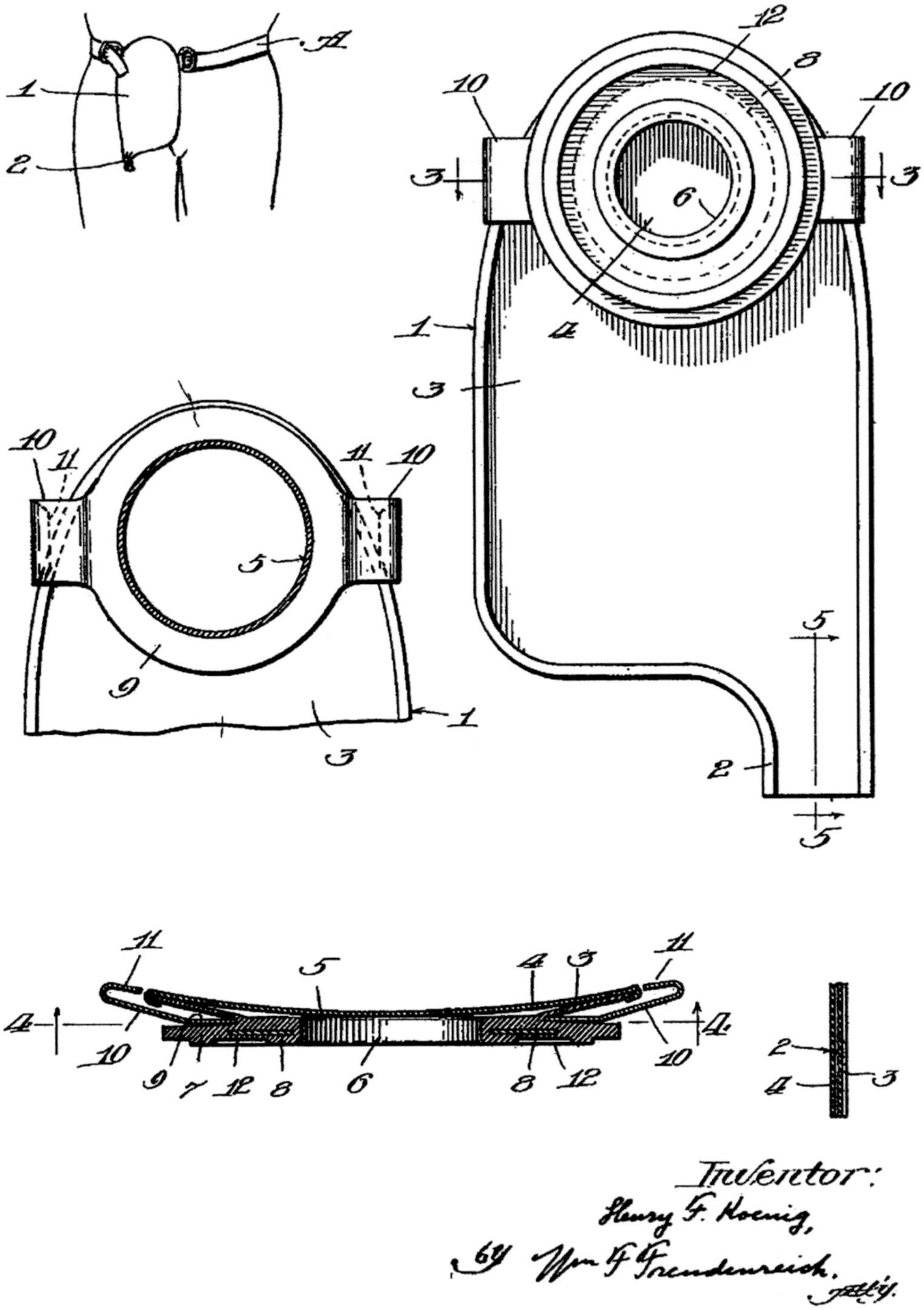

Fig. 1.21 The Koenig colostomy appliance as submitted in the United States Patent Office application, March 19, 1934

Anastomosis of the ureters to an isolated segment of terminal [ileum] is now practiced. This appears to be the simplest way to convey the urine from both kidneys to an external stoma conveniently located for the use of a Rutzen bag.

Eugene M. Bricker
St. Louis, 1950 [129]

It would be a grave injustice, however, not to remind all patients requiring surgical intervention and all surgeons doing ileostomies how much they and we are indebted to Mr. H. W. Rutzen who, with an ileostomy himself, was a pioneer in developing the idea of the fitted ileostomy bag with a collar cemented to the skin.

Frank H. Lahey
Boston, 1951 [107]

Since the introduction in 1945 of the Koenig-Rutzen bag or some modification of it, the outlook for patients with ileostomy has been revolutionised.

T. L. Hardy
Birmingham, 1955 [140, 141]

> The last quarter century has seen the gradual development of ileostomy from an unmitigated disaster to a stoma brought to a level of efficiency that has made it acceptable not only as a gastrointestinal but also as a urinary conduit, thanks to the invention by Rutzen of the adherent bag and its subsequent development.
>
> B. N. Brooke
> London, 1975 [119]

Sorenson's Disposable Ostomy Appliance

In the 1950s, the rise of plastic disposable ostomy appliances occurred in Denmark. [142] The following history of the Coloplast company is courtesy of Troels Nørgaard Laursen, Head of Professional Partnerships, Coloplast A/S, Holtedam 3 3050 Humlebæk, Denmark:

> In 1954, 50-year-old Elise Sorensen was known by her colleagues as a very dedicated visiting nurse. This dedication took on added meaning when her younger sister, Thora, got cancer on the colon and underwent colostomy surgery.
>
> Like others in her situation, Thora was devastated not only by her future physical limitations—she was only 32—but the perceived social rejection she faced.
>
> The physical limitations were not made easier by the appliances then available. They were cumbersome, unhygienic and costly. But most seriously, they failed to offer reliable protection against odor and leakage. It is not surprising that many outgoing men and women dropped out of social activities they formerly enjoyed.
>
> The hardships faced by colostomists were not lost on Elise Sorensen. In a 1955 interview she said: 'Actually, I have been preoccupied by the psychological difficulties of patients since my student days. I have especially felt empathy for those who have had a colostomy. The psychological stress and anxiety caused by the inability to control bowel movements has forced many people to change their lives completely, because they simply could not lead normal lives.'
>
> Moved by her sister's predicament, Elise Sorensen went about developing an appliance that would overcome the drawbacks of available devices. The new bag was 'non-porous, thin and elastic,' according to her patent application. And as a revolutionary breakthrough, it was disposable and equipped with an adhesive for direct application to the body—no need for cumbersome straps.
>
> As her idea had been dismissed by many manufacturers of products for the handicapped, Elise Sorensen turned to Dansk Plastic Emballage, a small but successful plastic bag company owned by Aage Louis-Hansen.
>
> Louis-Hansen had achieved early success by developing innovative welding methods that made his bags absolutely tight. However, he had not planned on medical applications, so naturally he was somewhat skeptical when Elise Sorensen made her initial approach. Fortunately for a world of ostomists, Johanne Louis-Hansen, his wife, interceded. Having been a student nurse herself, she fully understood the potential of the new bag for relieving a great deal of human distress. [143]

Dansk Plastic Emballage subsequently became the Coloplast Company in 1957. [144]

Karaya

Karaya is a vegetable gum produced by the tropical Asian trees, genera *Sterculia* [145]. Improved methods of protecting the skin included the application of materials used as denture fixatives. The possible use of karaya was identified by Turnbull in Cleveland, by chance:

> In 1952, he was cleaning out the desk of his former chief, Tom Jones, and accidently knocked over a small cannister of Jones' dental powder into spilled coffee on the desk. The karaya immediately absorbed the coffee and stuck to Turnbull's wet hand. He thought that the powder might also absorb ileostomy effluent and protect the skin from the excoriating effects of the liquid stool. He contacted Leonard Fenton, an engineer and brother-in-law of one of Turnbull's patients. [146]

With Turnbull's medical knowledge and Fenton's manufacturing and engineering skills, karaya was produced by the Marlen Company, named after the founders Marvin Magar and Leonard Fenton. Mr. Gary Fenton:

> My father, Leonard Fenton, was an engineer who in the late 1940s was working at the Cleveland Clinic Foundation with Dr. Willem J. Kolff [147] designing a kidney dialysis machine. While there, the young Dr. Rupert Turnbull approached my father and asked for his help to design a better ostomy appliance. At the time skin excoriation from the ileostomy effluent was a major problem. Patients were using all kinds of receptacles such as rubber gloves and kidney basins. After an initial meeting at the clinic, Dad set the project aside and did not think about it further until one evening, there was a knock on the front door, and there stood Dr. Turnbull who asked once again for Dad's help. The first ostomy appliance designs were done on our front door step. It turns out that the two families lived only three blocks away from each other in Shaker Heights. The Fentons and the Turnbulls became close both professionally and personally. My father became Godparent to the Turnbull children, and Dr. Turnbull in turn was Godfather to us. Dad and Dr. Turnbull were joined by Ms. Norma Gill on the stoma appliance work and came to be known as the 'Three Musketeers.' The business was run by my uncle, Marvin Magar. Combination of Marvin and Leonard eventually led to the company name: Marlen. Contributions that we are particularly proud of include the application of karaya for skin protection and the addition of convexity to pouch face-plates. Type A and Type B rubber cement (then used as glue for carpets) was the method used to adhere pouches to the skin. This unfortunately resulted in significant skin problems around the stoma. Karaya was used as the first type of barrier that is applied directly onto the skin to give protection to the skin against the adhesives used to attach the appliance. The second contribution that our company is particularly proud of is the addition of convexity to pouches. People come in all shapes and sizes, and sometimes a flat plate just does not fit properly. Convexity helped to solve this problem for many patients.

The Marlen Company continues today, 50 years later, in Bedford Heights, Ohio, under the direction of Leonard and Marvin's sons: Gary Fenton and Michael Magar.

Hydrocolloids

In 1963, Gilman Cyr and James Chen, assignors, by mesne assignments, to E. R. Squibb & Sons, Inc, New York, N.Y., submitted an application for a patent: 3,312,594 Longlasting Troche:

> This invention relates to longlasting troches or pastilles. By longlasting troche is meant one which does not disintegrate or lose its integrity for 30 minutes or more. According to this invention, troches or pastilles are prepared which provide a vehicle for various medicaments used in treating the oral cavity or for sublingual or transbuccal administration lasting for periods of 30 minutes to about 8 hours. [148]

Orahesive™ is a hydrocolloid made from a blend of gelatin, pectin, and sodium CMC in polyisobutylene (PIB) developed by J. L. Chen of E. R. Squibb and Sons, Inc. Dr. Chen's invention of hydrocolloid adhesive technology enabled a variety of medical devices to be securely attached to the body [149]. In 1964, Sircus [150] described the use of "Orabase" in the management of abdominal wall digestion by ileostomy and fistulas:

> Sir,
> Despite the use of barrier creams, pastes, and paints of various kinds, excoriation and digestion of the skin around ileostomies, small-bowel fistulas, and, occasionally, colostomies often persist. The problem becomes aggravated when the epithelium is denuded and oozing serum prevents the application from coming into contact with the ulcerated areas. 'Orabase' (Squibb) has the property of sticking to the wet mucosal surfaces of the buccal cavity. Through the courtesy of the manufacturers we were given for trial supplies of orabase gel, which is the base of the preparation marketed in the United Kingdom for the treatment of mouth ulcers as 'Adcortyl-A in Orabase' and 'Orahesive' (the same compound in powder form).
>
> For some months patients in our wards with fistulas and leakage around ileostomies have had the surrounding skin protected or treated with either a coating of the gel or (when excoriated) with powder sprayed on with an insufflator. In the opinion of the nursing staff and the patients, the applications have been uniformly successful. The skin heals rapidly and is protected against further ulceration.
>
> W. Sircus
> Western General Hospital, Edinburgh

The application of Orahesive™ to bond an appliance to a patient's abdomen is attributed to Sister Elinor Kyte and Sir E. S. R. Hughes of Australia in 1970 [151, 152]. Stomahesive was subsequently introduced to protect the parastomal skin in 1972 and is still manufactured today by ConvaTec.

Nu-Hope

The following history of the Nu-Hope company is courtesy of Mr. Bradley J. Galindo and Ms. Estelle Galindo:

> Mr. Edmund Galindo suffered from chronic kidney disease that in 1958 was treated by irrigation of an isolated segment of small intestine with a dialysis-type of solution through an intestinal stoma. At that time, ostomy products were crude and ineffective, and their use caused frustration and anguish because of leakage, skin breakdown, and soiling of clothing and bed linen. On his own, Ed created new appliance designs. He proved the worthiness of a new appliance system on himself and was able to return to an active life of business, golf and swimming. His doctors in Los Angeles were so impressed with his success that they urged him to manufacture and market his appliances so that others might benefit. At first, supplies and appliances were freely handed out. However, it soon became apparent that in order to continue, a company would have to be formed. In 1959, Nu-Hope Laboratories was founded. The name was derived from Mrs. Galindo's first name 'Hope' and the feeling that they were offering 'new hope' to others in need. Custom appliances is an area they are particularly proud of. Following the untimely death of the founder in 1959, the company was managed by Hope Galindo, and her children, Eugene and Louise.
>
> Eugene had a keen mind like his father. He obtained six patents and was the innovator of many new developments in ostomy products in use today. He further developed the means for customization of the appliances to manage challenging pouching situations; a contribution of which they are particularly proud.
>
> Nu-Hope continues to thrive as a family business for more than 50 years, with Edmund Galindo's grandson Bradley, President/CEO, Granddaughter, Debbie Director of Administration. Eugene's wife Estelle, RN, CWOC Nurse Consultant and great granddaughters Chanelle and Kathleen, office support.

Hollister

The following history of the Hollister company is provided by courtesy of Ms. Diane M. Owen, Professional Relations Liason, Hollister Inc. and Ms. Bobbi Micale of Hollister Inc.:

> Hollister began simply as the dream of one man: John Dickinson Schneider. In 1921, he opened a one-man print shop, JDS Printer Craftsman. In 1948, Mr. Schneider acquired the Franklin C. Hollister Company, which printed birth certificates. In 1964 the company entered the new field of ostomy care when an employee approached Mr. Schneider about the need for a colostomy bag. The employee's father was an ostomate with a colostomy and expressed the need for a colostomy bag that would work. At the time, the products used were relatively ineffective and included a bag with a cardboard gasket. Mr. Schneider thought that he could design a first class product; so he dedicated employees to investigating a karaya and glycerin formula that would allow the bag to be placed directly on the body. He had learned of karaya from an article on karaya powder by Dr. Rupert Turnbull of the Cleveland Clinic. Mr. Schneider had his engineers experiment with glycerin, karaya, and propylene glycol until a formula was developed. The result was the solid state Karaya Seal Ring—first marketed on disposable appliances and later patented by Hollister. [153, 154]
>
> The great success enjoyed by this product occurred in large measure because it provided effective skin protection. Mr. Schneider worked closely with colostomy clubs, founded by ostomates to support other ostomates. At the clubs, many ostomates shared their problems, and Mr. Schneider was interested in learning about them. At the time, Hollister was selling retail directly from the Hollister office in Chicago, so he would invite ostomates to visit Hollister and share their experiences in order to develop ideas to solve their issues. In the early days, people didn't talk

openly about their ostomies. Hollister ran one of the first advertisements in a retail publication, *McCall's*, bringing ostomates out into the open. Suddenly people who had undergone ostomy surgery could do more with life than just cope with it. User feedback contributed to the development of the opaque bag and original stoma cap. User feedback continues to drive Hollister product innovation today. [154]

Ostomy Support Groups

Dr. Albert Lyons records that the first organized ostomy support group in the world was formed in 1950 at The Mount Sinai Hospital, in New York [155]. Support groups had two major functions:

- Psychological: reassurance and understanding from other ostomates before and after the operation; advice on how to deal with oneself and others.
- Educational: instruction on the details of stoma management; information for surgeons on the proper location and other details of fashioning a stoma; information to the public on the existence and needs of ostomates.

Dr. Lyons recalled:

> Since the patients were admitted to Wards Q and/or T, the new group called themselves 'QT Alumni.' The choice of the term 'QT' avoided using the word 'stomas.' Elsewhere, other groups began to form. For instance, in recognition of the fact that the pioneering work was done in New York, the Boston group called themselves QT Boston and the Detroit group, QT Detroit. Years later, people no longer felt it necessary to use the term 'QT' and groups became known as ileostomy, colostomy, or ostomy associations.

From this seed have grown ostomy associations representing regions, nations, and the world [156].

Enterostomal Therapy Education

Before there were schools, enterostomal therapy education involved learning at the side of a Master clinician. The bond between the surgeon and the patient was close and often reached beyond the operating room, into the home. Mr. Robert W. Turnbull, recalls how his own education began one day at the side of his father.

> My father, Rupert B. Turnbull, Jr. was a gifted pianist, amateur botanist, champion swimmer, prolific reader, and avid writer. Memories of him are so plentiful, rich, and varied, it is hard to select just one story for the second rendition of his original *Atlas of Intestinal Surgery.* To my mind, perhaps the one that best symbolizes my father's compassion, dedication, and energy for life centers around a visit to a patient's home I made with him when I was 12. To me, he had always been 'Dad' but this visit revealed an entirely different facet of him I'd never seen—one that completely changed my perception of him forever—launching me into a lifelong career dedicated to ostomy care—the speciality he developed, which continued to consume his mind and energies until the day he died.
>
> One Saturday afternoon, he asked me if I wanted to see what he did for a living. I knew he was a surgeon at the Cleveland Clinic, but little more. With some trepidation, I accepted his invitation. In the days before Home Health Care, Enterostomal Therapists, ET Schools, and United Ostomy Association Visitor programs, my father would occasionally go to a recently discharged patient's home to follow up, especially if he had particular concerns about how the patient was progressing—physically and emotionally. This day, Dad wanted to follow up and check the patient's peristomal skin, incision, stoma, his overall mood and that of his family. He seemed to sense that things were not going well.
>
> As we pulled up to the house on Shaker Boulevard, the patient's wife greeted us at the front door with a somber face. She quietly escorted us to her husband's bedroom. We entered a dark, seemingly airless room without any sign of life—a scary scene for a young boy. My father asked the patient how he was feeling, receiving only a mumbled response in return. Dad then strode to the window, pulled back the curtains, and opened the window to allow light and air to pour in. Understanding the patient's progress was being hampered more by his emotional state than his physical condition, Dad reassured the patient things were healing well and that his spirits would improve in time. In a kind but stern voice, Dad told him it was time to stop hiding. Life was out there waiting for him—a life which had been given back to him—A gift—and it was time to get out of bed and enjoy this gift. After checking the patient and talking to the patient's wife, the atmosphere seemed brighter and laced with more hope than despair. I will never forget the smiles and expression of relief on the faces of the patient and his wife as we left. They were both at the front door waving good-bye. There was going to be life for them, it would just be a little different.
>
> That moment comes back to me when I have a difficult day. I open the curtains, let the sun shine in, and remember my father, and marvel at how much light and hope he and his teachings and innovations brought to so many people around the world.

In 1961, Rupert B. Turnbull Jr. created the first school dedicated to the training of experts in the field of enterotomal therapy with the assistance of Mrs. Norma Gill, herself an ostomate who had undergone surgery for colitis by Turnbull. Mrs. Gill then became the school's first director. Enterostomal therapy has since grown into an international nursing specialty [157].

The following history of the beginning of the Cleveland Clinic Foundation School of Enterostomal Therapy is courtesy of Ms. Sally J. Thompson, ET:

> For five years beginning in 1948, my mother, Norma Gill, suffered the wraths of ulcerative colitis along with the associated complication of pyoderma gangenosum. Unsure if she would survive, she vowed that if she did recover she would help others who were suffering as she had. Finally in 1954, she was referred to Rupert Turnbull, MD, at the Cleveland Clinic, who determined her need for an ileostomy. After her recovery, she acted on her desire to help others as she began visiting doctors in her hometown offering to help them with their ostomy patients. In a follow-up visit with Dr. Turnbull in May of 1958, she informed him of her assistance with these patients. A few months later, Dr. Turnbull contacted her and in October of 1958 she began her career at the Cleveland Clinic assisting with the rehabilitation of ostomy patients. Word of this new "specialty" soon spread, and Dr. Turnbull was contacted by other surgeons asking to send their assistants to the Cleveland Clinic to observe and to

be educated in the care and rehabilitation of ostomy patients, thus beginning the specialty of Enterostomal Therapy.

At present there are nine nursing education programs accredited by the Wound Ostomy and Continence Nurses (WOCN) society [158].

Summary

The current state of modern gastrointestinal ostomies is the culmination of work performed over the last two and a half centuries. The intentional exteriorization of the gut to the skin was introduced as a drastic measure to save life. The earliest ostomies were used to relieve intestinal obstruction from colorectal cancer, hernia, or imperforate anus. Intestinal stomas subsequently have served other roles, acting as the artificial end of the gastrointestinal, urinary, and hepatobiliary tracts. Life with a stoma, previously dreaded, is now manageable thanks to steady advances in surgery, medicine, nursing, industry, patient support groups, and education. Ultimately, the prime force that drives progress is the commitment of one individual person to care for another. Paula Toth recalls meeting Norma Gill shortly after she had received an ileal conduit as a young child:

> I was fortunate to meet Norma in 1965, a few days after having an ileal conduit. Norma lived in Akron (Ohio) and took the bus every day to work in Cleveland. She came to see me after work on a hot August day. I was 10 years old and scared. I vividly remember Norma's decisive, calm and optimistic approach. She had an ostomy herself. The equipment at that time was archaic and not designed for pediatric patients. Norma got me through that most difficult time and always helped me to find a solution to the many challenges of life with an ostomy. She became part of my life that day, and I cherished her like a second mother.
>
> Paula Erwin-Toth, ET
> Director, The Rupert B. Turnbull,
> Jr. School of Enterostomal Therapy

Acknowledgments The author gratefully acknowledges the following: the Cleveland Clinic Foundation and the Department of Colorectal Surgery for their unreserved support of this work; Mr. Joe Pangrace and the staff of the Cleveland Clinic Department of Art and Photography for their superb illustrations and photographs; the staff of the Cleveland Clinic Library for providing access to the medical literature; Mr. Peter Inglin and Ms. Jill Pinto, H-I Translation Services; Mr. John Holland, The Latin Translator; Major Kenneth M. Koyle, AMEDD office of Medical History; Mr. Earl Ruzen, W.H. Rutzen and son; Mr. Troels Nørgaard Laursen and Mr. Michael C. Davidsen, Coloplast A/S; Mr. Gary Fenton, The Marlen Company; Ms. Punny Donohoe, Mr. George Fattman, Ms. Annette Lee, The ConvaTec Company; Mr. Bradley Galindo and Ms. Estelle Galindo, Nu-Hope Laboratories; Ms. Bobbi Z. Micale and Ms. Diane M. Owen, Hollister International; Mr. Robert W. Turnbull, Vice President, Genairex; Ms. Sally J. Thompson, ET; Mr. Jack B. Chalker, Hon MA., ARCA., RWA., Hon FMAA., RMIP., medical artist and military historian; and Ms. Joyce Balliet and Ms. Marty Hodgson of the Department of Colorectal Surgery, Digestive Disease Institute, The Cleveland Clinic Foundation for their selfless support of this work. Special thanks are expressed to Mr. John B. Small and Mr. Gerard LeTendre of the Taft School, Watertown, Connecticut, who instilled in the author a love of the German and French languages years ago.

References

1. Merriam-Webster. Online dictionary of the English language. Accessed 5 May 2010.
2. Long CW. An account of the first use of sulphuric ether by inhalation as an anæsthetic in surgical operations. South Med Surg J. 1849;5:705–13.
3. Simpson JY. On a new anæsthetic agent, more efficient than sulphuric ether. Lancet. 1847;2:549–50.
4. Macewen W. Clinical observations on the introduction of tracheal tubes by the mouth instead of performing tracheotomy or laryngotomy. Br Med J. 1880;2:122–4, 163–5.
5. Röntgen WC. Über eine neue Art von Strahlen. Sitzungsberichte der Physikalischmedizinischen Gesellschaft zu Würzburg. 1895;137.
6. Stanton A. Translation: concerning. On a new type of rays by W. C. Röntgen. Nature. 1896;53:274–6.
7. Bier A. Versuche über Cocainisirung des Rückenmarkes. Dtsch Z Chir. 1899;51:361–9.
8. Landsteiner K. Ueber agglutinationserscheinungen normalen menschlichen Blutes. Wien Klin Wochenschr. 1901;14:1132–4.
9. Meltzer SJ, Auer J. Continuous respiration without respiratory movements. J Exp Med. 1909;11:622–5.
10. Fischer AW. Über eine neue Röntgenologische Untersuchungsmethode des Dickdarms-Kombination von Kontrasteinlauf und Luftaufblähung. Klin Wochenschr. 1923;2:1595–8.
11. Fleming A. On the antibacterial action of cultures of a penicillium, with special reference to their use in the isolation of *B. influenzae*. Br J Exp Pathol. 1929;10:226–36.
12. Griffith HR, Johnson GE. The use of curare in general anesthesia. Anesthesiology. 1942;3:418–20.
13. Thorn GW, Forsham PH, Frawley TF, Hill Jr SR, Roche M, Staehelin D, et al. The clinical usefulness of ACTH and cortisone (continued). N Engl J Med. 1950;242:824–34. The authors credit DuToit and Bauer with the first two cases of ulcerative colitis in which ACTH induced a favorable response.
14. Truelove SC, Witts LJ. Cortisone in ulcerative colitis. Preliminary report on a therapeutic trial. Br Med J. 1954;2:375–8.
15. Dudrick SJ, Vars HM, Rawnsley HM, Rhoads JE. Total intravenous feeding and growth in puppies. Fed Proc. 1966;25:481, abstract 1632.
16. Larson MD. History of anesthetic practice. In: Miller RD, editor. Miller's Anesthesia, vol. 1. 6th ed. Philadelphia: Churchill Livingstone; 2004. p. 3–52.
17. Wangensteen OH, Wangensteen SD. The rise of surgery. Minneapolis: The University of Minnesota Press; 1981, 3rd printing.
18. Anus praeternaturalis, künstlichen Afters, and anus artificiel are terms in Latin, German, and French respectively that have been used to describe colostomy. Anus praeternaturalis refers to the anus beyond the natural. Künstlichen Afters and anus artificiel specify the artificial anus.
19. Caelius Aurelianus. On acute diseases and on chronic diseases (Drabkin IE, edited and trans). Chicago: The University of Chicago Press; 1950. p. 2.
20. Caelius Aurelianus. On acute diseases and on chronic diseases (Drabkin IE, edited and trans). Chicago: The University of Chicago Press; 1950. Acute diseases; Book III, XVII,138; p. 388.
21. Caelius Aurelianus. On acute diseases and on chronic diseases (Drabkin IE, edited and trans). Chicago: The University of Chicago Press; 1950. p. 3.
22. Caelius Aurelianus. On acute diseases and on chronic diseases (Drabkin IE, edited and trans]). Chicago: The University of Chicago Press; 1950. Acute diseases; Book III, XVII,138; p 389.
23. Caelius Aurelianus. On acute diseases and on chronic diseases (Drabkin IE, edited and trans). Chicago: The University of Chicago Press; 1950. In his introduction (p. 11), Drabkin writes that Caelius Aurelianus is recognized the foremost translator of the medical works of Soranus of Ephesus, a physician who practiced in Rome

during the time of Trajan and Hadrian, from Greek into Latin. It is proposed that Caelius probably lived in the fifth century.
24. Caelius Aurelianus. On acute diseases and on chronic diseases (Drabkin IE, edited and trans). Chicago: The University of Chicago Press; 1950. Acute diseases; Book III, XVII, 146–63, pp. 392–405
25. Sudhoff K. Zur operativen Ileusbehandling des Praxagorus. Quellen Stud Gesch Naturwiss. 1933;3:359–62.
26. Caelius Aurelianus. On acute diseases and on chronic diseases (Drabkin IE, edited and trans). Chicago: The University of Chicago Press; 1950. Acute diseases; Book III, XVII, 163, pp. 400–2.
27. Caelius Aurelianus. On acute diseases and on chronic diseases (Drabkin IE, edited and trans). Chicago: The University of Chicago Press; 1950. Acute diseases; Book III, XVII, 163; p. 401.
28. Caelius Aurelianus. On acute diseases and on chronic diseases (Drabkin IE, edited and trans). Chicago: The University of Chicago Press; 1950. Acute diseases, Book III, XVII, 165; p. 402.
29. Caelius Aurelianus. On acute diseases and on chronic diseases (Drabkin IE, edited and trans). Chicago: The University of Chicago Press; 1950. Acute diseases; Book III, XVII, 165; p. 403.
30. Cromar CDL. The evolution of colostomy. Dis Colon Rectum. 1968;11:256–80.
31. Cheselden W. The anatomy of the human body. Case report of Margaret White. C. Hitch and R Dodsley, London, 1750. p. 324.
32. Amussat JZ. Mémoire sur la possibilité d'établir un anus artificiel dans la région lombaire sans pénétrer dans le péritoine. Acad R Méd, Germer-Baillière, Paris, 1 Oct 1839.
33. Littre. Diverses observations anatomiques II. Histoire de l'Academie R Sci (France). 1710:36–7.
34. Translation by H-I Translation Service; www.hitranslation.com.
35. Amussat JZ. Mémoire sur la possibilité d'établir un anus artificiel dans la région lombaire sans pénétrer dans le péritoine. Acad R Méd, Germer-Baillière, Paris, 1 Oct 1839, pp. 84–8.
36. Pillore H. Opération d'anus artificiel, pratiquée en 1776. L'Expérience J Méd Chir. 1840;5:73–5.
37. Amussat JZ. Mémoire sur la possibilité d'établir un anus artificiel dans la région lombaire sans pénétrer dans le péritoine. Acad R Méd Paris, Germer-Baillière, Paris, 1 Oct 1839, p. 84–8.
38. Amussat JZ. Mémoire sur la possibilité d'établir un anus artificiel dans la région lombaire sans pénétrer dans le péritoine. Acad R Méd, Germer-Baillière, Paris, 1 Oct 1839, p. 85–7.
39. Amussat JZ. Mémoire sur la possibilité d'établir un anus artificiel dans la région lombaire sans pénétrer dans le péritoine. Acad R Med, Germer-Baillière, Paris, 1 Oct 1839, p. 88.
40. Duret C. Observation sur un enfant né sans anus, et auquel il a été fait une ouverture pour y suppléer. Rec Périod Soc Méd Paris. 1798;4:45–50.
41. Dinnick T. The origins and evolution of colostomy. Br J Surg. 1934;22:142–54.
42. Verneuil, Reclus P. Des anus artificiels iliaque et lombaire. Congrès Français Chir. 1886;431–41.
43. Amussat JZ. Mémoire sur la possibilité d'établir un anus artificiel dans la région lombaire sans pénétrer dans le péritoine. Acad R Med, Germer-Baillière, Paris, 1 Oct 1839, pp. 91–4. The report was written by Leveillé, a student of Desault.
44. Dumas CL. Observations et réflexions sur une imperforation de l'anus. Rec Périod Soc Méd Paris. 1797;3:46–57.
45. Amussat JZ. Mémoire sur la possibilité d'établir un anus artificiel dans la région lombaire sans pénétrer dans le péritoine. Acad R Med, Germer-Baillière, Paris, 1 Oct 1839, p. 108.
46. Amussat JZ. Mémoire sur la possibilité d'établir un anus artificiel dans la région lombaire sans pénétrer dans le péritoine. Acad R Med, Germer-Baillière, Paris, 1 Oct 1839, p. 109.
47. Translation with the assistance of H-I Translation Service: www.hitranslation.com.
48. Amussat JZ. Mémoire sur la possibilité d'établir un anus artificiel dans la région lombaire sans pénétrer dans le péritoine. Acad R Med, Germer-Baillière, Paris, 1 Oct 1839, p. 114.
49. Callisen H. Chirurgia imperforationis ani. Systema Chirurgiae Hodiernae in Usum Publicum Et Privatum Adornatum. Hafniae. 1800;688–9.
50. Translation: Mr. John Holland, www.thelatintranslator.com.
51. Amussat JZ. Mémoire sur la possibilité d'établir un anus artificiel dans la région lombaire sans pénétrer dans le péritoine. Acad R Med, Germer-Baillière, Paris, 1 Oct 1839, p. 4.
52. Amussat JZ. Mémoire sur la possibilité d'établir un anus artificiel dans la région lombaire sans pénétrer dans le péritoine. Acad R Med Paris, Germer-Baillière, Paris, 1 Oct 1839.
53. Kelsey CB. The formation and closure of artificial anus. Surgery of the rectum and pelvis. New York: E. R. Pelton; 1897. p. 315.
54. Amussat JZ. On an operation of enterotomia, successfully performed without opening the peritonæum. Med Times. 1844;10:401–3, 425–6, 441–2.
55. Amussat JZ. Mémoire sur la possibilité d'établir un anus artificiel dans la région lombaire sans pénétrer dans le péritoine. Acad R Med, Germer-Baillière, Paris, 1 Oct 1839, p. 1.
56. Amussat JZ. Mémoire sur la possibilité d'établir un anus artificiel dans la région lombaire sans pénétrer dans le péritoine. Acad R Med, Germer-Baillière, Paris, 1 Oct 1839, p. 34.
57. Amussat JZ. Notes on the possible establishment of an artificial anus in the lumbar region without entering the peritoneal cavity. Dis Colon Rectum. 1983;26:483–7.
58. Amussat JZ. Mémoire sur la possibilité d'établir un anus artificiel dans la région lombaire sans pénétrer dans le péritoine. Acad R Med, Germer-Baillière, Paris, 1 Oct 1839, p. 47.
59. Erichsen J. On the formation of artificial anus in adults, for the relief of retention of the faeces. Lond Med Gaz. 1841;2(189–92): 223–7.
60. Avery. Extraordinary displacement and twisting of the cæcum and ascending colon, producing obstruction of the bowels, in which an operation for artificial anus in the left lumbar region was performed. Lancet. 1850;1:607.
61. Mason E. Six cases of lumbar colostomy, with remarks upon this operation, and a table of eighty cases in which it was performed. Am J Med Sci. 1873;66:354–92.
62. Pring D. History of a case of the successful formation of an artificial anus in an adult; Freer G. Account of an analogous Operation in two cases. Med Phys J. 1821;45:1–15.
63. Luke J. A case of obstruction of the colon, relieved by an operation performed at the groin. Med Chir Trans. 1851;34:263–76.
64. Schinzinger. Über Operationen am Darme. Centralblatt Chir. 1881;48:767–8.
65. Madelung. Über eine Modifikation der Colotomie wegen Carcinoma recti. Centralblatt Chir. 1884;11:68–9.
66. Knie A. Zur Technik der Kolotomie. Centralblatt Chir. 1885;25:433–6.
67. Allingham HW. Inguinal colotomy; its advantages over the lumbar operation, with special reference to a method for preventing fæces passing below the artificial anus. Br Med J. 1887;2:874–8.
68. Reclus P. Anus artificiel iliaque. Bull Mém Soc Chir. 1887;13:685–7.
69. Maydl K. Zur Technik der Kolotomie. Centralblatt Chir. 1888;24:433–9.
70. Pfaar O. Karl Maydl. Dis Colon Rectum. 2001;44:280–3.
71. Kelsey CB. An improvement in the technique of inguinal colotomy. Med Rec (NY). 1889;36:398.
72. Reeves HA. Sigmoidostomy simplified. Br Med J. 1892;1:66–7.
73. Hartmann H. Technique de la colostomie dans le traitement de certaines tumeurs inopérables du rectum. Rev Chir. 1900;22: 613–20.
74. Davies-Colley N. On three cases of colotomy with delayed opening of the intestine. Trans Clin Soc Lond. 1885;18:204–9.

75. Bloch O. Extraabdominal resektion af hele Colon descendens og et Stykke af Colon transversum for Cancer. Hospitalstidende 1894;4: Række, Bd II, Nr 43; 1053–61.
76. Bloch O. Om extra-abdominal behandling af cancer intestinalis (Rectum derfra undtaget). Nord Med Ark 1892;2(1):1–74 & 2(8):1–10.
77. Paul FT. Colectomy. Br Med J. 1895;1:1136–9.
78. Mikulicz J von. Chirurgische Erfahrungen über das Darmcarcinom. Arch klin Chir. 1903;69:28–47.
79. Mikulicz J von. Surgical experiences with intestinal carcinoma. Med Classics. 1937;2:210–29.
80. Sistrunk WE. The Mikulicz operation for resection of the colon. Its advantages and dangers. Ann Surg. 1928;88:597–606.
81. Mayo CH. Cancer of the large bowel. Med Sentinel. 1904;12:466–73.
82. Schede. Zur Operation des Mastdarmkrebses. Dtsch Med Wochenschr. 1887;13:1048–9.
83. Kraske P. Zur Exstirpation hochsitzender Mastdarmkrebse. Dtsch Ges Chir. 1885;14:464–74.
84. Hartmann H. Nouveau procédé d'ablation des cancers de la partie terminale du colon pelvien. Congrès Français Chir. 1921;30: 411.
85. Heister L. A general system of surgery in three parts. W. Innys and J. Richardson, J. Clarke, R. Manby, J. Whiston and B. White, H.S. Cox and L. Davis and C. Reymers: London: 1757. pp. 72–3.
86. Daguesceau. Artificial anus. Med Times (Lond). 1844;10:446.
87. Fraser J, Drummond H. A clinical and experimental study of three hundred perforating wounds of the abdomen. Br Med J. 1917;1(2932):321–30.
88. Welch CE. War wounds of the abdomen. N Eng J Med 1947;237:156-94.
89. Ogilvie WH. Abdominal wounds in the western desert. Surg Gynecol Obstet. 1944;78:225–38.
90. A copy of the original Circular Letter 178 from 1943 was kindly provided by Major Kenneth M. Koyle, AMEDD Office of Medical History, US Army Medical Department, Directorate of Strategic Communications, Falls Church.
91. Colcock BP. Traumatic perforation of the colon as seen in a general hospital. Surgery. 1945;17:1–10.
91. Patey DH. Primary epithelial apposition in colostomy. Proc R Soc Med. 1951;44:423–4.
93. Butler C. Some observations on the treatment of carcinoma of the rectum. Proc R Soc Med. 1952;45:41–50.
94. Lemmer KE, Mehnert JH. Colostomy, advantages of establishing an immediate mucotaneous suture. Arch Surg. 1954;68:463–8.
95. Sames CP. Extaperitoneal colostomy. Lancet. 1958;1:567–8.
96. Goligher JC. Extraperitoneal colostomy or ileostomy. Br J Surg. 1958;46:97–103.
97. Turnbull Jr RB, Weakley FL. Atlas of intestinal stomas. St. Louis: Mosby; 1967. p. 161–5.
98. Henrotin F. Enterostomy and drainage in the treatment of diffuse septic peritonitis. Am J Obstet Dis Women Child. 1893;28: 199–205.
99. Maydl K. Zur Technik der Kolotomie. Centralbl Chir. 1888;24:434.
100. Pfaar O. Karl Maydl. Dis Colon Rectum. 2001;44:280–283.
101. Smith JG. Enterostomy in intestinal obstruction. Br Med J. 1892;1(1628):554–5.
102. Lund FB. The value of enterostomy in selected cases of peritonitis. J Am Med Assoc. 1903;41:74–80.
103. Brown JY. The value of complete physiological rest of the large bowel in the treatment of certain ulcerative and obstructive lesions of this organ. Surg Gynecol Obstet. 1913;16:610–3.
104. Arn ER. Chronic ulcerative colitis: surgical treatment of refractory cases. Ohio State Med J. 1931;27:121–7.
105. Corbett RS. A review of the surgical treatment of chronic ulcerative colitis. Proc R Soc Med. 1944;38:277–90.
106. Bargen JA, Lindahl WW, Ashburn FS, Pemberton J deJ. Ileostomy for chronic ulcerative colitis (end results and complications in 185 cases). Ann Intern Med. 1943;18:43–56.
107. Lahey FH. Indications for surgical intervention in ulcerative colitis. Ann Surg. 1951;133:726–42.
108. Brooke BN. The management of an ileostomy including its complications. Lancet. 1952;2:102–4.
109. Brooke BN. The surgery of ulcerative colitis. Ann R Coll Surg Engl. 1951;8:440–56.
110. Rankin FW. Total colectomy; its indication and technic. Ann Surg. 1931;94:677–704.
111. Bargen JA, Brown PW, Rankin FW. Indications for and technique of ileostomy in chronic ulcerative colitis. Surg Gynecol Obstet. 1932;55:196–202.
112. Cattell RB. The surgical treatment of ulcerative colitis. J Am Med Assoc. 1935;104:104–9.
113. Cave HW, Nickel Jr WF. Ileostomy. Ann Surg. 1940;112:747–62.
114. Warren R, McKittrick LS. Ileostomy for ulcerative colitis: technique, complications, and management. Surg Gynecol Obstet. 1951;93:555–67.
115. Crile Jr G, Turnbull Jr RB. The mechanism and prevention of ileostomy dysfunction. Ann Surg. 1954;140:459–65.
116. Beahrs OH. The acceptability of ileostomies. Dis Colon Rectum. 1971;14:460–3.
117. Dragstedt LR, Dack GM, Kirsner JB. Chronic ulcerative colitis. A summary of evidence implicating bacterium necrophorum as an etiologic agent. Ann Surg. 1941;114:653–62.
118. Monroe CW, Olwin JH. Use of an abdominal flap graft in construction of a permanent ileostomy. Arch Surg. 1949;59:565–77.
119. Brooke B. Ileostomy diarrhea. Arch Surg. 1975;110:781–2.
120. Turnbull Jr RB. Management of the ileostomy. Am J Surg. 1953;86:617–24.
121. Turnbull Jr RB, Crile Jr G. Mucosal-grafted ileostomy in the surgical treatment of ulcerative colitis. J Am Med Assoc. 1955;158:32–4.
122. Beaumont W. Experiments and observations on the gastric juice and the physiology of digestion. F.P. Allen, Plattsburgh, 1833; pp. B, 10, C.
123. Verneuil. Observation de gastro-stomie pratiquée avec succès pour un rétrécissement cicatriciel infranchissable de l'œsophage. Bull Acad Med. 1876;2:1023–38.
124. Nélaton. Union Med Paris. 1851;5:344.
125. Witzel O. Zur Technik der Magenfistelanlegung. Centralbl Chir. 1891;32:601–4.
126. Stamm M. Gastrostomy by a new method. Med News. 1894;65:324–6.
127. Chalker JB. Burma railway artist. The war drawings of Jack Chalker. Viking. Victoria: Penguin Books Australia Ltd.; 1994. p. 70.
128. Chalker JB. Burma railway. Images of war. The original war drawings of Japanese POW Jack Chalker. United Kingdom: Mercer Books; 2007. p. 90.
129. Bricker EM. Bladder substitution after pelvic evisceration. Surg Clin North Am. 1950;30:1511–21.
130. Bishop HC, Koop CE. Management of meconium ileus: resection, Roux-en-Y anastomosis and ileostomy irrigation with pancreatic enzymes. Ann Surg. 1957;145:410–4.
131. Kock NG. Intra-abdominal "Reservoir" in patients with permanent ileostomy. Arch Surg. 1969;99:223–31.
132. Suruga K, Nagashima K, Kohno S, Miyano T, Kitahara T, Inui M. A clinical and pathological study of congenital biliary atresia. J Pediat Surg. 1972;7:655–9.
133. Feustel H, Hennig G, Filler D. Zur kontinenten Kolostomie durch Erlanger Magnetverschluß. Therapiewoche. 1976;26:4095–6.
134. Angevine RW. Fat excretion. VI. Excretion by Thiry-Vella Fistulas. J Biol Chem. 1929;82:559–65.

135. Thiry L. Über eine neue Methode, den Dünndarm zu isoliren. Sitzungsber Akad Wissensch (Wien). Abt. 1, 1864. pp. 77–96.
136. Davidson W, Fischer J. History of ostomy products manufacturers. In: Erwin-Toth P, Krasner D, editors. Enterostomal therapy nursing: growth & evolution of a nursing specialty worldwide: a Festschrift for Norma N. Gill-Thompson, ET. Baltimore: Halgo, Inc.; 1996. p. 55–73.
137. United States Patent Office, 2,048,392, Colostomy appliance, Henry F. Koenig, Chicago. Application 19 Mar 1934, Serial No. 716, 235.
138. Strauss AA, Strauss SF. Surgical treatment of ulcerative colitis. Surg Clin North Am. 1944;24:211–24.
139. Dennis C. Ileostomy and colectomy in chronic ulcerative colitis. Surgery. 1945;18:435–52.
140. Hardy TL. Notes on recent trends in gastroenterology in the United Kingdom. Gastroenterologia. 1955;83:321–9.
141. Hardy TL, Brooke BN, Hawkins CF. Ileostomy and ulcerative colitis. Lancet. 1949;2:5–9.
142. The history of the Coloplast company was obtained from and reproduced with permission courtesy of Mr. Troels Nørgaard Laursen and Mr. Michael C. Davidsen, Coloplast A/S, Holtedam 3 3050 Humlebaek, Denmark.
143. Coloplast Company. Helios. 40th Anniversary Article. 13.8.1997 Revised, pp. 2–3.
144. Coloplast Company. How it all began. Humlebaek, Sept 1997.
145. Merriam-Webster Unabridged Medical Dictionary. http://unabridged.merriam-webster.com/cgi-bin/medical?book=Medical&va=karaya+gum. Accessed 5 May 2010.
146. Turnbull RW, Turnbull GB. The history and current status of paramedical support for the ostomy patient. Sem Colon Rectal Surg. 1991;2:131–40.
147. Hartwell Jr SW, editor. "…to act as a unit." The story of the Cleveland Clinic. Philadelphia: Saunders; 1985. p. 71.
148. Cyr GN, Chen JL. United Patent Office 3,312,594 Longlasting Troche. Filed, 21 June 1963.
149. Fattman G. Hydrocolloids: designed to provide reliable adhesion and security; past, present, and future. Poster FAC# GO-06-771(B), 2006 WCET Conference. Presentation courtesy of Mr. George Fattman, Ms. Punnie Donohue, and Ms. Annette Lee of the ConvaTec Company.
150. Sircus W. 'Orabase' in the management of abdominal-wall digestion by ileostomy and fistulas. Lancet. 1964;2:762.
151. Kyte EM, Hughes ESR. Peristomal skin protection with "Orahesive". Med J Aust. 1970;2:186–7.
152. Killingback M. Sir Edward Hughes and colorectal surgery. Aust N Z J Surg. 2000;70:137–9.
153. With appreciation to Ms. Diane M. Owen, Professional Relations Liason, Hollister Incorporated.
154. Hollister. The karaya story. Courtesy of Ms. Bobbi Micale, Hollister, Incorporated.
155. Lyons AS. Ileostomy and colostomy support groups. Mt Sinai J Med. 2001;68:110–2.
156. See International ostomy association; www.ostomyinternational.org, Accessed 5 May 2010.
157. d'E Stevens PJ. Development of enterostomal therapy as an international nursing specialty. In: Erwin-Toth P, Krasner D, editors. Enterostomal therapy nursing: growth & evolution of a nursing specialty worldwide, a Festschrift for Norma N. Gill-Thompson, ET. Baltimore: Halgo, Inc.; 1996. p. 45–54.
158. Wound, Ostomy and Continence Nurses Society. www.wocn.org. Accessed 5 May 2010.

Gastrointestinal Anatomy

2

Richard L. Drake and Jennifer M. McBride

Introduction

An ostomy is an opening in the abdominal wall to which a portion of the gastrointestinal tract is attached. Its purpose is to provide a pathway for digested material to leave the body when the normal pathway is blocked due to a variety of situations. It can involve a part of the small intestine, i.e. an ileostomy, or a part of the large intestine, i.e. a colostomy. Thus, an overview of the anatomy of the gastrointestinal tract is a logical place to begin.

Small Intestine

The small intestine consists of the duodenum, the jejunum, and the ileum and extends from the pyloric sphincter to the ileocecal junction (Fig. 2.1). It is 6–7 m in length and narrows from beginning to end.

Duodenum

The duodenum is the first part of the small intestine and is 20–25 cm in length. It is C-shaped, formed around the head of the pancreas and is the widest portion of the small intestine (Fig. 2.2). Due to changes that occur during development, the duodenum is retroperitoneal except for the first or superior part that is connected to the liver by the hepatoduodenal ligament, the lateral part of the lesser omentum.

R.L. Drake (✉)
Cleveland Clinic Lerner College of Medicine of Case Western Reserve University, Cleveland, OH, USA
e-mail: draker@ccf.org

J.M. McBride
Cleveland Clinic Lerner College of Medicine of Case Western Reserve University, Cleveland, OH, USA

The duodenum is divided into four parts (Fig. 2.3):

- The superior or first part begins at the pyloric sphincter and ends in the area of the neck of the gallbladder. It is located to the right of vertebra L1 and lies anterior to the bile duct, gastroduodenal artery, portal vein, and inferior vena cava.
- The descending or second part passes from the neck of the gallbladder to the inferior edge of vertebra L3. It is posterior to the transverse colon, anterior to the medial portion of the right kidney and just lateral to the head of the pancreas (Fig. 2.2). Associated with this part of the duodenum is the major duodenal papilla, the entrance of the bile and major pancreatic ducts into the small intestine, and the minor duodenal papilla, the entrance of the accessory pancreatic duct into the small intestine. Just below the major duodenal papilla in this section of the duodenum is the junction between the foregut and midgut.
- The inferior or third part passes anterior to the inferior vena cava, the abdominal aorta and the vertebral column. Its anterior surface is crossed by the superior mesenteric artery and vein.
- The ascending or fourth part is to the left of the abdominal aorta, and passes upward ending at the duodenojejunal junction. The ligament of Treitz, or suspensory muscle (ligament) of the duodenum, is associated with this junction.

The arterial supply to the duodenum is extensive. It receives branches directly from the gastroduodenal artery, the supraduodenal artery from the gastroduodenal artery, duodenal branches from the anterior and posterior superior pancreaticoduodenal arteries, duodenal branches from the anterior and posterior inferior pancreaticoduodenal arteries and the first jejunal branch from the superior mesenteric artery (Fig. 2.4).

Jejunum

The jejunum follows the duodenum and represents about two-fifths of the small intestine (Fig. 2.1). Located primarily in the left upper quadrant of the peritoneal cavity, it has a

V.W. Fazio et al. (eds.), *Atlas of Intestinal Stomas*,
DOI 10.1007/978-0-387-78851-7_2, © Springer Science+Business Media, LLC 2012

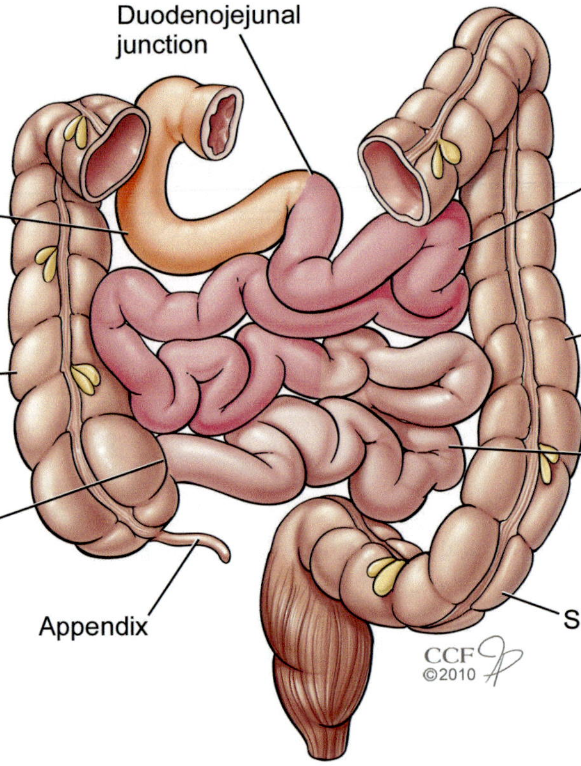

Fig. 2.1 Small intestine, duodenum, jejunum and ileum, surrounded by components of the large intestine (Illustration © CCF)

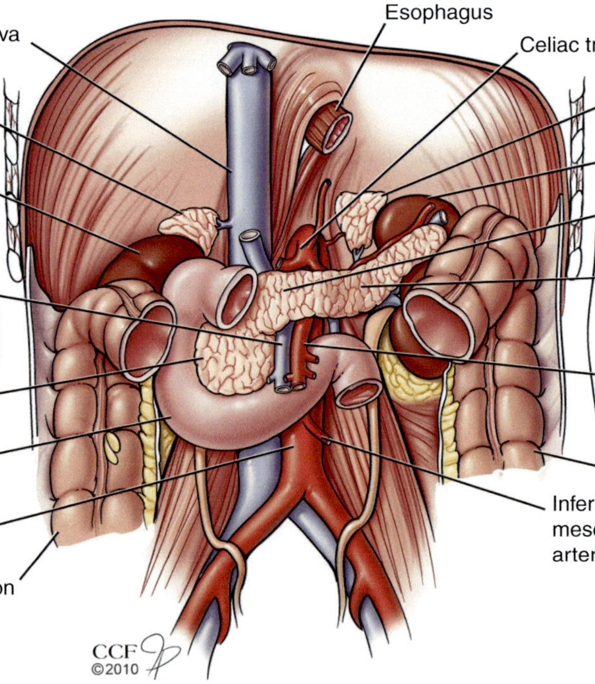

Fig. 2.2 Duodenum in its typical location (Illustration © CCF)

larger diameter and thicker walls than the final portion of the small intestine, the ileum. Also, large folds, plicae circulares, surround the lumen.

The arterial supply to this portion of the small intestine consists of jejunal arteries that are branches of the superior mesenteric artery (Fig. 2.5).

Ileum

The ileum is the final portion of the small intestine and represents about three-fifths of this structure (Fig. 2.1). Located primarily in the right lower quadrant of the peritoneal cavity, it has thinner walls and fewer and smaller plicae circulares

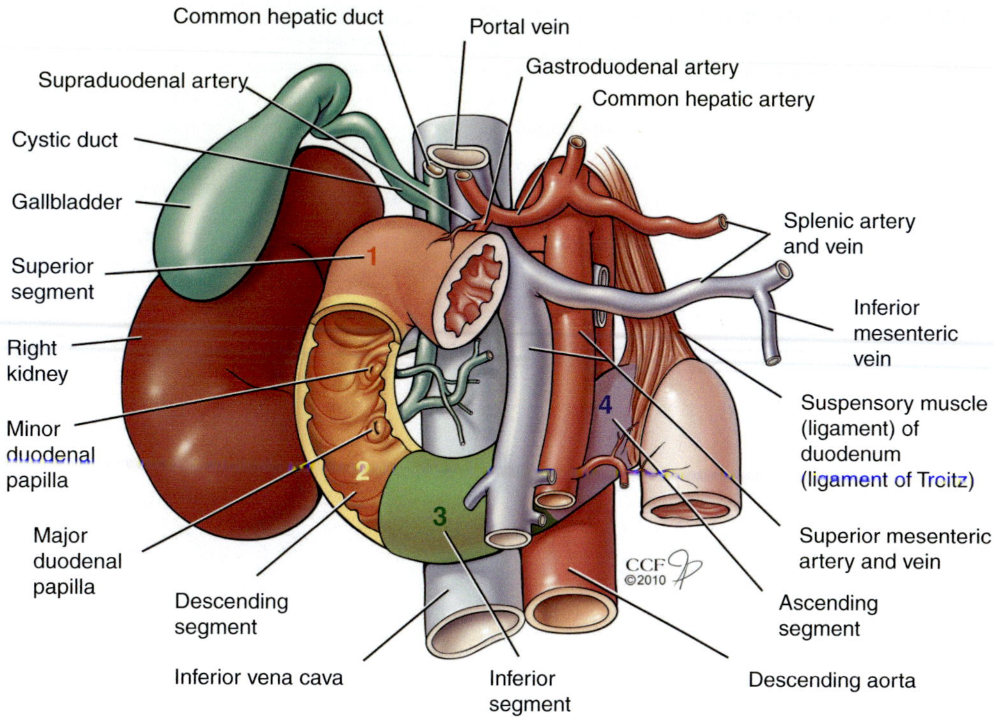

Fig. 2.3 Different segments of the duodenum and various other structures (Illustration © CCF)

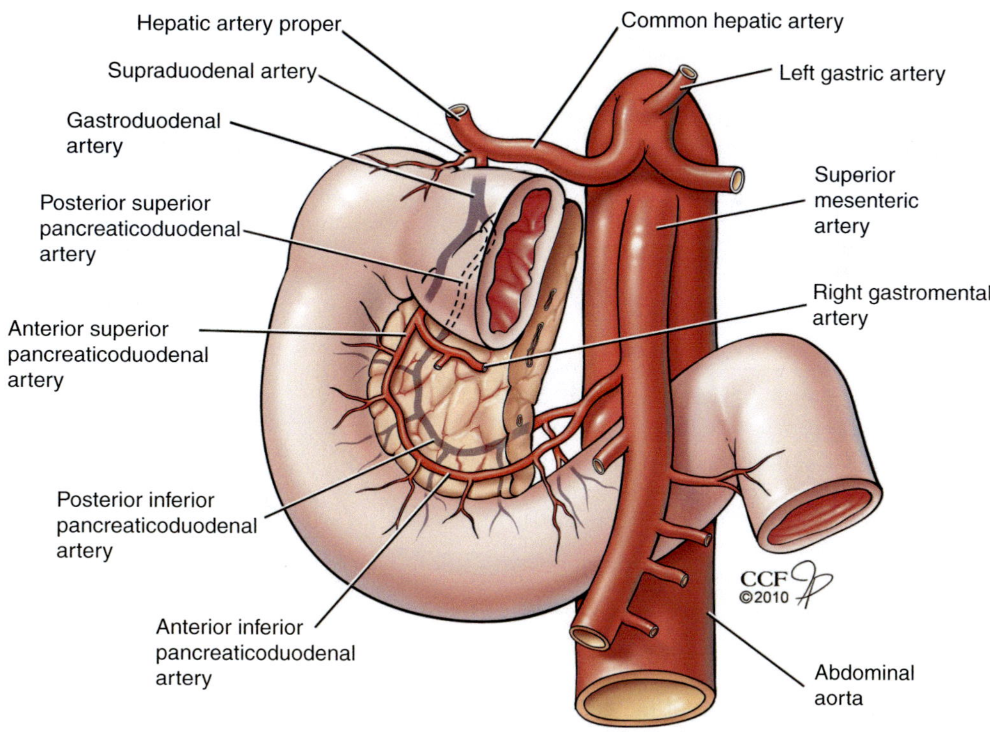

Fig. 2.4 Arterial supply to the duodenum (Illustration © CCF)

when compared to the jejunum. The ileum joins the large intestine at the junction of the cecum and the ascending colon. At this location, two flaps, the ileocecal fold, are visible on the wall of the large intestine (Fig. 2.6).

The arterial supply to this portion of the small intestine consists of ileal arteries from the superior mesenteric artery and an ileal branch from the ileocolic artery (Fig. 2.5).

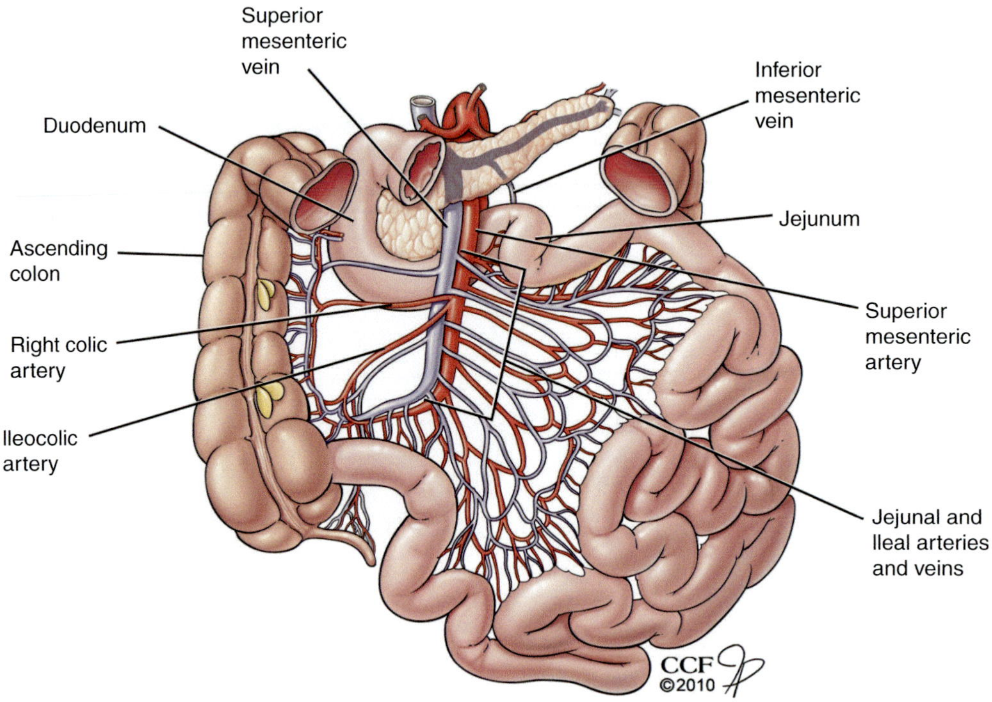

Fig. 2.5 Small intestine moved laterally to demonstrate the superior mesenteric vessels (Illustration © CCF)

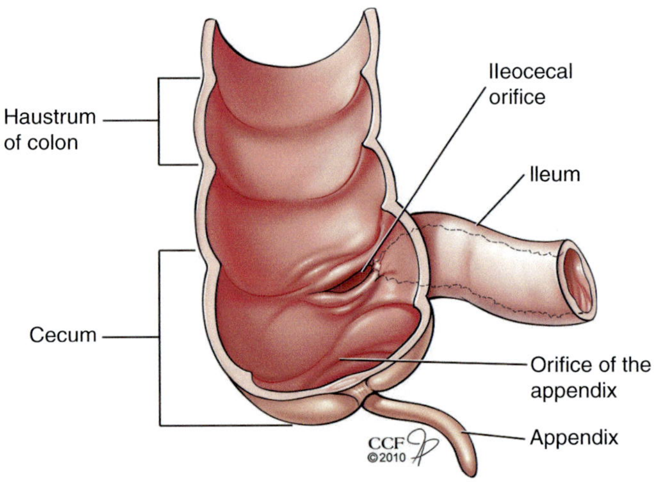

Fig. 2.6 Junction of the ileum and the cecum and the ileocecal fold (Illustration © CCF)

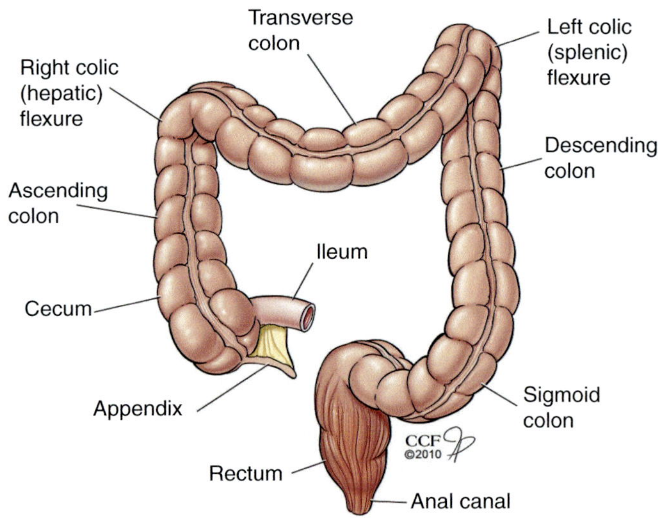

Fig. 2.7 Anterior view of the large intestine (Illustration © CCF)

Large Intestine

The large intestine consists of the cecum, appendix, colon, rectum and anal canal (Fig. 2.7). Starting in the lower right quadrant with the cecum (Fig. 2.8), and its attached appendix, it continues superiorly as the ascending colon with the right colic flexure (hepatic flexure) in the right upper quadrant, just inferior to the liver (Fig. 2.9). At this point the large intestine moves to the left as the transverse colon turning inferiorly at the left colic flexure (splenic flexure) in the left upper quadrant immediately below the spleen. It then continues inferiorly as the descending colon to the lower left quadrant (Fig. 2.10). Entering the lower abdominal/upper pelvic cavity as the sigmoid colon, the large intestine moves inferiorly into the pelvic cavity as the rectum and anal canal. Unique aspects of the large intestine include (Fig. 2.7):

- A larger internal diameter than the small intestine
- The presence of omental appendices (appendices epiploicae) – "bags" of fat

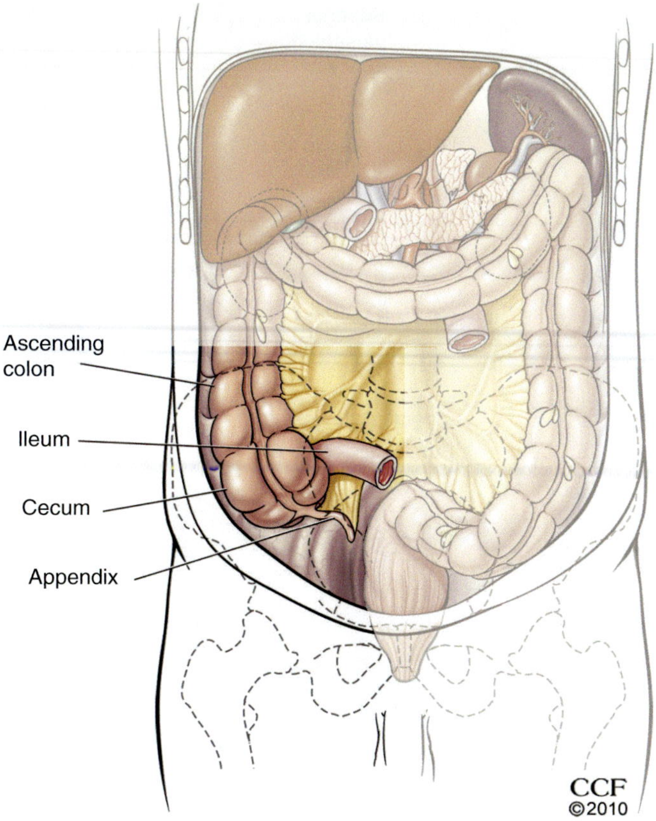

Fig. 2.8 Cecum and appendix (Illustration © CCF)

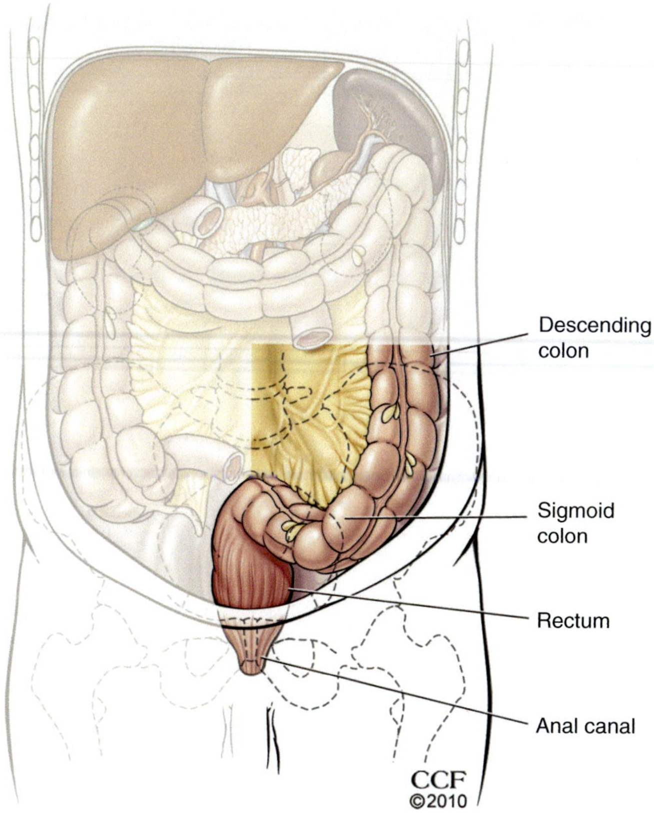

Fig. 2.10 Descending colon, sigmoid colon, rectum, and anal canal (Illustration © CCF)

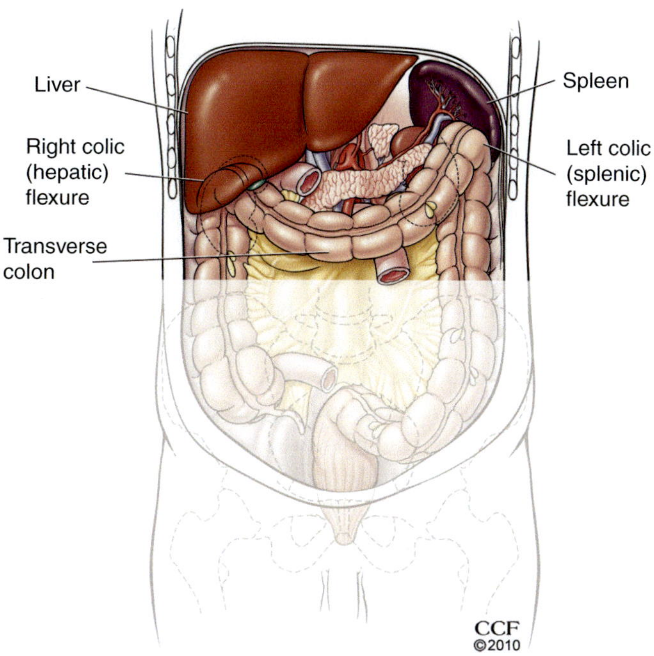

Fig. 2.9 Right and left colic flexures (Illustration © CCF)

- Three narrow bands of longitudinal muscle, taeniae coli, visible on the walls of primarily the cecum and colon
- The appearance of haustra or sacculations

Cecum and Appendix

The first part of the large intestine, inferior to the ileocecal opening, is the cecum (Fig. 2.8). Typically located in the lower right quadrant, it is continuous with the ascending colon, may be in contact with the anterior abdominal wall and, at times, part of it may descend into the pelvic cavity.

Attached inferiorly to the cecum is the appendix. This narrow, hollow, blind-ended tube has accumulations of lymphoid tissue in its wall and is attached to the most distal portion of the ileum by a mesentery, the mesoappendix (Fig. 2.11). This fold of tissue contains the appendicular vessels. Positioning of the appendix varies considerably and the structure has been described as being pre-ileal, postileal, subcecal, retrocecal and pelvic.

The arterial supply to the cecum and appendix originates from the superior mesenteric artery. It consists of the anterior and the posterior cecal arteries and the appendicular artery, which are all branches of the ileocolic artery (Fig. 2.12).

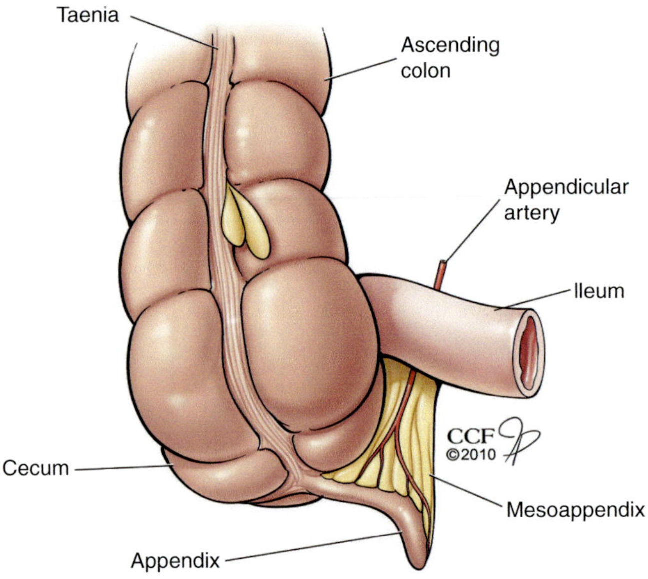

Fig. 2.11 Mesoappendix and appendicular vessels (Illustration © CCF)

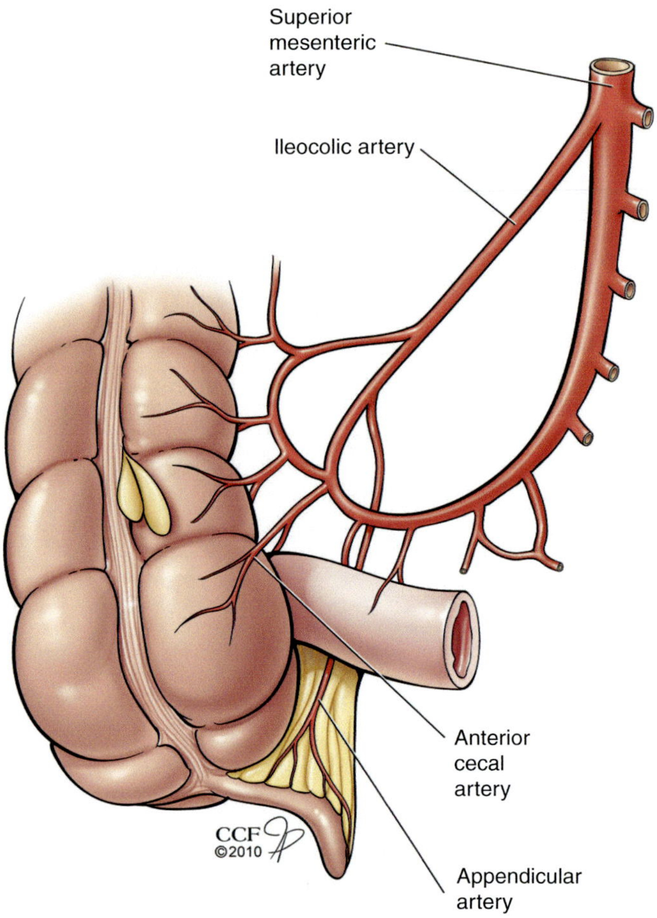

Fig. 2.12 Arterial supply to the cecum and appendix (Illustration © CCF)

Colon

Ascending Colon

Beginning at the superior end of the cecum, the ascending colon continues superiorly to the right colic flexure just inferior to the liver (Fig. 2.7). It has no mesentery and is fixed, to varying degrees, to the posterior abdominal wall. The upper portion of the ascending colon is covered anteriorly by the small intestine, while the lower portion may come into direct contact with the anterior abdominal wall. Posterior to this structure is the lower pole of the right kidney, the iliacus muscle and the aponeurotic portion of the transversus abdominis muscle. The right kidney and parts of the lumbar plexus separate the ascending colon from the quadratus lumborum muscle.

Immediately lateral to the ascending colon is the right paracolic gutter. This depression, formed as the peritoneum passes from the ascending colon to the posterior abdominal wall, passes from the appendix to the hepatorenal recess superiorly and from the liver to the pelvic cavity inferiorly. Since blood vessels are located in the retroperitoneal tissue on the medial/posteromedial border of the ascending colon, surgeons can mobilize this structure along its lateral avascular border, an area referred to as the "white line of Toldt." When this is done, the ascending colon along with the connective tissue containing its blood vessels can be moved towards the midline.

The arterial supply to the ascending colon consists of the colic branch of the ileocolic artery (from the superior mesenteric artery), the anterior and posterior cecal arteries from the ileocolic artery (from the superior mesenteric artery) and the right colic artery from the superior mesenteric artery directly (Fig. 2.13).

Transverse Colon

Beginning at the right colic, or hepatic, flexure and continuing to the left colic, or splenic, flexure is the transverse colon (Fig. 2.7). Unlike the ascending colon, this structure is intraperitoneal and suspended from the posterior abdominal wall by the transverse mesocolon. Because of this mobility, its posterior relationships may vary, but it is usually regarded as being anterior to the hilus of the right kidney, the descending part of the duodenum and the head of the pancreas. Cranially, it contacts the liver, gallbladder, greater curvature of the stomach and spleen. Caudally, it is against the small intestine, and its anterior surface is against the greater omentum and abdominal wall.

The arterial supply to the transverse colon consists of the right colic artery and the middle colic artery from the superior mesenteric artery, and the left colic artery from the inferior mesenteric artery (Fig. 2.13).

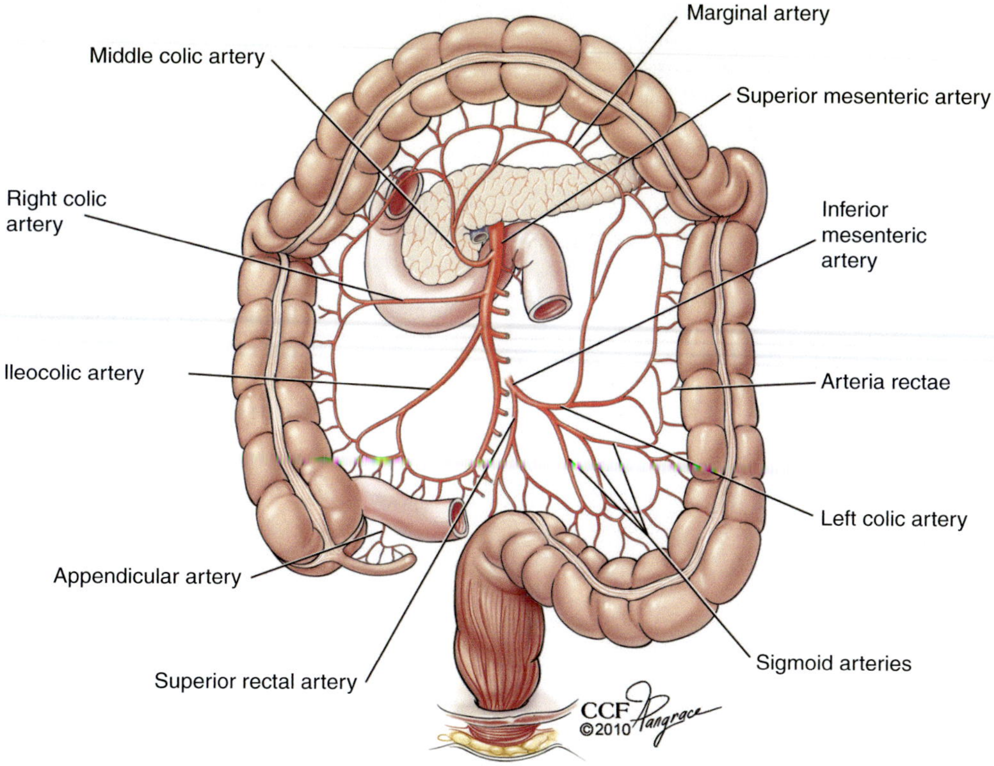

Fig. 2.13 Colon arterial supply (Illustration © CCF)

Descending Colon

Beginning at the left colic flexure, where the intestine loses its mesentery, and extending to the area of the crest of the ileum is the descending colon (Fig. 2.7). It, like the ascending colon, has no mesentery and is fixed, to varying degrees, to the posterior abdominal wall. Superiorly the descending colon has the transverse colon and loops of small intestine separating it from the anterior abdominal wall, while inferiorly it may contact the wall. Posteriorly is the lower pole of the left kidney, the iliacus muscle and the aponeurotic portion of the transversus abdominis muscle. As was the case with the ascending colon, the left kidney and parts of the lumbar plexus separate the descending colon from the quadratus lumborum muscle, but it is in contact with the left psoas major muscle posteromedially.

As was the case with the ascending colon, immediately lateral to the descending colon is the left paracolic gutter. Again, due to the fact that the major blood vessels approach the descending colon from the medial or posteromedial side, a relatively bloodless plane exists laterally. Thus, mobilization of the descending colon towards the midline is possible through incisions of the peritoneum along the gutter.

The arterial supply to the descending colon consists of the left colic artery from the inferior mesenteric artery (Fig. 2.13).

Sigmoid Colon

Near the crest of the ileum, the sigmoid colon begins as the descending colon acquires a mesentery (Fig. 2.7). It continues inferiorly until the mesentery is lost, usually anterior to vertebra S3. This location may also be indicated by a slight constriction, a functional rectosigmoid sphincter that marks the beginning of the rectum.

The sigmoid colon is attached where it begins and ends, but is mobile throughout its length. It is suspended by a mesentery, the sigmoid mesocolon, which is a peritoneal attachment that is shaped like an inverted V. In this configuration the apex of the V is located adjacent to where the left common iliac artery divides into its internal and external iliac branches, with the right stem of the V passing inferiorly into the pelvic cavity ending at vertebra S3 and the left stem along the medial edge of the left psoas major muscle.

Important structures posterior to the sigmoid colon and the sigmoid mesocolon, which must be considered in any surgical dissection in this area, include the left external and internal iliac vessels, the left gonadal vessels, the left ureter and the roots of the sacral plexus. Anteriorly, the sigmoid colon is separated from the bladder in the male and the bladder and uterus in the female by loops of small intestine.

The arterial supply to the sigmoid colon consists of several sigmoidal arteries from the inferior mesenteric artery (Fig. 2.13).

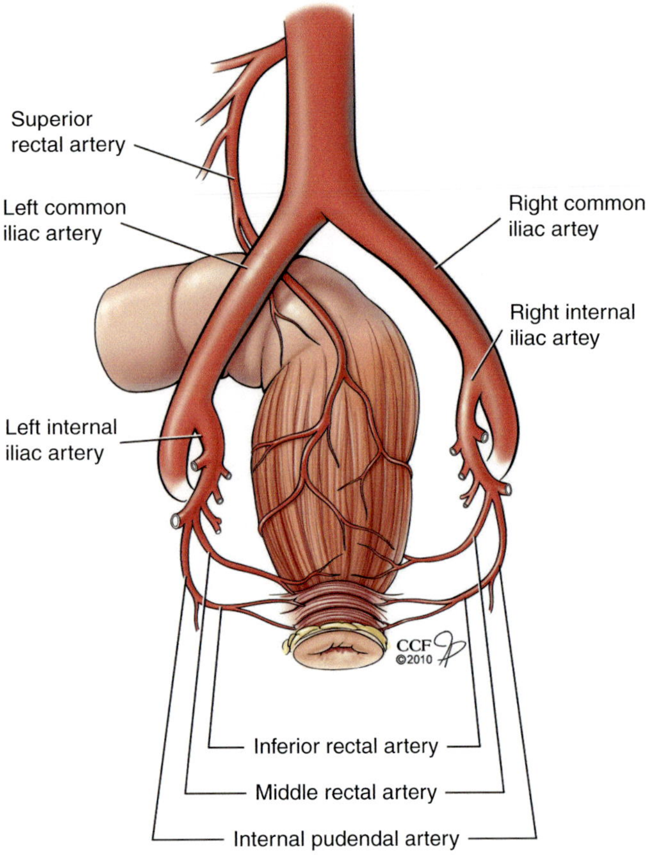

Fig. 2.14 Rectum and anal canal arterial supply (Illustration © CCF)

Rectum

The rectum extends from the sigmoid colon with the recto-sigmoid junction defined as either the level of vertebrae S3 or at the end of the sigmoid mesocolon (Fig. 2.7). It is a retroperitoneal structure and is immediately anterior to the sacrum. The rectum lacks distinct taeniae coli, omental appendices and sacculations (haustra of the colon). It does have three lateral curves and ends in the rectal ampulla before becoming the anal canal.

The arterial supply to the rectum consists of the superior rectal artery from the inferior mesenteric artery, the middle rectal artery from the internal iliac artery and the inferior rectal artery from the internal pudendal artery, a branch of the internal iliac artery (Fig. 2.14).

Anal Canal

The anal canal is the final portion of the large intestine (Fig. 2.7). It begins at the terminal end of the rectal ampulla as it narrows to pass through the pelvic floor. The anal canal ends as the anus after it has passed through the perineum. The anal canal is surrounded throughout its length by the internal and external anal sphincters.

The arterial supply to the anal canal consists of the inferior rectal artery from the internal pudendal artery, a branch of the internal iliac artery (Fig. 2.14).

Suggested Reading

Drake RL, Vogl AW, Mitchell AWM. Gray's anatomy for students. 2nd ed. Philadelphia: Churchill Livingstone/Elsevier; 2010.

Drake RL, Vogl AW, Mitchell AWM, Tibbits R, Richardson P. Gray's atlas of anatomy. Philadelphia: Churchill Livingstone/Elsevier; 2008.

Structure and Function of the Large Bowel

3

Ann E. Brannigan and James M. Church

Introduction

Knowledge of the anatomy and an understanding of the physiology of an organ are basic to an awareness of the diseases of that organ, and underlie a successful approach to their diagnosis and treatment. Several misconceptions about the structure and function of the large bowel have become commonplace, and new surgical techniques have produced unnatural structures with poorly understood functions. This chapter reviews the basic anatomy and physiology of the large bowel including anus, rectum, and colon. Areas of common misunderstanding will be pointed out, and emphasis will also be given to important clinical applications.

The Large Intestine

The large intestine comprises the colon, rectum, and anus. It can be viewed as a muscular tube whose basic role is to process the end products of digestion into a form appropriate for elimination, to store these processed products, and to allow elimination to take place at a convenient time and place. In a broad sense, the right colon (splenic flexure and all points proximal) is the processing unit, the left colon is the storage unit, and the rectum and anus comprise the elimination unit.

A.E. Brannigan (✉)
Mater Misericordiae University Hospital,
Dublin, Ireland
e-mail: aebrannigan@gmail.com

J.M. Church
Department of Colorectal Surgery,
Digestive Diseases Institute, Cleveland Clinic Foundation,
Cleveland, OH, USA

The Colon: Its Structure, Position in the Abdomen, and Relations

The colon extends from the ileocecal valve in the right lower quadrant of the abdomen to the rectosigmoid junction at the pelvic brim. Here it becomes the rectum. It measures approximately 135 cm (53 in.) although it tends to be about 12 in. longer in women than in men. Its caliber is largest at the cecum and is narrowest at the distal sigmoid. The colon is variably retroperitoneal in that parts are often fixed by a peritoneal reflection (usually the ascending and descending colon). The cecum, the transverse colon, and the sigmoid have free mesenteries. Slim people tend to have unzygosed ascending and descending colons, with the entire colon having a mesentery. This phenomenon makes for a more difficult colonoscopy but an easier colectomy [1].

The colon has the same basic wall structure as the remainder of the gastrointestinal tract. The mucosa is supported by the submucosa but separated from it by the muscularis mucosae. There are two layers of smooth muscle: an inner circular layer and an outer longitudinal layer. The muscular tube is covered by serosa.

The longitudinal muscle layer of the colon differs from that of the small bowel in that it is condensed into three bundles: the *Taenia coli*. The taenia are shorter than the colon itself and this produces sacculations, obvious during endoscopy as haustral folds and causing the form of peristalsis known as segmentation. The taenia originates at the appendix, diverging from it to occupy mesenteric (1) and antimesenteric (2) positions. They are a means of identifying the appendix, and also the rectosigmoid junction, as here their muscle spreads out to provide a complete longitudinal coat for the rectum.

The colon is also characterized by fatty tags that are attached to the antimesenteric taenia: the appendices epiploicae. These tags can twist and infarct, causing abdominal pain and point tenderness.

V.W. Fazio et al. (eds.), *Atlas of Intestinal Stomas*,
DOI 10.1007/978-0-387-78851-7_3, © Springer Science+Business Media, LLC 2012

An Overview

The colon originates in the right iliac fossa at the ileocecal valve. Here the terminal ileum enters the ascending colon, defining the cecum as that part of the right colon below the valve. Externally, the ileocecal valve is identified by a triangular fold of fat on the antimesenteric border (ligament of Treves), running from a narrow attachment on the ileum to a broad base on the colon. Internally, the valve has a variable appearance depending on how much ileal mucosa is prolapsing through it. There is almost always a yellowish hue because of intramural fat, and the lips of the valve may be plainly seen or may be tucked under a haustral fold. Endoscopic identification of the valve is crucial to assuring complete colonoscopy, as it is an unequivocal landmark. At the base of the cecum, the appendix can be found at the confluence of the taenia. The mesoappendix attaches it to the fat on the inferior aspect of the cecum and contains the appendiceal artery and vein, branches of the ileocolic vessels.

From the ileocecal valve the ascending colon passes upward, lateral to psoas, the vertebra, and the inferior vena cava, to the right upper quadrant of the abdomen. The right kidney and duodenum lie behind the upper ascending colon. Below the liver and gallbladder the colon makes a turn to the left and continues across the abdomen as the transverse colon. This turn, the hepatic flexure, is of variable complexity and is rarely a simple right angle. The transverse colon is typically V-shaped as it drops toward the pelvis before ascending toward the left upper quadrant and the splenic flexure. The transverse colon provides an attachment for the greater omentum – an apron of fat and lymphatics that originates from the inferior border of the stomach. Endoscopically, the transverse colon has a triangular cross section, perhaps due to the omentum pulling on one side of the bowel. At the splenic flexure, the colon may undergo one or more spiral turns before passing inferiorly to become the descending colon. The colonic mesentery is sometimes attached to the spleen and traction on the colon during mobilization may cause disruption of the splenic capsule. The descending colon lies laterally to the aorta and left psoas muscle, and in front of the left kidney. It passes caudally to the left iliac fossa, where it becomes the sigmoid colon. The sigmoid colon is a loop of variable size and configuration. It occupies the pelvis but may extend into the upper abdomen. During colonoscopy, sigmoid loops can reach the diaphragm. The sigmoid joins the rectum at the pelvic brim. The high-pressure zone of the rectosigmoid is not related to any external landmarks as its position is quite variable. However, the spreading taeniae allow it to be defined. The rectum is usually fixed to the hollow of the sacrum and encapsulated by its fascia propria. It passes through the pelvis to the pelvic floor. Here, there is the anorectal junction, defined by a backward angulation that is created by the levator ani muscle. The anus passes through the levator ani and the overlapping anal sphincter complex to the anal verge.

The Cecum

Structure

The cecum extends from the appendicular orifice to the ileocecal valve, and is about 7.5 cm long. It rests upon the lateral cutaneous nerve of the thigh, the iliacus, and the psoas muscles. It is sometimes retroperitoneal in location but its peritoneal attachment is incomplete posteriorly, allowing it a variable degree of mobility. Anteriorly, it usually contacts the abdominal wall and/or the omentum.

Function and Pathophysiology

The cecum appears to act as a sump, allowing heavier objects in the stool to collect as the liquid stream passes on by. Endoscopists frequently note tablets, chewing gum, and other particles here. When the solid objects attain a critical mass they are passed up into the ascending colon. The intermittent peristalsis is analogous to that of the rectum and may be the reason why both parts of the bowel tend to develop flat, carpet-like neoplasms. The tendency for the cecum to be unzygosed and its lack of a broad-based mesentery means that it is occasionally prone to twist or flip, as seen in volvulus and bascule.

The Appendix

Structure

The appendix, which normally measures approximately 9 cm (range 2–20 cm), originates from the posteromedial cecal wall. The three taeniae coli diverge from the base of the appendix where they form a complete longitudinal muscle layer. The position of the appendix varies, but it is most often retrocecal or pelvic. The blood supply to the appendix is via the appendicular artery, an end artery originating from the ileocolic. It passes posterior to the terminal ileum to enter the mesoappendix at the base of the appendix. The appendix opens into the cecum approximately 3 cm below the ileocecal valve and occasionally a semilunar fold guards the appendiceal orifice.

Function and Pathophysiology

The appendix serves no obvious gastrointestinal function but is heavily infiltrated by lymphoid tissue. In fact, it is the apex of gut lymphoid tissue, which becomes more and more prominent from the jejunum to the terminal ileum. Childhood and adolescent hypertrophy of gut lymphoid tissue predisposes the appendix to blockage and inflammation.

The Ileocecal Valve

Structure

The ileocecal valve is the entry point of the small intestine into the colon. Its entry on the posteromedial wall of the large intestine defines the cecum and separates it from the ascending colon. The orifice is usually a horizontal slit, but when the ileum prolapses into the colon through the valve, it looks circular. A vertical cleft in the upper leaf of the valve ("buttock sign") is often seen when it is viewed from above through a colonoscope.

Function and Pathophysiology

The muscle layers of the small intestine form a nipple valve that prevents reflux of colonic contents into the ileum and controls the release of small intestinal content into the cecum. It is kept tonically contracted by sympathetic neural input. When the ileocecal valve is resected, bacterial counts in the terminal ileum rise. If total colectomy is indicated in a patient prone to incontinence, there may be some advantage to preserving the cecum and ileocecal valve and performing a cecorectal anastomosis. Endoscopically, prolapsing ileal mucosa can be confused for a villous adenoma, leading to attempts at snaring the valve.

The Ascending Colon

Structure

The ascending colon extends from the ileocecal valve to the hepatic flexure. It is approximately 15 cm long and of smaller caliber than the cecum. The ascending colon is largely intraperitoneal except posteriorly where it lies upon the perirenal fascia, iliolumbar ligament, quadratus lumborum, and iliac fascia. It leaves an impression on the undersurface of the right lobe of the liver where it turns medially, anteriorly, and inferiorly at the hepatic flexure to become the transverse colon. The ilioinguinal and iliohypogastric nerves, fourth lumbar artery and lateral femoral nerve cross behind it from medial to lateral.

The hepatic flexure overlies the inferolateral aspect of the anterior right renal (Gerota's) fascia, lies below and behind the right lobe of liver and gallbladder fundus, and is anterolateral to the second part of the duodenum.

Function and Pathophysiology

The ascending colon is the site of most of the water absorption from the colon. Approximately 1,500 cc of liquid stool enter daily through the ileocecal valve. By the time the stool reaches the transverse colon it is usually solid. The predominant forms of colonic motility in the right colon are segmentation and reverse peristalsis.

The Transverse Colon

Structure

The transverse colon extends intraperitoneally from the hepatic flexure to the left hypochondrium, where it turns inferiorly thus forming the splenic flexure. It is approximately 50 cm in length. The proximal transverse colon lies over the second part of the duodenum and the head of the pancreas, to which it is relatively closely fixed by peritoneum. Within its mesocolon it is suspended between both colonic flexures and descends into the abdominal cavity. The position of the transverse colon varies between individuals and also within the individual depending on whether the person is supine or recumbent. Its apex can reach the pelvis in the upright position.

Clinically, the transverse colon is the most superficial part of the colon in the supine patient. Colonic gas will tend to accumulate here, and on a flat AP X-ray the transverse colon will be magnified relative to the rest of the colon.

The mesentery of the transverse colon is fused with the greater omentum in its right half, and separated from it by the lesser sac of the peritoneum in its left half. In dissecting omentum from mesocolon, it is sometimes easy to damage mesenteric veins. In dissections for cancers of the right colon, omentum and mesentery are removed together.

The Splenic Flexure

Structure

The splenic flexure represents the junction of the transverse and descending colon. The angulation of the splenic flexure is markedly more acute than that of the hepatic flexure, and it is more complex. Sometimes the colon undergoes several spiral twists, making passage of a colonoscope difficult. Overlying the tail of the pancreas, the inferomedial aspect of the spleen, and lying anterolateral to the right kidney, the splenic flexure is higher and more posterior than the hepatic flexure. Often, the transverse colon overlaps the descending colon, with the bowel fused together by adhered omentum. The splenic flexure is attached to the diaphragm by the phrenicocolic ligament, which lies below the anteroinferior aspect of the spleen.

Clinically, the splenic flexure is recognized during colonoscopy because of the pool of liquid that always accumulates in the proximal descending colon, because it is the most posterior part of the colon when the patient is supine.

The Descending Colon

Structure

The descending colon runs from the splenic flexure inferiorly to the level of the iliac crest where it becomes the sigmoid colon. This junction is noticeable during colonoscopy as an acute elbow bend. The descending colon is approximately 25 cm in length and is more posterior than the ascending colon. The following structures pass posterior to it; left subcostal vessels and nerve, the iliohypogastric and ilioinguinal nerves, fourth lumbar artery, lateral femoral cutaneous nerve, femoral and genitofemoral nerves, the gonadal vessels, and the external iliac artery. The descending colon does not usually have a mesentery. Its posterior surface overlying the inferolateral aspect of the kidney, transverses abdominis, quadratus lumborum, iliacus, and psoas muscles is not invested in peritoneum.

The Sigmoid Colon

Structure

"Sigmoid" is derived from a root meaning "S-shaped." The sigmoid colon is a curved intraperitoneal segment of colon of variable length (average 40 cm). It is attached to the retroperitoneum by the sigmoid mesentery, which is maximal in length at its midpoint. The sigmoid colon occupies the upper pelvis as it snakes its way from the descending colon to the rectum. The more tortuous the sigmoid, the more acute the angles will be at either end. Sigmoid anatomy is often distorted by adhesions, either congenital or surgical. These adhesions need to be completely taken down at surgery or else the anatomy can be confused. The sigmoid colon is the narrowest part of the large bowel, and has the thickest muscle.

Function and Pathophysiology

The sigmoid and descending colons are the reservoir for stool. Stool passes along the transverse colon piece by piece, but builds up on the left side. There is a high pressure zone at the rectosigmoid that acts as a brake. The left colon empties by a mass movement, a concerted peristaltic wave that expels stool into the rectum. The mass movement is usually stimulated by a meal (gastrocolic reflex) or by activity.

Loss of the sigmoid produces multiple stools, as the reservoir function is lost. This function, along with high muscular tone and thick muscle, means that pressures within the sigmoid colon are high. This makes the sigmoid colon prone to diverticulosis, most likely to produce symptoms in patients with irritable bowel syndrome, and a likely cause of constipation.

Blood, Lymphatic, and Nerve Supply to the Colon

Arteries

Colonic arterial blood is delivered through a marginal artery (of Drummond) that runs around the entire colon and provides collateral supply in the event that one or more of the feeding arteries is absent (see Fig. 3.1). It also offers the opportunity for anatomic variants, which are common. The origin of the feeding arteries to the colon is determined by the embryological origin of the part of the bowel being supplied. The cecum, appendix, ascending colon, and proximal two thirds of the transverse colon, derived from the midgut, are supplied by the concave surface of the superior mesenteric artery (SMA). Its colonic branches include the ileocolic, right colic, and middle colic arteries. One or more of these branches are absent in up to 20% of people. In 50% of cases, the marginal artery of the right colon is deficient, making this part of the colon prone to ischemia [2].

The ileocolic artery is the last colonic branch of the SMA. It descends inferiorly toward the right iliac fossa where it divides into two branches. The superior ascends to anastomose with the right colic artery, and the inferior branch anastomoses with the end of the superior mesenteric artery. The inferior branch supplies four arteries. The colic branch passes upward to the ascending colon, the anterior and posterior cecal divisions travel to the cecum. The appendicular artery runs in the free edge of the mesoappendix and an ileal branch anastomoses with the SMA.

The right colic artery arises from the middle of the SMA and travels anterior to the gonadal vessels and the right ureter to the middle of the ascending colon. Here, it divides in two: an ascending branch anastomoses with the middle colic and the descending branch anastomoses with the ileocolic.

The middle colic artery arises from the SMA just distal to the pancreas and quickly divides into a right and left branch approximately 3 in. from the colonic edge. The right branch anastomoses through the collateral arcade with the right colic and the left with the left colic.

The distal third of the transverse colon and the left colon, including the sigmoid colon, are supplied by the inferior mesenteric artery (IMA) via the left colic, the sigmoid arteries and the termination of the inferior mesenteric – that is, the superior rectal artery (SRA) – supplying mainly the rectum. The IMA arises from the aorta 3–4 cm proximal to the aortic bifurcation just below the third part of the duodenum. Here, it is surrounded by nerve fibers of the superior hypogastric plexus. This corresponds to L3. The IMA runs on the anterior surface of the aorta and then passes to the left of the aorta crossing over the left common iliac artery, descending into the pelvis where it runs in the base of the sigmoid mesentery to the upper third of the rectum. As it crosses the pelvic brim, the IMA becomes the SRA. The left colic artery is the first branch of the IMA arising just distal to its origin and running to the left and upward within the colonic mesentery. It runs a short course dividing into an ascending and a descending branch. The former ascends to the transverse colon and anastomoses with the right branch of the middle colic artery while the descending branch anastomoses with the most proximal branch of the sigmoid artery. Two or three

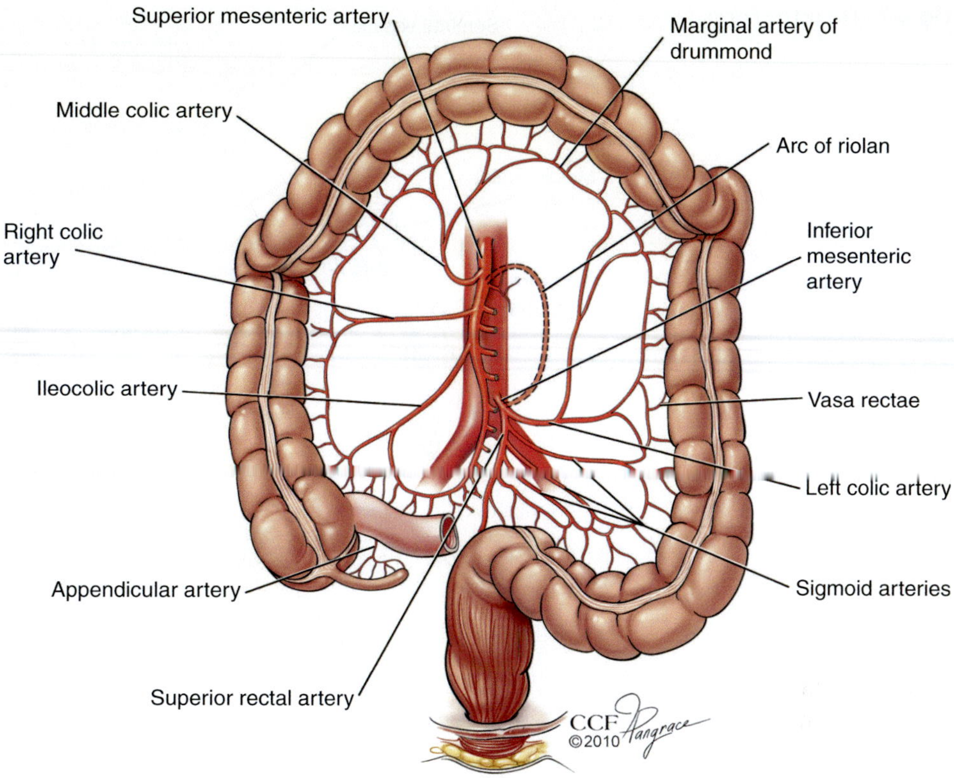

Fig. 3.1 Blood supply of the colon and rectum. Illustration © CCF

sigmoid arteries arise from IMA at the level of the aortic bifurcation. These vessels run directly toward the sigmoid colon and anastomose with the descending branch of the left colic and the SRA. Following the origin of the final branch, the IMA crosses over the left common iliac, becoming the SRA and descending into the pelvis supplying the upper third of the rectum.

The watershed in the marginal artery between the superior and inferior mesenteric arterial circulation is at the splenic flexure. This is called Griffith's point, and if the marginal artery is absent in this area (5% of people) [3] the splenic flexure and descending colon are prone to ischemic colitis. Approximately, 7% of people have another collateral artery running more proximally in the mesentery, carrying blood between superior and inferior circulations. If this "meandering mesenteric artery" (see Fig. 3.1) (Arc of Riolan) [4] is divided in the course of a colectomy, intestinal ischemia may result.

The watershed in the marginal artery between the sigmoid arteries and the rectum is known as Sudek's point. A devascularized sigmoid stump left on top of the rectum after sigmoid colectomy is prone to ischemia and is a reason to ensure that such resections encompass all the sigmoid colon.

The marginal artery (of Drummond) [4] runs at a variable distance from the colonic wall and has two types of branches: the short vasa recta that supply the mesenteric aspect of the colonic wall and the long vasa recta that supply the appendices epiploicae and the antimesenteric aspect of the colonic wall.

Veins

The venous drainage of the colon mirrors that of the arterial supply except that the superior and inferior mesenteric veins drain into the portal venous system. The inferior mesenteric vein runs past the origin of the IMA up to the lower border of the pancreas. It then joins the splenic vein, which in turn unites with the superior mesenteric vein to become the portal vein.

Lymphatics

Lymphatic drainage follows the blood supply. There are several tiers of lymphatics in the colon and its mesentery. Pericolic nodes lie on the colon, and pericolic lymphatics coalesce and drain directly into the epicolic nodes at the mesenteric edge. Further, lymphatic channels then pass to nodes located at the level of the marginal artery. This chain represents the paracolic nodes. Drainage then continues along intermediate chains of nodes distributed along the main arterial branches of the mesenteric vessels. Ultimately, the lymphatic drainage passes through the main nodes at the origin of the major mesenteric vessels along the aorta.

Nerves

The nerve supply to the colon is both sympathetic (inhibitory) and parasympathetic (excitatory). The sympathetic chains lie behind the inferior vena cava on the right and lateral to the aorta on the left. Preganglionic white fibers pass from the spinal cord at T6-12 to the sympathetic chains at the

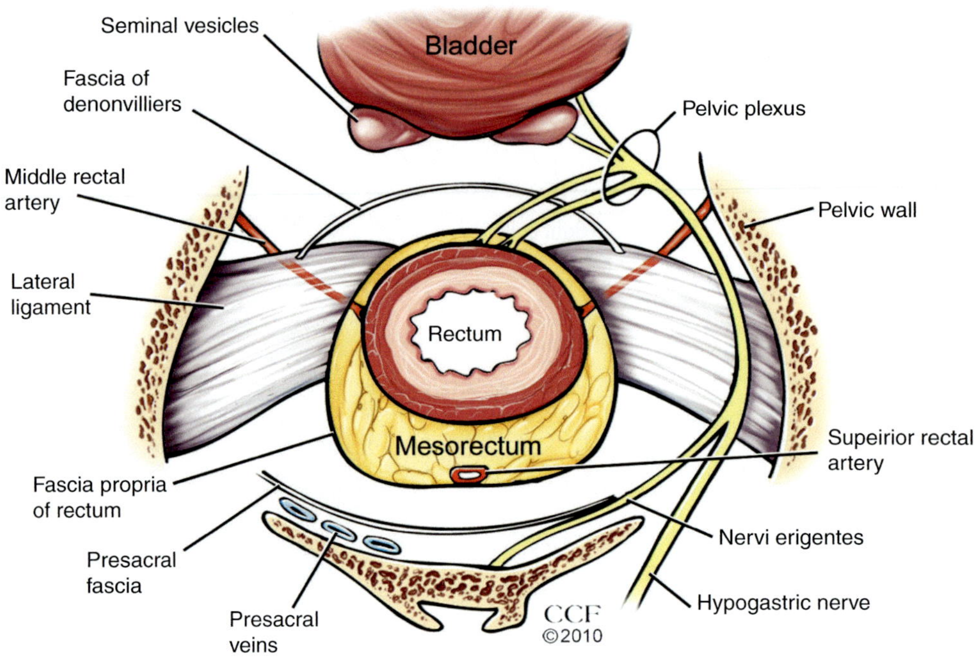

Fig. 3.2 The pelvic fascia. Illustration © CCF

celiac and superior mesenteric ganglia. Sympathetic fibers then run to that part of the colon derived from the midgut, namely, the cecum, ascending colon, and proximal two thirds of the transverse colon.

The sympathetic supply to that area of the colon derived from the hindgut is via the first three lumbar nerves. Nerve fibers coalesce at the superior hypogastric plexus and travel to the perivascular ganglia at which they synapse and run to supply the colon.

The parasympathetic supply to the midgut is via the posterior vagus through the superior mesenteric plexus and to the hindgut is via the second, third, and fourth sacral nerves. Having exited from the sacral foramina, they form the nervi erigentes, which lie behind the parietal endopelvic fascia and travel to the hypogastric and pelvic plexuses to supply the abdominal and pelvic viscera.

Rectum

Structure

The rectum is the last 12–15 cm of the large bowel, from the rectosigmoid junction above to the anorectal angle below. It lies in the hollow of the sacrum and is completely extraperitoneal posteriorly. In front, the rectum is extraperitoneal only in its lower one third where it is a direct posterior relation of the bladder, seminal vesicles, and the prostate in men and the cervix uteri and posterior wall of the vagina in women. The lumen of the rectum is S-shaped because of the rectal valves (valves of Houston). The upper and lower valves are convex to the right and the middle valve is convex to the left. The middle rectal valve is a landmark for the anterior peritoneal reflection.

The Pelvic Fascia

The extraperitoneal rectum is surrounded by endopelvic fascia that support and define rectal and perirectal structures. This fascia has visceral and parietal components (see Fig. 3.2).

The Parietal Endopelvic Fascia

The parietal endopelvic fascia lines the walls and the floor of the pelvis, covering obturator internus, piriformis, levator ani, and coccygeus muscles. It is continuous with the transversalis fascia and is fused with the periosteum of the linea terminalis of the hip bones.

The Presacral Fascia

The presacral fascia is an adherent, tough, gray-white membrane plastered to the cavity of the sacrum, covering nerves and vessels. It is a thickened part of the parietal endopelvic fascia and is deficient in the midline. The fascia is thinner laterally, where it overlies piriformis and the upper part of coccygeus. From here, it swings medially as part of the lateral ligament of the rectum to become continuous with the posterior part of the rectal fascia propria. Wilson [5] claims that anteroinferiorly it becomes continuous with the rectovesical septum. It forms part of the uterosacral, infundibulopelvic, and transverse (cardinal) ligaments. Its upper part contains the superior hypogastric plexus, continuous with the hypogastric nerves. An additional component of the presacral fascia reaches the anorectal junction, covering the rectococcygeus muscle and anococcygeal ligament.

The Rectosacral Fascia

The rectosacral fascia was described by Crapp and Cuthbertson as a fascial layer of variable thickness passing anteriorly from the level of the fourth sacral vertebra to blend with the posterior layer of the fascia propria about 3–5 cm above the anorectal junction [6]. It attaches the rectum to the hollow of the sacrum. It must be deliberately divided during rectal mobilization and this division allows the rectum to be lifted out of the hollow of the sacrum.

Waldeyer's Fascia

Waldeyer originally described all pelvic fascia without referring to any specific component [7]. However, his name has been used for the presacral fascia, the fascia between the sacrum and the anorectal junction, the fascia investing the superior rectal artery, or to the entire fascia behind the rectum. Waldeyer's fascia is currently taken to represent that part of the pelvic fascia anchoring the sacrum to the anorectal junction.

Visceral Endopelvic Fascia

This invests the pelvic organs and blood vessels, and forms the perineural sheaths. Its important components in rectal anatomy are the fascia propria of the rectum and Denonvilliers fascia.

The Fascia Propria of the Rectum

The fascia propria of the rectum is a fibrous capsule that envelops the rectum and its associated nerves, blood vessels, and lymphatics. It is continuous with the parietal fascia of the pelvic floor from which it extends upward to the rectosigmoid junction.

The Retrorectal Space

This avascular plane lies between the presacral fascia and fascia propria and is filled with loose areolar tissue. Superiorly, it begins at the sacral promontory, is limited laterally by the lateral ligaments and piriformis fascia and inferiorly by the rectosacral fascia. Entry to this space is gained immediately behind the superior rectal artery.

The lateral relations of this space are the internal iliac vessels, the pelvic plexuses, and the pelvic splanchnic nerves. These nerves are generally buried behind endopelvic fascia and are only injured during pelvic dissection if the plane is carried beyond the retrorectal space.

Denonvilliers' Fascia

Denonvilliers described a fascial layer separating the anterior wall of the rectum from the prostate and seminal vesicles in men, and from the vagina in women. This fascia is V-shaped, its caudal part being contiguous with the fascia overlying pubococcygeus and inserting into the pelvic floor in the region of the perineal body. It fuses with the caudal part of the posterior vaginal wall in the female and with the base of the bladder in the male. The arms of the "V" extend over the seminal vesicles and curve posterolaterally to merge with the parietal endopelvic fascia. Superiorly, it inserts into the rectovesical pouch.

Denonvilliers' fascia can be a thick tough layer, or a thin and translucent membrane. It is prominent in young men and becomes less so with advancing age. It is generally more substantial than the fascia propria of the rectum, containing dense collagen, smooth muscle fibers, and coarse elastic fibers. Posteriorly, the septum is loosely applied to the rectum, but there is a more vascular attachment anteriorly because the mesenchyme surrounding the prostate and seminal vesicles is derived from the rectovesical peritoneum. Resection of anteriorly located rectal tumors requires dissection anterior to Denonvilliers' fascia, despite the risk of injury to the nervi erigentes. Dissection for posterolateral and posterior rectal cancers can spare Denonvilliers' fascia, staying posterior to it.

The Lateral Ligaments

The lateral ligaments are structures that are only defined during rectal dissection, when mobilization of the rectum unearths condensations of connective tissue running between the lateral endopelvic fascia of the lower pelvis and the lateral aspect of the fascia propria. These condensations contain nerves and, in 25% of patients, an accessory middle rectal artery. Division of the lateral ligaments, performed just after division of the rectosacral fascia, allows the rectum to be completely lifted out of the pelvis.

The Rectal Mesentery

The mesorectum is the block of fatty tissue on the posterior two thirds to three quarters of the circumference of the rectum. It is not a "mesorectum" in the true sense of a mesentery but common usage has validated the term. It contains the terminal branches of the inferior mesenteric artery and is invested by the fascia propria of the rectum. It ends 1 or 2 cm above the pelvic floor, and is clinically significant because it may contain tumor deposits up to 5 cm away from the intrarectal tumor.

Blood Supply to the Rectum

The arterial blood supply is via the superior, middle, and inferior rectal arteries. The SRA is a caudal extension of the IMA and acquires its name as it traverses the left common iliac artery. It passes forward to the bowel in the base of the sigmoid mesentery and enters the mesorectum at the rectosigmoid junction. Before its terminal division, it gives rise to a rectosigmoid branch that bifurcates – one branch passing superiorly to anastomose with the distal sigmoid branch of the IMA and the other inferiorly to anastomose with the upper rectal branch of the SRA. The upper rectal branch supplies the upper third of the rectum. In 80% of patients, the IMA bifurcates into right and left terminal branches, while in 17% of cases there are multiple branches [7]. The right branch is usually dominant and is the continuation of the IMA [8]. Each branch of the SRA has two to four major divisions and a number of smaller ones, which descend as far as the pelvic floor.

The anatomy of the middle rectal artery is controversial as it is absent in as many as 80% of cases [9]. The presence of a middle rectal artery (MRA) can be predicted from the size of the SRA [7]. The MRA is derived from the internal iliac artery, and approaches the lower third of the rectum at the level of the levator ani. Boxall and colleagues showed that it courses anteriorly, and is closely related to the seminal vesicles and the apex of the prostate [10]. The importance of the contribution of the MRA to rectal blood supply is disputed and is probably dependant on the integrity of the SRA [11]. Because it does not run in the lateral ligaments, these structures can usually be divided without ligation.

The inferior rectal artery (IRA) is a branch of the internal pudendal artery that pierces the wall of the anal canal in the region of the external sphincter. The entire course of the IRA is extrapelvic below levator ani, where it is encountered during abdominoperineal excision of the rectum running across the roof of the ischiorectal fossa.

It has intramural anastomoses with the SRA.

Rectal venous drainage exists as a dense plexus of veins draining upward (superior rectal veins) to the portal system and downward (inferior rectal veins) to the systemic venous system. There is a potential portal-systemic shunt that is clinically significant in patients with portal hypertension. Rectal varices may be mistaken for hemorrhoids and excision under these circumstances causes disastrous bleeding.

Pelvic Nerves

The pelvic autonomic nervous system is intimately related to the rectum, lying in the plane between the peritoneum and the endopelvic fascia. There are three major complexes: the superior hypogastric plexus (SHP), the hypogastric nerves (HN), and the pelvic plexus (PP).

The superior hypogastric plexus is a network of sympathetic pre- and post-ganglionic fibers mixed with visceral afferent fibers that occupy the interiliac trigone just below the bifurcation of the aorta. Cephalad it is continuous with sympathetic preaortic trunks that are closely applied to the aorta and surround the origin of the IMA. Sympathetic fibers leave the SHP caudad to form the hypogastric plexus.

The hypogastric plexus is an extension of the sympathetic nervous system that unites the SHP and the PP. There are two or three trunks, which run medial and parallel to the ureters bilaterally along the pelvic sidewall. The left hypogastric nerve originates posterior to the superior rectal artery and is at risk during proctectomy. These sympathetic trunks join the pelvic parasympathetic nerves to become the PP. The PP runs toward the bladder, prostate, and upper urethra. Some fibers pass posteromedially to the rectum.

The pelvic parasympathetic nerves contributing to the PP arise from the second, third, and fourth sacral nerve roots and pierce the endopelvic fascia from behind to enter the plane of the plexus. The plexus lies laterally in the pelvis at the level of the distal third of the rectum. It appears to be arranged in layers. Some fibers pass superficially to the rectum, but those components of the PP that supply the sexual organs and the bladder lie deep within the endopelvic fascia around the iliac vessels. These fibers pass along the levator muscle to the bladder and prostate. The deepest layer of pelvic nerves consists of proximal portions of the visceral arm of the pudendal plexus and the sacral plexus. The lowermost fibers of the PP pass to the rectum and the prostate gland concentrating at their termination just anterior to the fascia of Denonvilliers. They are at highest risk of injury during dissection for anterior rectal cancers. Having incised transversely in the plane between the vesicles and the rectum, the incision should not be carried beyond the lateral border of the vesicle on either side, in order to protect the neurovascular bundle. The incision should be carried inferiorly at this point, thus avoiding injury, which may result in erectile dysfunction in men.

The Pudendal Nerve

The pudendal nerve arises from the sacral plexus, containing fibers from S2, S3, and S4. It passes out of the pelvis through the greater sciatic foramen and reenters the pelvis through Alcock's canal. Its major branches are the inferior rectal nerve, the perineal nerve, and the dorsal nerve of the penis/clitoris. The inferior rectal branch accompanies the inferior rectal artery across the ischiorectal fossa to innervate the external sphincter muscle and supply sensation to the anal canal. The puborectalis is supplied by a direct pelvic branch of S3 and S4, while the rest of the levator is innervated by S4 and branches of the perineal nerve.

Rectal Lymphatics

Rectal nodes are mostly in the mesorectum, where lymphatics from the upper two thirds drain to the inferior mesenteric nodes. Lymph from the lower third of the rectum can drain either upward to the inferior mesenteric nodes or sideways to the internal iliac nodes.

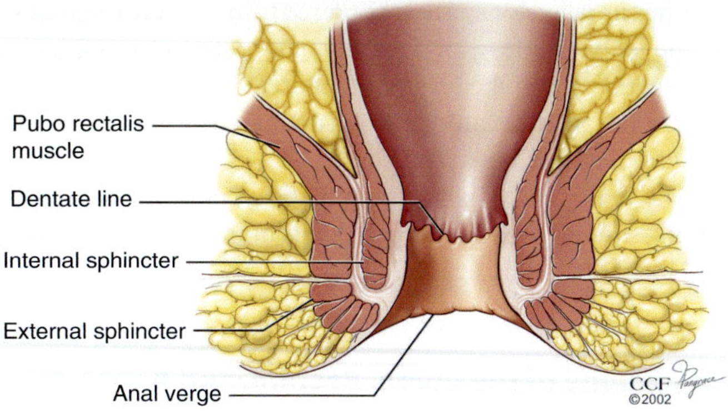

Fig. 3.3 The anus. Illustration © CCF

The Anal Canal

This canal is 2.5–4 cm long and represents the terminal portion of the gastrointestinal tract. It begins at the level of the levator ani and terminates at the anal verge. It forms an inferoposterior angle with the lower aspect of the rectum, the angle being created by the puborectalis component of the levator ani and varying with its activity. Rectal examination must take this anorectal angle into account as it governs the direction in which the examining finger or scope is inserted.

The anus appears as an anteroposterior slit because of the tonic contraction of its muscles. It is surrounded by overlapping tubes of muscle: the internal anal sphincter and the external anal sphincter (see Fig. 3.3).

Posterior to the anal canal is the anococcygeal body, comprised of a mass of fibromuscular tissue. Anteriorly lies the perineal body, separating the anus from the vagina in women and from the membranous urethra in men.

Interior of the Anal Canal

The upper half of the anal canal is lined by a mucous membrane, while the lower half is lined by squamous epithelium. The upper anal canal is characterized by the presence of 6–14 longitudinal mucosal folds called anal columns (of Morgagni). At the apex of these columns the rectum joins the anal canal at the anorectal line. Anal columns are linked at their base by anal valves, which form the wavy line of separation of anoderm and rectum known as the dentate line. The anal valves are the site of opening of the 4–10 anal glands, which penetrate the extra-anal tissue to varying degrees. One or two glands reach the intersphincteric plane. The dentate line is the embryologic junction of the hindgut and the proctodeum. This different embryologic origin of the upper and lower halves of the anal canal means that their blood supply and lymphatic drainage differ.

The Anal Transitional Zone

The anal transitional zone is the zone of epithelium between the pure columnar epithelium of the rectum above and the modified squamous epithelium of the anal canal below. This transitional extends for 1–3 cm above the dentate line, and contains a variety of cellular types including columnar, squamous, cuboidal, melanocytes, and endocrine cells. The zone is not uniform but is penetrated by tongues and islands of columnar epithelium [12]. The modified squamous epithelium of the anal canal extending about 1.5 cm below the dentate line is the anoderm. It is modified in that it has no hair follicles or sebaceous glands. These appear toward the anal verge.

Blood Supply and Lymphatic Drainage of the Anal Canal

The superior rectal artery supplies the anal canal above the dentate line. The venous drainage from this area is via the superior rectal vein, which drains into the inferior mesenteric vein. Below the level of the dentate line, the arterial supply and venous drainage are via the inferior rectal artery and vein, which originate from the internal iliac vessels. The anal canal therefore represents an area of portosystemic anastomosis.

The lymphatic drainage above the dentate line is to the internal iliac lymph nodes and from there to the common iliac and lumbar region, or along the superior rectal nodes to the aorta. From below the dentate line, lymph drains to the superficial inguinal nodes.

Above the dentate line, the sympathetic nerve supply to the anal canal is via branches of the inferior hypogastric plexus. Parasympathetic nerve supply is via the pelvic splanchnic nerves. Below the dentate line, somatic innervation is via the inferior rectal nerves, which are branches of the pudendal nerve.

The External Anal Sphincter

This striated muscle surrounds the distal two thirds of the anal canal and is composed of three parts: subcutaneous, superficial, and deep. The subcutaneous part of the sphincter is inferior and surrounds the canal in a circular fashion. These fibers are not anchored to bone. The superficial part of the sphincter is oval in shape and its fibers extend from the coccyx circumferentially around the anal canal to the perineal body, anchoring the anal canal in the midline. The fibers of the deep aspect of the external anal sphincter arise from the perineal body, merge laterally with some of the fibers of the superficial transverse perineal muscle and blend into the puborectalis part of the levator ani muscles.

The EAS is innervated by fibers from S2 and S3 via the inferior rectal branch of the pudendal nerve and the perineal branch of S4.

The Internal Anal Sphincter

The internal anal sphincter is composed of involuntary smooth muscle and forms a cylinder investing the upper two thirds of the anal canal. It is a thickening and an extension of the circular muscle of the rectum. The lower edge of the internal anal sphincter is located approximately 1.2 cm distal to the dentate line. A groove is palpable here, between the internal and external sphincters (the intersphincteric groove). Running in the intersphincteric plane is the conjoined longitudinal muscle, which arises from the longitudinal muscle of the rectum added to by fibers from levator ani. It descends in the intersphincteric space and some fibers spread out through the subcutaneous external sphincter and attach to the perianal skin. This muscle is often referred to as the corrugator cutis ani. The internal sphincter receives sympathetic innervation from L5 and parasympathetic innervation via S2, 3, and 4.

The Anal Spaces

A variety of potential spaces exist around the anus and are clinically significant in that they provide a potential pathway for the spread of sepsis.

1. The perianal space lies subcutaneously at the anal verge. Its boundaries are the anal mucosa medially, the fat of the buttocks laterally, and the perianal skin inferiorly. Superiorly it is limited by the mucosal suspensory ligament. This space contains the most inferior aspect of the external anal sphincter, branches of the inferior rectal vessels, the external hemorrhoidal plexus and lymphatics.
2. The intersphincteric space lies between the internal and external sphincters and is continuous inferiorly with the perianal space. It extends superiorly into the wall of the rectum. Two thirds of anal glands terminate here, making this a common site of cryptoglandular sepsis.
3. The ischiorectal space is a large pyramidal space whose inferior border is the perianal skin; the superior border is formed by the levator ani as it courses inferiorly from the obturator fascia. The lateral border is formed by the fascia overlying the obturator internus, which also contains the internal pudendal vessels and the pudendal nerve running in Alcock's canal. The medial boundary is the external sphincter and puborectalis muscles. The ischiorectal space contains fat, the inferior rectal nerve, inferior rectal vessels, nerves to the external genitalia, transverse perineal vessels, and the perineal branch of the fourth sacral nerve. The ischiorectal spaces on each side communicate contralaterally via the deep postanal space.
4. The deep postanal space lies between the anococcygeal ligament below and the levator ani above. Laterally, it is bordered by the ischioanal spaces. Anteriorly lies the external sphincter and posteriorly the inferior aspect of the fifth sacral body and the coccyx. This space is a communication between both ischioanal spaces. It should always be examined perioperatively in a patient with perianal pain and no obvious external source of evident sepsis.
5. The superficial postanal space allows posterior communication between both perianal spaces.
6. The supralevator space is bordered by the rectum medially, the pelvic side wall laterally, the peritoneal reflection superiorly, and the levator ani muscle inferiorly. The right and left supralevator spaces communicate posteriorly to form a horseshoe-shaped cavity.

The three spaces, which communicate posteriorly to form a horseshoe-shaped cavity, are the ischiorectal, supralevator, and intersphincteric spaces.

Physiology of the Colon, Rectum, and Anus

Colonic Absorption and Digestion

The function of the colon is to receive small bowel content through the ileocecal valve and to resorb salt and water as required. As it processes the stool, the colon propels it to the sigmoid colon where it is stored. At defecation, stool is emptied into the rectum where there is short-term storage via accommodation.

Metabolic Functions

The colon receives approximately 1,500 mL of fluid stool from the ileum daily, of which it resorbs 1,350 mL of water and excretes 150 mL in the stool. It absorbs sodium and chloride and secretes potassium and bicarbonate. The absorptive capacity is maximal in the right colon. Sodium passes into the colonocyte along a concentration and electrochemical gradient. The rate of sodium absorption is directly proportional to the luminal concentration. Water is passively absorbed along an osmotic gradient following sodium absorption. Once sodium reaches the intracellular area it is actively transported out of the cell at the basolateral membrane against a concentration gradient in exchange for potassium. The concentration of potassium within the colonocyte allows it to passively traverse the colonocyte and travel into the colonic lumen where it is excreted.

Chloride is actively resorbed at the luminal surface of the colonocyte in exchange for bicarbonate. Its absorption is increased by a low luminal pH.

Urea is delivered to the colon at a concentration of 0.4 g/day and is metabolized by colonic bacteria to approximately 300 mL of ammonia. The concentration of ammonia in feces is usually 1–3 mmol daily, therefore the majority of the ammonia produced must be reabsorbed across the colonocyte cell membrane. This most probably results from formation of ammonia and carbon dioxide.

Mucus production occurs throughout the length of the large intestine. In addition, the colon has a minor role in digestion. Protein digestion by anaerobic bacteria leads to the production of products (e.g., phenol, cresol, and hydrogen sulfide) that cause fecal odor. Metabolism of undigested carbohydrate into short-chain fatty acids (acetic, butyric, and proprionic acid) by colonic flora provides up to 70% of the energy requirement of the colon. In addition, short-chain fatty acids provide substrates for gluconeogenesis, lipogenesis, protein synthesis, and mucin production. Butyrate, in particular, is antitumorigenic and may account for some of the cancer-preventing benefits of a diet rich in resistant starch.

Patterns and Purposes of Colonic Motility

One of the main functions of the colon is to process the 1,500 cc of liquid stool it receives each day into a compact bolus that can be stored until defecation occurs. This process involves absorption of water, passage of the stool, and storage of the stool. Both the structure and the function of colonic muscle are suited to this task.

Normal colonic transit is dependent on a number of factors but is approximately 32 h for men and 41 h for women. The three patterns of colonic contraction determining transit are segmentation, mass movements, and retrograde peristalsis.

Segmentation is a form of non-propulsive movement in which the bowel content is moved between individual segments. The arrangement of muscle in the colonic wall is perfect for producing segmentation, which occurs through simultaneous contraction of the circular muscle of the colon and the taenia. Constant segmentation allows maximal exposure of stool to the colonic mucosa, facilitating absorption of fluid and electrolytes. Retrograde peristalsis occurs in the ascending colon and the transverse colon and facilitates absorption of water by prolonging exposure of stool to the mucosa.

Once stool reaches the sigmoid colon, a high pressure zone at the rectosigmoid junction prevents it from moving into the rectum until a mass movement occurs. The sigmoid colon acts as a fecal reservoir, storing its contents and allowing accumulation of stool until the next mass movement. The clinical implications of this reservoir function are related to the high pressures within the sigmoid and its thick muscle. It is the part of the colon most prone to developing pulsion diverticulae, and most prone to producing symptoms of bloating, cramping, and constipation when it is dysfunctional.

Colonic mass movements empty the contents of the left colon into the rectum. These are high amplitude, rapidly propagating contractions, which physically propel the fecal bolus toward the rectum. They often occur after meals, which are followed by a sensation of rectal fullness and the desire to defecate. During mass movement there are no visible haustrations. A segment of colon at least 20 cm in length sequentially contracts. These movements are maximal in the left and sigmoid colon, emptying the stored stool into the rectum.

Muscular Activity in the Colon

There are three types of muscular activity occurring in the colon: types I, II, and III. Type I contractions are monophasic and have an amplitude of 5–10 cm of water. Their frequency is 10/min and they are of short duration (5–10 s). Type II contractions occur every 2 min and last for 30 s with an amplitude of 15–30 cm of water. These movements account for more than 90% of normal colonic activity and correspond to haustral contraction and relaxation. Type III contractions override the other two types and have an amplitude of 10 cm of water, representing a change in basal pressure.

Defecation

The rectum is the organ of defecation and adaptation, conferring the ability to defecate or to postpone defecation. It is a compliant, capacious organ that has the ability to accommodate to increased pressure should that pressure not be relieved. Rectal resting pressure is approximately 5 mmHg. The entry of a fecal bolus into the rectum results in an awareness of the urge to defecate and an increase in intrarectal pressure. This rise in pressure triggers reflex relaxation of the internal anal sphincter. The external anal sphincter remains contracted to maintain continence. This reflex, named the rectoanal inhibitory reflex, is mediated by the autonomic nervous system. It is the mechanism by which rectal contents come into contact with the sensitive anal transitional epithelium, allowing discrimination between gas, liquid, and solid and selective passage of rectal contents when appropriate. When defecation is inappropriate the EAS stays contracted and the anus remains shut. The rectum accommodates, decreasing pressure while intrarectal volume stays the same. The call to stool temporarily wanes.

If defecation is appropriate, the individual sits and relaxes their pelvic floor. The anorectal angle straightens out and the external sphincter muscle relaxes. The rectum then contracts to expel the stool. Straining to increase intra-abdominal pressure may be necessary to evacuate stool if the rectum contracts ineffectively, or if the stool bolus is too large or too hard. On straining, the pelvic floor descends and acquires a funnel shape facilitating expulsion of rectal contents.

Following defecation, the EAS and the puborectalis contract in the closing reflex. The IAS resumes resting tone and the anal canal closes.

References

1. Church J. The unzygosed colon as a factor predisposing to difficult colonoscopy in slim women. Gastrointest Endosc. 2002;55:965–6.
2. Sonneland J, Anson LJ. Surgical anatomy of the arterial supply to the colon. Surg Gynecol Obstet. 1958;106:385–97.
3. Griffiths JD. Surgical anatomy of the blood supply of the distal colon. Ann R Coll Surg Engl. 1956;19:241–56.
4. Fisher DF, Fry WJ. Collateral mesenteric circulation. Surg Gynecol Obstet. 1987;164:487–92.
5. Wilson PM. Anchoring mechanisms of the anorectal region. S Afr Med J. 1967;141:1138–43.

6. Crapp AR, Cuthbertson AM. William Waldeyer and the rectosacral fascia. Surg Gynecol Obstet. 1974;138:252–6.
7. Waldeyer W. Das Becken. Bonn: Cohen, 1899.
8. Ayoub SF. Arterial supply to the human rectum. Acta Anat. 1978;100:317–27.
9. Michels NA, Siddarth P, Kornblith PL, Park WW. The variant blood supply to the small and large intestines: its import in regional resections. J Int Coll Surg. 1963;39:127–70.
10. Church JM, Raudkivi PJ, Hill GL. The surgical anatomy of the rectum – a review with particular relevance to the hazards of rectal mobilization. Int J Colorectal Dis. 1987;2:158–66.
11. Boxall TA, Smart PJ, Griffiths JD. The blood-supply of the distal segment of the rectum in anterior resection. Br J Surg. 1963;50: 399–404.
12. Ambroze Jr WL, Pemberton JH, Dozois RR, et al. The histological pattern and pathological involvement of the anal transition zone in patients with ulcerative colitis. Gastroenterology. 1993;104:514–8.

Physiologic and Metabolic Effects of Intestinal Stomas

4

John Rombeau

This chapter briefly reviews normal small bowel and colonic functions with particular relevance to intestinal stomas. The pathogenesis, diagnosis, and monitoring of physiologic and metabolic abnormalities in both ileostomies and colostomies are discussed. The treatment of high-output intestinal stomas is presented in Chap. 8.

Normal Jejunal and Ileal Absorption

Under normal conditions, approximately 90% of nutrients are absorbed within the first 150 cm of small intestine. In the intact gastrointestinal tract, 9–10 L of endogenous fluid enters the small bowel daily. This fluid is composed of saliva and bile (approximately 1 L each) and gastric and pancreatic juices (1.5–3 L combined). Nearly 6 L of enteric contents are absorbed in the jejunum and 2.5 L in the ileum. This absorptive pattern results in approximately 1.5 L of contents entering the colon daily. Ninety percent of the liquid entering the cecum is absorbed in the colon, leaving approximately 0.1 L of fluid in the feces.

The differences in absorption within intestinal segments depend, in part, on electrolyte transport processes and the permeability of the intercellular spaces. In the jejunum, sodium is absorbed actively and moves with bulk flow of water through relatively large mucosal pores. Sodium absorption is enhanced by intraluminal glucose, other actively absorbed monosaccharides, amino acids, and bicarbonate ions. Two main processes mediate the absorption of sodium and chloride. The first is coupled to the absorption of carbohydrates and amino acids and the second is isotonic sodium chloride absorption. The first occurs primarily in the jejunum, whereas the second occurs principally in the ileum and colon.

Water transport is passive and depends upon osmotic forces. Potassium also moves across the mucosa, following its concentration gradient between lumen and blood modified by a small electric potential of jejunal mucosa. Bicarbonate disappears rapidly from the lumen by mechanisms that involve active ion absorption and neutralization of bicarbonate by hydrogen ions in chyme.

The ileum absorbs vitamin B12 and bile salts. Normally, the hepatic synthesis of bile salts does not meet the demand for fat digestion. This need is met by ileal reabsorption of bile salts, which are then recycled into the jejunum. These functions are unique to this segment of the small intestine and have important implications in patients with either ileal disease or resection. Inadequate absorption of bile salts in the ileum alters digestion and absorption of fat in the jejunum and frequently causes diarrhea.

With ileal resection, recycling of bile salts decreases and hepatic synthesis increases. However, if a total ileectomy is performed, synthesis never increases sufficiently to meet the needs for fat absorption. Additionally, the malabsorption of bile acids results in increased bile salts entering the colon, which in turn impairs colonic absorption of water and sodium. Unabsorbed bile acids also cause fluid secretion, thus enhancing fluid and electrolyte losses from the colon. These events contribute to increased output in patients with colostomies.

The ileum significantly slows intestinal motility. Intestinal transit studies reveal that markers traverse the first 50% of the small bowel in one third the time as the ileum [1]. Thus, ileal resection in turn results in shortened small bowel transit time and increased ileostomy output. Since the motility of the jejunum is rapid and that of the distal ileum slow, jejunal resection alone does not result in a faster rate of intestinal transit. In contrast, the remaining bowel has a very rapid transit after ileal resection.

J. Rombeau
Department of Veterans Affairs,
Palo Alto Health Care System, Palo Alto, CA, USA
e-mail: john.rombeau@gmail.com

V.W. Fazio et al. (eds.), *Atlas of Intestinal Stomas*,
DOI 10.1007/978-0-387-78851-7_4,

Normal Postoperative Ileostomy Effluent: Volume and Composition

Recent meta-analyses of preferences among surgeons [2] reveal that a diverting ileostomy is preferable to a colostomy. Inasmuch as ostomies are often performed to provide proximal diversion of the fecal stream, it is projected that more ileostomies will be constructed in the future. It is therefore incumbent upon surgeons to understand both normal and abnormal ileostomy functions.

Volume of Ileostomy Effluent

There is a wide range in the volume of ileostomy excretion in patients with normal intestines. Approximately 200–700 mL of ileostomy effluent is ejected daily. Some individuals excrete consistently low (less than 500 mL/day) and others discharge inordinately high volumes (1,000–1,500 mL/day) of ileal excreta regardless of dietary intake. This variance may be due, in part, to the preoperative intrinsic motility of the gut; that is, irritable bowel versus chronic constipation. If the volume of ileostomy output exceeds 1,500 mL daily, possible causes should be investigated such as dietary indiscretion, Crohn's disease, previous intestinal resections, and a very proximal location of the stoma such as a jejunostomy. (See section on "Ileostomy Dysfunction".) Ileostomy patients occasionally excrete a considerable amount of water and sodium in the early postoperative period; however, high early postoperative ileostomy volumes are the exception rather than the rule. Typically, fluid and electrolyte losses decrease to approximately 600–700 mL daily 1–2 weeks postoperatively. Occasionally, output greater than 1 L/day may persist longer than 1–2 months during the period of postoperative adaptation of the remaining ileum in continuity. Although, few long-term follow-up studies of ileostomy volume are available, measurements in patients who have had ileostomies for 10 or more years show fecal volumes of the same magnitude of those in patients in whom the ileostomy has been present for only a year or two [3]. Early postoperative ileal contents are characterized by clumps of mucus and are often termed "rice water stools." If this appearance persists, investigation should be directed to rule out either an ileus or partial intestinal blockage.

A normal ileostomy empties at frequent intervals and with varying volumes. Usually there is frequent, small, slow seepage of fluid, with intermittent larger amounts of excreta or gas. Generally, these discharges are larger after eating and become minimal a couple of hours postprandially. As mentioned, the volume, composition, and time of emptying of the ileostomy effluent are influenced, in part, by dietary intake; however, a specific food that increases volume or causes abdominal symptoms in one patient may not affect another individual. Fasting may decrease the volume of ileostomy output to as low as 50–100 mL daily. Most patients with established low volume ileostomies have a surprisingly constant daily fecal volume varying only about 20% around a mean, regardless of eating habits [4]. Apart from dietary indiscretion, intestinal infection, or recurrent intrinsic disease, this constant volume excretion usually remains indefinitely. In one study after the ingestion of cream, the remains of the meal appeared at the ileostomy stoma within 1 h and 15 min; after a meat meal, the contents appeared 4 ½h later [5]. Fluid restriction delayed transit, whereas fluid ingestion accelerated the process, and the end products of a meal were completely discharged from the intestine 6 ½h to 10 h later. Food particles, particularly the remains of vegetables, appear normally in the ileostomy effluent. The transit time for dietary contents to be excreted through a normal ileostomy is longer (348 min) in patients with ileostomies versus 243 min in the control population with an intact ileum [6].

Interestingly, increased intake of free water has very little effect on the volume of ileostomy effluent and only causes larger urine output. Increased sodium intake directly correlates with ileostomy output. Fruit juices increase the wet weight of the stool and cooked cabbage increases both wet and dry weight [7]. Dietary fiber increases dry weight. A well-adapted ileostomy excretes very few nutrients to cause significant nutritional/metabolic deficits.

Composition of Ileostomy Effluent

The composition of normal ileostomy effluent is shown in Table 4.1. The normal ileostomy effluent is nearly 90% water with a sodium concentration of approximately 120 mL mmol/L. This is almost isotonic with normal saline. The normal amount of sodium lost in ileostomy effluent is approximately 60 mEq daily, significantly more than 2–10 mEq of fecal sodium losses in a person without a stoma. Stomal losses of sodium are approximately 1 mEq/h in a fasting patient and 3–4 mEq/h postprandially. The obligatory ileal sodium losses are normally overcome with the ingestion of a well-balanced diet. Approximately, 6–12 mEq of potassium are lost daily through the ileostomy effluent. These findings in turn are important when prescribing postoperative intravenous fluid. If chronic salt depletion occurs, ileostomy output decreases significantly to compensate for the sodium deficit, resulting in increased potassium concentrations in the effluent. When sodium chloride is liberally added to the normal diet such that 260 mEq (approximately 15 g) is consumed, there is increased water content of the ileostomy fluid and increased daily ileostomy volume [8]. Additionally, normal ileostomies excrete approximately 1.5 g of nitrogen daily.

Bacterial flora is significantly increased in ileostomy patients when compared to the normal ileum. There is approximately an 80-fold increase primarily due to an increased number of coliform organisms [9]. The ileostomy

Table 4.1 Composition of normal ileostomy effluent

	Daily excretion	Range	Concentration	Range
Wet weight	500 g	200–600 g	–	–
Dry weight	38 g	24–48 g	–	–
Water content	–	–	92%	88–94%
pH	–	–	6.3	6.1–6.5
Sodium	55 mEq	30–80 mEq	115 mEq/L	100–130 mEq/L
Potassium	4 mEq	3–6 mEq	8 mEq/L	5–11 mEq/L
Chloride	20 mEq	15–30 mEq	45 mEq/L	15–40 mEq/L
Calcium	18 mEq	15–40 mEq	25 mEq/L	10–64 mEq/L
Magnesium	8 mEq	7–9 mEq	15 mEq/L	10–28 mEq/L
Phosphorus	150 mg	122–202 mg	–	–
Nitrogen	1 g	0.6–2.4 g	–	–
Fat	2.2 g	1.5–3.8 g	–	–
Bile acids	–	–	0.9 mm/mL	??

Modified from [3]

flora has a quantity of 10^4–10^7 number of organisms per mL and the qualitative characteristics are intermediate between feces and normal ileal contents. Ileostomy effluent also contains large amounts of proteolytic enzymes, which in turn can attack the keratin layer of the epidermis and produce skin irritation and necrosis. These events in turn may cause adherence problems for stomal appliances.

Ileostomy Dysfunction

Metabolic-associated complications of ileostomies include diarrhea, cholelithiasis, urolithiasis, and nutrient deficiencies. The most important and frequent complication is ileostomy diarrhea. This topic has recently been the subject of a comprehensive review [10].

Ileostomy Diarrhea

Ileostomy diarrhea is defined as passage of greater than 1 L/day of output, with patients emptying the appliance six or more times daily [10]. In the author's experience, this definition is too restrictive. For example, some patients excrete up to 1.5 L of content daily without any adverse physiologic or metabolic sequelae. Additionally, many fastidious patients empty their appliances 10–12 times daily when the volume of effluent in the pouch is as little as 25–50 mL. Despite these varied patterns, ileostomy output less than 1 L/day rarely causes nutritional/metabolic deficits.

Etiology

The causes of ileostomy diarrhea are listed in Table 4.2. The most important determinants of ileostomy diarrhea are the length and quality of function of the intestine remaining in continuity. Persistently elevated ileostomy output is typically seen in patients who have had more than 50 cm of terminal ileum resected, however, increased output can occur with minimal ileal resection as well. The small intestine's total absorptive capacity is generally preserved up to removal of one half of its length; however, knowing how much bowel has been resected is not sufficient by itself to predict permanent dependence on total parenteral nutrition. Most importantly, the volume of ileostomy output following a resection depends on the remaining length of small bowel rather than the amount of intestine removed. Repeated resections of small amounts (6–8 in.) of small intestine, with prolonged intervals are better tolerated than a single massive resection.

Table 4.2 Etiology: ileostomy diarrhea

- Extensive enterectomy
- Medications – sudden discontinuation steroids or opiates
- Crohn's disease
- Dietary indiscretion
- Lactose intolerance
- Intra-abdominal sepsis
- Partial intestinal obstruction
- Enteritis (bacterial/viral/radiation)
- Intestinal ischemia
- Stress/anxiety
- Bacterial overgrowth

Diarrhea associated with limited ileal resection (less than 100 cm) tends to be secretory with minimal nutrient malabsorption, whereas diarrhea due to short bowel syndrome, typically seen with resections leaving less than 200 cm of remaining small intestine, is usually osmotically mediated [11].

Additional causes of output greater than 1 L/day include partial small bowel obstruction, ileostomy stenosis, adhesions, intra-abdominal sepsis, and recurrent Crohn's disease. Obstruction due to extrinsic (adhesions) or intrinsic (stricture) leads to increased ileostomy output due to reduced fluid and electrolyte absorption and increased proximal fluid secretion. Endoscopic balloon dilation of strictures may improve symptoms and help avoid or postpone surgery.

There are also anatomic and physiologic causes of increased ileostomy output. Output increases with increased body mass. For example, a daily output of 800 mL may be normal for someone weighing 80 kg, whereas an output of 400 mL is within normal limits for a 40-kg individual [12]. Overproduction of gastric acid may contribute to the volume of ileostomy output in patients with short bowel syndrome. This is thought to be due to rapid gastric emptying due to the lack of Peptide YY [13], present throughout the distal small bowel and colon, which normally acts as a "brake" to slow intestinal transit. Gastric hypersecretion is not a cause of ileostomy diarrhea in patients with otherwise intact small bowel. In one study, omeprazole decreased ileostomy output in patients with outputs of 2.6 L/day who had significant small bowel resection [14].

Emotional stress may increase ileostomy output. In a study involving direct visualization of the terminal ileum not only was motor activity increased during an emotionally stressful interview, but there was increased fragility and hyperemia of the ileal mucosa. Unlike the stomach and colon, these changes were observed with emotional tension of any type such as anger, resentment, and hostility [15].

Recently, methicillin-resistant *Staphylococcus aureus* (MRSA) was reported in six patients with high-output ileostomies [16]. It was hypothesized that prolonged usage of antibiotics and passage of a nasogastric tube through the nose, where *S. aureus* often resides, were important factors in the pathogenesis. A high index of suspension was advocated with appropriate cultures of the ileostomy effluent.

Symptoms

Patients with ileostomy diarrhea may not complain of an excessive volume of ileostomy output, but may mention frequent emptying of the stomal appliance (eight or more times per day), pouch leakage, skin irritation, lightheadedness, or fatigue. If there is abdominal pain, distention, fever, vomiting, or weight loss, studies should be performed to rule out intestinal obstruction, intra-abdominal infection, recurrent disease (e.g., Crohn's disease), infectious enteritis, and bacterial overgrowth.

Symptoms during the immediate postoperative period suggest diarrhea due to ileal resection, partial obstruction, or a preexisting condition unmasked by colectomy (e.g., lactose intolerance). Dietary history should be obtained to evaluate for lactose intolerance and use of artificial sweeteners. Recent medication changes (e.g., sudden discontinuation of steroids or opioids) should be assessed.

Evaluation

Following a detailed history to rule out the aforementioned causes, attention is directed to identifying anatomic abnormalities. The role of endoscopy in patients with ileostomy diarrhea is usually limited to the evaluation of cause of the increased ileostomy output. An ileoscopy may be required to exclude stricture or recurrent Crohn's disease. Obstruction is typically best diagnosed radiographically by retrograde injection of contrast through the stoma. This approach is better than upper gastrointestinal studies because it avoids inordinate amounts of contrast in the bowel proximal to the site of obstruction, which can be troublesome if urgent resection is needed.

Most patients with ileostomy diarrhea do not have an identifiable cause and must be treated empirically. A random urinary sodium concentration of 10 mM is a good indication of sodium depletion [17]. The initial management of ileostomy diarrhea should focus on evaluation and treatment of dehydration (see Chap. 8 see Chap. 8 (High Output Stoma Management).

Cholelithiasis

The incidence of cholelithiasis correlates with the time of ileostomy construction – 10% after 5 years, ~25% after 15 years, and 50% if the ileostomy has been present for more than 15 years [18]. Gallstone formation in patients with ileostomies is increased when greater than 10 cm of ileum has been resected [19]. The pathogenesis of cholelithiasis in this setting is presumably due to an increased loss of bile salts and a reduction in the bile salt pool, which in turn decreases the solubility of cholesterol [20]. These findings are exacerbated in patients with ileal Crohn's disease who have a five- to sevenfold increased incidence of gallstones when compared to a normal population [21]. Ursodeoxycholic acid may be therapeutic for these patients because of its ability to desaturate cholesterol in bile [22].

Urolithiasis

Urolithiasis occurs in a wide range (0.7–12%) of patients with ileostomies [23]. The type of antecedent surgery and duration from the time of surgery are important in the pathogenesis. In one report [24] urolithiasis occurred in 7% of patients if there was no loss of small bowel and in 15% where 20–300 cm of ileum had been resected.

Interestingly, a high incidence (60%) of uric acid stones exists in ileostomy patients with urolithiasis [25, 26]. High uric levels in the serum occur in these patients, which presumably contributes to this type of stone formation. If uric acid stones are identified, serum uric acid levels should be measured and allopurinol therapy prescribed when appropriate. Additionally, persistent acid urine predisposes to precipitation of uric acid. Most urolithiases are radiolucent, while a greater percentage of renal stones among ileostomy patients are radiopaque. This is probably due to uric acid crystals providing a nidus for calcium salt precipitation.

In summary, there are many causes of urolithiasis in ileostomy patients; however, an important variable is dehydration with decreased urine output. This is more common in warm climates.

Vitamin Deficiencies: B12 and Folic H+

Contrary to popular opinion, serum B12 levels are usually normal in ileostomy patients even when 30–40 cm of terminal ileum is removed. Additionally, both serum and red blood cell levels of folate remain normal. Despite normal serum B12 levels, decreased absorption of B12 has been demonstrated in Crohn's patients with ileostomies [23].

Jejunostomy

As the result of its proximal anatomic site, a jejunostomy is only created in unusual operative settings. In elective surgery jejunostomies are usually constructed as temporary stomas to "protect" anastomoses in the distal small bowel and colon. In rare circumstances, a permanent end jejunostomy is the only operative option in the presence of massive destruction to the distal small bowel and colon.

In both settings, physiologic and metabolic deficits mimic those of short bowel syndrome with high stomal volumes and increased risk for dehydration. These metabolic deficits frequently resolve upon closure of the stoma. Patients with high output permanent jejunostomies must be monitored carefully with frequent measurements of electrolytes and hydrational status. Most of these individuals require intravenous feeding indefinitely. In some instances, small bowel transplantation should be considered.

As mentioned, the jejunal mucosa is unable to concentrate the luminal contents and sodium diffuses freely into the lumen through leaky intercellular junctions. The concentration of sodium in jejunostomy fluid is about 100 mM (range 90–140 mM). Hypomagnesemia occurs in approximately 60% of patients as the result of secondary hyperaldosteronism (sodium absorbed in renal tubule in exchange for magnesium and potassium) with loss of magnesium-absorbing intestine and unabsorbed fatty acids binding free magnesium [27]. Hypokalemia is unusual and occurs only when less than 50 cm of jejunum remains [28]. A stomal output of greater than 2 L/day frequently leads to dehydration and sodium and magnesium depletion.

To help guide therapy and estimate prognosis, measurement of the remaining small bowel should be determined intraoperatively. This is performed by placing a moist, measured length of umbilical tape along the mesentery bowel junction (fixed portion of bowel more amenable to accurate measurements). Additionally, postoperative contrast X-ray of the small bowel can be performed and measurements obtained with the aid of fluoroscopy. Patients with less than 50 cm of remaining jejunum and no remaining small intestine or colon require permanent home parenteral nutrition.

Colonic Physiology

Contrary to the traditional teaching of most surgeons, the colon is indeed an important metabolic organ and is not solely for fecal storage. Its essential metabolic functions have been summarized in a scholarly review by Daniels [29] from which a portion of this section has been abstracted.

Colonic function differs as to the anatomic site. In the cecum and ascending colon, there is retention and mixture of the entering ileal effluent to permit bacterial fermentation and metabolism of residual dietary carbohydrate and a small amount of undigested protein. This dynamic process produces many important byproducts, which are either absorbed or metabolized in the cecum, ascending, and transverse colon. These functions are enhanced by retropulsive waves extending from the transverse colon back toward the cecum. The transverse colon in turn helps regulate intraluminal fluid volume by enhancing sodium and water absorption. Due to its intrinsic propulsive qualities, it also facilitates the efficient transfer of proximal colonic contents to the descending colon for final mixing of colonic contents before evacuation. The diminished rate of fluid and electrolyte transfer in the descending colon is a result of protein ion channels in the luminal (apical) and (serosal) basolateral membranes of mucosal cells, which have different biochemical and pharmacologic properties when compared to those of the ascending colon [29]. The most important physiologic/metabolic functions of the colon are bacterial fermentation, sodium and water absorption, and motility.

Bacterial Fermentation

The more than 400 species of bacteria in the human colon comprise 40–55% of fecal solids in individuals consuming a typical Western diet [30]. Although *Bacteroides* organisms (gram-negative rods) are the most common genera, the gram-positive *Eubacterium* and *Bifidobacterium* are also present in large numbers along with several gram-positive *cocci* and *Clostridium* species.

Bacterial fermentation is initiated by the colonic inflow of ingested non-starch polysaccharides and resistant dietary starch. Non-starch polysaccharides (e.g., dietary fiber) are resistant to upper gastrointestinal enzymatic digestion and are the primary substrates for colonic bacterial fermentation. These substances are the derivatives of plant material and

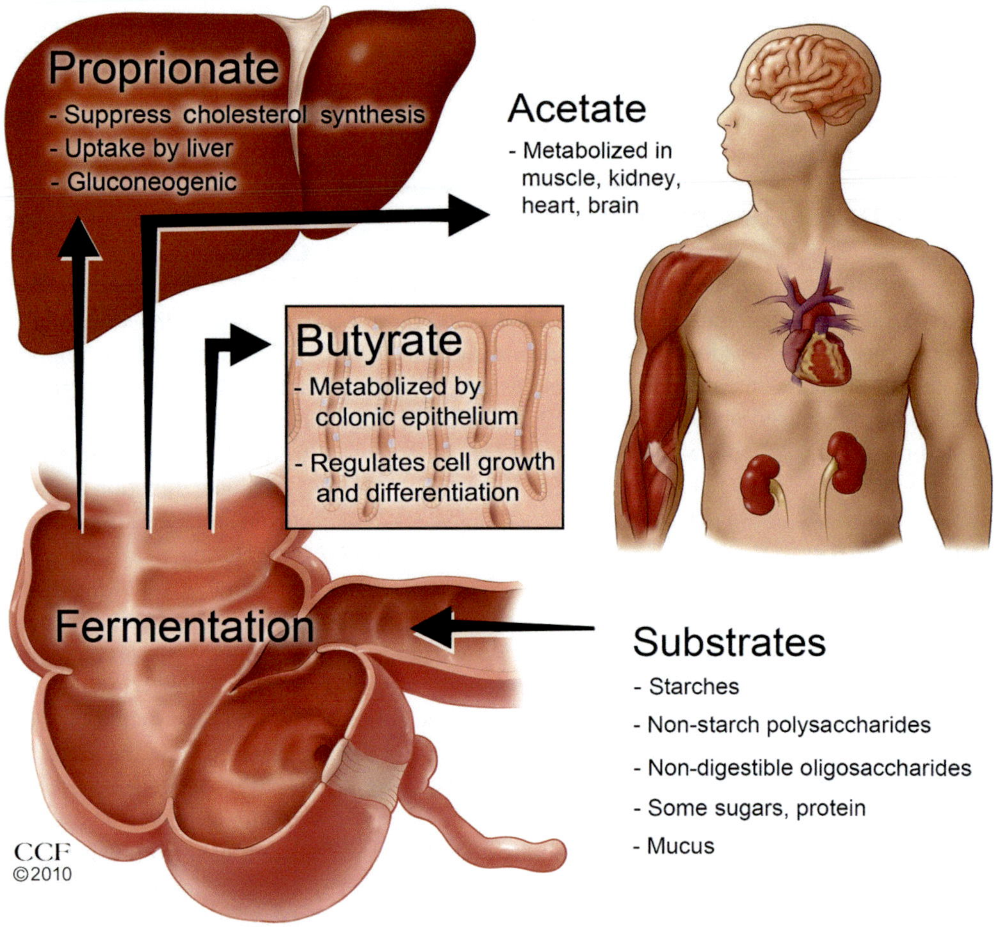

Fig. 4.1 Metabolic fate of the three principal short chain fatty acids (SCFA) produced by bacterial fermentation in the colon (Illustration © CCF)

include cellulose as well as non-cellulosic substrates. Approximately, 10% of ingested starch (resistant dietary starch) is not digested in the small bowel and enters the colon to serve as an additional substrate for fermentation. Overall, the daily ileal effluent provides 6–8 g of nitrogen-containing compounds and 8–40 g of carbohydrates daily for bacterial fermentation [31].

Once these substrates enter the cecum and ascending colon, they are acted upon by polysaccharidases in the cell walls of primarily anaerobic organisms such as bacteroides. This enzymatic process initiates bacterial fermentation including anaerobic glycolysis (Embden-Myerhof pathway) with the metabolism of pyruvate. The short chain fatty acids (SCFA) butyrate, propionate, and acetate, in addition to several gases, are important byproducts of this fermentation process. The metabolic fate of each of these SCFAs differs (Fig. 4.1). Despite being produced in the least amount quantitatively, butyrate is the primary oxidizable fuel for the colonocyte and provides an important stimulus for colonocyte growth and function. Moreover, it is estimated that normal, daily endogenous butyrate production is sufficient to provide nearly all the energy needs for the total colon [32].

More than 90% of SCFA produced by bacterial fermentation is absorbed by the colonic mucosa. Additionally, SCFAs are relatively weak acids; therefore, high concentrations lower the luminal pH, which in turn alters the growth of pH-sensitive pathogenic bacteria such as *E. coli* and *Salmonella*.

Absorption

Sodium and water absorption are important aspects of colonic function. This is especially significant in surgical patients because the colon assumes a major compensatory absorptive role in individuals with extensive resection of the small bowel.

Sodium transport in the colon is an active process. Two opposing forces must be overcome for this process to occur. First, a concentration gradient opposes the movement of sodium. This is due to the higher sodium concentration of plasma compared with the colonic lumen. Secondly, sodium transport is confronted by an electronegative lumen, which delays the movement of sodium across the basolateral membrane of the colonocyte. Despite these two opposing forces, normal daily fecal water only contains 1–5 mEq of sodium, thus confirming that more than 90% is absorbed of the 200 mEq of sodium in the ileal effluent [33].

Colonic sodium absorption is mediated by both the apical and basolateral membranes of the colonocyte. The permeability of sodium across the apical membrane depends on several physiologic factors such as the intracellular sodium concentration within the colonocyte, which is inversely related to apical membrane sodium permeability. In order to ensure an adequate concentration difference, this concentration must be kept relatively low compared with the amount of luminal sodium. This process is mediated in part by the sodium/potassium ATPase located on the basolateral aspect of the colonic epithelial cells. Therefore, the net movement of sodium across the colonic wall through this active mechanism is a combination of both apical and basolateral membrane activities. Thus, regulation of this method of transport can be targeted to either apical or basolateral processes.

Control of fecal water is a major function of the colon. As mentioned, the average ileocecal flow for a healthy individual is approximately 1,500–2,000 mL/day. From this amount, only 100–150 mL of water is normally present in the evacuated stool. Colonic water absorption is affected by the volume and flow of luminal contents and generally follows the osmotic gradient produced by the absorption of electrolytes. The colon, therefore, has a significant absorptive reserve and is capable of absorbing as much as 5–6 L over a 24-h period [34].

Similar to other colonic metabolic functions, potassium transport is segmental with mucosal cells in the proximal colon functioning differently from the distal colonocytes. Potassium absorption is mediated, in part, by a secretory mechanism, in which energy is used to drive a basolateral sodium/potassium or sodium potassium/chloride pump. This energy in turn enhances the diffusion of potassium ions down an electrochemical gradient into the lumen through apical, potassium permeable ion channels [35]. As a result of this process and other observations, potassium absorption is considered to be predominantly a function of the distal colon, which is electroneutral, sodium independent, and mediated through an apical potassium/hydrogen/ATPase and basolateral potassium ion channel.

Colonic Motility

Motility of the gastrointestinal tract is slowest in the colon. Transit of substrates through the colon varies between 24 and 150 h depending on the fat and fiber contents of the diet [36]. Similar to other colonic functions, motility differs within the anatomic segments of the colon. For example, the retrograde movement in the right colon delays the progression of contents in order to provide thorough mixing, microbial metabolism, and efficient absorption.

The smooth muscle wall of the colon produces strong propulsive contraction over a large surface area. Electrical slow waves are the result of the rhythmic alternations in smooth muscle membrane potentials and pacemaker cells predominantly in the circular muscle layer of the colonic wall [37]. Moreover, the interstitial cells of Cajal are thought to be pacesetters of the colon [38].

Colonic muscle contains cholinergic and noncholinergic excitatory nerves and adrenergic and nonadrenergic inhibitory nerves. Cholinergic innervation of the large bowel is provided by the vagus and sacral nerves. The main parasympathetic supply arises from the second and third sacral nerves innervating the distal colon and rectum. The vagus nerve carrying cranial parasympathetic supply is believed to innervate the ascending colon. An important component of this nerve carries the afferent supply from the colon. The sympathetic nervous system inhibits colonic motility as evidenced by disruption of pelvic sympathetic flow resulting in colonic contraction.

Normal Colostomy Function

Normal colostomy function varies as to the anatomic site, type, and amount of dietary intake, and duration of postoperative recovery. Ascending colon colostomies are seldom constructed because of the proximity to the ileum, marked liquidity of stool, and generally inferior function when compared to an ileostomy. The use of a transverse colon as a site for a loop colostomy has decreased in frequency due to frequent prolapse (usually of the distal stoma), peristomal hernia, and overall difficulty in management. Thus, most colostomies are constructed in either the sigmoid or descending colon.

The consistency of stool in the descending and sigmoid colon approximates normal defecation. Large amounts of colostomy effluent are usually discharged once or twice daily. The viscosity of the colostomy effluent increases with the amount of ingested dietary fiber. The increased ingestion of insoluble dietary fiber is often efficacious to thicken preexisting liquid output. This dietary modification often improves management of the stomal appliance and care of the peristomal skin. Initial postoperative colostomy output is usually liquid. As dietary intake increases and becomes more varied, the colostomy output becomes more viscous approximately 10–14 days postoperatively.

Colostomy Dysfunction

Fluid and electrolyte absorption and colostomy output depend largely upon both, the extent and site of concomitant intestinal resection, and the amount and the type of intestine remaining in continuity. Colostomy diarrhea is minimal as long as more than half of the small intestine remains and most of the colon is in continuity. Fluid and electrolyte losses generally are not excessive, unless either (1) the fluid delivered to the colon following a small bowel resection exceeds its reserve capacity, or (2) the contents of the entering small intestinal dejecta inhibit colonic absorption.

Proximal colectomy results in minimal diarrhea and does not significantly affect colostomy output because the ileum reabsorbs the increased fluid and electrolyte load with the remaining unabsorbed fluid absorbed by the colon. The reabsorption of bile salts by an intact ileum causes the colon to receive very few substances capable of impeding water and electrolyte absorption. In contrast, when the ileum is resected, the colon receives a larger fluid load because the contents are not isotonic and contain substances (bile salts, fatty acids, unabsorbed carbohydrate) that reduce the reabsorption of water and electrolytes, resulting in increased colostomy output.

If the small bowel and colon are resected either partially or completely, the colonic compensatory absorptive response is lost for the concomitantly resected small bowel. The importance of the colon in modulating the severity of diarrhea following resection has been emphasized in studies of patients with short bowel syndrome [39]. If both ileum and colon are resected, patients are left with bowel that cannot concentrate luminal contents. In such patients, isotonic water and salt loss is a major problem resulting in dehydration, hypokalemia, and hypomagnesemia. If a concomitant large amount of ileum is resected, this impairs absorption of bile salts and produces bile salt (cathartic)-induced diarrhea by stimulating increased colonic secretion of water and electrolytes.

Conclusion

The causes of preoperative physiologic and metabolic stomal complications are multifactorial, consisting of residual intestinal disease, the amount and site of remaining intestine, and the anastomotic site of the ostomy. Surgeons must have a thorough understanding of the normal physiologic and metabolic functions of the normal small and large intestine in order to provide the most efficacious treatments for stomal dysfunction.

References

1. Connell AM. Propulsion in the small intestine. Rend Gastroenterol. 1970;2:38–46.
2. Tilney HS, Parvinder SS, Lovegrove RE, et al. Comparisons of outcomes following ileostomy versus colostomy for defunctioning colorectal anastomoses. World J Surg. 2007;31:1142–51.
3. Hill GL. Ileostomy surgery, physiology and management. New York: Grune & Stratton; 1976. p. 68.
4. Hill GL, Mair WSJ, Goligher JC. Impairment of ileostomy adaptation in patients after ileal resection. Gut. 1974;15:982–7.
5. Landt H, Daum K. Physical characteristics of residues from the small intestines. Arch Intern Med. 1933;52:96.
6. Soper NJ, Orkin BA, Kelly KA, et al. Gastrointestinal transit after proctocolectomy with ileal pouch anal anastomosis or ileostomy. J Surg Res. 1989;46:300–5.
7. Kramer P, Kearney MM, Inglefinger FJ. The effect of specific foods and water loading on the ileal excreta of ileostomal human subjects. Gastroenterology. 1962;42:535–45.
8. Kramer P. The effect of varying sodium loads on the ileal excreta of human ileostomized subjects. J Clin Invest. 1966;45:1710–8.
9. Gorbach SL, Nahas L, Weinstein L. Studies of intestinal microflora. IV. The microflora of ileostomy effluent: a unique microbial ecology. Gastroenterology. 1967;53:874–80.
10. DuPont AW, Sellin JH. Ileostomy diarrhea. Curr Treat Options Gastroenterol. 2006;9:39–48.
11. Lennard-Jones JE. Review article: practical management of the short bowel. Aliment Pharmacol Ther. 1994;8:563–77.
12. Hill GL, Millward SF, King RF, et al. Normal ileostomy output: close relation to body size. BMJ. 1979;4:831–2.
13. Nightingale JM, Kamm MA, van der Sijp JR, Nightingale JM, Kamm MA, van der Sijp JR, et al. Gastrointestinal hormones in short bowel syndrome. Peptide YY may be the "colonic brake" to gastric emptying. Gut. 1996;39:267–72.
14. Jeppesen PB, Staun M, Tjellesen I, et al. Effect of intravenous ranitidine and omeprazole on intestinal absorption of water, sodium and macronutrients in patients with intestinal resection. Gut. 1998; 43:763–9.
15. Cummings AJ. Small intestine function in patients with an ilestomy. Am J Med. 1954;16:237–45.
16. Haq AI, Cook LJ. MSRA enteritis causing a high stoma output in the early postoperative phase after bowel surgery. Ann R Coll Surg Engl. 2007;89:303–8.
17. Tsao SKK, Baker M, Nightingale J. High-output stoma after small-bowel resections. Gastroenterol Hepatol. 2005;2:604–8.
18. Kretschmer KP. The intestinal stoma. Philadelphia: W.B. Saunders; 1978. p. 79.
19. Hill GL, Mair WS, Goligher JC. Cause and management of high volume output salt-depleting ileostomy. Br J Surg. 1975;62: 720–6.
20. Dowling RH, Bell GD, White J. Lithogenic bile in patients with ileal dysfunction. Gut. 1972;13:415–20.
21. Kurchin A, Ray JE, Bluth EI, et al. Cholelithiasis in ileostomy patients. Dis Colon Rectum. 1984;27:585–8.
22. Chadwick VS, Camilleri M. Pathophysiology of small intestine function and the effect of Crohn's disease. In: Allan RN, Keighley MRB, Alexander-Williams J, Hawkins C, editors. Inflammatory bowel disease. London: Churchill Livingstone; 1983. p. 29–42.
23. Keighley MRB, Williams NS. Surgery of the anus, rectum and colon. 2nd ed. Philadelphia: W.B. Saunders; 1999. p. 227.
24. Bambach CP, Robertson WG, Peacock M, et al. Effect of intestinal surgery on the risk of urinary stone formation. Gut. 1981;22:257–63.
25. Kennedy HJ, Fletcher EWL, Truelove SC. Urinary stones in subjects with a permanent ileostomy. Br J Surg. 1982;69:661–4.
26. Grotz RL, Pemberton JH. Stoma physiology. In: MacKeigan JM, Cataldo PA, editors. Intestinal stomas. St. Louis: Quality Medical Publishing, Inc; 1993. p. 43.
27. Hanna S, MacIntyre I. The influence of aldosterone on magnesium metabolism. Lancet. 1960;2:348–50.
28. Nightingale JMD, Lennard-Jones JE, Walker ER, et al. Jejunal efflux in short bowel syndrome. Lancet. 1990;336:765–8.
29. Daniels E. Colonic physiology. In: Corman MC, editor. Colon and rectal surgery. 5th ed. Philadelphia: Lippincott; 2005. p. 31–42.
30. Finegold SM, Sutter VL, Mathieson GE. Normal indigenous intestinal flora. In: Hentges DJ, editor. Human intestinal microflora in health and disease. London: Academic; 1983. p. 3.

31. Cummings JH, MacFarlane GT. The control and consequences of bacterial fermentation in the human colon. J Appl Bacteriol. 1991;70:443–59.
32. Cummings JH, Gibson GR, MacFarlane GT. Quantitative estimates of fermentation in the hindgut of man. Acta Veternaria Scand. 1989;86:76–82.
33. Rechkemmer G, Ronnau K, von Engelhardt W. Fermentation of polysaccharides and absorption of short-chain fatty acids in the mammalian hindgut. Comp Biochem Physiol. 1988;90A:563.
34. Debongnie JC, Phillips SF. Capacity of the human colon to absorb fluid. Gastroenterology. 1978;74:698–703.
35. Del Castillo JR, Sepulveda FV. Activation of a sodium/potassium/chloride cotransport system by phosphorylation in crypt cells isolated from guinea pig distal colon. Gastroenterology. 1995;109:387.
36. Jeejeebhoy KN. Short bowel syndrome. In: Kinney JM, Jeejeebhoy KN, Hill Gl, Owen OE, editors. Nutrition and metabolism in patient care. Philadelphia: W.B. Saunders; 1988. p. 259–65.
37. Caprilli R, Onri L. Origin, transmission and ionic dependence of colonic electrical slow waves. Scand J Gastroenterol. 1972;7:65–74.
38. Langton P, Ward SM, Carl A, et al. Spontaneous electrical activity of interstitial cells of Cajal isolated from canine proximal colon. Proc Natl Acad Sci USA. 1989;86:7280–4.
39. Byrne TA, Wilmore DW, Iyer K, et al. Growth hormone, glutamine, and an optimal diet reduces parenteral nutrition in patients with short bowel syndrome: a prospective, randomized, placebo-controlled, double-blind clinical trial. Ann Surg. 2005;242:655–61.

Quality of Life of the Ostomate

5

Meagan M. Costedio and James I. Merlino

Introduction

Patients faced with the prospect of bowel surgery are often anxious about the possibility of an ostomy. Frequently, ostomies are temporary, but occasionally patients require a permanent stoma. Patients rarely prefer an ostomy; however, there are circumstances when construction of an ostomy leads to significant improvement in quality of life and may be lifesaving.

Quality-of-life issues are an important component of the discussion regarding reestablishment of bowel continuity after resection. A patient with a low rectal cancer may be a candidate for sphincter-sparing operations to avoid a permanent ostomy, but poor sphincter function may worsen their quality of life. An elderly woman with a history of multiple vaginal deliveries and a pretreatment history of incontinence may well prefer the controlled incontinence of a colostomy to the multiple and unpredictable episodes of incontinence, or the fecal seepage with perianal skin excoriation. Both outcomes must be presented in a balanced way, although it is hard for a patient to appreciate the reality of something they have not yet experienced.

Subconsciously, patients are always evaluating quality of life. This is a complex judgment with multiple interacting factors, one of the most important of which is an inevitable comparison between recent, current, usual, and "ideal" health status. Thus, a patient with an asymptomatic, low rectal cancer may be devastated by the thought of having a permanent colostomy, while a patient with terrible urgency and incontinence may see a colostomy as a significant improvement in their life. Another factor weighing into quality of life is attitude toward the disease so that the patient with a low rectal cancer may readily accept a permanent colostomy as long as the cancer is completely resected. Quality-of-life measures are an important part of surgical decision-making. They also help patients by providing realistic expectations of surgical outcomes.

Preoperative Preparation

One of the keys to successful acceptance of an ostomy is the surgeon's ability to appropriately approach the topic. A realistic discussion of the possibility of a stoma, its likely permanence or otherwise, and the reasons for it helps patients to understand that creation of an ostomy is not a failure, nor is it the end of their lives. This discussion with the physician is followed by an appointment with an enterostomal nurse, who explains the practical issues raised by a stoma, allowing the patient to appreciate that they will not be alone. Families are an important part of these discussions as they will be an important part of postoperative support.

Multiple factors weigh into health-related quality of life (HR-QOL) measures during the preoperative discussion about a stoma, including age of the patient, cultural or geographic factors, comorbidities, preoperative performance status, personality, and expectations [1, 2]. For example, Siassi and colleagues showed that extroverted people with coherent families have improved QOL despite stoma construction [2]. Holzer and colleagues demonstrated that the presence of permanent colostomy is a social and cultural disaster for patients from southern Europe as well as Islamic origin [3]. Pittman et al. reported that patients who are currently working or whose income is less than $30,000 per year had severe difficulty adjusting to an ostomy [4]. It is important that surgeons are sensitive to these patient-specific factors when outlining an operative plan.

The first stoma therapist, Norma Gill, was trained by Dr. Rupert B. Turnbull at the Cleveland Clinic in 1961. Since that time, enterostomal therapy has become an essential part of patient education and a strong aid to patients' acceptance of an ostomy. All patients should be seen and evaluated by an enterostomal therapist (ET) prior to surgery where a stoma is

M.M. Costedio (✉) • J.I. Merlino
Department of Colorectal Surgery, Digestive Disease Institute, Cleveland Clinic Foundation, Cleveland, OH, USA
e-mail: costedm@ccf.org

V.W. Fazio et al. (eds.), *Atlas of Intestinal Stomas*,
DOI 10.1007/978-0-387-78851-7_5,

a possibility. Preoperative preparation allows the patient to learn about ostomies and their use and care, and determine suitable positioning for the ostomy. The ET should mark the patient either permanently with tattooing if the time of surgery is distant or with a permanent marker covered by an occlusive dressing if surgery is more imminent.

Bass and colleagues in Chicago reviewed complications in 593 patients, 292 of whom were marked by ET and 301 who were not. The group marked by ET preoperatively had a statistically significant decrease in complications (32% vs. 45%) postoperatively [5]. Two further studies addressed preoperative counseling and demonstrated that enterostomal therapy not only improves ostomy adjustment and QOL but is associated with decreased hospital stay and ostomy-related readmissions to the hospital [6–8]. These data reveal that preoperative ET visits not only improve adjustment to ostomy care, but also, in combination with expert surgery, decrease postoperative complications and decrease readmission, sparing the health care system further resources.

Quality of Life: Methods of Assessment

Quality of life is an important patient-specific outcome in medicine that is difficult to quantify. However, quality of life has become increasingly important as patients and physicians realize that morbidity and mortality alone underestimate the consequences of medical interventions. The World Health Organization defines health-related quality of life as "a patient perceived multidimensional construct that encompasses an evaluation of at least three basic aspects of quality of life; namely emotional, well-being, physical state and social functioning." [9]

Two types of instruments are used to compute quality of life: psychometric and utility-based measures. Psychometric measures attempt to quantify a range of symptoms, behaviors, or feelings by rating the individual items and assigning a summation of QOL [10]. Importantly, this assessment method compares many different groups of individuals on a functional continuum and detects changes in attitudes, feelings, and perceptions regarding certain interventions. Psychometric measures often ignore clinically important variables such as cancer recurrence or survival [11]. Examples of psychometric instruments are the Sickness Impact Profile, the Nottingham Health Profile, the Inflammatory Bowel Disease Questionnaire, the City of Hope Quality of Life Ostomy-specific, as well as the validated Cleveland Global Quality of Life Form based on the SF – 36 Quality of Life Questionnaire. [12, 13]

Utility-based measures are used as a model to predict individual preferences. It assigns personal value to outcomes using a scale from 0 = death to 1.0 = perfect health. This measure attempts to assign a weighted assessment of quality of life and therefore predict the amount of risk or time the patient would be willing to give up for normal health: quality-adjusted life years. This tool is useful in performing cost-utility studies, and the measured outcomes are usually clinically significant as they are predictive models. It also allows a direct comparison of a patient's life before and after a treatment, and so produces a measurement of the effect of the intervention. The concerns with utility-based measurements are the lack of sensitivity of perceptions to emotionally or socially significant changes, as well as the complexity of interpretation of the scores and the wide variety of perceptions, and lack of generalizability.

Quality of Life with an Ostomy

Many studies suggest that stoma construction has a significantly detrimental effect on QOL [14, 15]. Studies examining the psychosocial impact of a stoma reveal that up to one third of patients experience depression, social problems, and/or sexual problems [16, 17]. Recently, HR-QOL studies have included both the patient population receiving a stoma as well as the group maintaining continuity, and results have been mixed [2, 18, 19]. In other words, it may not be that the stoma itself that diminishes the psychosocial aspects of QOL, but the health condition leading to the stoma.

Ileostomy

A majority of patients presented with the possibility of a permanent ileostomy have ulcerative colitis (UC), while some have familial adenomatous polyposis (FAP) or Crohn's disease. Multiple options are available to patients with FAP or UC, such as end ileostomy, a continent ileostomy (CI), or ileoanal pouch anastomosis (IPAA). Decisions regarding these options are based not only on the disease process, but the likely effects of the choice on perceived QOL.

Comparing ileostomates to non-ileostomates is difficult with the current quality of life assessment tools available. It is difficult to compare stoma function, odor control, body image, and appliance adequacy in ostomates to stool frequency, incontinence, pad usage, and urgency in patients with bowel continuity [20]. Ko and colleagues compared these factors with a generic HR-QOL tool and showed that appropriately selected patients have equally high QOL whether they have an ileostomy or not. Seidel and colleagues support this notion, showing that not only do ileostomates have comparable QOL scores to those status post-IPAA, but that the majority of both groups have a "better" QOL since their operation [21]. Jimmo and Hyman demonstrated a 95% satisfaction rate with IPAA and 100% with ileostomy, and that, in retrospect, none of those patients would have chosen the other procedure [22].

Several studies show that ileostomates consider their health to be good or excellent, and this is likely due to the fact that people with UC recapture a sense of well-being postoperatively [10]. In other words, QOL is already satisfactory after the cure of UC, and maintenance of bowel continuity does not yield significant further improvement [23].

Despite these data showing equivalent QOL between ileostomy and IPAA patients, ileostomies present specific problems. At the Cleveland Clinic, 40–50% of ileostomates reported a moderate restriction in their diet, sports, recreational activities, and clothing selection [24]. Though many of these restrictions were improvements from their preoperative status, they still were present. Burnham et al. found that 12% of patients felt that their marriage was adversely affected by the ileostomy, and Rolsted reported 30–40% of ileostomates had physical or emotional difficulties with intercourse because of the ostomy [25, 26]. Berndtsson and Oresland demonstrated a significant (15%) improvement in role function, sexual relations, and improved body image after IPAA using the Osbrisch adjustment scale in patients who had previously had an ostomy [27]. While this study demonstrates a significant improvement in some aspects of QOL, IPAA also has consequences, and its complications make comparative QOL assessment difficult.

Continent Ileostomy

In 1969, Professor Nils Kock developed an ileal pouch with a nipple valve to maintain continence, which acts as a reservoir for stool [10]. The benefits of the continent ileostomy (CI) include no pouching and fewer restrictions in work activities, sports, and clothing selection [28]. Patients who were embarrassed by their ileostomy reported a significant resolution of these feelings with a continent ileostomy [29].

Despite the potential benefits of CI over conventional ileostomy, the complication rate of this procedure is high [30]. Complications include valve slippage, fistula formation, and prolapse, and patients report increased food and travel restrictions after CI [31]. Approximately 12–50% of patients require valve revision, and many others require readmission for inability to intubate the CI [32].

Overall, quality-of-life scores are similar between patients with a continent ileostomy and a conventional ileostomy due to trade-offs between different QOL improvements and increased complications after the continent stoma. Preoperative planning may identify those patients who would be negatively affected by the body image issues of an end ileostomy, and counseling regarding CI should be provided. On the other hand, patients that live a distance from a large medical center or ET may have more difficulty with a CI if they do not have the medical support to cope with the potential complications.

Colostomy

End colostomies are often performed following abdominoperineal resection in patients who would be incontinent if bowel continuity were restored. Unfortunately, QOL studies are difficult to generalize as there are significant changes in bowel function in patients with anastomoses in the lower third of the rectum versus higher in the rectum [10]. Engel et al. showed a consistently lower quality of life in patients with a permanent colostomy compared with those with ultralow anterior resections over a 4-year follow-up [33]. Consistent with these data, patients with a diverting ostomy have a significant improvement in the quality of life with time after reversal after the stoma. Yau et al. evaluated HR-QOL of rectal cancer patients with and without colostomy prospectively and found similar results of diminished role and social functioning in ostomates, though the measured HR-QOL results were similar [34]. Other studies have shown consistent results of similarly HR-QOL measures, but significantly lower body image scores, more sexual dysfunction, and diminished social function [35, 36].

Overall, there is a clear alteration in the social function of cancer patients with a colostomy versus a continent reconstruction. This is contrary data to the patients receiving an ileostomy for inflammatory bowel disease (IBD). This difference is likely due to the difference in preoperative status between groups. Often rectal cancer patients are asymptomatic at presentation; therefore, a colostomy is a drastic change. If a patient is experiencing life-limiting diarrhea or incontinence, an ostomy may be a welcome treatment for their symptoms. The prior data suggest that colostomy patients may require more pre- and postoperative counseling and support.

Temporary Defunctioning Stoma

A temporary defunctioning stoma is used to divert stool from an anastomosis, theoretically improving the outcome of anastomotic leaks [37]. Diversion is most often used for colo- or ileoanal anastomoses or in patients with complications during construction of an anastomosis, patients after radiation, on steroids, or in poor health [38]. A meta-analysis of loop ileostomy versus loop colostomy for diversion showed that both techniques provided adequate diversion with similar complication rates, except for a higher prolapse rate with loop colostomy [38].

Surprisingly diverting ostomies cause a significant worsening of QOL. Reasons for this are that patients with diverting stomas do not adapt themselves to a life with a stoma, and that patients with a diverting stoma may not have such severe preoperative symptoms as those needing a permanent stoma. Camilleri-Brennan and Steele illustrated an improvement in overall QOL after ostomy reversal, but identified a subgroup of patients with significant defecatory problems resulting in a poorer quality of life [39]. Gooszen et al. showed that more than half of the patients with temporary defunctioning stomas became socially restricted and experienced stoma care problems [40]. Issues of diminished QOL due to their new intestinal anatomy after stoma reversal were also found to be significant in this group. Siassi et al. demonstrated that for over a year up to 50% of patients reported incontinence, urgency, and a diminished QOL [41].

Because of the temporary nature of a diverting stoma, preoperative planning and support may be less than for permanent stomas. A similar phenomenon is liable to occur postoperatively in the form of support groups and preparation for altered bowel function. However, temporary stomas sometimes become permanent, and even if not permanent may not be closed for months or even years. Therefore, preoperative counseling is just as important as it is for a permanent stoma, and construction techniques should be just as meticulous.

Postoperative Adaptation to the Ostomy

Enterostomal therapists are currently a mainstay in pre- and postoperative ostomy care and planning. Karadag and colleagues in Turkey had patients complete a psychometric HR-QOL questionnaire before and 3 months after receiving stoma therapy. All types of ostomy patients showed a significant improvement in HR-QOL scores, from 60% prior to ET to 81.2% after. This study also reported that meeting with ET led to a significant improvement in frequency of problems: bathing, traveling, sports, bag evacuation, noise, and skin problems [15]. Marquis and colleagues also found that ET support led to improved QOL scores in the first 3–6 months with an ostomy [42]. Regular postoperative ET visits are essential in easing adaptation to an ostomy. ETs can often foresee difficulties and help prevent issues, leading to an easier adjustment and hopefully a transition back to normal social life.

Patient adaptation to an ostomy is primarily affected by the following factors: (1) the level of ostomy self-care, (2) psychological support, and (3) social support from family and significant others [43]. Many different organizations exist to further support these patients and help to circumvent some of the avoidable problems encountered by the ostomate. For example, the United Ostomy Associations of America is an association of affiliated, nonprofit support groups committed to improving the quality of life of ostomates of all kinds. If education is available – not only to the patient, but to their families and support networks – it can help to prevent social isolation.

Conclusion

Quality of life in patients with IBD or FAP is similar – regardless of the presence of an end ileostomy, continent ileostomy, or ileoanal pouch – as long as there is preoperative planning and education. Identification of personal cultures, values, and demographic factors is important. Enterostomal therapy, both pre- and postoperatively, not only improves the quality of life in ostomates, but helps to decrease postoperative complications and readmissions. Patients with both permanent colostomy and temporary diverting ostomy have decreased quality of life when compared with similar peer groups. These groups should be provided with education and counseling about their possible future difficulties preoperatively. Meetings with family stomal therapy and support groups perioperatively may help to ease this transition.

References

1. Wilson TR, Alexander DJ. Clinical and non-clinical factors influencing postoperative health-related quality of life in patients with colorectal cancer. Br J Surg. 2008;95:1408–15.
2. Siassi M, Weiss M, Hohenberger W, et al. Personality rather than clinical variables determines quality of life after major colorectal surgery. Dis Colon Rectum. 2009;52:662–8.
3. Holzer B, Matzel K, Schiedeck T, et al. Do geographic and educational factors influence the quality of life in rectal cancer patients with a permanent colostomy? Dis Colon Rectum. 2005;48:2209–16.
4. Pittman J, Rawl SM, Schmidt CM, et al. Demographic and clinical factors related to ostomy complications and quality of life in veterans with an ostomy. J Wound Ostomy Continence Nurs. 2008;35:493–503.
5. Bass EM, Del Pino A, Tan A, et al. Does preoperative stoma marking and education by the enterostomal therapist affect outcome? Dis Colon Rectum. 1997;40:440–2.
6. Colwell JC, Gray M. Does preoperative teaching and stoma site marking affect surgical outcomes in patients undergoing ostomy surgery? J Wound Ostomy Continence Nurs. 2007;34:492–6.
7. Chaudhri S, Brown L, Hassan I. Preoperative intensive, community-based vs. traditional stoma education: a randomized, controlled trial. Dis Colon Rectum. 2005;48:504–9.
8. Haugen V, Bliss DZ, Savik K. Perioperative factors that affect long-term adjustment to an incontinent ostomy. J Wound Ostomy Continence Nurs. 2006;33:525–35.
9. Power M, Harper A, Bullinger M. The World Health Organization WHOQOL-100: tests of the universality of quality of life in 15 different cultural groups worldwide. Health Psychol. 1999;18:495–505.
10. McLeod RS, Cohen Z. Quality of life with a stoma. In: Anonymous intestinal stomas: principles, techniques, and management. New York: Marcel Dekker, Inc; 2004. p. 91–109.
11. Revicki DA, Kaplan RM. Relationship between psychometric and utility-based approaches to the measurement of health-related quality of life. Qual Life Res. 1993;2:477–87.
12. Grant M, Ferrell B, Dean G, et al. Revision and psychometric testing of the City of Hope Quality of Life-Ostomy Questionnaire. Qual Life Res. 2004;13:1445–57.

13. Kiran RP, Delaney CP, Senagore AJ, et al. Prospective assessment of Cleveland Global Quality of Life (CGQL) as a novel marker of quality of life and disease activity in Crohn's disease. Am J Gastroenterol. 2003;98:1783–9.
14. Nugent KP, Daniels P, Stewart B, et al. Quality of life in stoma patients. Dis Colon Rectum. 1999;42:1569–74.
15. Karadag A, Mentes BB, Uner A, et al. Impact of stomatherapy on quality of life in patients with permanent colostomies or ileostomies. Int J Colorectal Dis. 2003;18:234–8.
16. Bekkers MJ, van Knippenberg FC, van den Borne HW, et al. Psychosocial adaptation to stoma surgery: a review. J Behav Med. 1995;18:1–31.
17. Wade BE. Colostomy patients: psychological adjustment at 10 weeks and 1 year after surgery in districts which employed stoma-care nurses and districts which did not. J Adv Nurs. 1990;15:1297–304.
18. Camilleri-Brennan J, Munro A, Steele RJ. Does an ileoanal pouch offer a better quality of life than a permanent ileostomy for patients with ulcerative colitis? J Gastrointest Surg. 2003;7:814–9.
19. Grumann MM, Noack EM, Hoffmann IA, et al. Comparison of quality of life in patients undergoing abdominoperineal extirpation or anterior resection for rectal cancer. Ann Surg. 2001;233: 149–56.
20. Ko CY, Rusin LC, Schoetz DJ, et al. Using quality of life scores to help determine treatment: is restoring bowel continuity better than an ostomy? Colorectal Dis. 2002;4:41–7.
21. Seidel SA, Newman M, Sharp KW. Ileoanal pouch versus ileostomy: is there a difference in quality of life? Am Surg. 2000;66:540–6; discussion 546–7.
22. Jimmo B, Hyman NH. Is ileal pouch-anal anastomosis really the procedure of choice for patients with ulcerative colitis? Dis Colon Rectum. 1998;41:41–5.
23. Weinryb RM, Gustavsson JP, Liljeqvist L, et al. A prospective study of the quality of life after pelvic pouch operation. J Am Coll Surg. 1995;180:589–95.
24. McLeod RS, Lavery IC, Leatherman JR, et al. Factors affecting quality of life with a conventional ileostomy. World J Surg. 1986; 10:474–80.
25. Burnham WR, Lennard-Jones JE, Brooke BN. Sexual problems among married ileostomists. Survey conducted by The Ileostomy Association of Great Britain and Ireland. Gut. 1977;18:673–7.
26. Rolstad BS, Wilson G, Rothenberger DA. Sexual concerns in the patient with an ileostomy. Dis Colon Rectum. 1983;26:170–1.
27. Berndtsson I, Oresland T. Quality of life before and after proctocolectomy and IPAA in patients with ulcerative proctocolitis – a prospective study. Colorectal Dis. 2003;5:173–9.
28. McLeod RS, Fazio VW. Quality of life with the continent ileostomy. World J Surg. 1984;8:90–5.
29. Nilsson LO, Kock NG, Kylberg F, et al. Sexual adjustment in ileostomy patients before and after conversion to continent ileostomy. Dis Colon Rectum. 1981;24:287–90.
30. Nessar G, Fazio VW, Tekkis P, et al. Long-term outcome and quality of life after continent ileostomy. Dis Colon Rectum. 2006; 49:336–44.
31. Kohler LW, Pemberton JH, Zinsmeister AR. Quality of life after proctocolectomy. A comparison of Brooke ileostomy, Kock pouch, and ileal pouch-anal anastomosis. Gastroenterology. 1991;101:679–84.
32. Ojerskog B, Kock NG, Nilsson LO, et al. Long-term follow-up of patients with continent ileostomies. Dis Colon Rectum. 1990;33: 184–9.
33. Engel J, Kerr J, Schlesinger-Raab A, et al. Quality of life in rectal cancer patients: a four-year prospective study. Ann Surg. 2003;238: 203–13.
34. Yau T, Watkins D, Cunningham D, et al. Longitudinal assessment of quality of life in rectal cancer patients with or without stomas following primary resection. Dis Colon Rectum. 2009;52:669–77.
35. Krouse R, Grant M, Ferrell B, et al. Quality of life outcomes in 599 cancer and non-cancer patients with colostomies. J Surg Res. 2007;138:79–87.
36. Bartha I, Hajdu J, Bokor L, et al. Quality of life of post-colostomy patients. Orv Hetil. 1995;136:1995–8.
37. Dehni N, Schlegel RD, Cunningham C, et al. Influence of a defunctioning stoma on leakage rates after low colorectal anastomosis and colonic J pouch-anal anastomosis. Br J Surg. 1998;85:1114–7.
38. Guenaga KF, Lustosa SA, Saad SS. Ileostomy or colostomy for temporary decompression of colorectal anastomosis. Systematic review and meta-analysis. Acta Cir Bras. 2008;23:294–303.
39. Camilleri-Brennan J, Steele RJ. Prospective analysis of quality of life after reversal of a defunctioning loop ileostomy. Colorectal Dis. 2002;4:167–71.
40. Gooszen AW, Geelkerken RH, Hermans J. Quality of life with a temporary stoma: ileostomy vs. colostomy. Dis Colon Rectum. 2000;43:650–5.
41. Siassi M, Hohenberger W, Losel F, et al. Quality of life and patient's expectations after closure of a temporary stoma. Int J Colorectal Dis. 2008;23:1207–12.
42. Marquis P, Marrel A, Jambon B. Quality of life in patients with stomas: the Montreux Study. Ostomy Wound Manage. 2003;49: 48–55.
43. Piwonka MA, Merino JM. A multidimensional modeling of predictors influencing the adjustment to a colostomy. J Wound Ostomy Continence Nurs. 1999;26:298–305.

Wound, Ostomy, and Continence/Enterostomal Therapy (WOC/ET) Nursing

6

Paula Erwin-Toth, Barbara Hocevar, and Linda J. Stricker

The specialty of enterostomal therapy nursing (ET), now known as wound, ostomy, and continence nursing (WOC), was founded in 1958 at Cleveland Clinic, Cleveland, Ohio. Pioneering colorectal surgeon Rupert B. Turnbull, M.D., joined forces with former patient Norma Gill to improve care and rehabilitate people with ostomies and enterocutaneous fistulae [1].

Advances in medicine, surgery, pouching technology, and skin and wound therapies led to the expansion of the ET nurse role to include wound and continence care as well as ostomy and fistulae management. A holistic approach to the care of patients with wound, ostomy, and incontinence needs along with collaboration between the surgeon and WOC/ET nurse promotes cost-effective care with optimal patient outcomes [2].

Preoperative Care

Successful postoperative management of the patient undergoing ostomy surgery begins with comprehensive preoperative care. Counseling and stoma site selection are key services the WOC/ET nurse provides to patients and their families. Information regarding basic ostomy function and self-care, lifestyle issues, body image, and sexuality can help prepare the patient for living with an ostomy. Optimum stoma placement and stoma construction are essential in obtaining a reliable, secure pouching system seal after surgery. Even in an emergency situation, basic counseling and stoma site marking should be completed. The prospect of a temporary or permanent stoma can be overwhelming. Comprehensive preoperative preparation lays the foundation for achieving long-term ostomy rehabilitation [3, 4].

Including a trained ostomy visitor can help facilitate this process. The United Ostomy Association of America (UOAA) and the International Ostomy Association (IOA) offer training sessions that enable people with established ostomies help new ostomates cope with their stomas [5, 6].

Selection of the stoma site will depend on the type of stoma to be constructed. Siting below the level of the umbilicus is preferred and will minimize clothing adjustments. Locating the stoma site on the summit of the infraumbilical fat mound of the abdomen and within the body of the rectus muscle will promote visualization of the stoma by the patient and provide a sound base of support, thus reducing the incidence of peristomal hernia. Avoiding scars, creases, and bony prominences will ensure a smooth pouching surface around the stoma. Evaluating the patient supine, sitting, and standing allows the clinician to see how the abdominal topography alters with position changes [3, 7]. This evaluation, coupled with an assessment of the patient's ability to see the chosen site, is essential to selecting the best site, optimize postoperative pouch security, and facilitate self-care. For patients with a protuberant abdomen or those requiring long-term use of a wheelchair, the upper abdomen provides better visualization for stoma management.

Once the site is determined, a mark can be made using a surgical marker to draw a small circle or "X," then covering the site with a transparent dressing. Another, long-standing method is the use of a sterile 26-gauge needle and India ink to create a small indelible tattoo in the shape of a triangle. In both cases, these marks serve as a guide to the surgeon for stoma placement during the operative procedure.

Ideally, the mark should represent the apex of the stoma; deviation from the site even by 1 cm can have an adverse effect on securing a good seal postoperatively [3]. Application of a properly sized pouching system in the operating room is also important.

P. Erwin-Toth (✉)
The Rupert B. Turnbull School of WOC/ET, Cleveland Clinic/ET, Cleveland, OH, USA
e-mail: erwinp@ccf.org

B. Hocevar
Nursing Institute/Digestive Disease Institute, Cleveland Clinic/ET, Cleveland, OH, USA

L.J. Stricker
WOC Nursing Education, Cleveland Clinic/ET, Cleveland, OH, USA

V.W. Fazio et al. (eds.), *Atlas of Intestinal Stomas*,
DOI 10.1007/978-0-387-78851-7_6, © Springer Science+Business Media, LLC 2012

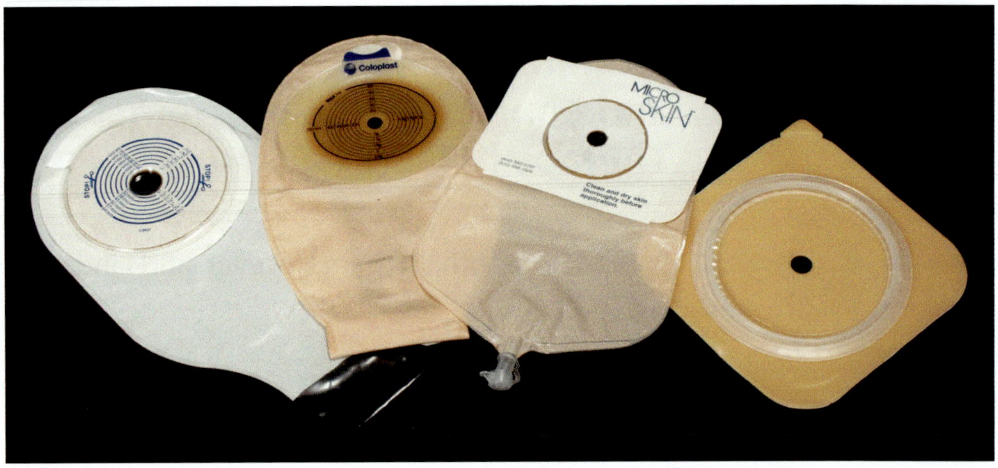

Fig. 6.1 Assorted flat skin barriers. From left, flat one-piece drainable pouch, flat one-piece drainable pouch, flat one-piece urinary spout pouch, flat skin barrier with flange for two-piece pouches

Postoperative Patient Care, Education, and Counseling

Postoperatively, the role of the WOC/ET nurse complements the care rendered by other members of the healthcare team. Depending on the setting, the WOC/ET nurse will provide individualized fitting, self-care education, and counseling for the patient with a new ostomy. Direct care staff needs to possess the knowledge and skill to reinforce the teaching provided by the WOC/ET nurse. Patient needs should be addressed along all aspects of the healthcare continuum. Changes in stoma size and abdominal contours post-discharge will require modification of the pouching system to ensure maintenance of peristomal skin integrity and a secure, odor-proof seal [7–9]. Additional education, counseling, and support are needed to assist the patient during his or her recuperation. Modifying information to meet an individual's needs is integral to successful rehabilitation.

Management Principles

Scientific and technological advances have allowed vast improvements to be made in the skin barriers, pouching systems, and odor-controlling agents used in ostomy care. A few reusable systems, consisting of a stoma plate and vinyl pouch requiring the use of a double-faced adhesive disc or skin cement and separate skin barrier, are still available. Disposable ostomy systems and accessories dominate modern ostomy management. These products are designed to maintain or restore peristomal skin integrity and provide individuals with a secure, comfortable, odor-proof seal, and are integral to successful adjustment following ostomy surgery.

Skin barriers prevent peristomal skin irritation and breakdown due to exposure to ostomy effluent. These products also create an environment for healing if damage to the skin has occurred. Depending on the composition and form, skin barriers can be used by themselves or combined to maintain or restore the integrity of peristomal skin (Fig. 6.1). Intact peristomal skin is necessary to obtain a secure and reliable seal.

The first skin barrier to be used in ostomy care was karaya. Originally used as dental powder, karaya gum was the primary skin barrier used by clinicians and patients from the 1950s through the 1970s. Karaya products are hydrophilic and help maintain the skin's acid mantle. Disadvantages of karaya products include rapid meltdown of the barrier with high-volume output and a burning sensation when applied to denuded skin.

In the 1970s, the introduction of sodium carboxymethyl cellulose (CMC) combined with pectin and gelatin began a new era in skin protection and spawned the development of a wide array of disposable ostomy products [10, 11]. Although hydrophilic, CMC does not erode as rapidly as karaya, maintains the skin's acid mantle, and does not sting denuded skin.

Synthetic skin barrier products include a wide array of skin sealants, films, and solid barriers. These products tend to be hydrophobic. Sealants containing alcohol may cause a stinging sensation when applied, but alcohol-free products are now available to avoid this effect. Since moisture will be trapped and not absorbed, adherence of solid skin barriers to denuded skin may be compromised, and patients may be vulnerable to fungal infections [7, 12, 13].

Skin barriers are manufactured in a variety of forms including wafers, rings, strips, powders, pastes, wipes, and films (Fig. 6.2). These products are not only useful in protecting peristomal skin, but many can be used to even out the topography around an ostomy, fistulae, or a draining wound. Use of these products can increase the wear time of a pouching system by minimizing the undermining and skin irritation associated with leakage where irregular skin contours are present [7, 11, 13].

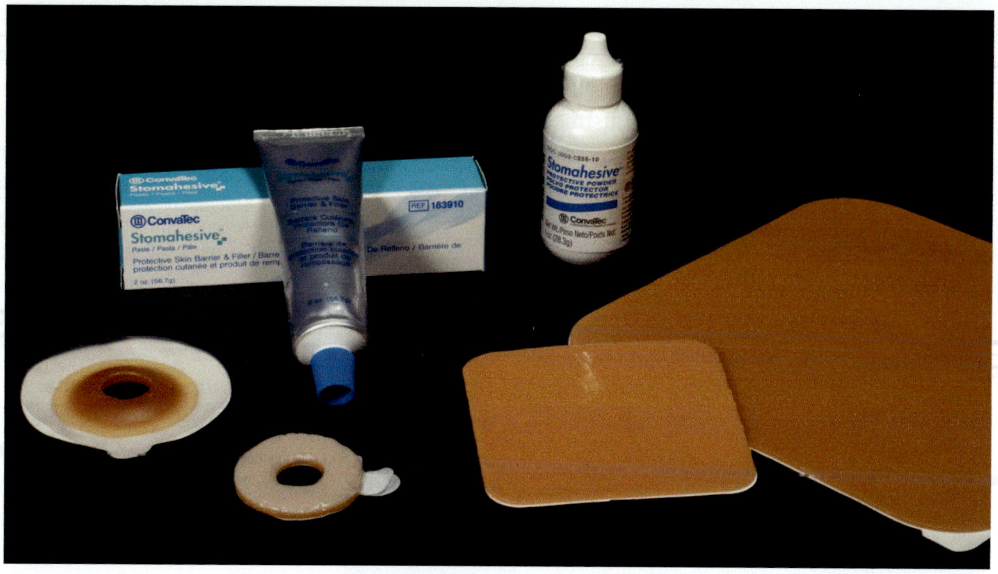

Fig. 6.2 Accessory products for pouching systems including skin barrier paste, skin barrier powder, skin barrier rings, and flat solid skin barriers

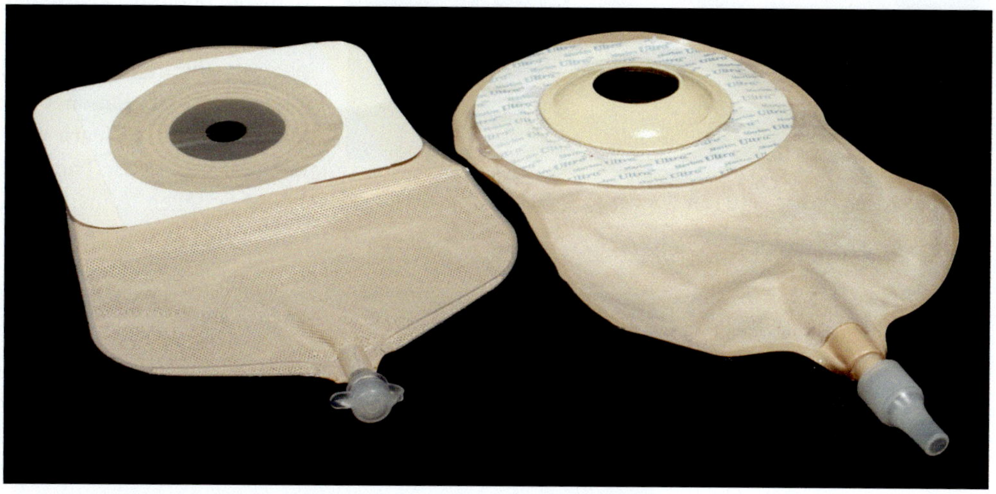

Fig. 6.3 One-piece urinary pouches. From left, flat and flexible, convex

Disposable pouching systems are available in one- and two-piece varieties (Fig. 6.3). One-piece pouches integrate a solid skin barrier and a pouch into one product. They are either pre-sized or require using scissors to cut the aperture to the appropriate size. Two-piece systems consist of a solid skin barrier and a separate pouch that is attached with a coupling mechanism. Two-piece systems are available in precut, cut-to-fit, and a type that enables customization of the opening by molding the pliable barrier to the exact shape of the stoma [13]. The properties of the two-piece systems are unique to the specific manufacturer and are not interchangeable from one brand to another.

Both one- and two-piece pouching systems are available in flat and convex shapes. Convexity is especially useful in patients with flush or retracted stomas and those with soft abdominal tissue around the stoma. The types of systems available include different degrees of convexity (shallow, medium, and deep) and varying degrees of firmness of the barrier (flexible or rigid, localized or gradual). Care must be taken to select the appropriate degree of convexity; too little will not be effective; too much may cause pressure necrosis [7, 9, 11, 14, 15].

Pouches are made with a wide opening at the bottom to drain stool or are equipped with a small spout to empty urine. Drainable pouches require an external clip to secure the bottom of the pouch or use an integrated closure that allows the bottom to be folded and secured by a self-locking mechanism. Urinary pouches have adaptors available to facilitate attachment to a bedside drainage bag or leg bag. Drainable pouches are made odor proof while urinary pouches are generally odor resistant. Both drainable and urinary pouches are available in either transparent or opaque materials.

Patient Education

Proper selection of the pouching system is an important part of the patient's rehabilitation. Adjustment to an ostomy is optimized with the attainment of a secure, reliable, and odor-proof pouch. This is best achieved with a well-sited, well-constructed, budded stoma. Consideration of visual acuity, manual dexterity, and patient preference should be included in the selection of the pouching system (Figs. 6.4 and 6.5).

Positional changes can have a significant impact on pouch adhesion. Patients should be evaluated sitting, supine, and standing to ensure a secure, comfortable fit. Stoma edema decreases significantly the first 4–6 weeks following surgery, and abdominal firmness and contours change as well. The aperture of the pouch should fit closely to the base of the stoma without impinging the mucosa.

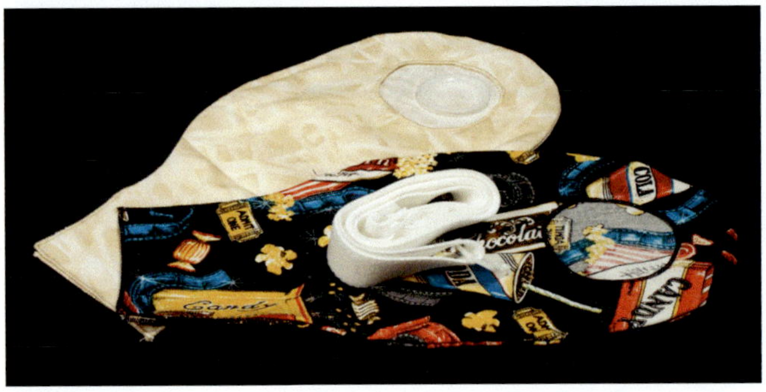

Fig. 6.4 Pouch covers and a belt

Learner readiness is a key component of adult education [16]. Limited preoperative contact, reduced hospital stays, and decreased home-care visits pose significant challenges to patients and their healthcare providers. Mastering self-care is a major factor in successful adjustment. The clinician needs to consider psychosocial development, culture, social support, and individual patient needs when establishing a plan of care [7]. Although emptying and changing a pouch is not a complex procedure, acquisition of self-care skills requires time, practice, and patience.

Pouch emptying is usually the first task taught to patients. The pouch should be emptied when a third half full. Care should be taken to avoid overfilling since the weight of the pouch may weaken the seal. In addition, there is a risk of spilling the contents of an over-full pouch while emptying.

Viewing the stoma for the first time can be overwhelming to many patients. Calm reassurance and reinforcement of preoperative information is important. Patients need time to integrate the changes brought about by a stoma into their concept of self. Patients need to examine their stoma and peristomal skin to learn what is normal and how to identify potential problems. Then, when the pouch is removed, care should be taken to inspect the peristomal skin as well as the

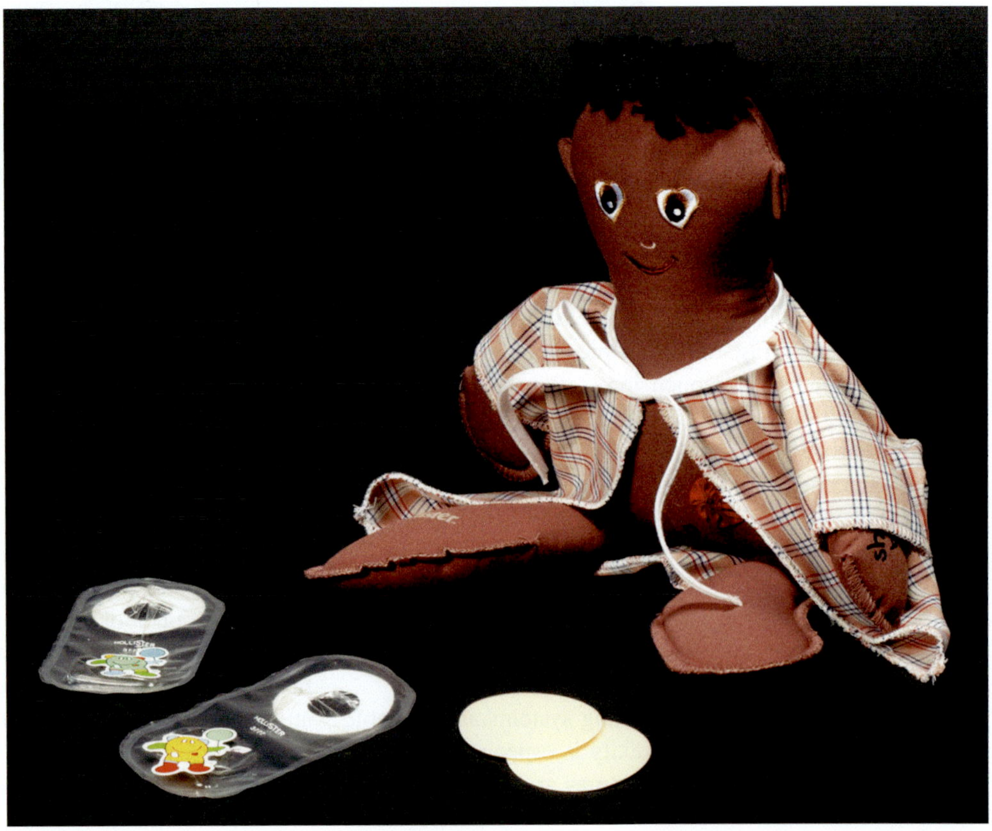

Fig. 6.5 Pediatric pouches and a doll with a stoma for use as pediatric teaching aids

back of the pouch upon removal. The underside of the pouch can reveal tracking, melting, or undermining of the seal. Prevention of skin breakdown and early identification and treatment of complications are important [7, 9, 14]. Frequency of pouch changes varies; patients should not wait for leakage to occur before changing the pouch.

Dermatologic conditions occurring in the peristomal skin can be challenging to manage. Treatments must be tailored to the specific skin complication yet not interfere with adherence of the pouching system. Common causes of peristomal skin complications include chemical, mechanical, infectious, immunologic, and disease related [7, 9, 14] (Table 6.1). Early identification and treatment are essential to minimize the physical and psychological effects of peristomal skin conditions.

Ideally, patients should be seen by a WOC/ET nurse within 4–6 weeks after discharge to ensure the patient is using the appropriate pouching system and is adjusting psychologically. In addition to making any modifications to the pouching system, further education or psychological support can be provided. Once ostomy management has been mastered, annual visits with a WOC/ET nurse are recommended. This will ensure the patient is properly fitted, educated about new products that are available, and provided additional support and information where needed.

Wound Management

Wound care is an integral part of modern WOC/ET nursing practice. Typical wound care therapies are intended to create a physiologic environment to promote healing, enhance patient comfort, and improve patient outcomes in a cost-effective manner that complements the entire plan of care. Principles of topical wound care include removal of nonviable tissue in well-vascularized wounds, noncytotoxic cleansing of the wound bed, identifying and eliminating infection, and filling dead space without over packing [8, 17]. A holistic approach to patient care is essential; nursing care addresses the needs of the entire patient and not just the stoma. Taking into consideration the intrinsic and extrinsic factors affecting the patient helps the clinician create a healing environment to improve patient outcomes. The PET Model for Wound Care (see Table 6.2) represents a framework of care for managing patients with wounds.

Table 6.1 Stoma and peristomal skin conditions

Conditions	Characteristics	Treatment
Folliculitis	Traumatic removal of hair during pouch change results in inflammation and infection of hair follicles. Lesions are painful and moist	Topical antimicrobial powder as needed. Once healed, carefully shave area. Use of adhesive remover and skin sealant is advised. Instruct patient on proper pouch removal
Candidiasis	Warm, moist area creates an environment for growth of *Candida albicans*. Generally diffuse red patches with characteristic advancing border and satellite lesions. Severe itching is common	Topical antifungal powder. Assess system for leakage or undermining of seal. Refit pouching system
Irritant dermatitis	Chemical destruction of the skin caused by topical products or leakage. Area appears red, moist, and painful. May be localized to a specific area of pouch undermining or leakage	Review product usage and techniques to determine cause. Correct/revise pouching system
Pseudoverrucous lesions (formerly called PEH)	Overgrowth of tissue caused by overexposure to moisture. Appears as raised, moist lesions with a wart-like appearance. Lesions are painful	Assess equipment for proper aperture and convexity. Refit as needed. In severe cases, sharp debridement of the tissue may be required
Mechanical trauma	External item or force causing damage to the stoma and/or skin from pressure, laceration, friction or shear	Assess equipment and technique. Modify to prevent re-injury
Allergic contact dermatitis	Allergic response generated by patient sensitivity to a particular product. Skin appears red, swollen, eroded, weepy, or bleeding. Generally corresponds to the exposed area	Remove the allergen, avoid other irritants, and protect the skin. Patch test with other products as needed. Refer to dermatologist for multiple allergies
Peristomal abscess	One or more painful lesions surrounded by a halo of redness. Not uncommon in patients with Crohn's disease in the distal bowel	Unroofing of ulcer or incision and drainage of abscess. Management depends on size. Review options, including non-adherent dressings, hydrogel, astringent solution, calcium alginate, hydrofiber or hydrocolloid wafer. Antibiotics. A non-adherent pouching system can be fashioned with a one-piece pouch with belt tabs, an extra gasket and a solid skin barrier wafer
Pyoderma gangrenosum	Associated with IBD, arthritis, leukemia, polycythemia vera, and multiple myeloma. Red open lesions with irregular purplish margins. Exquisitely painful	Systemic treatment of underlying disease including steroids or immunomodulator therapy. Local ulcer treatment: intralesional or topical steroid, dressings and pouching the same as with an abscess

(continued)

Table 6.1 (continued)

Conditions	Characteristics	Treatment
Radiation injury	Red, thinned skin. Easily traumatized by removal of skin adhesives	Gently cleanse skin with cool water. Be cautious in use of solvents or skin sealants due to frequent sensitivities and risk of chemical trauma. Use a skin barrier that is easy to remove
Caput medusa	In patients with portal (liver) hypertension, the pressure at the portal systemic shunt in the mucocutaneous junction increases, creating venous engorgement. With trauma, profuse bleeding can occur	Apply pressure and/or use hemostatic agents (e.g., silver nitrate). Cautery or surgical ligation may be necessary. Remove pouch carefully. Avoid aggressive skin barriers and skin sealants. If stoma is relocated, varices will eventually recur around the new stoma unless underlying liver disease is treated (e.g., liver transplant)
Necrosis/ ischemia	Dark, red to black mucosa may appear dry, mottled	Distal necrosis – if superficial, conservative management – tissue allowed to demarcate, slough
	Stoma may be firm or flaccid	• Stoma will then be flush or slightly retracted; stenosis may occur
	Ischemia usually noticeable within 12–24 h; it can be evident up to 3–5 days postop	Necrosis extending below fascial level • Run risk of perforation and subsequent peritonitis • Surgeon immediately notified • Usually requires re-operation with construction of new stoma • Mucocutaneous separation occurs
	Results from:	Intervention
	(a) Excessive tension on the mesentery with resultant compromise to arterial inflow, venous outflow, or both. Can be a result of abdominal distension, obesity, excessive edema	• Ongoing mucosal assessment
	(b) Interruption of blood supply to the stoma (e.g., embolus, clot)	• Prompt notification of surgeon of mucosal changes
	(c) Excessive devascularization	• Utilization of clear pouches in postoperative period, proper sizing of equipment, frequent pouch changes
	(d) Narrowly spaced sutures; sutures tied snugly around stoma, or continuous constricting sutures	• Odor control as tissue sloughs • Psychological support
Mucocutaneous separation	Separation of the suture line at the junction of the stomal mucosa and skin. May be superficial or deep: may be partial or circumferential	Interventions: (a) Gently probe with swab to determine depth, undermining (b) Irrigate with normal saline to clean (c) Deep wounds: use calcium alginate rope packing; two-piece pouching system may be beneficial (d) Shallow wounds: use skin barrier powder to fill defect, then cover and pouch (e) If separation is draining large amounts of fluid, it may need to be included in pouch opening (f) If peritoneal contamination is a concern, the surgeon may resuture the stoma to the skin, either locally or under anesthesia
Prolapse	Telescoping of bowel through the stoma	Interventions: (a) Surgery (b) Conservative management: reduce prolapse with use of a binder or prolapse belt (c) Modify pouching system as needed to avoid trauma to bowel mucosa
Retraction	Stoma resting at or below skin level. Can be due to weight changes. Recession may be indicative of recurrent Crohn's disease due to scarring and contracting of bowel	Modify pouching system: maintain seal between pouch and skin without undermining: (a) Use of convexity (b) Accessory products Surgery as needed
Stenosis	Narrowing or stricture of the stoma. Often associated with scarring due to ischemia	Possible local revision of stoma or, if recurrent or severe, more extensive stoma revision

Table 6.1 (continued)

Conditions	Characteristics	Treatment
Parastomal hernia	Most common with colostomies. Appears as a bulge around the stoma; the bulge represents loops of intestine that have protruded through fascial defect around the stoma and into subcutaneous tissue Results from: • Stoma placed outside of rectus muscle • Increased intra-abdominal pressure with lifting and straining • Defect in abdominal musculature, loss of muscle tone (as with weight gain or aging) • Excessively large fascial defect • Placement of stoma in midline incision • Wound infection	Avoid colostomy irrigation If hernia can be reduced, apply hernia belt/binder If obstructed or incarcerated, seek immediate medical care

Table 6.2 The PET Model for holistic care

Intrinsic	Topical therapy
Intrinsic means originating from within the body. As the WOC nurse begins to assess the patient with a wound, a careful accounting must be made of factors from within the patient that can create a barrier to healing. While reviewing the medical record, consider how the patient's comorbid conditions can have an effect on healing. For example, uncontrolled diabetes can lead to other chronic conditions such as peripheral vascular disease, coronary artery disease, and even tissue ischemia. Lower extremity venous insufficiency interferes with venous blood returning to the heart, which leads to pooling of blood in the ankle and calf area of the affected leg. Skin damage can be a result of many causes. Radiation, for example, is a conventional treatment for some types of cancer, but also has the capability to damage the skin cells in the adjacent area. This damage can extend deep into the nucleus of the cell and reach DNA, which can change the cell's physiology. This can also lead to loss of sebaceous glands, loss of elasticity with atrophy, and discoloration [1]. Bacterial, fungal, and viral organisms have the ability to overcome the body's immune system and either appear as skin complications such as a fungal rash within skin folds or impair the healing process of any wound. The important part in this phase of assessment is to recognize when an infection is present and treat according to organism type. Skin and wounds require adequate perfusion and nutrition for normal physiological maintenance and tissue repair. Wounds complicated by perfusion problems have the risk of becoming devitalized and develop nonviable or necrotic tissue. Patients who have poor nutritional reserves are likely to have delayed healing times. A thorough assessment of any patient with delayed wound healing includes investigating for adequate perfusion and nutritional stores. Other intrinsic factors can include the type(s) of medications the patient may be taking. Anti-inflammatory agents or chemotherapeutic agents in particular have the capability to interfere with tissue repair because they have an effect on the wound-healing cascade [1]. Finally, consider the impact of the aging process and the effects of stress when working through the assessment process. As part of the normal aging process, the immune system starts to diminish in its ability to protect the person from outside factors. Skin repair is slowed, and there is a greater incidence of chronic illness. As the WOC nurse develops a plan of care to manage the wound, optimizing all internal factors will provide the best chance for successful healing.	The selection of a specific wound treatment can be a daunting task if the wound assessment is incomplete. This is not just a process of making decisions based on depth of tissue injury, but based on: • Sound understanding of how wounds heal • How different categories of wound care products work • Thorough assessment of the wound • Managing intrinsic and extrinsic factors Before a treatment is decided, everything impacting the patient must be considered first. Simply put, select a dressing based on creating an optimal environment for healing.

(continued)

Table 6.2 (continued)

Extrinsic	Plan of care
Extrinsic means an outside factor having an impact on the whole. Many types of extrinsic factors can impact a person, but also impact each person differently. The WOC/ET nurse needs to consider the outside factors significant to each patient situation. Environmental factors are a priority management issue. For example, consider if the patient has a pressure ulcer: • What support surface will offer the most optimal pressure redistribution while at the same time be covered by the payer source? • What if there is no payer source? • How can we offer each patient safe and effective care while working within organization policies, predetermined insurance coverage, and the patient's own psychosocial concerns? The answers to these questions come from a careful look at each person and including the appropriate interdisciplinary team member in the planning process Functional deficits are also an important consideration. Patients with a combination of pressure ulcers and ambulatory problems will require more than simply adding a support surface to the bed Think about how activities of daily living impact the wound • Does the patient require a seating device in addition to a specialized bed? • What about transferring a patient from one department or one facility to the next? • What type of repositioning schedule will meet the needs of the patient and be realistic for the caregivers?	The nursing process involves the use of assessment, planning, implementation, documentation, evaluation, and reassessment. The goal of this process is to alleviate, minimize, or prevent actual or potential problems. The nursing process can be applied in any interaction that involves a nurse and a patient. The process can take place in a variety of settings, including a hospital, community setting, private home, or long-term care facility

A holistic approach by definition considers the patient as a whole system. WOC/ET nurses take a holistic view of the patient when determining the best approach to wound management. Using the PET Model includes effective management of wounds through careful assessment of the patient's intrinsic environment, extrinsic environment, topical wound care, and a complete plan of care based on all these factors. To begin the holistic approach, consider the type of wound and the origins of the wound. This is accomplished by analyzing the patient's intrinsic and extrinsic environment.

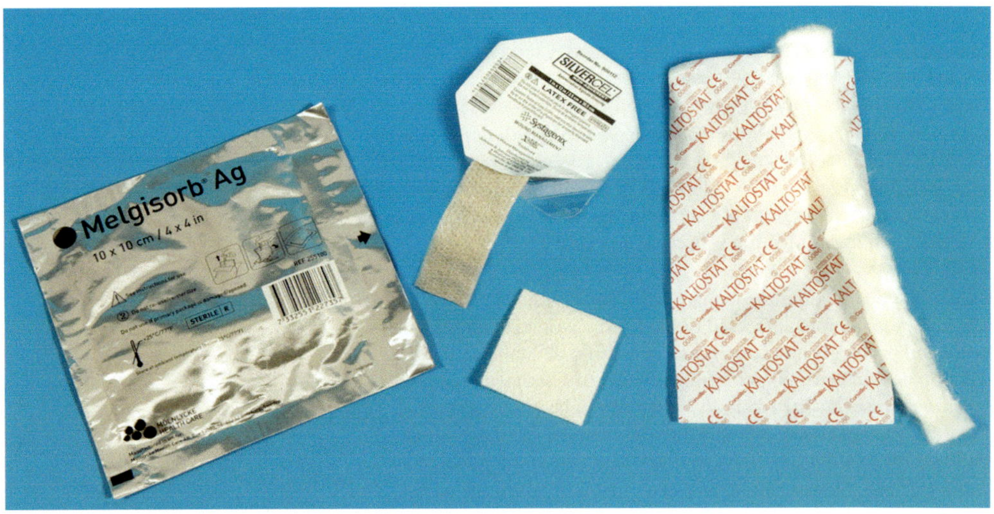

Fig. 6.6 Calcium alginate wound care products

Maintaining moisture balance in the wound by absorbing excess exudate without drying out the wound bed is critical. Care should be taken to preserve or restore the integrity of the periwound skin. Topical therapies range from a variety of dressings and debriding agents as well as adjunct therapies such as negative pressure wound therapy, hyperbaric oxygen, ultrasound, and electrical stimulation. Categories of wound dressings include transparent films, foams, hydrocolloids, calcium alginates (Fig. 6.6), hydrofiber, collagen-based, biologic, and antimicrobial agents. Combination dressings are available to accommodate special wound needs (Table 6.3) [8, 17].

Table 6.3 Dressing categories

Dressing category	Properties	Examples
Transparent films	• Adhesive, semipermeable, clear polyurethane material • Maintain moist wound environment • Non-absorptive • Can be used as primary or secondary dressing	Op-Site™, Tegaderm™, Bioclusive™
Foams	• Hydrophilic, polyurethane layer • May have transparent film outer covering • Non-adherent; available in adhesive version • Absorb small/moderate exudate • Can be used as primary or secondary dressing	Allevyn™, Lyofoam®
Hydrocolloids	• Composed of carboxymethylcellulose, gelatin, and pectin • Occlusive • Promote autolytic debridement • Maintain moist wound environment • Absorb small to moderate amount of exudate	DuoDERM®, Restore™, Tegasorb™, Comfeel®, Replicare®
Calcium alginates	• Composed of polysaccharide material derived from brown seaweed • Absorb moderate/large amounts of exudate • Form a gel • Biodegradable • Require secondary dressing	Kaltostat®, Tegagen™, Restore™, Sorbsan®, Curasorb®
Collagens	• Composed of purified bovine or avian collagen • Optimum results obtained in wounds with slough/eschar removed • Absorb minimal to moderate exudate • Indicated for recalcitrant wounds	FIBRACOL®, Medifil®, Promogran®
Hydrogels	• Composed of water or glycerin-based hydrophilic polymers • Maintain moist wound environment • Most absorb minimal amounts of exudate • Can be used to soften eschar • Most require secondary dressing	Carrasyn®gel, DuoDERM®gel, Elasto-Gel™, Intrasite™gel, CURASOL®gel
Biologicals/biosynthetics	• Derived from bioactive materials from human, bovine, porcine, or other sources • Create an interactive wound environment to enhance/promote healing in recalcitrant wounds • Optimum results with a wound bed free of slough or eschar • Require a secondary dressing	Regranex™, Hyalofill®, Apligraf®
Enzymatic agents	• Topical agents derived from animal or plant enzymes • Digest, lift, or liquefy nonviable tissue • Need interface with moist tissue • Some require protection of periwound skin • Require secondary dressing • September 2008 FDA banned all enzymatic agents containing papain	Santyl®
Gauze	• Dressings composed of cotton wool, cellulose, or rayon • Variety of forms, shapes, and sizes • Plain and impregnated • Absorb minimal to moderate exudate • Provide nonselective debridement	Kerlix®, Kling®, Mesalt®, ADAPTIC®
Combination dressings	• Combines two or more dressing properties • Wound fillers • Layered dressings	CombiDERM®, Alldress®, TIELLE®

Enterocutaneous Fistula

WOC/ET-nursing management of patients with enterocutaneous fistula (ECF) requires knowledge, skill, and creativity. Goals of therapy require a holistic approach that will enhance the entire plan of care. Efforts to contain and quantify the output, control odor, and protect the surrounding skin in a cost-effective manner are key elements of fistula care. Ostomy pouches, skin barriers and accessories, fistula pouches, wound drainage collection devices, and wound care products may all be used to manage an ECF [7, 17].

Several pouching modifications may be required while managing an ECF to achieve optimal results. There is greater potential for skin breakdown around a fistula as opposed to an ostomy. Oftentimes, the pouching system needs to be changed more frequently secondary to high fistula output and challenges with maintaining seals in extremely uneven perifistular tissue planes. Achieving a predictable wear time and ensuring adequate patient/family education and support are important to factor into the plan of care [7, 17]. In most cases, patients will require assistance to manage at home. Follow-up visits with a WOC/ET nurse are desirable.

Reimbursement for supplies used in fistula management varies widely. Writing letters of medical necessity may be required to support coverage of supplies, but this is no guarantee that the supplies will be covered by insurance [10, 18, 19]. The physical, emotional, and economic impact of an ECF cannot be underestimated. Patient and family support throughout the process are key components of effective management.

Conclusion

Pouch security and maintenance of peristomal skin integrity provide a foundation for long-term success for the patient's rehabilitation following ostomy surgery. Ostomy surgery is not a handicapping procedure. By individualizing patient preparation, counseling, postoperative fitting, self-care education, and integrating the stoma into follow-up care, the patient's self-concept and lifestyle can be enhanced.

The past 50 years have seen the practice of colorectal surgeons and WOC/ET nurses evolve. What has remained constant is the partnership between these two healthcare professionals to improve the quality of life for patients with ostomies, wounds, and fistulae.

References

1. Erwin-Toth P, Krasner D, editors. Enterostomal therapy nursing growth & evolution of a nursing specialty worldwide. A festschrift for Norma Gill-Thompson, ET. Baltimore: Halgo, Inc.; 1996.
2. Wound Ostomy and Continence Nurses Society. www.wocn.org (2009). Accessed 5 Mar 2009.
3. Erwin-Toth P, Barrett P. Stoma site marking: a primer. Ostomy Wound Manage. 1997;43(4):18–25.
4. Lavery I, Erwin-Toth P. Stoma therapy. In: MacKeigan J, Cataldo P, editors. Intestinal stomas: principles, techniques, & management. St. Louis: Quality Medical Publishing; 1993. p. 60.
5. The International Ostomy Association. www.ostomyinternational.org (2009). Accessed 5 Mar 2009.
6. The United Ostomy Association of America. www.uoaa.org (2009). Accessed 5 Mar 2009.
7. Colwell J, Goldberg M, Carmel J. Fecal & urinary diversions: management principles. St. Louis: Mosby; 2004.
8. Krasner D. Chronic wound care. 4th ed. Malvern: HMP Communications; 2007.
9. Rolstad B, Erwin-Toth P. Peristomal skin complications: prevention and management. Ostomy Wound Manage. 2004;50(9):68–77.
10. Turnbull G. The evolution, current status, and regulation of ostomy products in the United States. J Wound Ostomy Continence Nurs. 2001;28(1):18–24.
11. Turnbull G. The ostomy assessment inventory: a data-gathering process to enhance appropriate pouching system selection. Ostomy Wound Manage. 1998;44(2):28–37.
12. Fazio V, Erwin-Toth P. Stoma therapy. In: Corman M, editor. Colon and rectal surgery. 4th ed. Philadelphia: Lippincott-Raven; 1998. p. 1320–48.
13. Felice P. The many parts of ostomy collection systems. What are your options? Ostomy Wound Manage. 1985;9:31.
14. Erwin-Toth P. Prevention and management of peristomal skin complications. Adv Skin Wound Care. 2000;13:175–81.
15. Turnbull G. The convexity controversy. Ostomy Wound Manage. 2003;49(1):16–7.
16. Russell S. An overview of adult-learning processes. Urol Nurs. 2006;26:349–52.
17. Bryant R, Nix D. Acute and chronic wounds: current management concepts. 3rd ed. St. Louis: Mosby; 2007.
18. Kesselman P. Orthotics billing: an update. Podiatr Manage. 2007;26(7):139–46.
19. Turnbull G. New HCPCS codes for ostomy supplies. Ostomy Wound Manage. 2002;48(4):12–5.

Ileostomy

7

Luca Stocchi

Introduction

An ileostomy can be a very effective substitute to anal function and is compatible with an excellent quality of life. However, an appropriate construction is paramount to manage the potentially corrosive enteric content that exits from the stoma spout. The appropriate location of an ileostomy on the abdominal wall may be the most important factor in allowing optimal function of the stoma and should be appropriately planned and selected preoperatively. The ideal location for most ileostomies is in the right lower quadrant through the rectus muscle, sufficiently away from the midline incision to allow proper placement of the stoma appliance. The infraumbilical fat mound over the rectus muscle sheath is generally an ideal location because it is away from the umbilicus, skin creases, or bony prominences (Figs. 7.1 and 7.2). In fact, it is particularly important to avoid any skin creases that may cause breaking of the appliance-to-skin seal when the patient sits down. Similarly, an ostomy placed on an irregular surface may make it impossible to maintain an effective seal between the appliance and skin and predisposes to frequent leaks. Adjustments in the location of the ileostomy may become necessary depending on changes in body habitus or scars from subsequent operations. It is critical to select the stoma site with the patient standing, bending, and sitting, ensuring the planned site is visible to the patient for appropriate stoma management. The creation of an ostomy site below the belt line to facilitate hiding of a stoma bag with clothing may be desirable but unrealistic in the obese patient or when previous stomas have been created. Under these circumstances, alternative locations, such as the upper quadrants, may become preferable to achieve a flat abdominal surface. Especially in difficult cases, it is advisable to mark multiple stoma sites in case the ideal stoma site cannot be used due to adverse intraoperative findings.

The marking of the stoma site can involve the drawing of an "X" with a marking pen covered by transparent occlusive dressing if the operation involving the stoma creation is anticipated in the short term. In this case, it is important to create a superficial scar with a needle when the patient has

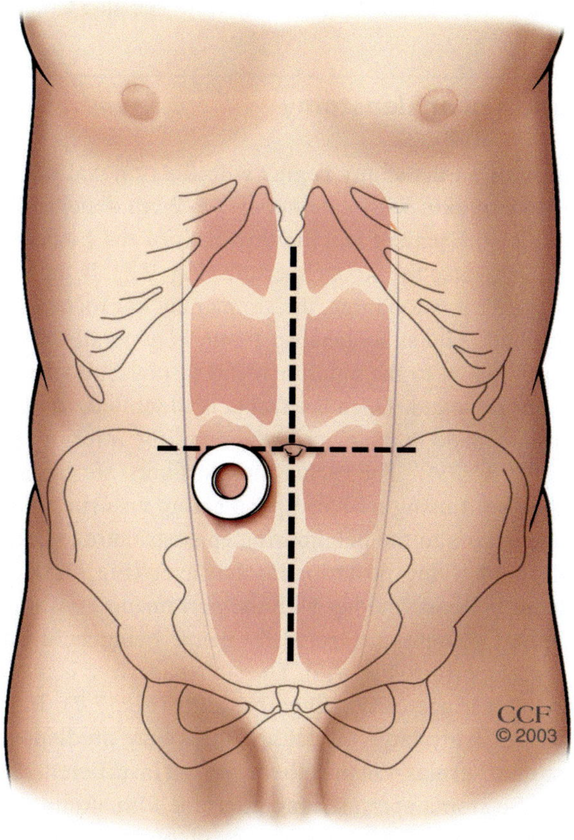

Fig. 7.1 The optimal stoma site is located over the rectus sheath, on the flat surface of the infraumbilical fat mound, away from irregular surfaces such as scars, incisions, umbilicus, and bony prominences (Illustration © CCF)

L. Stocchi
Department of Colorectal Surgery, Digestive Disease Institute, Cleveland Clinic Foundation, Cleveland, OH, USA
e-mail: stocchl@ccf.org

V.W. Fazio et al. (eds.), *Atlas of Intestinal Stomas*,
DOI 10.1007/978-0-387-78851-7_7, © Springer Science+Business Media, LLC 2012

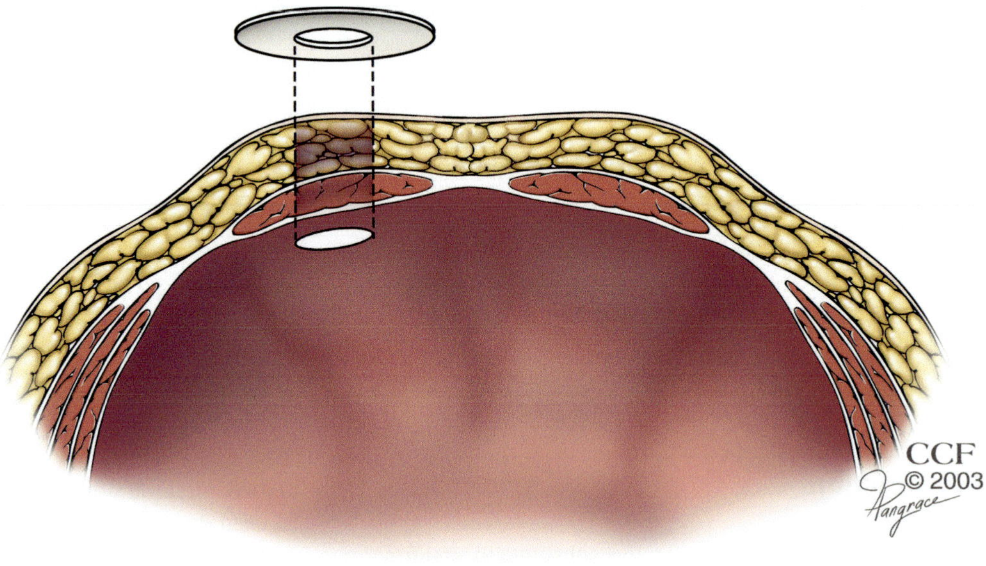

Fig. 7.2 Cross-sectional view showing the position of the intestine, traversing the rectus muscle and the rectus sheath (Illustration © CCF)

been anesthetized and prior to cleansing of the abdomen for surgery to prevent the marking from being deleted. Alternatively, a more permanent marking of the abdominal wall can be achieved with subcutaneous injection of methylene blue to create visible dots in the skin (see also Chap. 6).

Creation of an Ileostomy

Creation of an ileostomy begins with the removal of a circular disk of skin with a radius of 1.5–2 cm depending on the size of the patient and the thickness of the bowel loop that will traverse the stoma aperture (Fig. 7.3). If the opening in the skin is too large, the stoma may not form a satisfactory bud. The subcutaneous tissue is generally divided vertically down to the anterior rectal fascia. Subcutaneous fat is not removed. Once the fascia is identified, a vertical incision is made in the anterior fascia of the inferior rectus muscle (Fig. 7.4). The rectus muscle fibers are identified and then split using a blunt-tipped clamp ensuring that no damage occurs to the neighboring epigastric artery, exposing the underlying posterior fascial layer (Fig. 7.5). This last layer is divided along with the peritoneum, with intra-abdominal contents protected by gauze being held under the stoma aperture (Fig. 7.6). The stoma aperture is made to allow the passage of two fingerbreadths (Fig. 7.7). In general, excessively large fascial apertures may predispose to parastomal hernias. On the other hand, an insufficient diameter of the stoma aperture may interfere with stoma perfusion or cause a postoperative bowel obstruction. When faced with the specific circumstances of an obese patient and/or edematous bowel, it is therefore preferable to use larger openings than typically employed in an elective surgical case performed in a normally sized individual. The muscle-splitting aperture reduces the risk of injury to the epigastric vessels, which typically course along the lateral edge of the rectus muscle. Occult injuries to the inferior epigastric vessels may be detected by placing a clean laparotomy sponge through the stoma aperture. The sponge is then left in place for a few minutes while the intra-abdominal portion of the procedure is completed prior to abdominal fascial closure. Following this, the sponge is removed and checked for bleeding before the stoma loop is passed through the stoma aperture. At this stage, the ileum should also be examined to ensure that it is not ischemic. A pink intestinal serosal color with a palpable pulse in the corresponding mesentery generally indicates appropriate blood supply. However, if bowel viability is in question, the ileal edge should be trimmed to ensure appropriate bleeding. Brisk or "nuisance" bleeding, which requires hemostasis, indicates viable ileum. Once bowel viability is confirmed, it is necessary to ensure appropriate orientation of the ileal stoma loop. An appropriate mesenteric orientation is important for intestinal viability. In the case of an end ileostomy, many surgeons secure the edge of the intra-abdominal mesentery of the stoma loop to the anterior abdominal wall from the stoma aperture to the falciform ligament to prevent mesenteric twisting and internal herniation (Fig. 7.8). This technique is not universally adopted, especially in the course of minimally invasive procedures, and its importance has not yet been rigorously tested. While technically more demanding than in open surgery, suturing of the stoma mesentery to the anterior abdominal wall may also be possible laparoscopically. After closure of the abdomen, the ileostomy is matured. The techniques for maturing an ileostomy may differ slightly depending on the ostomy type. However, all the various techniques share the same principle of avoiding the creation of an ileostomy flush with the skin, which could be extremely difficult to manage due to the semisolid or liquid nature of the ileostomy effluent.

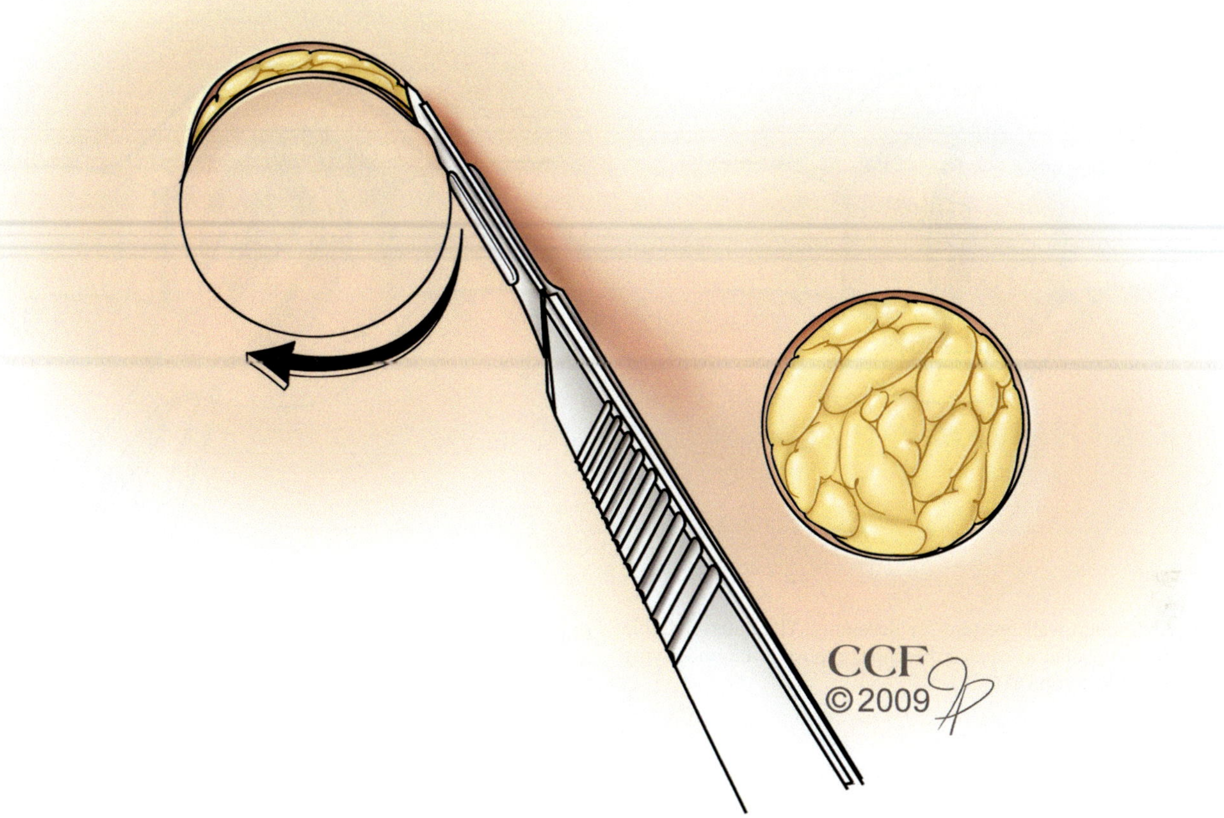

Fig. 7.3 Ostomy skin aperture. A circular skin incision is made with a diameter of approximately 1.5 cm (Illustration © CCF)

End Ileostomy

This type of ileostomy may be created after total proctocolectomy or total abdominal colectomy with preservation of a rectal or colorectal stump of variable length. The maturation of the stoma is carried out using slightly different techniques, all of which allow appropriate eversion of the ileostomy. Some surgeons prefer not to use any stitches in the seromuscular layer of the bowel at the base of the stoma loop in the belief that any suturing of the ileum may be predisposing to the onset of enterocutaneous fistulas. Others pass three to four everting stitches, which include a full-thickness passage of the stoma edge, seromuscular bite at the skin level, and a subcuticular bite. Following that, other sutures between the full-thickness edge of stoma loop and the subcuticular layer are added in a staggered fashion through different points along the stoma circumference to accomplish ileostomy eversion. Other surgeons only place these stitches and avoid any seromuscular bites. These various techniques are equivalent and only depend on the individual surgeon's preferences.

When maturing the ileostomy, there may be times when the small bowel mesentery requires trimming to facilitate stoma eversion. Under these circumstances, it may be convenient to suture the cut edge of the mesentery to the subcutaneous fat to maintain protrusion of the ileostomy (Fig. 7.9). Most surgeons agree on placement of the sutures in the subcuticular layer rather than through the epidermis as this might promote mucosal skin implants with subsequent mucus secretion that breaks the seal of the skin protective barrier (Fig. 7.10). Absorbable sutures are generally preferred. The final result should be a circumferentially everted ileostomy protruding 2–3 cm above the skin level (Fig. 7.11).

Diverting Loop Ileostomy

The creation of a loop ileostomy allows reversible diversion of the gastrointestinal contents and is used after ileal pouch–anal anastomosis or low anterior resection with ultra-low colorectal or coloanal anastomosis. A diversion by means of a loop ileostomy is generally preferable to diverting colostomy when both options are available [1–3]. A meta-analysis

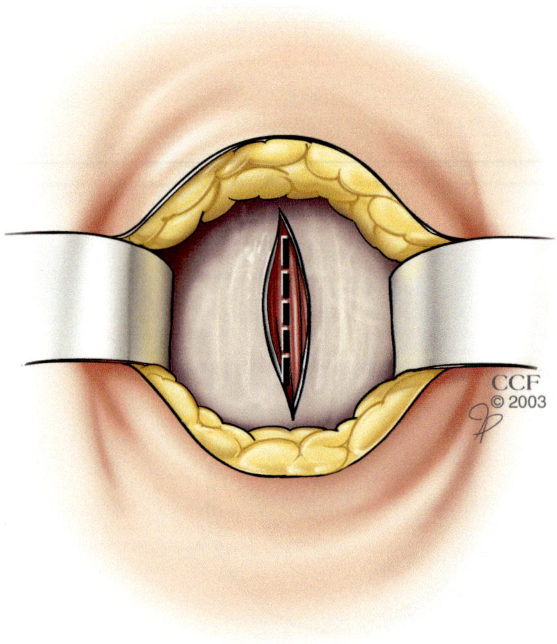

Fig. 7.4 Abdominal wall aperture for ileostomy. The anterior fascia is divided in a cephalad to caudad direction, exposing the underlying rectus muscle (Illustration © CCF)

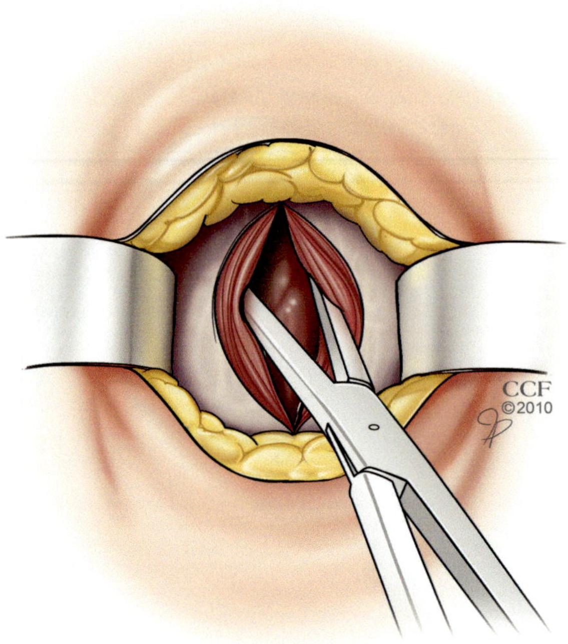

Fig. 7.5 Abdominal wall aperture for ileostomy. The rectus muscle fibers are separated with the tips of a blunt clamp, taking care to avoid injury to the epigastric artery (Illustration © CCF)

on 12 studies comparing diverting ileostomy and diverting colostomy showed that while an ileostomy may predispose more easily to dehydration and bowel obstruction after takedown, these downsides are offset by a reduced risk of prolapse and sepsis [4]. In addition, an important advantage in favor of a loop ileostomy – compared to other ileostomy types – is that it predisposes to a technically easier closure, as both the proximal and distal intestinal limbs are located at the skin surface. The selection of an appropriate site for a diverting ileostomy and the creation of the stoma aperture are comparable to what was described for the creation of an end ileostomy and other types of ileostomies. However, a slightly larger stoma aperture may be indicated for a diverting loop ileostomy than for an end ileostomy as two limbs of small bowel are passed through the aperture. The selected loop is marked with an umbilical tape passed through the mesentery very close to the bowel at the apex of the loop. Proper orientation of the ileostomy is facilitated by placing sutures of different color on the afferent and efferent loops of bowel (Fig. 7.12). Typically, a blue-dyed suture is placed on the proximal aspect ("blue is the sky") whereas a brown suture, typically chromic, is placed in the distal limb ("brown is the earth"). The appropriately oriented loop is then passed through the stoma aperture, and the umbilical tape encircling the bowel may be substituted with a stoma rod, which is typically left in place for 3 days (Fig. 7.13). Following placement of the stoma rod, fascial closure of the abdomen may begin. After closure of the midline wound or exteriorization site in case of minimally invasive procedures, the distal stomal limb is open transversally at skin level, from one mesenteric margin to the other on its anti-mesenteric aspect. The distal bowel edge is secured to the subcuticular tissue located just caudally with interrupted 3–0 stitches, generally chromic or Vicryl (Fig. 7.14). The proximal lip of the opened small bowel wall is then everted with full-thickness stitches, which may be passed more proximally through the seromuscular layer of the bowel and then also passed through the subcuticular layer of the skin at the upper border of the stoma aperture. A diverting loop ileostomy should be well budded so that the highly corrosive, semiliquid, enteric fluid may be appropriately collected into a stoma bag, and any direct contact with the skin minimized. The everted, dominant, diverting portion of the stoma should occupy approximately two-thirds of the aperture circumference with the remaining third occupied by the diminutive, defunctionalized distal portion of the diverting ileostomy (Figs. 7.15 and 7.16). If appropriately constructed, a loop ileostomy should be effective in diverting the enteric content. Bleeding from a pelvic ileal pouch may become visible in the stoma bag, and it is important to identify the source of bleeding from the distal, defunctionalized limb of the diverting loop ileostomy rather than from the more proximal gastrointestinal tract.

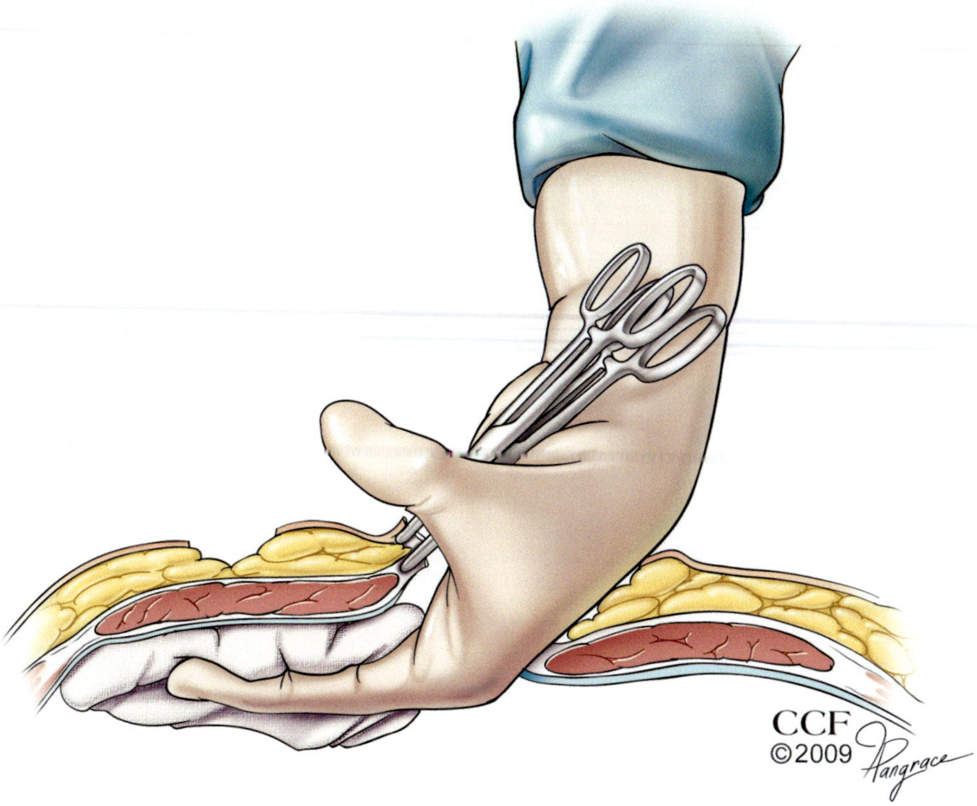

Fig. 7.6 Abdominal wall aperture for ileostomy. Alignment of the skin, fascia, and muscle is maintained by Kocher clamps placed on the dermis and the fascia. The surgeon's hand and intra-abdominal structures are protected by placing a gauze sponge beneath the fascia (Illustration © CCF)

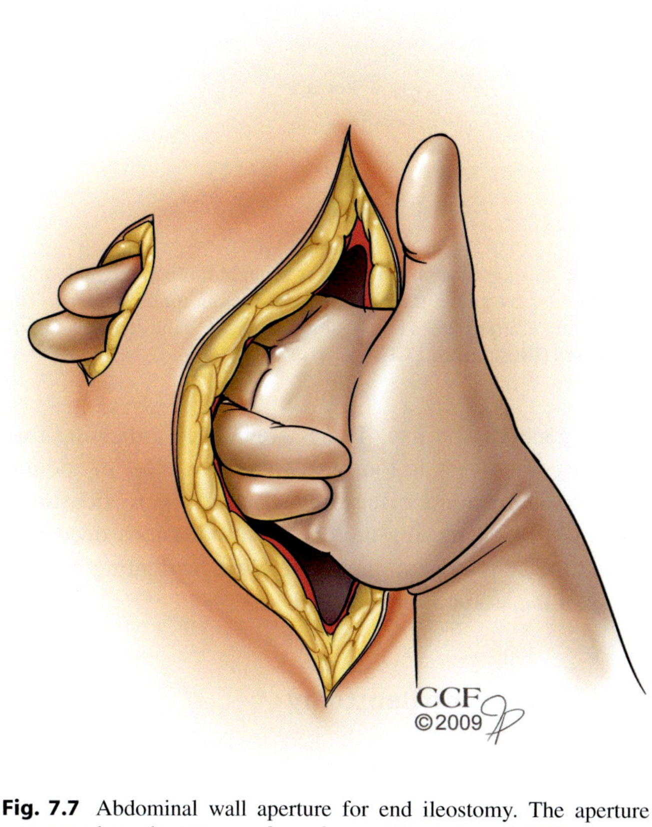

Fig. 7.7 Abdominal wall aperture for end ileostomy. The aperture accommodates the passage of two fingers (Illustration © CCF)

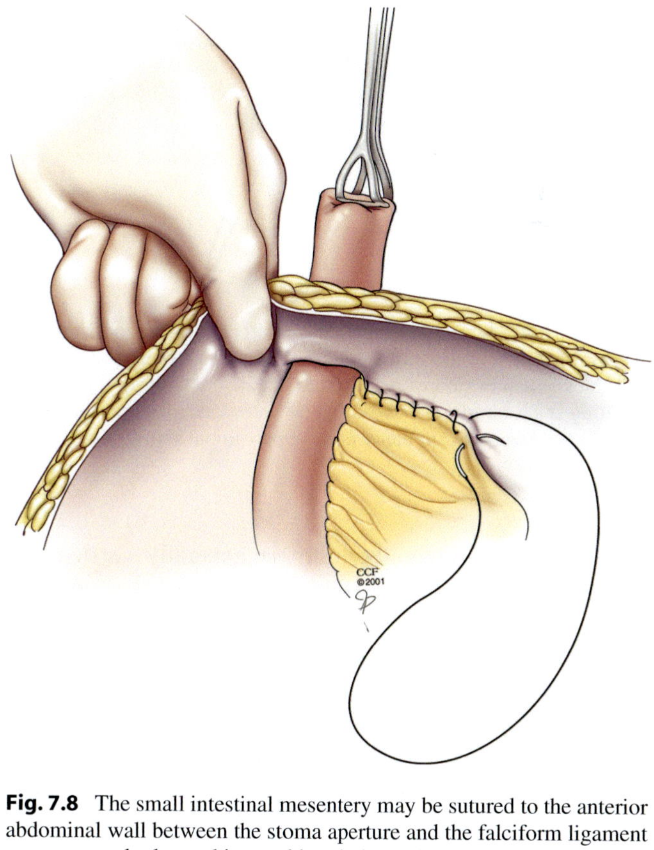

Fig. 7.8 The small intestinal mesentery may be sutured to the anterior abdominal wall between the stoma aperture and the falciform ligament to prevent volvulus and internal herniation (Illustration © CCF)

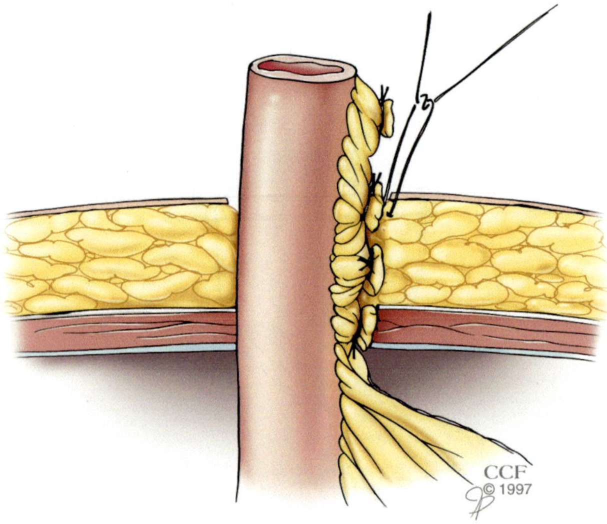

Fig. 7.9 End ileostomy. The ligated vascular pedicles of the terminal ileal mesentery may be sutured to the subcutaneous fat to provide stoma support (Illustration © CCF)

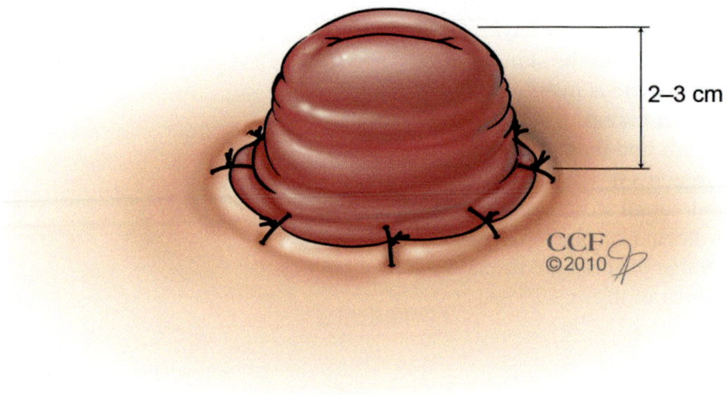

Fig. 7.11 Primarily matured stoma. Ideally, the stoma protrudes 2–3 cm above the skin to prevent contact of the corrosive stoma effluent with the skin (Illustration © CCF)

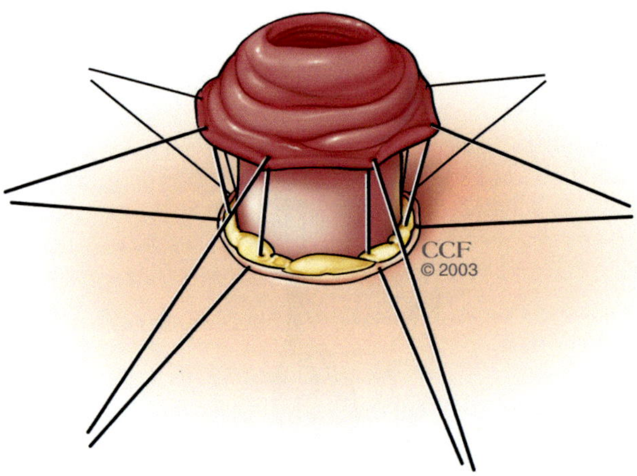

Fig. 7.10 Primary stoma maturation. Absorbable sutures pass through the full thickness of the bowel wall but only through the skin dermis. Full-thickness skin sutures may lead to needle tracts lined with mucus secreting small intestinal mucosa. These secretions may prevent secure adherence between an appliance and the peristomal skin (Illustration © CCF)

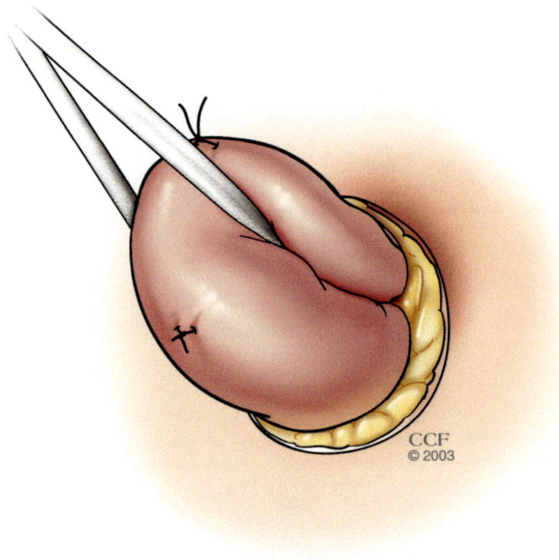

Fig. 7.12 A loop of terminal ileum is brought through the abdominal wall aperture by gentle traction on an encircling umbilical tape. The afferent and efferent limbs of intestine have been identified with different sutures (Illustration © CCF)

Closure of a loop ileostomy is generally carried out 3 months after its creation unless intervening courses of chemotherapy or postoperative complications mandate further delay. Three months generally allows sufficient time for the postoperative adhesions to decrease to a minimum, rendering the ileostomy takedown easier and reducing perioperative morbidity [5]. The use of laparoscopic surgery might reduce the time to closure of an ileostomy by reducing the number and degree of adhesions, although this has not been proven. If postoperative chemotherapy is necessary, a waiting period of 1 month following completion of all courses should generally suffice. There is evidence indicating that wrapping the diverting loop ileostomy in a sheet of sodium hyaluronate membrane may reduce the time to ileostomy takedown by decreasing the degree of adhesions occurring around the stoma aperture and therefore facilitating mobilization of the stoma limbs [6, 7].

Closure of a Loop Ileostomy

A water-soluble contrast enema is generally performed prior to takedown of a diverting loop ileostomy to demonstrate absence of any anastomotic leaks or other abnormalities in the downstream anastomosis [8, 9]. The takedown of the

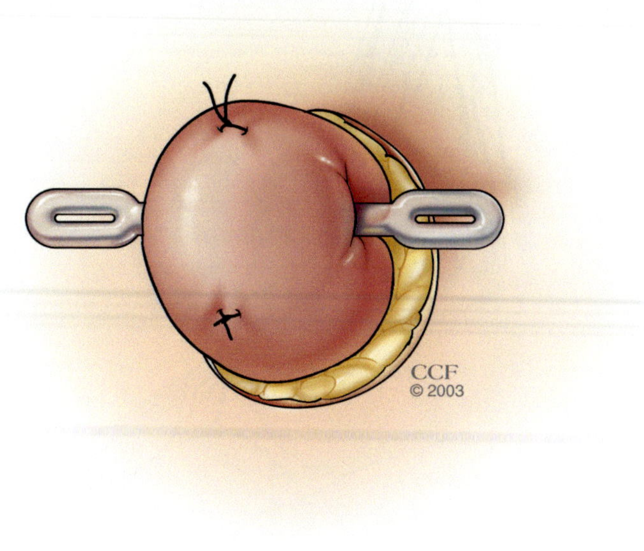

Fig. 7.13 Loop ileostomy. The intestine is secured at the skin level with a stoma rod (Illustration © CCF)

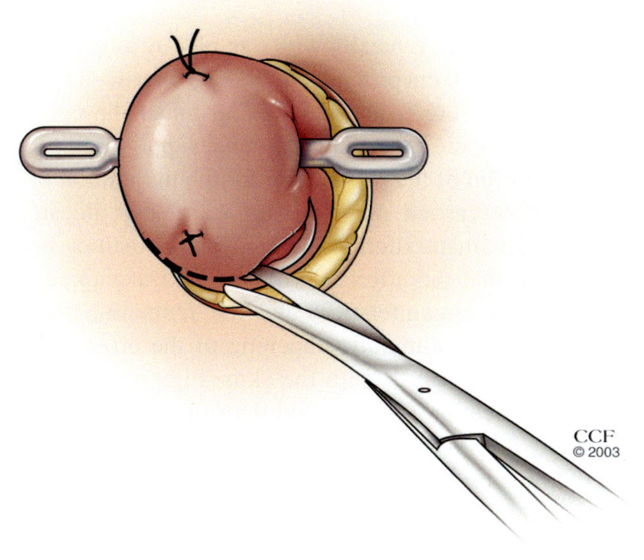

Fig. 7.14 Loop ileostomy. The distal aspect of the intestinal loop is opened from one mesenteric margin to the other (Illustration © CCF)

ileostomy is possible in the vast majority of cases through a local circumferential incision at the level of the stoma itself. Only in the most extreme cases of tenacious adhesions is it necessary to use a midline incision. A circumferential incision is carried out, encompassing 1–2 mm of skin surrounding the diverting loop ileostomy (Fig. 7.17). Both the proximal and distal limbs are then dissected off the surrounding tissues all the way down into the peritoneal cavity. The rim of excised skin may be grasped with clamps to provide traction without causing injury to the intestine (Fig. 7.18). If

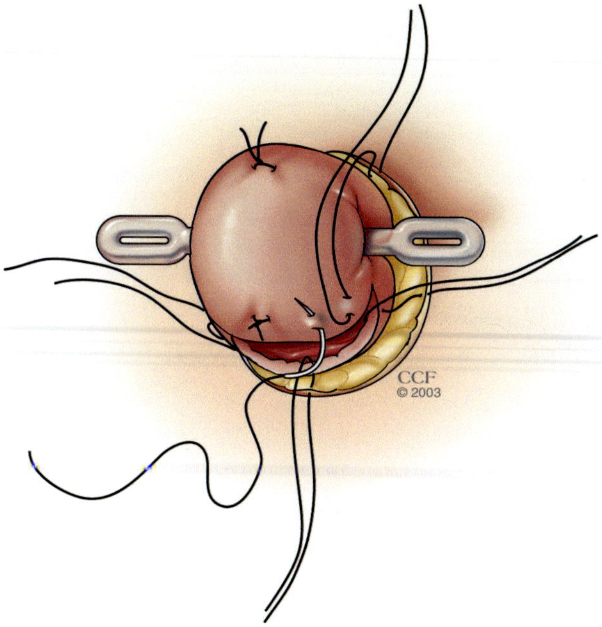

Fig. 7.15 Loop ileostomy. Sutures used to mature the active half of the ileostomy occupy two-thirds of the skin aperture circumference while sutures used to mature the inactive half occupy only one-third of the circumference (Illustration © CCF)

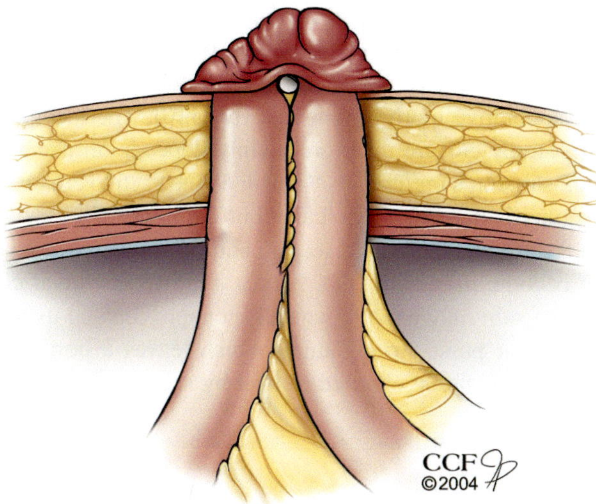

Fig. 7.16 Matured loop ileostomy. The efferent limb opening is small and flush with the skin while the everted afferent limb occupies most of the aperture and protrudes above the skin (Illustration © CCF)

dense adhesions are encountered during this portion of the procedure, it is advisable to lengthen the skin incision cephalad or caudad to improve exposure before resorting to a midline laparotomy. Serosal tears should be immediately sutured as continued traction on the bowel may transform an unrepaired serosal tear into an enterotomy. Following complete bowel mobilization, the tip of the proximal limb is re-inverted, and the lumen of each of the limbs is injected under

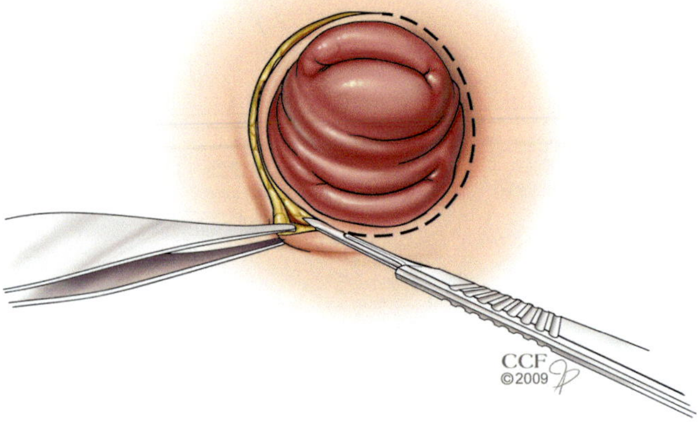

Fig. 7.17 A skin incision is made approximately 2 mm away from the intestine (Illustration © CCF)

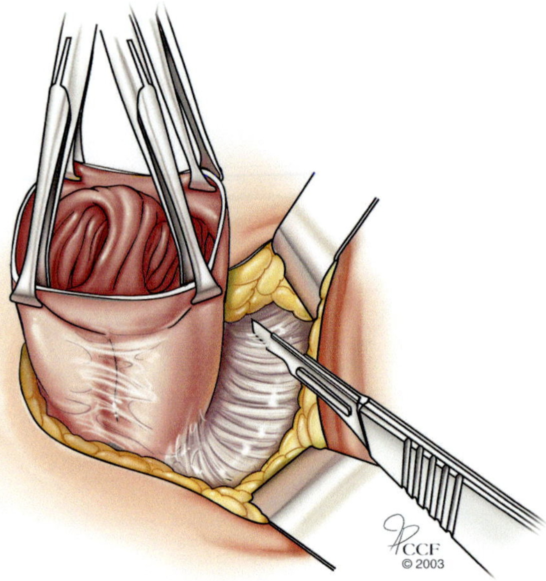

Fig. 7.18 Loop ileostomy closure. Using the peristomal cuff of skin as a handle, the intestine is carefully dissected free of the surrounding subcutaneous fat and fascia (Illustration © CCF)

pressure with diluted Betadine solution or similar colored liquids mixed with air to check for occult leaks from inadvertent enterotomies (Fig. 7.19). Once this has been addressed, the edges of the stoma are trimmed, excising any residual skin and subcutaneous fat. The ileostomy is then closed, either by suturing the resulting anti-mesenteric defect in one or two layers or by performing a side-to-side stapled enteroenteric anastomosis (Fig. 7.20a, b). Studies comparing these two techniques have not demonstrated any differences in postoperative morbidity or recovery [10]. The technique of ileostomy closure therefore mainly depends on the individual surgeon's preference. If the intestine used to create the ileostomy is not suitable to carry out the ileostomy closure, then a short small bowel resection and primary anastomosis may become necessary (Fig. 7.20c). Following fascial closure, the skin may be only partially reapproximated using a subcuticular purse-string suture, which leaves a portion of subcutaneous tissue exposed to heal by secondary intention (Fig. 7.21).

Loop–End Ileostomy

This type of ileostomy may become necessary when the ileum cannot comfortably reach the skin level because of a short mesentery, a thick abdominal wall, or a combination thereof. To create a loop–end ileostomy, the bowel is transected distally, typically with a stapler. A loop of bowel approximately 10 cm proximal to the edge is passed through the stoma aperture while maintaining intact the common mesenteric arcade, providing vascular supply (Fig. 7.22). The orientation of the bowel loop for the maturation of the ileostomy is carried out similarly to a loop ileostomy. Similarly, the maturation of the loop–end ileostomy is carried out so that the afferent proximal limb occupies two-thirds of the circumference, and the remaining third is occupied by the diminutive opening of the efferent limb, which is sutured flush with the skin (Fig. 7.23). Another possible indication for loop–end ileostomy is when a loop ileostomy is converted to permanent ileostomy by dividing the efferent limb of intestine. On rare occasions, a split ileostomy may become necessary to effectively separate the proximal diverting limb from the distal defunctionalized counterpart. In this technique, the bowel is transected, and the proximal end is matured as an end ileostomy. The distal bowel is placed intra-abdominally just underneath the abdominal wall (Fig. 7.24) and oftentimes sutured to the peritoneum to facilitate future retrieval at a time of a possible stoma takedown.

Fig. 7.19 The mobilized intestine is tested for unrecognized enterotomies by irrigating each intestinal limb with a diluted colored liquid and air (Illustration © CCF)

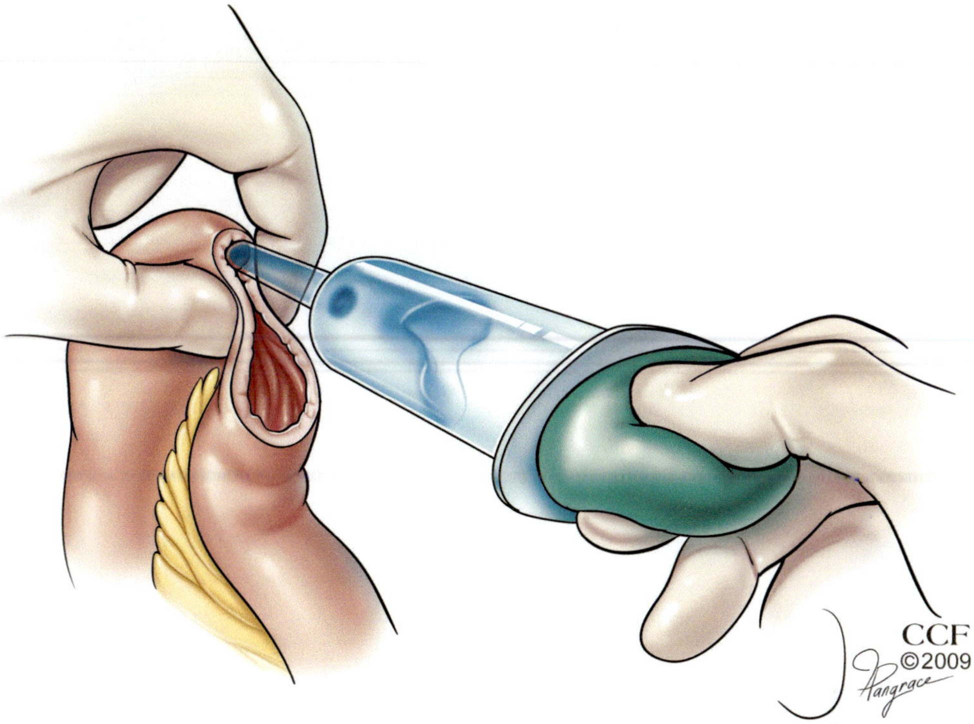

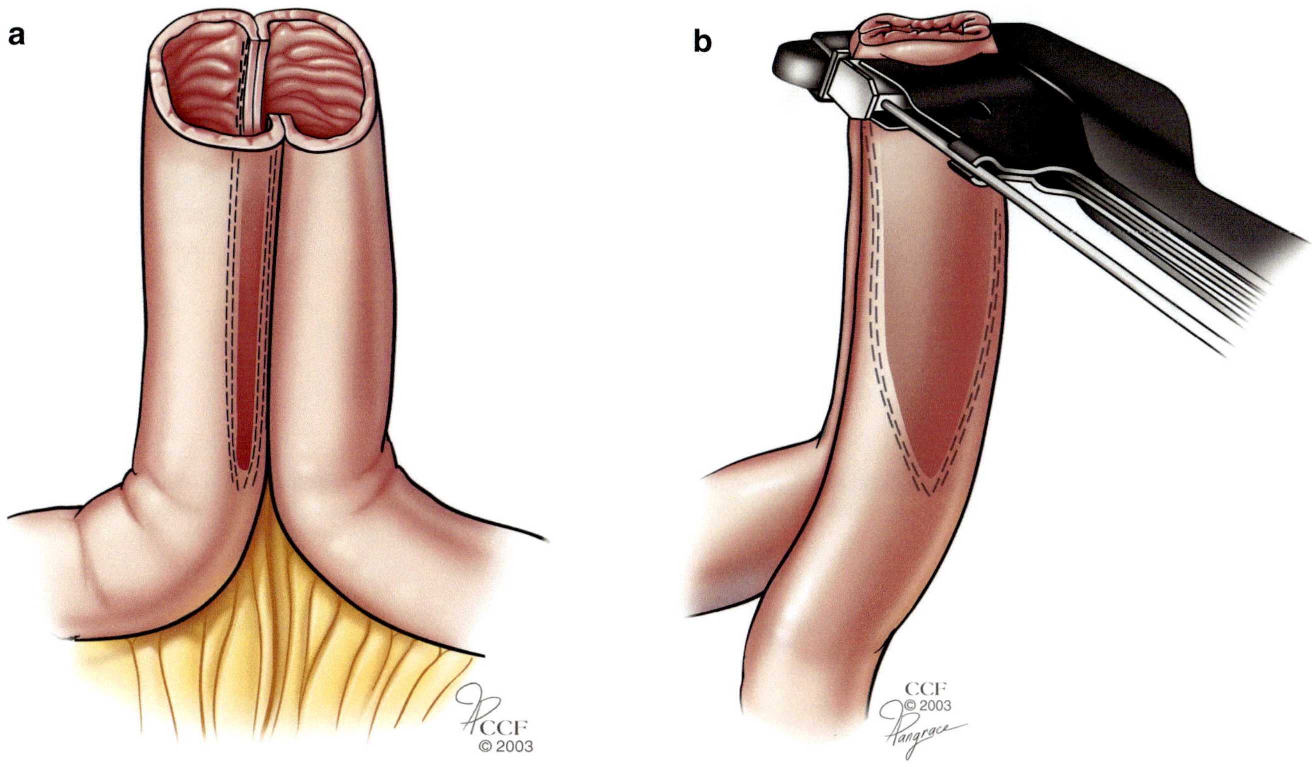

Fig. 7.20 (**a**) A functional end-to-end anastomosis created with a GIA stapling device. (**b**) The enterotomy is closed with a linear stapling device. (**c**) Sewn end-to-end anastomosis (Illustrations © CCF)

Fig. 7.20 (continued)

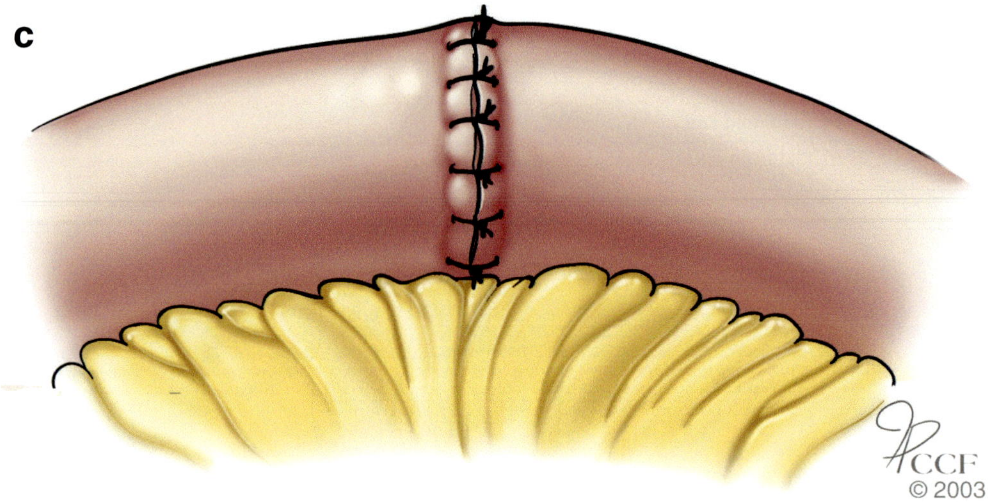

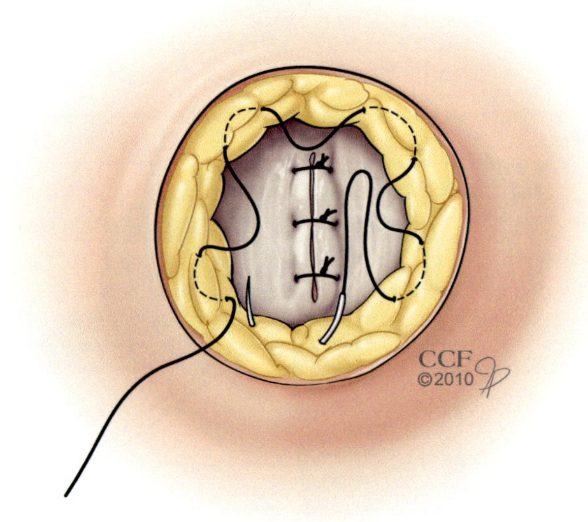

Fig. 7.21 Following fascial closure, the subcutaneous fat may be approximated. The skin is left open to close by secondary intention (Illustration © CCF)

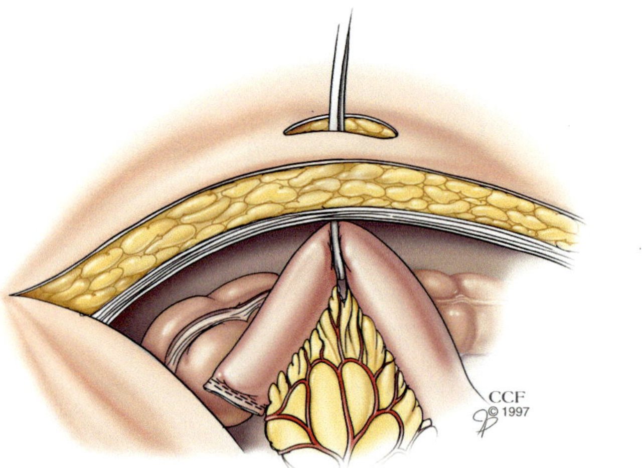

Fig. 7.22 Loop–end ileostomy. The loop of intestine is elevated out of the abdomen with an umbilical tape. Intestinal ischemia is avoided by preserving the terminal vascular arcade (Illustration © CCF)

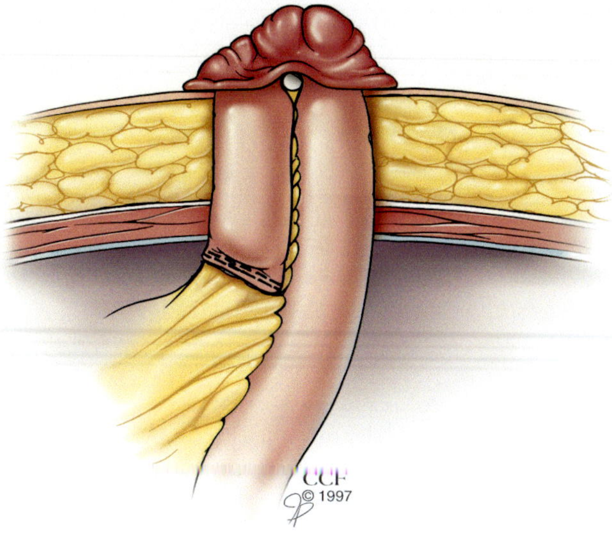

Fig. 7.23 Loop–end ileostomy. The stoma is matured so that the afferent limb occupies two-thirds of the skin aperture while the efferent limb occupies one-third (Illustration © CCF)

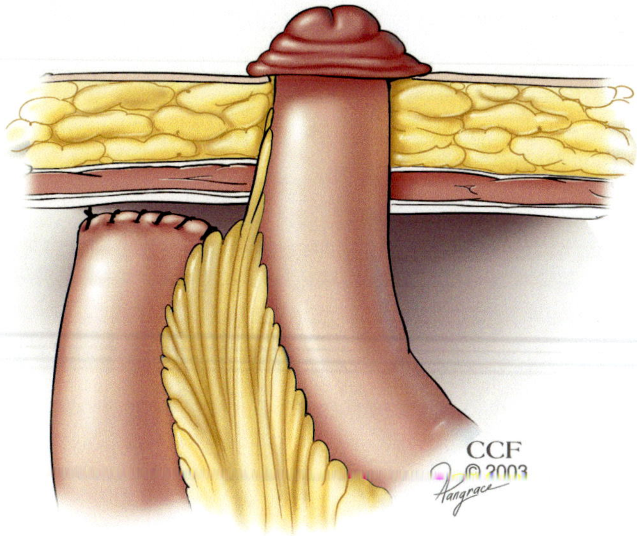

Fig. 7.24 Split ileostomy. The afferent limb is matured using the technique described for end ileostomy. The efferent limb is secured in close proximity to the afferent limb to facilitate identification at the time of stoma closure (Illustration © CCF)

References

1. Rullier E, Le Toux N, Laurent C, et al. Loop ileostomy versus loop colostomy for defunctioning low anastomoses during rectal cancer surgery. World J Surg. 2001;25(3):274–7; discussion 277–8.
2. Guenaga KF, Lustosa SA, Saad SS, et al. Ileostomy or colostomy for temporary decompression of colorectal anastomosis. Cochrane Database Syst Rev. 2007(1):CD004647.
3. Tilney HS, Sains PS, Lovegrove RE, et al. Comparison of outcomes following ileostomy versus colostomy for defunctioning colorectal anastomoses. World J Surg. 2007;31(5):1142–51.
4. Rondelli F, Reboldi P, Rulli A, et al. Loop ileostomy versus loop colostomy for fecal diversion after colorectal or coloanal anastomosis: a meta-analysis. Int J Colorectal Dis. 2009;24:479–88.
5. Perez RO, Habr-Gama A, Seid VE, et al. Loop ileostomy morbidity: timing of closure matters. Dis Colon Rectum. 2006;49(10):1539–45.
6. Tang CL, Seow-Choen F, Fook-Chong S, Eu KW. Bioresorbable adhesion barrier facilitates early closure of the defunctioning ileostomy after rectal excision: a prospective, randomized trial. Dis Colon Rectum. 2003;46(9):1200–7.
7. Tjandra JJ, Chan MK. A sprayable hydrogel adhesion barrier facilitates closure of defunctioning loop ileostomy: a randomized trial. Dis Colon Rectum. 2008;51(6):956–60.
8. Hrung JM, Levine MS, Rombeau JL, et al. Total proctocolectomy and ileoanal pouch: the role of contrast studies for evaluating postoperative leaks. Abdom Imaging. 1998;23(4):375–9.
9. Dolinsky D, Levine MS, Rubesin SE, et al. Utility of contrast enema for detecting anastomotic strictures after total proctocolectomy and ileal pouch-anal anastomosis. AJR Am J Roentgenol. 2007;189(1):25–9.
10. Wong KS, Remzi FH, Gorgun E, et al. Loop ileostomy closure after restorative proctocolectomy: outcome in 1,504 patients. Dis Colon Rectum. 2005;48(2):243–50.

Medical Management of the High-Output Enterostomy and Enterocutaneous Fistula

8

Neha Parekh and Douglas L. Seidner

Introduction

Medical management of the high-output enterostomy or enterocutaneous fistula (ECF) requires an understanding of mechanisms behind the malabsorption associated with short bowel syndrome (SBS) and intestinal failure (IF). A traditional definition of SBS is <200 cm of remaining viable jejunum and ileum following surgical resection for disease, trauma, infarction, or congenital defect. A more functional definition involves consideration of the quality of the bowel in continuity and the clinical status of the patient, both of which may further interfere with absorptive capacity of the bowel.

A thorough examination of remaining functional and structural anatomy can reveal potential causes of persistent malabsorption. Inflammation or infection within the bowel can result from a fistula, abdominal abscess, anastomotic leak, or active disease and can contribute to bowel dysfunction and IF. Injury and destruction of the cells lining the gastrointestinal (GI) tract reduce the mucosal surface area available for absorption leading to an excessive and frequent watery fecal output. Basic principles of nutrient and fluid absorption within the healthy and compromised GI tract should be fully understood in order to formulate the most effective plan of care for patients with SBS and IF.

Normal Gastrointestinal Function

An intact and disease-free intestinal tract is remarkably efficient at digesting and absorbing a wide variety of foodstuffs. The small bowel in an adult can range from 350 to 650 cm long and has a surface area of 3,300 cm^2, while the colon is approximately 150 cm in length [1]. Nearly all nutrient absorption takes place within the first 150 cm of the small bowel, with more than 75–80% of dietary carbohydrate and lipid absorption occurring in the first 70 cm [2]. Up to 9 L of fluid are orally consumed and secreted by the bowel over the course of a day, with the majority secreted and reabsorbed in the first 100 cm of the jejunum (see Fig. 8.1). Gastric emptying is primarily regulated by input from the vagus nerve and the release of neurohumoral factors from the duodenum in response to a meal, while intestinal transit time is prolonged by neurohumoral factors secreted by the distal small bowel. The ileocecal valve and colon also play an important role in prolonging transit time [3]. Bile salts, which emulsify dietary fat and complement the activity of pancreatic lipases, are absorbed in the distal 100 cm of ileum to maintain a normal concentration of these compounds in the enterohepatic circulation [4].

The colon also performs a wide range of functions vital to maintaining adequate absorptive capacity of the gastrointestinal (GI) tract. In addition to prolonging intestinal transit, the colon may absorb up to 5 L of fluid each day (see Fig. 8.1) [5]. Oligopeptides that are not absorbed by the small bowel may be salvaged in the colon through upregulation of the mucosal transport protein PepT1 [6]. Unabsorbed carbohydrates and soluble fiber are fermented by bacteria in the colon to produce short-chain fatty acids (SCFA), which provide an additional source of energy and act to enhance salt and water absorption in the distal colon [7].

Physiology of Intestinal Failure

Intestinal failure (IF) can result in extensive nutrient, fluid, and electrolyte losses. Whether intestinal failure occurs or not depends on the length of remaining bowel, the presence or absence of mucosal disease, and the segments of bowel that are in continuity with the upper digestive tract and thus exposed to oral intake [8]. While reduced absorptive surface

N. Parekh (✉)
Intestinal Rehabilitation and Transplant Nutrition, Digestive Disease Institute, Cleveland Clinic Foundation, Cleveland, OH, USA
e-mail: parekhn@ccf.org

D.L. Seidner
Division of Gastroenterology, Hepatology and Nutrition, Vanderbilt Center for Human Nutrition, Vanderbilt University Medical Center, Nashville, TN, USA

V.W. Fazio et al. (eds.), *Atlas of Intestinal Stomas*,
DOI 10.1007/978-0-387-78851-7_8, © Springer Science+Business Media, LLC 2012

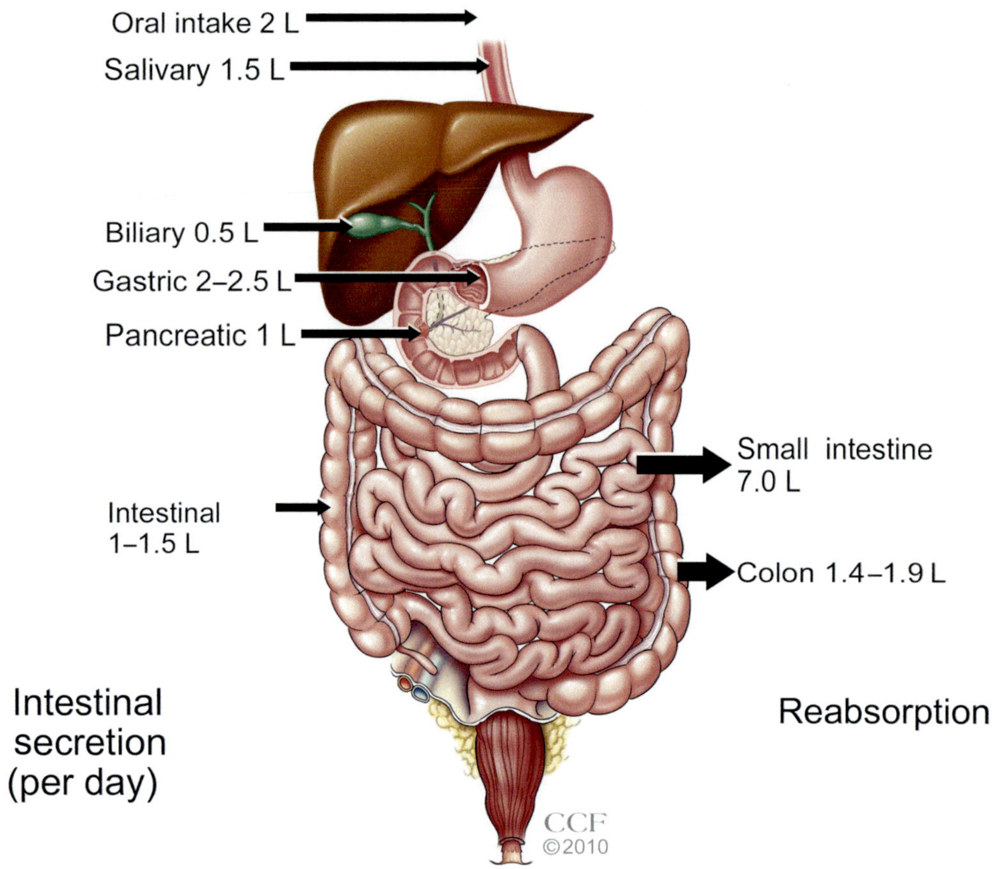

Fig. 8.1 Intestinal fluid secretion and absorption. Digestive secretions range from 6 to 7 L in addition to a typical oral intake of 2 L each day. Almost all of this is reabsorbed by the small bowel leaving 1–2 L to be absorbed by the colon. This leaves a fecal wet weight of approximately 0.1 L. While the normal small bowel can nearly double its capacity to absorb fluid, this is not possible after small intestinal resection. On the other hand, colon fluid absorption can increase two to three times above normal to compensate for the malabsorption of fluid seen after small intestinal resection (Illustration © CCF)

area is predominantly responsible for malabsorption in SBS, other factors may play a role in the development of IF. These factors include gastric acid hypersecretion, inactivation of pancreatic enzymes, diminution of the bile salt pool, rapid intestinal transit, and small bowel bacterial overgrowth. In some cases, these factors can result in severe malabsorption even when remaining bowel length is not exceedingly short. Conversely, the absorptive capacity of the colon and intestinal adaptation may allow patients with short bowel syndrome to absorb an adequate amount of their oral intake and transition off of parenteral nutrition. Therefore, an understanding of these factors is necessary when developing a treatment plan. Complications such as gallstone formation, renal calculi, liver dysfunction, and metabolic bone disease can develop over time. Knowledge of these problems, including their pathogenesis, prevention, and treatment, is important when caring for patients with IF as well [9].

In a study of 148 patients who underwent intestinal resection, Nordgaard and colleagues found that the colon could salvage as much as 4.2 MJ/day (1,000 kcal/day) of energy from SCFA, depending on the extent of bowel resection [10]. Jeppesen and Mortensen studied parenteral energy requirements in a group of home parenteral nutrition (PN) patients who had varying degrees of remaining bowel length [11]. In the 24 patients with <100 cm small bowel (mean, 50 cm) remaining, the amount of energy delivered parenterally was reduced by half if 50% or more of the colon was functional. Therefore, preservation of the colon is of key importance during surgery, and all available bowel should be placed back into continuity as soon as clinically safe in order to maximize absorptive potential.

There are three anatomical configurations, depicted in Fig. 8.2, that can remain following intestinal resection. The first configuration shows a jejunal resection with intact terminal ileum and colon, which, for example, may follow an intestinal volvulus. This configuration is generally well tolerated due to the ability of the remaining bowel to compensate by increasing absorptive function, prolonging intestinal transit time, and maintaining bile salt concentrations. The second configuration occurs after ileocolonic resection for Crohn's disease. A terminal ileal resection of <100 cm may lead to a chronic bile-salt (cholerrheic) diarrhea, whereas a more extensive ileal resection will provoke an initial large volume, watery diarrhea due to loss of bile salts, followed by chronic steatorrhea when the bile salt pool is depleted. The third configuration is seen following acute occlusion of the superior mesenteric artery with resection of much of the jejunum and ileum and most if not all of the colon. In this

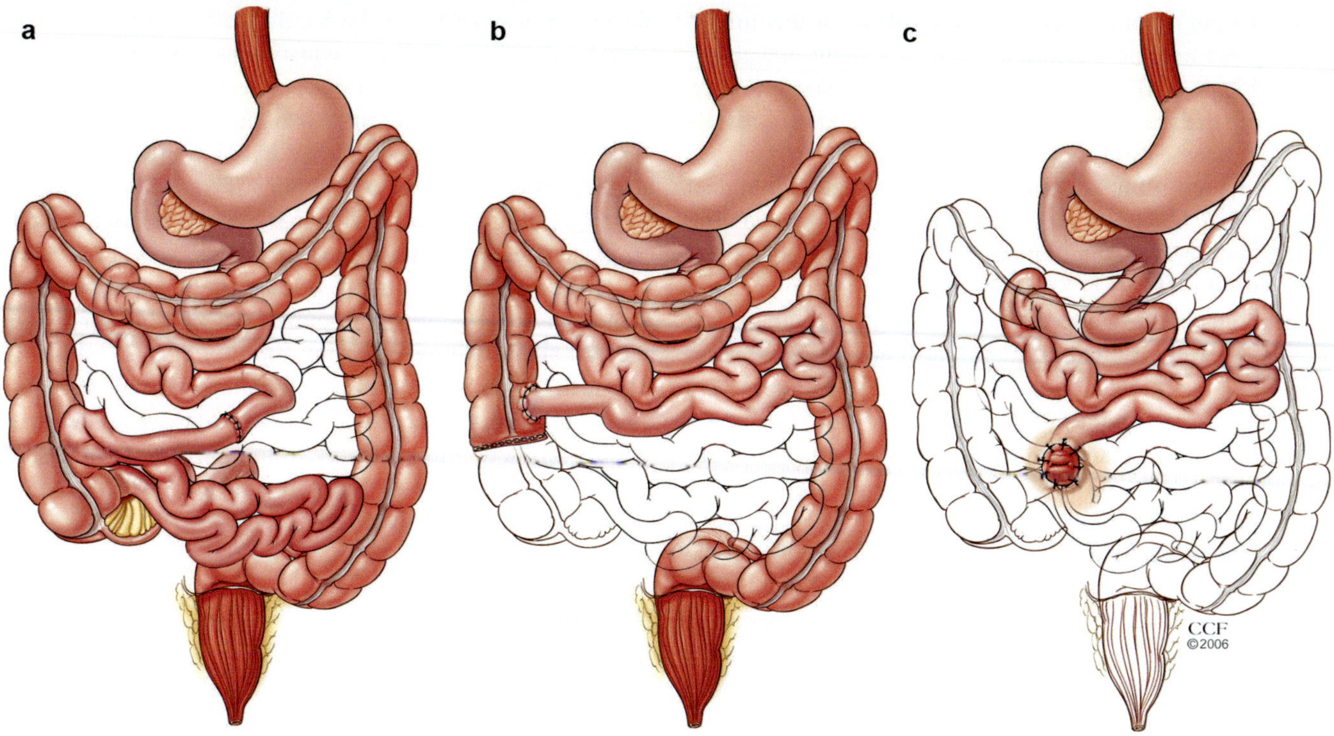

Fig. 8.2 Remnant anatomy following extensive intestinal resection. (**a**) Jejunal resection with intact terminal ileum and colon. (**b**) Ileal and proximal colon resection with intact jejunum and distal colon. (**c**) Jejunoileal and colonic resection with intact proximal jejunum (Illustration © CCF)

case, nutrient, fluid, and electrolyte balance can be severely impaired. A similar situation may be seen if the anastomosis from the first or second configuration leaks and develops into an enterocutaneous fistula.

After extensive small bowel resection, adaptation of the remaining intestine begins quickly and proceeds for up to 2 years, with the main response occurring within a few months of resection. The adaptive process can be divided into three clinical stages. The first stage occurs during the immediate postoperative period when the loss of GI secretions can be extraordinarily high. During this stage, fluid, electrolytes, and nutrients are provided parenterally until the patient is stabilized. During the second stage, there is a gradual transition from PN to enteral nutrition (EN) or oral feedings as adaptation occurs. In the third stage, there is the realization of complete independence from PN in patients with sufficient intestinal absorptive capacity and adequate enteral or oral intake. In patients with high volume GI losses who are scheduled to undergo bowel reconnection within 3 months of their initial surgery, PN or intravenous fluids (IVF) should be given without regard to adaptation because this process takes at least a few months for most individuals.

Unfortunately, definitive guidelines do not exist on whether any particular patient will require PN, IVF with electrolytes, EN, or an oral diet to replace losses in the setting of IF. In general, patients with <100 cm jejunum-ileum proximal to the fistula or enterostomy will likely require PN support until bowel reconnection [12]. Patients with 100–150 cm of functional jejunum-ileum may be supported with diet and a combination of IVF and/or EN until reconnection. Those with more than 150 cm of jejunum-ileum are often able to maintain adequate nutrition and hydration through oral measures alone after the initial surgical trauma and/or infectious process subsides. It is important to emphasize that therapy is individualized, outcomes are closely monitored, and interventions are routinely modified based on patient progress.

Assessment of the Anatomical Configuration and Function of the GI Tract

The first step in forming a treatment plan for a patient with a high-output enterostomy or fistula is an assessment of the anatomy of the remaining bowel. The best way to determine intestinal length is by measuring along the antimesenteric border from the ligament of Treitz at the time of surgery. Remaining small bowel lengths and colonic proportions have been shown to correlate with parenteral energy requirements in patients receiving home PN [13]. Although bowel length is an important factor in determining mode of therapy for IF, a measurement of remnant bowel length is sometimes difficult to obtain at the time of surgery. Radiologic techniques such as a small bowel follow through (SBFT) give a qualitative estimate; however, even with the use of instruments like the opisometer, results have not been entirely accurate [14].

Plasma citrulline appears to be a simple biological marker that has been shown to correlate with remaining bowel length, intestinal enterocyte mass, and absorptive function [15–18]. It is a readily measured amino acid not incorporated into endogenous or exogenous proteins and produced primarily within small bowel enterocytes. Crenn et al. studied plasma citrulline levels of 57 SBS patients and found that a threshold of 20 μmol/L was able to discern transient from permanent intestinal failure, defined as continued dependence on PN 2 years post-final digestive circuit modification [15].

It is important to note that citrulline levels are low in the immediate post-extensive bowel resection phase, and levels increase over time with adaptation. We recently evaluated plasma citrulline levels of 30 PN-dependent patients with SBS in the post-adaptation phase and were able to confirm the ability of post-absorptive plasma citrulline to estimate small bowel length [18]. A citrulline cutoff of 26 μmol/L had a sensitivity of 80% and a specificity of 75.6% in predicting the need for long-term PN in our SBS population.

Once bowel length is established, an assessment of intestinal function is necessary as treatment options for patients with malabsorption vary with both the extent and condition of the remaining intestine. A contrast-enhanced computer tomography scan can provide insight into fistula or enterostomy location and the presence of abscesses, leaks, or obstructions. The pathology of any resected anatomic specimens should be evaluated for the presence of active mucosal disease such as Crohn's disease or radiation enteritis and other conditions that can adversely affect absorption. Small bowel fistula and stoma output should be cultured to rule out *Clostridium difficile* enteritis, a rare but potentially fatal infection [19]. Celiac disease that may not have been apparent prior to intestinal resection should be considered when diarrhea cannot be completely explained by the surgical history and can be evaluated by measuring anti-tissue transglutaminase (tTGA) and IgA anti-endomysium antibodies (EMA) in the blood, and duodenal mucosal biopsy on upper endoscopy.

Both simple and complex measures of intestinal absorptive capacity exist to help make therapeutic decisions and track progress for patients with IF. Net nutrient absorption can be quantitatively measured by subtracting the nutrient content of fecal collections from the nutrient content of oral intake over the same period of time. In a meticulously performed balance study, Jeppesen and Mortensen found that patients with SBS were able to avoid parenteral fluid and nutrients if fluid absorption was ≥1.4 kg/day and energy absorption was ≥84% of the basal metabolic rate as calculated by the Harris Benedict equation [20]. Clinically available testing includes a 72-h stool collection for fecal fat and the D-xylose absorption test. When malabsorption is severe, these tests are generally not necessary. They are occasionally helpful when one needs to determine if transition from parenteral therapy to an oral diet is feasible or when one considers placement of an enteral feeding device.

Rapid motility of effluent through the GI tract is common in patients with a high-output enterostomy or fistula and can signal the need for anti-motility agents. Intestinal transit time can be measured radiographically by SBFT or by the time to appearance of an ingested dye in stool or ostomy effluent. Ingestion of a colored dye to measure intestinal transit time requires monitoring of fecal output for appearance of the dye.

Nutrition Assessment

The decision of whether to replace lost fluids and nutrients via PN or maintain the patient on oral supplementation with EN and/or IVF and electrolytes hinges on an accurate nutrition assessment. Malnutrition has an adverse effect on nearly every organ of the body including the GI tract. It can impair GI function by delaying gastric emptying and thereby prolong time to resumption of normal oral intake after surgery. Absorption is impaired by atrophy of the intestinal mucosa following prolonged periods of inadequate oral nutrition as well. Malnourished patients are also more prone to the development of fistulas postoperatively with an increased mortality rate and a decreased rate of spontaneous fistula closure [21, 22].

Simple clinical measures of nutritional status and intestinal function include dietary intake and daily fluid balance, changes in body weight, and laboratory values. Each of these parameters should be evaluated as a whole since many individual measures are not specific for intestinal function, have a high level of variance, and may take time to reflect changes in nutrition and bowel function. Hospitalized patients should be taught how to record total daily oral, enteral, and parenteral fluid intake, and both urinary and all GI output, so that this practice may continue in the home setting. In general, maintenance of a positive fluid balance with at least 500 mL more fluid intake than total daily output is desired in order to ensure sufficient hydration. Patients with consistently more fecal output than oral intake will require at least intravenous fluid for replacement of losses until absorptive improves. Adults with <1 L of urine output per day are usually dehydrated and will also require extra fluid that often must be given intravenously.

Body weight may be assessed as a change in weight over time or as an expression of weight for height known as body

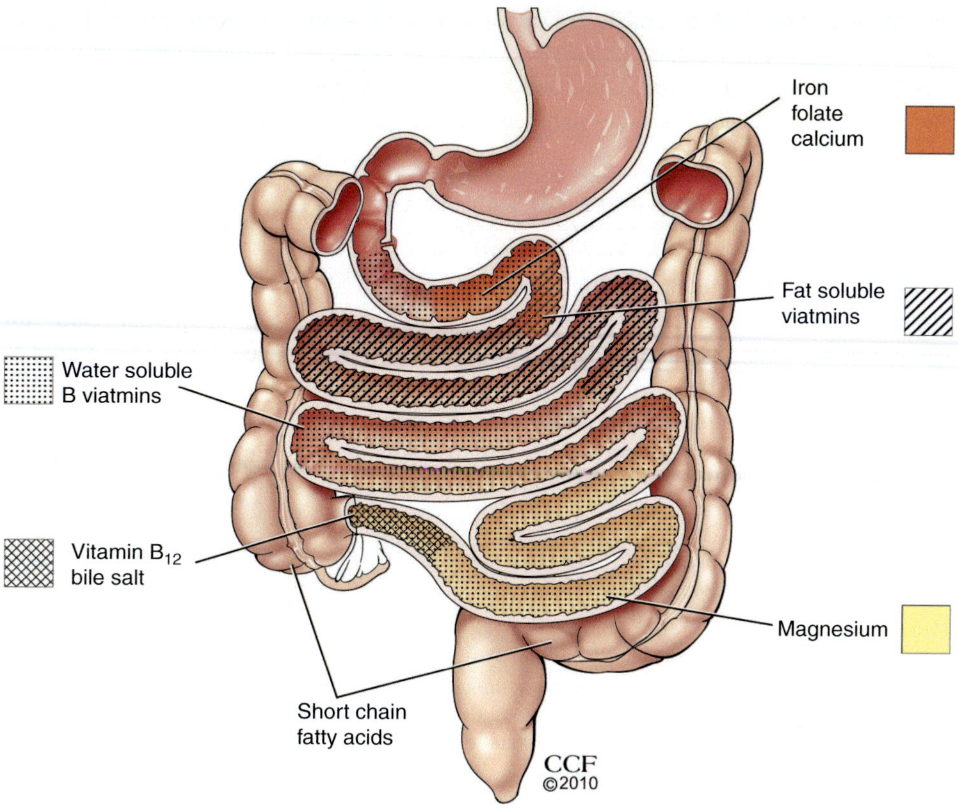

Fig. 8.3 Sites for nutrient absorption in the intestinal tract. Iron, folate, and calcium are best absorbed in the duodenum and proximal jejunum. Fat soluble vitamins are usually absorbed in the first 100–150 cm of small bowel, while the water soluble B vitamins are absorbed throughout the small bowel. Vitamin B12 and bile salts are predominantly absorbed in the terminal ileum. Magnesium is absorbed throughout the small bowel, but maximal absorption occurs in the distal small bowel (Illustration © CCF)

mass index (BMI). The weight maintained over the longest period of time in good health is considered the usual body weight (UBW). Weight fluctuations are common in patients with bowel disease due to changes in hydration and in the ability to eat. Patients experiencing a loss of more than 10% UBW over 1–2 months or more than 20% UBW over 6–12 months have lost a significant amount of lean body mass beyond fluid fluctuations and will likely require PN for repletion. Similarly, those with a BMI below 15 are considered severely malnourished and often require PN until adequate absorption can be established through the oral or enteral route.

Patients with IF commonly become deficient in magnesium, calcium, zinc, and certain vitamins depending on the area of bowel resection (see Fig. 8.3). Laboratory testing should consist of a comprehensive metabolic panel that includes electrolytes, blood sugar, renal, and liver function tests. Electrolytes and minerals to be measured include serum calcium, magnesium, phosphorus, and, when serum albumin is low, ionized calcium. Trace elements, fat-soluble vitamins, parathyroid hormone, and vitamin B12 should be measured when a prolonged history of malabsorption or severe diarrhea exists. A careful examination should be performed for clinical signs of deficiency such as diminished stores of fat and muscle, cheilosis, glossitis, dermatitis, alopecia, and edema (see Table 8.1). Patients should be questioned regarding signs of fluid and electrolyte deficiencies including excess thirst and the development of weakness and paresthesias.

Visceral proteins such as albumin, prealbumin, and transferrin are important predictors of morbidity and mortality in patients with ECFs. In a study of 79 patients with gastrointestinal cutaneous fistulas, a serum transferrin above 175 mg/dL at the start of PN therapy was shown to be predictive of spontaneous closure; however, transferrin levels did not increase with parenteral repletion in patients achieving fistula closure [23].

Nutrient and Fluid Requirements

Many factors contribute to malnutrition in patients with high-output enterostomies or fistulas. Oral intake is often limited for prolonged periods of time due to a fear of increased output or a general disinterest in food associated with uncontrolled abdominal pain, high-dose narcotics, and a chronic state of dehydration. There is also a significant loss of ingested nutrients and fluid and electrolyte-rich small bowel secretions due to abnormal absorption and reabsorption. Lastly, ongoing sepsis and inflammation can result in a catabolic state in which protein and energy demands are increased.

Initial daily energy requirements for patients with high-output ECFs or enterostomies should be estimated at 25–30 kcal/kg/

day. Many patients with extreme losses and/or hypercatabolism associated with sepsis require up to 45 kcal/kg/day (1.5–2.0 times their resting energy expenditure) and 1.5–2.5 g protein/kg/day in order to achieve positive nitrogen balance [24–26]. A recent prospective, observational, cohort study evaluating nitrogen losses in patients with open versus closed abdomens found that nitrogen loss through the open abdomen may be accounted for by using the following equation [27]:

$$\text{Nitrogen balance} = \text{Nitrogen intake} - (24\text{ h urine urea nitrogen} + 4\text{ g nitrogen} + 2\text{ g nitrogen / L daily abdominal fluid output}).$$

Caloric and protein provisions should be periodically adjusted based on patient response to therapy with progress evidenced by wound healing, weight gain toward goal, and improved functional status.

Daily fluid requirements for patients with high-output ECFs or enterostomies are based on the patient's total daily intake from oral, enteral, and intravenous sources subtracted by the patient's daily urinary and GI losses with provision of an additional 500 mL/day for insensible fluid loss (see Table 8.2). Initial daily electrolyte provisions are estimated using a typical daily requirement with additional sodium, chloride, bicarbonate, and potassium per liter of daily enteric loss (see Table 8.3). Fluid and electrolytes are subsequently adjusted according to laboratory values, change in weight, change in oral intake versus fluid loss, and the presence of signs and symptoms found with deficiencies that have already been discussed.

Clinical guidelines for vitamin and mineral supplementation in patients with high-output fistulas and enterostomies have been published, although the supporting research to establish evidence-based standards of practice is lacking (see Table 8.4). Many supplements are incompletely absorbed due to rapid transit, altered pH, and reduced endogenous production of factors enhancing absorption of micronutrients in

Table 8.1 Nutrition-focused physical exam

Possible deficiency	Body system	Symptoms/signs
Protein, protein-calorie, zinc, copper, biotin	Hair	Lackluster, thinness, sparseness, dryness, dyspigmentation, easy pluckability, texture change
Riboflavin, niacin, pyridoxine, iron	Face	Paleness, facial swelling, greasy, scaling around nostrils (nasolabial seborrhea)
Iron, vitamins A, C, and B12, riboflavin, pyridoxine, folate	Eyes	Pale whites of eyes and eyelid lining (pale conjunctivae), redness and fissuring of eyelid corners, dullness and dryness (Bitot's spots)
Riboflavin, niacin, pyridoxine, iron	Mouth	Redness, lesions, or scars at corners of mouth (angular stomatitis), swelling and redness of lips and mouth (cheilosis)
Niacin, pyridoxine, riboflavin, vitamin B12, folate, iron	Tongue	Smoothness, slickness, beefiness, redness, pain (glossitis), swollen magenta color
Vitamin C	Gums	Swelling, sponginess, bleeding, receding
Vitamins A, C, and K, zinc, essential fatty acids, protein	Skin	Dryness, scaling, lightening of color (diffuse pigmentation), rough, "goose-flesh" (follicular hyperkeratinosis), small hemorrhages (petechiae), excessive bruising, flaking, edema, delayed wound healing
Iron	Nails	Spoon-shaped (koilonychias), pale, brittle, ridged
Protein-calorie, vitamins C and D, calcium	Musculoskeletal	Enlarged joints, hemorrhages, muscle and fat wasting, myalgias, arthralgias, tetany
Thiamin, vitamin B12	Neurological	Mental confusion, irritability, psychomotor changes, motor weakness, sensory loss

Table 8.2 Daily parenteral fluid requirement for adults

Normal requirements are usually based on weight

30–35 mL/kg/day × 80 kg = 2,400–2,800 mL

Requirements for high gastrointestinal output focus on enteral I/O

Calculation uses normal urine output rather than actual output, which can be abnormal in the postoperative period, and solve equation for all parenteral fluid (TPN, antibiotics, etc.)

First, calculate total output based on daily average

Output = urine + stoma + insensible losses

5,400 ml = 1,700 ml + 3,200 ml + 500 ml

Next, calculate the average of the measured oral intake for the last few days

Oral intake = 1,500 mL

Finally, calculate the parenteral fluid requirement

Parenteral fluid requirement = total output − oral intake

3,900 ml = 5,400 ml − 1,500 ml

Table 8.3 Approximate electrolyte composition of various body fluids (mEq/L)

Source		Na	K	Cl	HCO_3
Gastric	pH<4	60	10	90	
	pH>4	100	10	100	
Pancreas		140	5	75	90
Bile		140	5	100	35
Small bowel		100	15	100	25
Colon		60	30	45	45

Table 8.4 Common oral vitamin and mineral supplements for adults with severe malabsorption

Micronutrient[a]	Strength[b]	Dose[c]
Vitamin A	5,000 IU	1–2 tabs daily
Vitamin D_2	50,000 IU	2–3 times/week
Vitamin E	400 IU	1–2 tabs daily
Vitamin K	5 mg	1–2 tabs daily
Calcium carbonate	500 mg tab	1–2 tabs TID
Magnesium lactate	84 mg tab	1–3 tabs TID
Potassium chloride	20 mEq tab	1–2 tabs daily
Sodium bicarbonate	1 mL = 1 mEq $NaHCO_3$	10 mL TID
Chromium picolinate	200 μ[micro]g tab	1 tab TID
Copper sulfate	3 mg tab	1–2 tabs daily
Zinc sulfate	220 mg tab	1–3 tabs daily

[a]Dosage forms given for tablets and capsules. Liquid formulation and alternative salts are available
[b]Other strengths are available
[c]Laboratory monitoring is necessary to assure adequate dosing and to avoid excess

the remaining bowel. In general, patients with malabsorption sustained without PN should receive up to three divided doses of the recommended daily allowance (RDA) for vitamins and trace minerals in tablet, powder, chewable, or liquid form.

Monitoring of serum electrolytes (weekly to monthly), vitamins, trace elements, and essential fatty acids (every 3–6 months), as well as annual bone densitometry should be performed on all patients with SBS until stable [28]. Additional calcium supplementation is routinely given to these patients in divided doses of 1,000–3,000 mg/day. Vitamin D should be given in doses of 1,200 IU daily to 50,000 IU three times weekly if serum 25-hydroxy vitamin D levels are below 30 mg/dL. Vitamin B12 absorption is interrupted in patients who have had >60 cm of terminal ileum resected. Supplementation of B12 is generally given by subcutaneous or intramuscular injection of 1,000 mcg/month. A nasal gel is also available that provides 500 mcg/dose and should be taken once weekly to maintain remission after parenteral repletion. Patients lose approximately 12 mg zinc/L of small bowel effluent, and often require more than that provided through standard IV multiple trace element preparations or standard multivitamins with minerals [29].

Magnesium deficiency is very common in patients with extensive fistula or stoma output, and certain forms of oral magnesium replacement can further aggravate GI losses. Hypomagnesemia may be a product of secondary hyperaldosteronism, and sodium depletion should be corrected prior to initiation of magnesium repletion. Oral supplementation with magnesium lactate or gluconate taken 1 h away from meals and at bedtime in total doses of up to 4,000 mg elemental Mg/day may be most effective [30]. If oral repletion at maximum doses is not successful, IVF with sodium chloride and magnesium sulfate (2–4 g Mg sulfate in 500–1,000 mL of 0.45–0.9% normal saline infused over 8 h 3–7 times/week) may be required [31, 32]. Magnesium infusion should be over no <8 h as more rapid infusion can result in increased renal wasting.

Medical Management of the High-Output Enterostomy

Once the patient has been thoroughly evaluated, an informed decision may be made as to what mode of therapy to undertake. Medical management of high-output enterostomies and ECFs is directed toward minimizing GI symptoms and maximizing absorptive capacity to maintain fluid, electrolyte, and nutrient balance. Treatment options are nutritional, pharmaceutical, and surgical, with many patients requiring a combination of treatments. This section will focus on nutritional and pharmacologic measures.

Nutrition Therapy

The primary goal of nutrition therapy is to prevent malnutrition and dehydration by maintaining adequate nutrient and fluid balance. A secondary goal of luminal nutrition is to promote bowel adaptation and improved absorption following extensive intestinal resection. Oral nutrients, EN, PN, or a combination of the three may be used depending on the length and anatomy of remaining bowel and the patient's absorptive capacity.

Patients with <100 cm jejunum-ileum in an end enterostomy or ECF, <65 cm jejunum anastomosed to colon or <30 cm jejunum-ileum anastomosed to colon will likely require long-term PN or IVF to maintain nutrient and fluid balance [33]. Those with preexisting malnutrition will require PN for at least 7–10 days following an extensive small bowel resection regardless of remaining anatomy and bowel lengths [31]. Thereafter, all attempts should be made to transition the patient onto an oral or enteral diet when clinically feasible.

Specific alterations in diet can lead to a significant reduction in fecal losses and should be considered the first line of therapy in most patients with high-output enterostomies. Gradual transition from clear liquids to a low-residue, low-sugar diet of small, frequent meals is generally appropriate for patients with an enterostomy in the postoperative setting. Within 4–6 weeks post-resection, patients with an enterostomy should gradually resume fibrous foods and begin soluble fiber supplementation as tolerated to add bulk and slow transit time through the remaining bowel. Those with difficulty maintaining fluid balance should be instructed on the liberal use of salt, starch, and 1–2 L of oral rehydration solution (ORS) sipped between meals.

Sodium and fluid transport across the upper intestinal membrane occurs through a sodium-glucose cotransport system, whereby active sodium absorption and subsequent water absorption is achieved through solvent drag. Isotonic glucose-electrolyte solutions (oral rehydration solutions or ORS) with approximately 90 mEq sodium/L (1 tsp NaCl/L) and 20 g glucose/L are used to maximize absorption and minimize additional losses [34]. Hypotonic, sodium-free fluids (such as water and tea) and hypertonic fluids (such as fruit juices, regular sodas, and sugary sports drinks) should be avoided as these may provoke additional loss of fluids and electrolytes.

In a carefully conducted nutrient balance study, Jeppesen et al. found that SBS patients who absorbed less than half of their daily intake were able to avoid the need for home PN through hyperphagia [20]. However, hyperphagia may lead to exceptionally high outputs in patients with preexisting fecal losses above 4 L/day. In these cases, oral intake should be limited to several extremely small meals per day (i.e., one serving starch per meal), and fluid intake may need to be restricted to no more than 1 L of ORS sipped daily. This type of restriction is imposed in order to reduce losses to the point where IV replacement can occur safely in the home setting. The IV solution is slowly weaned off as small portions of appropriate foods and fluids are reintroduced with the goal of maintaining urine output above 800 mL/day [20].

All patients with large fecal losses will generally benefit from a diet divided into several small meals per day and limited in simple sugars in order to minimize the osmolar load to the GI tract. For SBS patients with colon, a diet high in complex carbohydrates (50–60% of total calories) and low in fat (20–30% of total calories) with isotonic or hypotonic fluids sipped between meals is recommended. In SBS patients without colon, a moderate carbohydrate (40–50% of total calories), moderate fat (30–40% of total calories), and calorically dense diet is most optimal (see Table 8.5) [35].

Patients unable to consume adequate nutrition orally may benefit from EN infused at a slow rate into the bowel through a nasogastric feeding tube or a percutaneous endoscopic gastrostomy (PEG) tube [36, 37]. A standard, isotonic formula with intact protein, glucose polymers, and primarily long-chain fats is generally well tolerated and may have a favorable effect on bowel adaptation [38]. If a gradual advancement of polymeric feeds (in increments of 10 mL/h in an 8-h nursing shift) leads to increased output, trial feeding with a semi-elemental, isotonic, peptide-based formula should be attempted [39].

Murine models of SBS have found that soluble fibers (i.e., pectin, guar gum) and prebiotics (i.e., fructooligosaccharides or FOS) can enhance bowel adaptation and absorption, so many standard and elemental enteral formulas are now available with these compounds [40]. Fluid balance may be enhanced with the infusion of ORS through an enteral feeding tube by overnight continuous drip or by intermittent bolus as a replacement for the traditional water flush. Nauth et al. described three SBS patients who were weaned off of PN by optimizing enteral fluid absorption through the use of nocturnal enteral rehydration [41].

Table 8.5 Diet prescription for short bowel syndrome

Diet	Colon	No colon
Carbohydrate	50–60% of total calories (limit simple sugars)	40–50% of total calories (restrict simple sugars)
Protein	20–30% of total calories	20–30% of total calories
Fat	20–30% of total calories (primarily as essential fats)	30–40% of total calories (primarily as essential fats)
Fluid	Isotonic or hypo-osmolar fluids	Isotonic, high-sodium oral rehydration solutions
Soluble fiber	5–10 g/day (if stool output is >3 L/day)	5–10 g/day (if stool output is >3 L/day)
Oxalates	Limit intake	
Meals/snacks	5–6 meals/day	4–6 meals/day

Adapted from Byrne et al [35]., with permission

Patients unable to maintain their weight near an ideal level with oral or enteral nutrition and medical/surgical management alone will require PN to meet daily nutrient needs. Parenteral nutrient provisions should be initiated at 15–20 kcal/kg/day and 1.0–1.5 g protein/kg/day and advanced carefully as required to meet clinical goals of feeding. Those demonstrating maintenance of nutrient status but unable to attain fluid balance considering gastrointestinal, urine, and insensible losses will require IV hydration with a variable mix of electrolytes. In general, small bowel electrolyte losses can be replaced by using 0.45–0.9% normal saline with 10–20 mEq potassium chloride/L, 25–30 mEq sodium acetate/L, 5 mEq calcium gluconate/L, and 5–10 mEq (8.2 mEq = 1 g) magnesium sulfate/L [42].

Pharmacotherapy

Medical therapy for patients with high gastrointestinal losses is often initiated empirically and adjusted based on GI symptoms (Table 8.6). Gastric acid hypersecretion occurs in most patients for up to 6 months following extensive bowel resection, warranting treatment with histamine-2 blockers or proton pump inhibitors [43]. Antidiarrheal medications should be taken at least 30 min before meals in order to slow gastric and intestinal transit in patients free of ileus or obstruction. A trial of oral pancreatic enzyme preparations may also be attempted to enhance digestion by allowing food to mix with enzymes in the stomach prior to entering the shortened bowel [44].

Patients with an ileal resection of <100 cm attached to some portion of colon may benefit from bile-acid binding

Table 8.6 Antidiarrheal medications for high GI losses

Medication	One dose	Starting dose	Maximum daily dose
Loperamide tab	2 mg	2–4 mg PO QID	16 mg (4–8 tabs)
Loperamide liquid	1 mg (5 mL)	2–4 mg PO QID	80 mL (16 mg)
Diphenoxylate-atropine tab	2.5 mg	2.5–5 mg PO QID	20 mg (4–8 tabs)
Diphenoxylate-atropine liquid	2.5 mg (5 mL)	2.5–5 mg PO QID	40 mL (20 mg)
Codeine tab	15 mg	15–30 mg PO QID	240 mg (60 mg PO QID)
Codeine elixir	15 mg/5 mL, 30 mg, 60 mg	15–30 mg PO QID	240 mg (80 mL)
Paragoric 0.4 mg morphine/1 mL paragoric (45% alcohol)	5 mL (2 mg)	5 mL PO QID	37.5 mL PO QID (150 mL/day)
Opium tincture 10 mg morphine/1 mL opium (19% alcohol)	0.3 mL	0.3–1 mL PO QID	1.5 mL PO QID (6 mL/day)

All antidiarrheals should be given 30–60 min before meals and at bedtime
PO per os, *QID* four times daily

resins such as cholestyramine to reduce the irritation of bile acid contact with the colonic mucosa. Use of octreotide or clonidine to inhibit GI secretions and delay small bowel transit is best reserved for patients with large volume secretory diarrhea refractory to standard antidiarrheal and antisecretory therapy [45, 46].

Efforts in developing new treatment modalities for PN-dependent patients with enterostomies have centered on the use of growth factors, which are proposed to enhance intestinal mucosal structure and promote return of absorptive function post-resection [47]. At the end of 2003, the US Food and Drug Administration (FDA) approved the use of recombinant human growth hormone (GH) as an adjunctive pharmacological therapy for the treatment of SBS-induced malabsorption and malnutrition [48]. Debate still exists over whether the reduction in PN observed within the GH literature is a result of the GH or of intensive diet modification alone [49]. A phase II trial on the use of the glucagon-like peptide 2 (GLP-2) analogue teduglutide in SBS patients documented safety, tolerance, and increased intestinal wet weight absorption after 21 days of treatment [50]. Phase III, multicentered, controlled trials are in progress to assess the optimal dosage and administration and to evaluate long-term clinical benefits of teduglutide in SBS.

Medical Management of the High-Output Enterocutaneous Fistula

Identification of the location of the fistula within the bowel (proximal versus distal) and the extent of the fistulous tract (> or <2 cm) is essential in determining the appropriate medical regimen. A proximal ECF may be defined as one with <150 cm of small bowel proximal to the fistula opening, whereas a distal ECF may have more than 150 cm small bowel proximal to the fistula opening. An ECF is known as high output if the volume of drainage is >500 mL/24 h [51]. Spontaneous closure is more likely to be achieved if the fistulous tract is >2 cm in length, if the fistula is low output, and if the patient is well nourished and free of an intra-abdominal abscess and local infection. Therefore, all attempts should be made to treat any evidence of underlying infection through broad-spectrum IV antibiotics and percutaneous drainage to promote spontaneous fistula closure. On occasion, this approach is not successful and open surgical drainage of an abscess may be necessary. One should keep in mind that even the most aggressive medical and nutritional regimens will not allow for repletion and reduction of GI losses until sepsis is resolved [26].

Nutrition Therapy

Nutrition support should begin within 24–48 h after the appearance of an ECF in order to prevent malnutrition in patients with increased GI losses [52]. Parenteral nutrition and bowel rest have been utilized for years as modes to treat malnutrition, correct fluid and electrolyte disturbances, and allow skin lesions to heal through a reduction in caustic GI secretions. Although there is no clear evidence that PN and bowel rest can promote spontaneous ECF closure, the use of PN and bowel rest can facilitate nutritional homeostasis in patients expected to spontaneously close within 1–2 months [53].

The exact definition of bowel rest differs among healthcare providers and may vary with the medical condition of the individual patient. Ideally, it is recommended that all forms of oral intake be stopped as the nutrient composition of standard oral diets can stimulate further losses of fluids, electrolytes, and protein via the fistula and can hinder upper GI fistula healing [24]. Patients unable to avoid oral intake for the period of time required to allow fistula healing may trial sips of ORS (up to 500 mL/day) and three very small meals of low-residue items. Those with >200 cm of small bowel proximal to a fistula in the distal ileum or colon should be encouraged to take a low-residue, low-sugar, high-salt, high-starch diet of small, frequent meals as this should not significantly increase GI secretions.

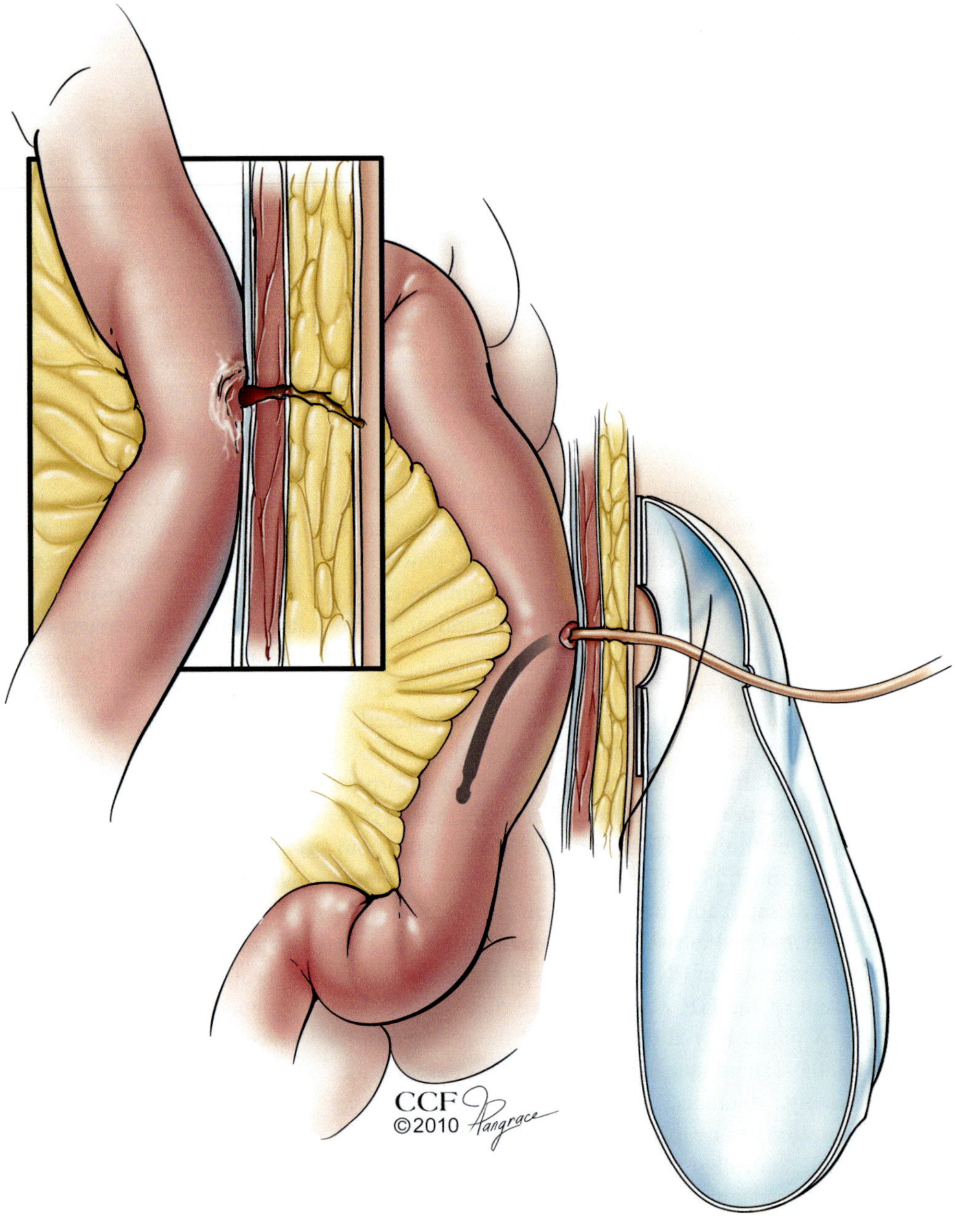

Fig. 8.4 Fistuloclysis permits the delivery of enteral tube feeding and fluid into the bowel beyond a proximal enterocutaneous fistula. There must be a sufficient amount of bowel distal to the fistula for this approach to be successful. The illustration depicts a feeding tube passing through a stoma collection appliance, into the distal opening of the fistula, and then advanced into the bowel in an aboral direction (Illustration © CCF)

Enteral Nutrition and Fistuloclysis

If feasible, all attempts should be made to use EN instead of PN, as the long-term use of PN is associated with multiple complications including catheter-related blood stream infection, liver dysfunction, and thromboses. Enteral diets contain nutrients such as arginine, glutamine, fish oils, and nucleotides, which have shown to help enhance enteric mucosal integrity and support immune function [24]. A retrospective review of 335 patients with a high-output small bowel ECF revealed that 285 patients (85%) were able to be fed solely with continuous EN using an elemental formula [54]. In general, at least 120 cm of intact, unobstructed, and disease-free bowel should be present either proximal or distal to the ECF in order to facilitate absorption of enteral feedings.

Historically, enteral feedings have been accomplished by the passage of a tube through a proximal fistula and into the distal bowel [22]. This has allowed for the provision of up to 3,000 cal/day in combination with intravenous feedings [22]. Fistuloclysis is a similar version of enteral feeding involving the insertion of a catheter or balloon-retention feeding tube through the fistula/stoma collection appliance and 5–10 cm into the distal opening of the fistula (see Fig. 8.4).

A case report describes the use of fistuloclysis in a male patient with hepatosplenomegaly and rising liver function tests while being supported on PN [55]. A jejunostomy tube was inserted by interventional radiology into the ECF, and semi-elemental feedings were gradually advanced to goal with subsequent discontinuation of PN. Liver function tests improved and nutritional parameters such as visceral proteins and weight increased during fistuloclysis to allow for successful surgical repair of ECF.

Teubner et al. attempted fistuloclysis in 12 patients with high-output small bowel ECF who were free from active infection and had a minimum of 75 cm small bowel available for absorption [56]. Fistuloclysis was deemed successful if body weight was maintained or increased and serum biochemistries remained normal without the need to resume PN. A standard polymeric formula was continuously infused over 12–16 h nightly with a low-residue oral diet and a 1,500 mL/day oral fluid restriction taken during the day.

In order to control proximal fistula output and diarrhea associated with fistuloclysis, patients were given oral omeprazole 40 mg twice daily, loperamide 4 mg four times daily, and codeine phosphate 30–60 mg four times daily. The feeding regimen was changed from a polymeric to semi-elemental or elemental formula if diarrhea or abdominal pain persisted. PN was discontinued only after patients achieved a goal feeding rate of 90 mL/h for at least 5 days without adverse symptoms, and PN was resumed if fistuloclysis with elemental feeding was not tolerated.

Fistuloclysis was found to be successful in 11 of the 12 patients within a median of 28 days from start of the feeding. The elemental and semi-elemental formulas appeared to be better tolerated than the polymeric feeds; however, no correlation was observed between the length of small bowel and colon available for absorption and the type of feed tolerated. Notably, only 100 cm or less of small bowel attached to colon was available for absorption in six of the successfully fed patients, and only 100 cm of small bowel without colon was present in two patients sustaining nutritional and metabolic parameters with fistuloclysis alone.

Enteral Nutrition and Vacuum-Assisted Closure

Medical management of high-output enterocutaneous fistulas should include an effective fistula skin protection plan to avoid breakdown from caustic enzymes within the fistula effluent. The leakage of enteric contents can lead to persistent tissue inflammation, infection, and sepsis in the worst of cases. Vacuum-assisted closure (VAC) therapy applies high levels of negative subatmospheric pressure in a vacuum tight system to pull effluent away from the fistula site into a self-contained canister. The negative pressure dressing can increase rates of granulation formation and wound contracture to thereby control fistula effluent [57].

A case study describes the use of a VAC system to completely close a lateral fistula presenting with eversion of the mucosa but without complete diversion of the bowel ends [58]. As soon as suction is introduced to the system, the drape of synthetic polymer compresses against the wound bed to create a semipermeable barrier over the fistula. Enzymatic effluent is readily sucked and directed through the barrier and to the collection flasks, but stool content is kept inside the lumen to restore normal enteral transit. Nasojejunal enteral feedings may be used to supplement oral feedings and can allow for discontinuation of PN within 10 days of initiating VAC therapy as shown in the case study [58].

Pharmacotherapy

Medical therapy for patients with high-output ECFs follows the same principles of symptom management as therapy for high-output enterostomies (see Table 8.6). Antidiarrheals are used to slow bowel motility for improved absorption, broad spectrum antibiotics may aid in controlling the inflammation associated with an open abdomen, and antisecretory medications can reduce excessive GI and pancreatic secretions. Octreotide is a powerful gastrointestinal hormone capable of inhibiting GI exocrine and endocrine secretions to thereby slow gut motility, increase intestinal water and electrolyte absorption, and reduce effluent through intestinal fistulas or stomas [59].

Octreotide may be administered subcutaneously (100 mcg every 8 h), intramuscularly (10–30 mg monthly), or via the PN solution. Subcutaneous octreotide and PN begun within 48 h of fistula onset were able to achieve a 94% mean reduction in ECF output and a 78% ECF closure rate within the first month of administration in a review of 40 patients with postoperative ECFs [60]. Although subcutaneous octreotide injection was shown to induce a 50% mean reduction in ECF output within 24 h of administration, a significant effect on spontaneous ECF closure was not observed in a retrospective analysis of 21 PN-dependent patients [61]. Sancho et al. conducted a multicenter, prospective, randomized, double-blind, placebo-controlled trial to compare administration of PN plus subcutaneous octreotide within 8 days of fistula onset with PN alone [62]. Fourteen patients received octreotide while 17 patients were studied in the control arm. The mean reduction in fistula output over the first 3 days of treatment and the frequency of fistula closure at 20 days were no different between the two study groups. Overall, these results suggest that the main effect of octreotide is to reduce the volume of fluid and quantity of electrolytes lost through an ECF.

Studies have not been done evaluating the clinical utility of adding octreotide to PN solutions; however, it appears to be safe and efficacious in doses of up to 900 mcg/day [63]. Possible adverse reactions to octreotide include cholelithiasis and biliary sludge formation, especially when used for

1 year or more. More frequently, hyperglycemia or abdominal distention and constipation are seen with short-term use of high doses of octreotide. General guidelines call for the use of octreotide in non-septic, non-obstructed patients with ECFs unresponsive to 7 days of conservative treatment [20, 26]. Octreotide should be discontinued after 2–3 weeks of treatment if there is no response, and long-term use should be routinely reevaluated for development of biliary tract abnormalities.

Fibrin Glue

Fibrin glue has been shown to lead to a more rapid closure of low-volume-output ECFs in a small randomized controlled trial. In 13 patients who had failed medical therapy after 2–4 weeks of fistula formation, those patients treated with fibrin glue experienced ECF closure within 4 days, while patients continuing conservative medical management closed after 1–2 weeks [64]. The ECFs in these patients were in a variety of locations including the stomach, small bowel, and colon. In a small case series of patients with chronic, high-output ECFs following surgical repair of gastroduodenal ulcers due to peptic ulcer disease, fibrin glue was shown to reduce ECFs draining as much as 500–1,000 mL each day [65]. These results suggest that in a select group of patients, fibrin glue may be useful in closing ECFs without surgical intervention.

Conclusion

Medical management of the high-output enterostomy or ECF is largely based on a working knowledge of the anatomy and physiology of the remaining GI tract. Nutrition and pharmacotherapy is tailored to treat patients with varying bowel lengths in continuity. Fistuloclysis has been shown to be a successful way to enterally feed patients with at least 100–120 cm of small bowel distal to the ECF. When GI losses remain exceptionally high despite optimal dietary and pharmacologic intervention, patients will often require intravenous nutrient and/or fluid support until further surgery can safely be performed. Further research is needed to investigate the role of probiotics and soluble fibers in improving sodium and fluid balance in patients with high-output enterostomies or ECFs.

References

1. Thompson JS. Management of the short bowel syndrome. Gastroenterol Clin North Am. 1994;23(2):403–20.
2. Borgstrom B, Dahlqvist A, Lundh G, Sjovall J. Studies of intestinal digestion and absorption in the human. J Clin Invest. 1957;36(10): 1521–36.
3. Nightingale JM, Kamm MA, van der Sijp JR, et al. Disturbed gastric emptying in the short bowel syndrome. Evidence for a 'colonic brake'. Gut. 1993;34(9):1171–6.
4. Hofmann AF, Poley JR. Role of bile acid malabsorption in pathogenesis of diarrhea and steatorrhea in patients with ileal resection. I. Response to cholestyramine or replacement of dietary long chain triglyceride by medium chain triglyceride. Gastroenterology. 1972; 62(5):918–34.
5. Debongnie JC, Phillips SF. Capacity of the human colon to absorb fluid. Gastroenterology. 1978;74(4):698–703.
6. Ziegler TR, Fernandez-Estivariz C, Gu LH, et al. Distribution of the H+/peptide transporter PepT1 in human intestine: up-regulated expression in the colonic mucosa of patients with short-bowel syndrome. Am J Clin Nutr. 2002;75(5):922–30.
7. Royall D, Wolever TM, Jeejeebhoy KN. Evidence for colonic conservation of malabsorbed carbohydrate in short bowel syndrome. Am J Gastroenterol. 1992;87(6):751–6.
8. Parekh N, Seidner D, Steiger E. Managing short bowel syndrome: making the most of what the patient still has. Cleve Clin J Med. 2005;72(9):833–8.
9. Buchman AL, Scolapio J, Fryer J. AGA technical review on short bowel syndrome and intestinal transplantation. Gastroenterology. 2003;124(4):1111–34.
10. Nordgaard I, Hansen BS, Mortensen PB. Importance of colonic support for energy absorption as small-bowel failure proceeds. Am J Clin Nutr. 1996;64(2):222–31.
11. Jeppesen PB, Mortensen PB. Colonic digestion and absorption of energy from carbohydrates and medium-chain fat in small bowel failure. JPEN J Parenter Enteral Nutr. 1999;23 Suppl 5:S101–5.
12. Wilmore DW. Indications for specific therapy in the rehabilitation of patients with the short-bowel syndrome. Best Pract Res Clin Gastroenterol. 2003;17(6):895–906.
13. Jeppesen PB, Mortensen PB. Significance of a preserved colon for parenteral energy requirements in patients receiving home parenteral nutrition. Scand J Gastroenterol. 1998;33(11):1175–9.
14. Nightingale JM, Bartram CI, Lennard-Jones JE. Length of residual small bowel after partial resection: correlation between radiographic and surgical measurements. Gastrointest Radiol. 1991 Fall;16(4):305–6.
15. Crenn P, Coudray-Lucas C, Thuillier F, Cynober L, Messing B. Postabsorptive plasma citrulline concentration is a marker of absorptive enterocyte mass and intestinal failure in humans. Gastroenterology. 2000;119(6):1496–505.
16. Jianfeng G, Weiming Z, Ning L, et al. Serum citrulline is a simple quantitative marker for small intestinal enterocytes mass and absorption function in short bowel patients. J Surg Res. 2005;127(2): 177–82.
17. Rhoads JM, Plunkett E, Galanko J, et al. Serum citrulline levels correlate with enteral tolerance and bowel length in infants with short bowel syndrome. J Pediatr. 2005;146(4):542–7.
18. Parekh NR, Natowicz M, Lopez R, Seidner DL, Su L, Steiger E. Plasma citrulline is a marker of home parenteral nutrition dependence in patients with short bowel syndrome. Clin Nutr Suppl. 2008;3(1):71–2.
19. Kim KA, Wry P, Hughes Jr E, Butcher J, Barbot D. Clostridium difficile small-bowel enteritis after total proctocolectomy: a rare but fatal, easily missed diagnosis. Report of a case. Dis Colon Rectum. 2007;50(6):920–3.
20. Jeppesen PB, Mortensen PB. Intestinal failure defined by measurements of intestinal energy and wet weight absorption. Gut. 2000;46(5):701–6.
21. Fazio VW, Coutsoftides T, Steiger E. Factors influencing the outcome of treatment of small bowel cutaneous fistula. World J Surg. 1983;7(4):481–8.
22. Chapman R, Foran R, Dunphy JE. Management of intestinal fistulas. Am J Surg. 1964;108:157–64.

23. Kuvshinoff BW, Brodish RJ, McFadden DW, Fischer JE. Serum transferrin as a prognostic indicator of spontaneous closure and mortality in gastrointestinal cutaneous fistulas. Ann Surg. 1993;217(6):615–22; discussion 22–3.
24. Meguid MM, Campos AC. Nutritional management of patients with gastrointestinal fistulas. Surg Clin North Am. 1996;76(5): 1035–80.
25. Dudrick SJ, Maharaj AR, McKelvey AA. Artificial nutritional support in patients with gastrointestinal fistulas. World J Surg. 1999; 23(6):570–6.
26. Makhdoom ZA, Komar MJ, Still CD. Nutrition and enterocutaneous fistulas. J Clin Gastroenterol. 2000;31(3):195–204.
27. Cheatham ML, Safcsak K, Brzezinski SJ, Lube MW. Nitrogen balance, protein loss, and the open abdomen. Crit Care Med. 2007; 35(1):127–31.
28. Staun M, Pironi L, Bozzetti F, et al. ESPEN guidelines on parenteral nutrition: home parenteral nutrition (HPN) in adult patients. Clin Nutr. 2009;28(4):467–79.
29. Wolman SL, Anderson GH, Marliss EB, Jeejeebhoy KN. Zinc in total parenteral nutrition: requirements and metabolic effects. Gastroenterology. 1979;76(3):458–67.
30. Matarese LE, Steiger E. Dietary and medical management of short bowel syndrome in adult patients. J Clin Gastroenterol. 2006;40 Suppl 2:S85–93.
31. Buchman AL. Etiology and initial management of short bowel syndrome. Gastroenterology. 2006;130(2 Suppl 1):S5–15.
32. Martinez-Riquelme A, Rawlings J, Morley S, Kendall J, Hosking D, Allison S. Self-administered subcutaneous fluid infusion at home in the management of fluid depletion and hypomagnesaemia in gastrointestinal disease. Clin Nutr. 2005;24(1):158–63.
33. Messing B, Crenn P, Beau P, Boutron-Ruault MC, Rambaud JC, Matuchansky C. Long-term survival and parenteral nutrition dependence in adult patients with the short bowel syndrome. Gastroenterology. 1999;117(5):1043–50.
34. Lennard-Jones JE. Oral rehydration solutions in short bowel syndrome. Clin Ther. 1990;12(Suppl A):129–37; discussion 38.
35. Byrne TA, Veglia L, Camelio M, et al. Clinical observations: beyond the prescription: optimizing the diet of patients with short bowel syndrome. Nutr Clin Pract. 2000;15:306–11.
36. Nightingale J. Gastrostomy placement in patients with Crohn's disease. Eur J Gastroenterol Hepatol. 2000;12(10):1073–5.
37. Joly F, Dray X, Corcos O, Barbot L, Kapel N, Messing B. Tube feeding improves intestinal absorption in short bowel syndrome patients. Gastroenterology. 2009;136(3):824–31.
38. Kollman KA, Lien EL, Vanderhoof JA. Dietary lipids influence intestinal adaptation after massive bowel resection. J Pediatr Gastroenterol Nutr. 1999;28(1):41–5.
39. Parekh NR, Seidner DL. Advances in enteral feeding of the intestinal failure patient. Support Line. 2006;28:18–24.
40. Welters CF, Dejong CH, Deutz NE, Heineman E. Intestinal adaptation in short bowel syndrome. ANZ J Surg. 2002;72(3):229–36.
41. Nauth J, Chang CW, Mobarhan S, Sparks S, Borton M, Svoboda S. A therapeutic approach to wean total parenteral nutrition in the management of short bowel syndrome: three cases using nocturnal enteral rehydration. Nutr Rev. 2004;62(5):221–31.
42. Jeejeebhoy KN. Short bowel syndrome: a nutritional and medical approach. CMAJ. 2002;166(10):1297–302.
43. American Gastroenterological Association medical position statement. Short bowel syndrome and intestinal transplantation. Gastroenterology. 2003;124(4):1105–10.
44. Seidner DL. Short bowel syndrome: etiology, pathophysiology and management. Pract Gastroenterol. 2001;25:63–72.
45. Nehra V, Camilleri M, Burton D, Oenning L, Kelly DG. An open trial of octreotide long-acting release in the management of short bowel syndrome. Am J Gastroenterol. 2001;96(5):1494–8.
46. McDoniel K, Taylor B, Huey W, et al. Use of clonidine to decrease intestinal fluid losses in patients with high-output short-bowel syndrome. JPEN J Parenter Enteral Nutr. 2004;28(4):265–8.
47. Yang H, Teitelbaum DH. Novel agents in the treatment of intestinal failure: humoral factors. Gastroenterology. 2006;130(2 Suppl 1): S117–21.
48. Byrne TA, Wilmore DW, Iyer K, et al. Growth hormone, glutamine, and an optimal diet reduces parenteral nutrition in patients with short bowel syndrome: a prospective, randomized, placebo-controlled, double-blind clinical trial. Ann Surg. 2005;242(5): 655–61.
49. Scolapio JS. Short bowel syndrome: recent clinical outcomes with growth hormone. Gastroenterology. 2006;130(2 Suppl 1):S122–6.
50. Jeppesen PB, Sanguinetti EL, Buchman A, et al. Teduglutide (ALX-0600), a dipeptidyl peptidase IV resistant glucagon-like peptide 2 analogue, improves intestinal function in short bowel syndrome patients. Gut. 2005;54(9):1224–31.
51. McIntyre PB, Ritchie JK, Hawley PR, Bartram CI, Lennard-Jones JE. Management of enterocutaneous fistulas: a review of 132 cases. Br J Surg. 1984;71:293–6.
52. Rose D, Yarborough MF, Canizaro PC, Lowry SF. One hundred and fourteen fistulas of the gastrointestinal tract treated with total parenteral nutrition. Surg Gynecol Obstet. 1986;163(4):345–50.
53. Visschers RG, Olde Damink SW, Winkens B, Soeters PB, van Gemert WG. Treatment strategies in 135 consecutive patients with enterocutaneous fistulas. World J Surg. 2008;32(3):445–53.
54. Levy E, Frileux P, Cugnenc PH, Honiger J, Ollivier JM, Parc R. High-output external fistulae of the small bowel: management with continuous enteral nutrition. Br J Surg. 1989;76(7):676–9.
55. Ham M, Horton K, Kaunitz J. Fistuloclysis: case report and literature review. Nutr Clin Pract. 2007;22(5):553–7.
56. Teubner A, Morrison K, Ravishankar HR, Anderson ID, Scott NA, Carlson GL. Fistuloclysis can successfully replace parenteral feeding in the nutritional support of patients with enterocutaneous fistula. Br J Surg. 2004;91(5):625–31.
57. Hyon SH, Martinez-Garbino JA, Benati ML, Lopez-Avellaneda ME, Brozzi NA, Argibay PF. Management of a high-output postoperative enterocutaneous fistula with a vacuum sealing method and continuous enteral nutrition. ASAIO J. 2000;46(4):511–4.
58. Goverman J, Yelon JA, Platz JJ, Singson RC, Turcinovic M. The "Fistula VAC," a technique for management of enterocutaneous fistulae arising within the open abdomen: report of 5 cases. J Trauma. 2006;60(2):428–31; discussion 31.
59. Torres AJ, Landa JI, Moreno-Azcoita M, et al. Somatostatin in the management of gastrointestinal fistulas. A multicenter trial. Arch Surg. 1992;127(1):97–9; discussion 100.
60. Spiliotis J, Briand D, Gouttebel MC, et al. Treatment of fistulas of the gastrointestinal tract with total parenteral nutrition and octreotide in patients with carcinoma. Surg Gynecol Obstet. 1993;176(6):575–80.
61. Alivizatos V, Felekis D, Zorbalas A. Evaluation of the effectiveness of octreotide in the conservative treatment of postoperative enterocutaneous fistulas. Hepatogastroenterology. 2002;49(46):1010–2.
62. Sancho JJ, di Costanzo J, Nubiola P, et al. Randomized double-blind placebo-controlled trial of early octreotide in patients with postoperative enterocutaneous fistula. Br J Surg. 1995;82(5): 638–41.
63. Seidner DL, Speerhas R. Can octreotide be added to parenteral nutrition solutions? Point-counterpoint. Nutr Clin Pract. 1998; 13:84–8.
64. Hwang TL, Chen MF. Randomized trial of fibrin tissue glue for low output enterocutaneous fistula. Br J Surg. 1996;83(1):112.
65. Huang CS, Hess DT, Lichtenstein DR. Successful endoscopic management of postoperative GI fistula with fibrin glue injection: report of two cases. Gastrointest Endosc. 2004;60(3):460–3.

9 Intestinal Stomas and the Biliary Tree

Michael D. Johnson and John Fung

The use of intestinal stomas in hepatobiliary surgery has traditionally been limited to use in hepatolithiasis and refractory biliary strictures. Surgical management of complex bile duct pathology often involves bile duct exploration followed by creation of a Roux-en-Y hepaticojejunostomy. The Roux limb acts as a defunctionalized conduit that maintains flow of bile into the intestine. When there are no residual stones or a stricture has been successfully bypassed, this can represent a definitive operation by itself. However, there are often more proximal intrahepatic strictures and stones requiring repeated therapy sessions. A Roux-en-Y reconstruction precludes easy endoscopic access to the biliary tree.

Hepaticocutaneous jejunostomy has been used in situations that require permanent, easy access to the biliary tree (Figs. 9.1 and 9.2). Many variations have been employed in Asia where hepatolithiasis is much more prevalent compared to North America. The Roux limb is left long, such that the end can be brought out as an intestinal stoma, or left closed but secured subcutaneously and marked with metal clips for later percutaneous access. Fan et al. reported a series of 41 patients undergoing hepaticocutaneous jejunostomy for hepatolithiasis. Sixty-six percent underwent postoperative choledochoscopy for recurrent symptoms anywhere from 1 to 15 times [1]. Patient comfort was much better compared to choledochoscopy performed through a T-tube tract. Drawbacks to this technique include inconvenience to the patient related to the presence of a stoma and development of Roux limb varices in patients with longstanding liver disease and portal hypertension. The latter have potential to cause dangerous variceal bleeding. Alternatives to a hepaticocutaneous jejunostomy include a classic Roux limb construction and simultaneous duodenojejunostomy or jejunal interposition between the duodenum and biliary tree. Both of these maintain endoscopic access to the biliary tree via the duodenum [2, 3].

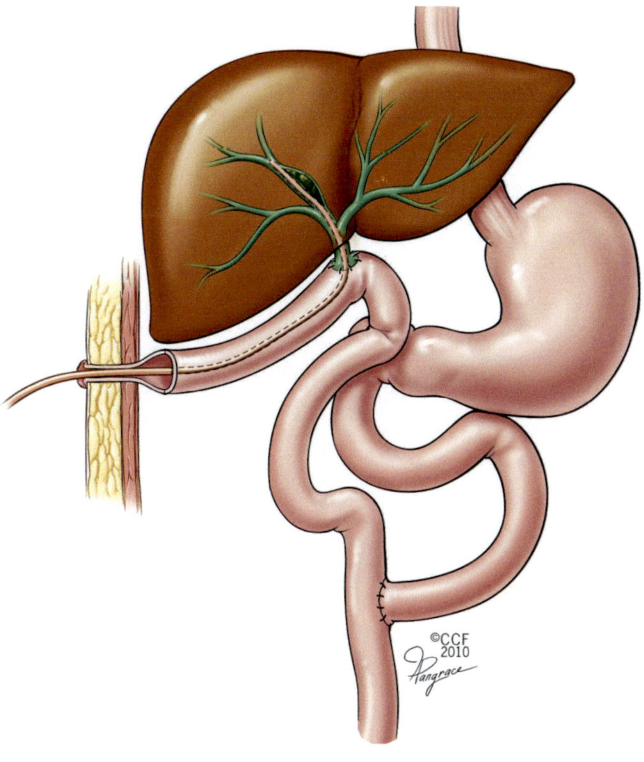

Fig. 9.1 Roux-en-Y hepaticojejunostomy with hepatocutaneous stoma for access to biliary tree (Illustration © CCF)

M.D. Johnson (✉)
The Nebraska Medical Center,
Surgical Services of the Great Plains, P.C., Omaha, NE, USA
e-mail: mdj2003@yahoo.com

J. Fung
Digestive Disease Institute, Transplant Center, Cleveland Clinic
Lerner College of Medicine, Cleveland Clinic Foundation,
Cleveland, OH, USA

V.W. Fazio et al. (eds.), *Atlas of Intestinal Stomas*,
DOI 10.1007/978-0-387-78851-7_9, © Springer Science+Business Media, LLC 2012

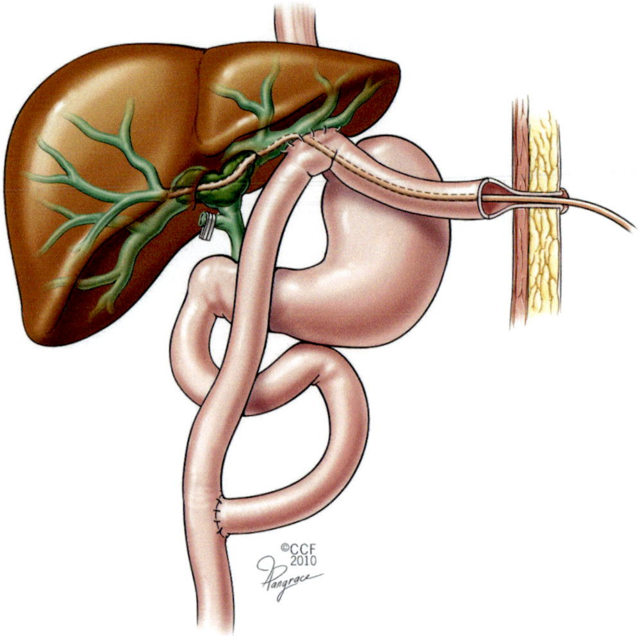

Fig. 9.2 Roux-en-Y access limb to left segmental bile ducts with hepaticocutaneous stoma (Illustration © CCF)

References

1. Fan ST, Mok F, Zheng SS, et al. Appraisal of hepaticocutaneous jejunostomy in the management of hepatolithiasis. Am J Surg. 1993;165(3):332–5.
2. Ramesh H, Prakash K, Kuruvilla K, et al. Biliary access loops for intrahepatic stones: results of jejunoduodenal anastomosis. ANZ J Surg. 2003;73:306–12.
3. Cunha JEM, Herman P, Machado MCC, et al. A new biliary access technique for the long-term endoscopic management of intrahepatic stones. J Hepatobiliary Pancreat Surg. 2002;9:261–4.

Continent Ileostomy

10

Ravi Pokala Kiran and Victor W. Fazio

Introduction

The ileoanal pouch (IPAA) is the procedure of choice in patients requiring proctocolectomy, as it provides control of colitis or polyposis but maintains normal per anal defecation. For certain groups of patients, however, IPAA may not be technically feasible or advisable. Expectations of poor functional outcomes due to sphincter compromise, risk of perianal sepsis in patients with preexisting perianal disease, and patients with cancer of the lower rectum where an adequate oncologic resection may not be achieved with a restorative proctocolectomy are examples of such circumstances. Further, some patients who develop pouch failure may not be candidates for a redo pouch procedure, or this may not be technically feasible. These patients face a permanent end ileostomy and may want to consider the merits of a continent ileostomy as an alternative [1–3]. Although the continent ileostomy is technically challenging and may be associated with a variety of complications, its advantages over an end ileostomy include continence for feces and flatus, better body image, and improved quality of life (QOL) [4–8].

Historical Perspective

The continent ileostomy was developed by Nils Kock in 1969 [9] based on previous reports by Tasker who first described the use of detubularized parts of the bowel for urinary diversion. A nipple valve was subsequently designed by adding an intussuscepted length of ileum as an efferent limb. Over the years, the continent ileostomy has shown itself to be prone to several complications, mostly related to the nipple valve. Numerous modifications have been made to circumvent these problems, but there continues to be a high incidence of pouch revision and excision.

R.P. Kiran (✉)
Department of Colorectal Surgery, Digestive Disease Institute, Cleveland Clinic Foundation, Cleveland, OH, USA
e-mail: kiranp@ccf.org

V.W. Fazio
Department of Colorectal Surgery, Digestive Diseases Institute, Cleveland Clinic Lerner College of Medicine of Case Western Reserve University, Cleveland Clinic Foundation, Cleveland, OH, USA
e-mail: faziov@ccf.org

Indications

The most common indication for the procedure is removal of the large intestine for ulcerative colitis and indeterminate colitis in patients who are not candidates for IPAA, or when the creation of an IPAA may be technically impossible due to difficulties with reach of the pouch to the anal canal. Some patients with an ileostomy are unable to cope with the demands of life with an external appliance, while others suffer complications of a conventional ileostomy including hernia, fistula, prolapse, recession, and leakage resistant to revisional surgery. In addition, some patients seek conversion of an end ileostomy to a continent ileostomy to circumvent psychological, social, and sexual problems associated with the wearing of an external appliance. In patients who experience failure of IPAA, and a redo IPAA is not possible, due consideration may be given to a continent ileostomy. In this case, the IPAA can be modified for use as a continent ileostomy pouch, offering the additional advantage of preservation of small bowel since pouch excision would otherwise have been performed.

In recent times, the procedure has been extended for use in a select group of patients with cancer of the colon and rectum, Crohn's disease confined to the large bowel and perineum, and patients with colonic inertia. In these situations, careful consideration is given to the relative risk of recurrence of disease, its effect on function of the pouch and small bowel, survival of the patient, and the risk of development of a short bowel syndrome were the patient to develop failure of the K-pouch, thus, requiring subsequent excision of the pouch. Patients in whom these risks are considered to be minimal, the procedure may be offered after due and thorough discussion of the potential risks involved.

V.W. Fazio et al. (eds.), *Atlas of Intestinal Stomas*,
DOI 10.1007/978-0-387-78851-7_10,

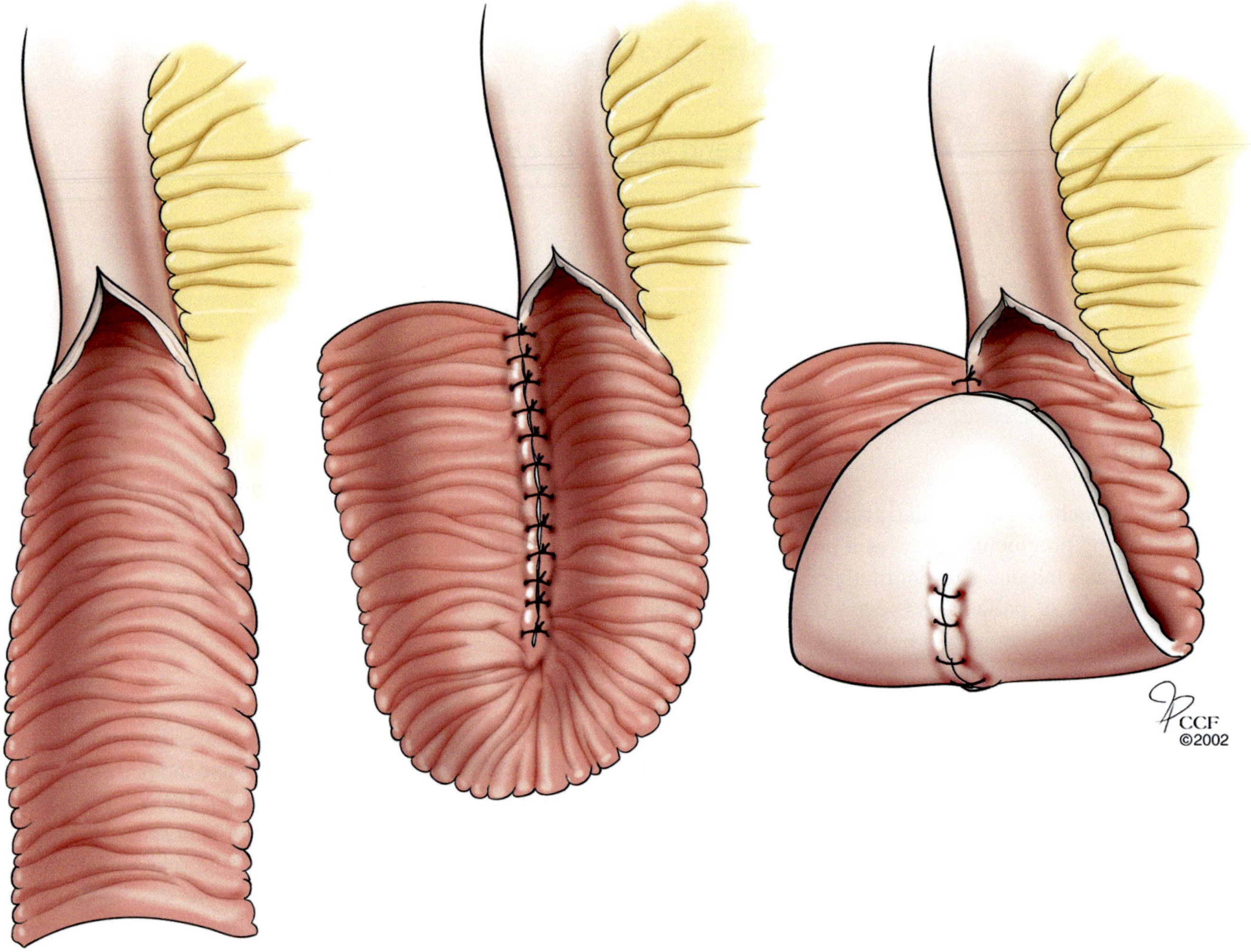

Fig. 10.1 Double-folded reservoir in the shape of a "U" as described by Nils Kock (Illustration © CCF)

Contraindications

It is crucial that patients understand the importance of timely catheterization of the continent ileostomy when full since the reservoir will not drain itself spontaneously. Patients need to have on their person at all times the drainage tube required to empty the pouch. Thus, patients lacking adequate mental competence required to master intubation are not candidates for the procedure. Obesity is a relative contraindication owing to several factors. In addition to the technical difficulty associated with delivery of the exit conduit through a thick abdominal wall, a foreshortened fatty mesentery may preclude creation of an adequate nipple valve and predispose to valve slippage. Patients with marginal small-bowel length and those who are deemed to be at a higher risk of failure of the continent ileostomy due to recrudescent Crohn's disease or desmoid disease in FAP are at risk of developing short bowel syndrome due to the potential loss of 50 cm of small-bowel length that is utilized in the creation of a continent ileostomy.

Original Surgical Technique

The continent ileostomy was originally designed by Nils Kock based on the two fundamental principles of creation of a low-pressure reservoir by detubularization of the bowel and use of intermittent catheterization to empty the reservoir. The double-folded reservoir, which was created by splitting a segment of ileum longitudinally at its antimesenteric border and folding it in the shape of a "U", was a modification of the original J-pouch design of Tasker (Fig. 10.1). The two limbs of the "U" were sutured together, and the pouch formed by a second fold. The double-folded design circumvented the problem of high pressures that developed at large volumes in the original J-pouch design. The reservoir initially had an opening at its corner through which it was emptied. Subsequently, a segment of intestine was interposed between the pouch and the skin. Since several patients suffered incontinence, an intussuscepting outlet ("nipple") was subsequently added to the design to prevent leakage (Fig. 10.2). The pouch was subsequently modified by Fazio to a 3-limb

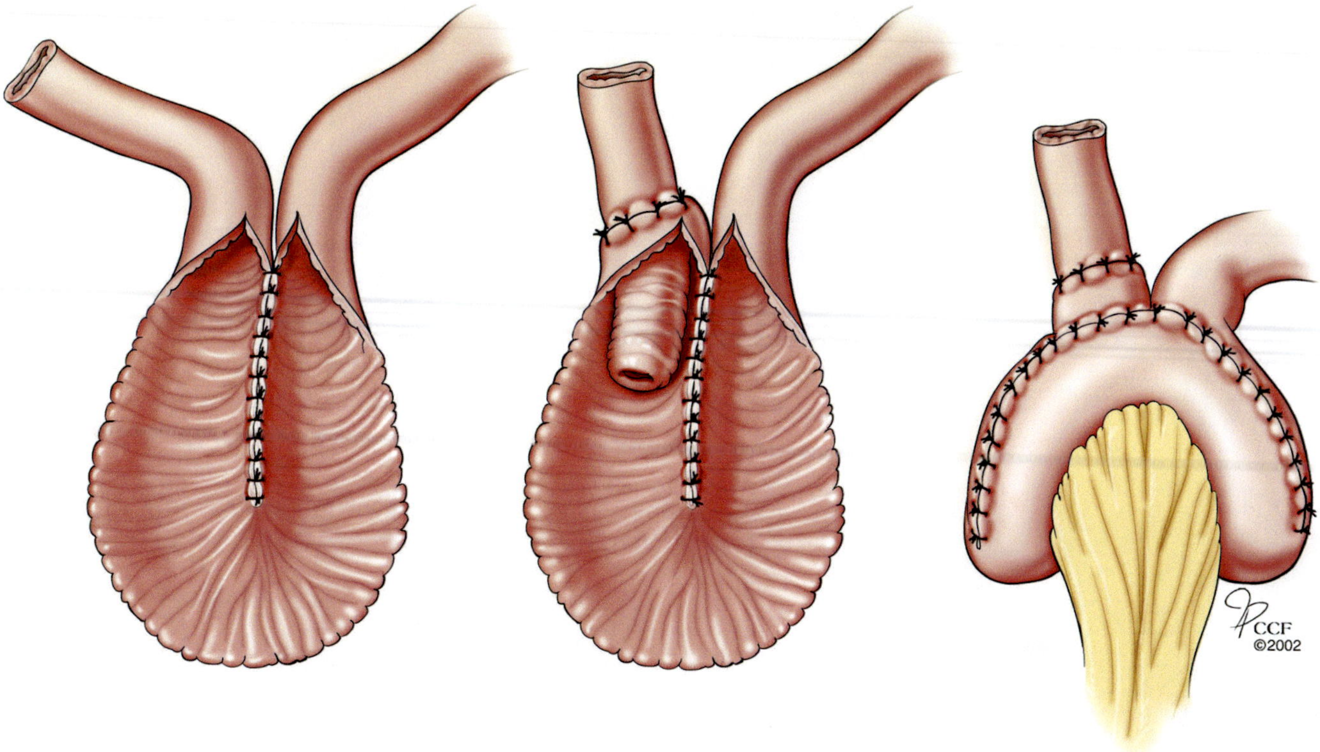

Fig. 10.2 Addition of an intussuscepting outlet ("nipple") to prevent leakage (Illustration © CCF)

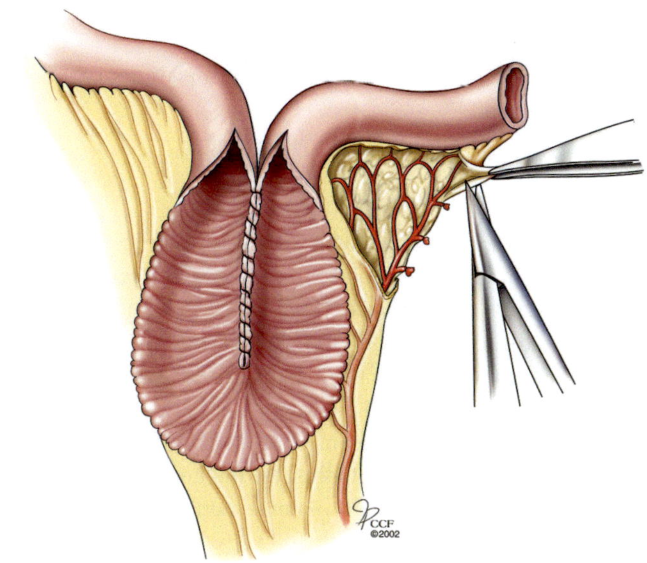

Fig. 10.3 Excision of mesenteric fat to reduce valve slippage (Illustration © CCF)

S-shape made of three 12–15-cm limbs of small bowel and a nipple segment that is created by intussuscepting the penultimate 12 cm into itself, followed by the last 8 cm forming the exit conduit and ileostomy segment.

There is, however, a high complication rate associated with the original design, the commonest being slippage of the nipple valve. The commonest portion of the valve that predisposes to dessusception is the mesenteric aspect, where one limb of the nipple valve tends to slip on the other. Although various modifications have been described to prevent slippage, the complication rate continues to remain high. The modifications that have been described include the use of a sling made of fascia, marlex, or prolene to support the base of the nipple [10, 11]; anchorage of the nipple valve to the pouch wall by sutures [12]; peritoneal stripping and mesenteric fat excision [12]; scarification of the serosa [13] (Figs. 10.3 and 10.4); and staple stabilization of the nipple valve [14–16]. Barnett described a modification of the procedure designed to stabilize the base of the nipple valve using a segment of the efferent limb to form a living collar [17] (Fig. 10.5). Stapler fixation of the nipple to the pouch wall and biomechanical stabilization have also been described [18, 19]. Unfortunately, the stabilizing procedures themselves can lead to complications [20].

Complications

The different modifications have reduced the complication rate [19, 21], but there continues to be a diverse spectrum of complications associated with the Kock pouch (Table 10.1). Early complications that have been described include anastomotic leak, necrosis of the nipple valve, fistula, pouchitis, wound sepsis, dehiscence, and intestinal obstruction. Late

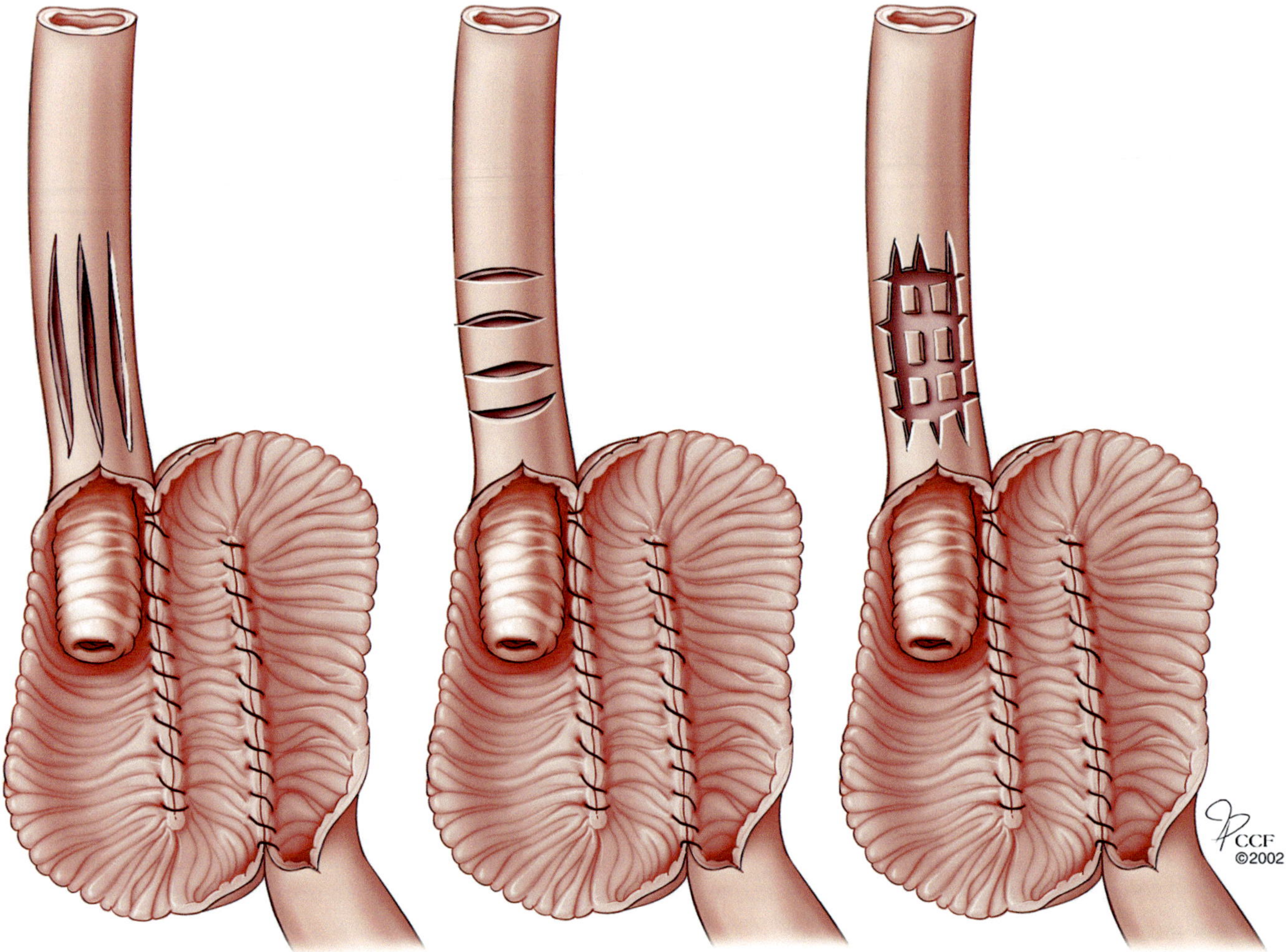

Fig. 10.4 Scarification of the serosa to reduce nipple valve slippage (Illustration © CCF)

complications include pouchitis, inability to intubate, incontinence, peristomal sepsis, fistula, anemia, stomal sepsis, parastomal hernia, redundant stoma, and skin level stricture.

Current Technique

The operative technique currently practiced at the Cleveland Clinic Foundation has gradually evolved based on increasing experience with the procedure. The procedure involves the construction of an ileal reservoir from three 12–15-cm loops of terminal ileum using a hand-suture technique. The terminal 20 cm of the ileum are used to create the nipple valve and the exit conduit, with 12 cm devoted to the valve, and 8 cm devoted to the exit conduit and stoma. Thus, by intussuscepting the 12-cm segment of the efferent limb, a 6-cm nipple is created.

After identifying and freeing the terminal ileum, the terminal 20 cm of the small bowel and the 3 12–15-cm length segments are measured and marked with stay sutures (Fig. 10.6a, b). Seromuscular sutures are placed to appose adjacent loops of bowel forming the S-pouch (Fig. 10.7). An enterotomy is made on adjacent limbs of the pouch (Fig. 10.8a, b), and mucosal approximation of the back wall of the pouch is completed (Fig. 10.9a, b). The 12-cm segment of ileum adjacent to the pouch is then intussuscepted on itself to form a nipple valve (Fig. 10.10a–c). Prior to this, the thickness of the mesentery supplying this segment of ileum is reduced by the application of coagulation current to the fat between the vasa recta.

Using the transverse stapler, two parallel rows of staples are then placed on the inner aspect of the nipple valve on either side of the folded mesentery of the intussuscepted segment (Fig. 10.11a, b). The fundus of the pouch is then sewn onto the base of the exit conduit to strengthen the intussusception. These "fundoplication-like" sutures help stabilize the valve, maintaining an adequate length of nipple valve intussuscepted into the pouch. Since these sutures could

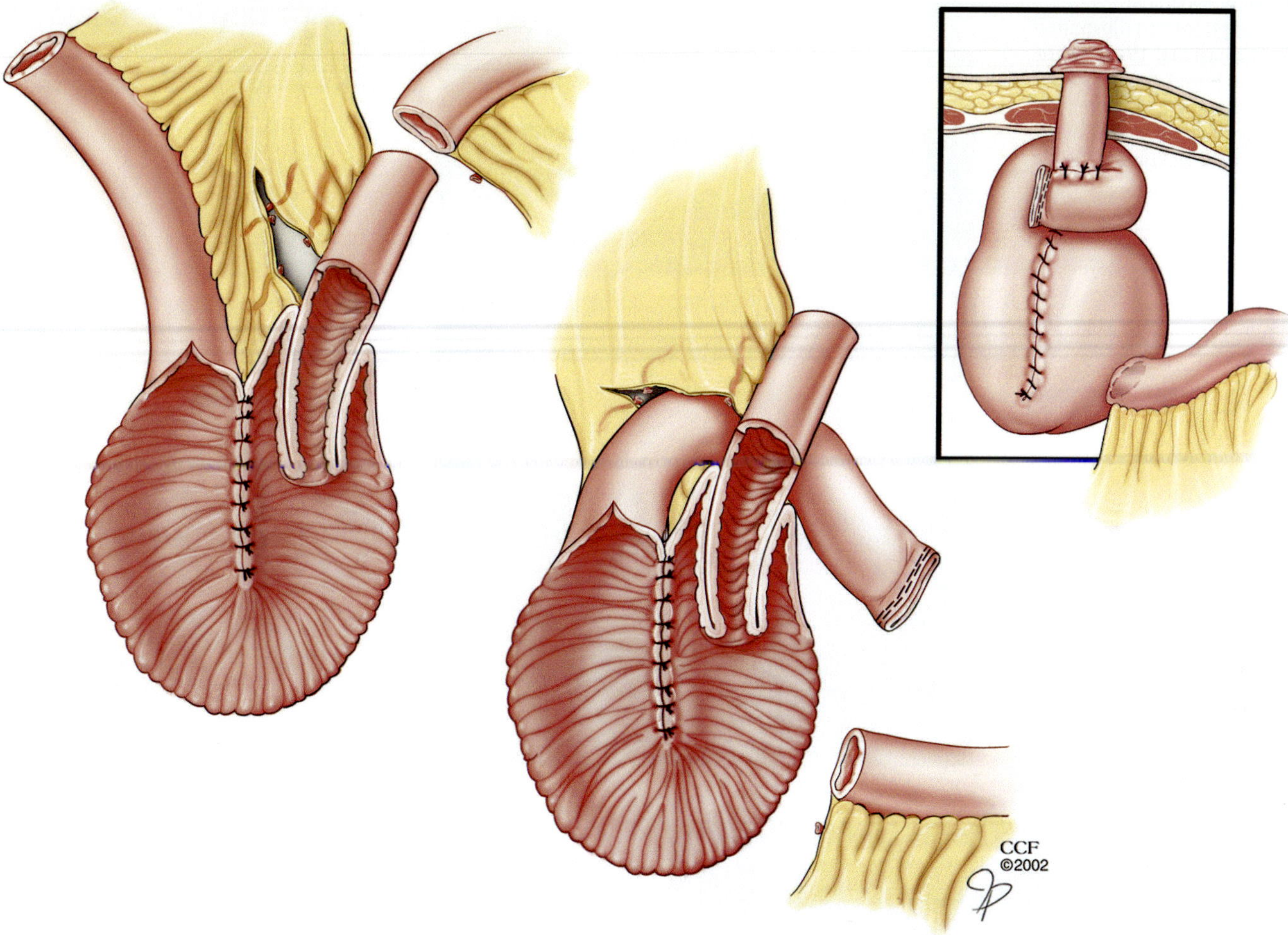

Fig. 10.5 Stabilization of the nipple valve with the use of a segment of the efferent limb to form a living collar (Illustration © CCF)

Table 10.1 Late complications of the Kock pouch

I. Abnormalities of Continence-Providing Valve and Efferent Ileal Segment
Sliding
Eversion
Detachment of the reservoir from the abdominal wall
Sliding hernia
Valve-shunting fistulas
II. Abnormalities of the Reservoir
Pouchitis
Relapse of Crohn's disease
Fistulas: internal or external
III. Abnormalities of the Afferent Ileal Segment
Ileitis
Stenosis and dilatation
Antireflux valve
Miscellaneous: stenosis resulting from misalignment between the afferent ileal segment and the reservoir.

potentially jeopardize the blood supply to the pouch/nipple valve (exit conduit), these are used selectively when the blood supply is felt to be good, and additional fixation sutures are felt necessary for maintaining the conformation of the nipple valve in relation to the pouch.

Closure of the anterior wall of the pouch is then commenced, starting from the apex of the pouch at its junction with the base of the nipple. Some of these sutures deliberately include a portion of the nipple valve in order to appose the nipple wall to the suture line. When the apex of the nipple has been reached, the transverse stapler is inserted into the lumen of the nipple valve, and the device deployed to form a row of staples that overlap the previously placed suture line (Fig. 10.12a–c) and providing additional fixation of the nipple valve to the pouch.

Closure of the anterior wall of the pouch is then completed and the pouch tested for integrity and continence (Fig. 10.13a–c). The exit conduit is brought through the abdominal wall and

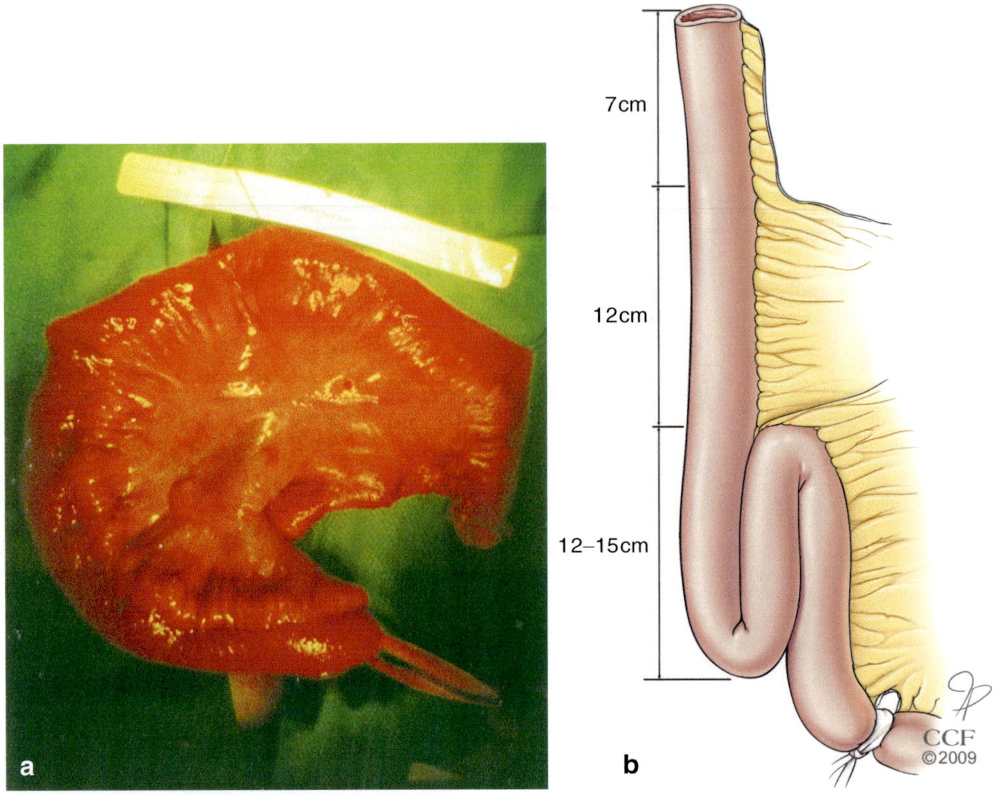

Fig. 10.6 Operative photograph (**a**) and illustration (**b**). The terminal 19–20 cm of the small bowel and the three 12–15 cm length segments are measured and marked with stay sutures (Illustration © CCF)

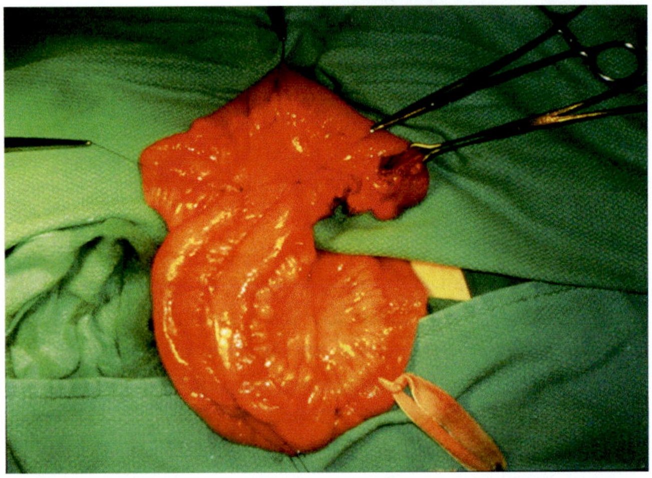

Fig. 10.7 Seromuscular sutures are placed to appose adjacent loops of bowel forming the S-pouch

anchoring sutures placed to secure the pouch to the inside of the abdominal wall. The lateral para-ileostomy space is obliterated and a drainage catheter secured safely in the pouch before the abdomen is closed (Fig. 10.14a, b).

Postoperative Care

The drainage catheter is left in the pouch for 4 weeks to allow complete healing of the pouch. The tube is connected to a drainage bag that is strapped to the patient's leg. The tube is irrigated with 30 mL of saline every 2–3 h postoperatively (Table 10.2). After the return of bowel activity, the frequency of irrigation is reduced to twice daily. The patients are normally discharged 5–7 days after surgery and scheduled for the first outpatient visit at 3 weeks. At that time, the pouch is tested, and intermittent catheterization begins at two hourly intervals, with a gradual reduction to a frequency of intubation as required by the patient within the subsequent 4 weeks (Table 10.3). Routine follow-up is scheduled at 3 months from the discharge day and at yearly intervals thereafter.

Conversion of the Ileoanal Pouch to Continent Ileostomy

The pouch is mobilized, disconnected, and detached from the anal anastomosis by either an abdominal or combined abdomino-anal approach. When a decision is made to preserve the entire, or a portion of, the pelvic pouch prior to the performance of the continent ileostomy, the mobilized pouch is disconnected from the proximal bowel segment to achieve pouch rotation, and a nipple valve about 6 cm long created by intussuscepting the afferent limb of the pelvic pouch into itself. A pouchotomy is created through which the transverse stapler is introduced and the valve stabilized with three firings of the stapler, the last one including the anterior pouch wall as previously described. Thus, in such cases, a two-loop continent ileostomy is created. When the

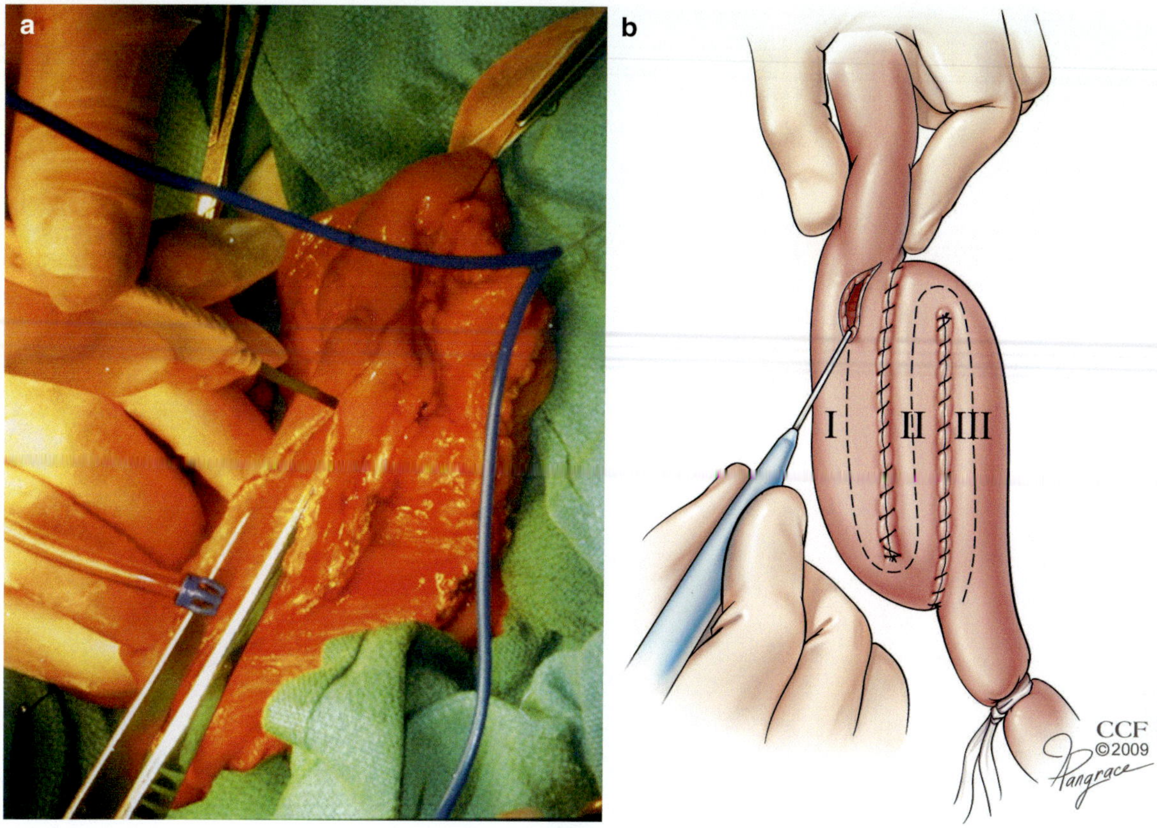

Fig. 10.8 Operative photograph (**a**) and illustration (**b**). Creation of enterotomy on adjacent limbs of the pouch (Illustration © CCF)

pelvic pouch is not utilized for the continent reservoir, a three-limb S-shaped continent ileostomy is constructed using a new bowel segment.

Long-Term Results

Though continence can be maintained in a significant number of patients, the reoperation rates are high. The mean number of revisions in one study [22] was 2.8 during a mean observation period of 7 years. The cumulative probability of revision of a newly created Kock pouch at 2–15 years was 52% and 57%, respectively, and pouch excision rate was 15%. Other studies have also reported high rates of revision [23, 24] and excision of the Kock pouch. Outcomes for 330 patients undergoing the continent ileostomy procedure between 1974 and 2001 at the Cleveland Clinic were recently reported [25]. Over a median patient follow-up of 11 years (range, 1–27 years), the median revision-free pouch interval was 14 months (95% confidence interval, 11–17 months). The 10-year and 20-year pouch survival was 87% and 77%, respectively. Patients had an average of 3.7 (range, 1–28) complications and 2.9 (range, 1–27) pouch revisions during follow-up. On multivariate analysis, Crohn's disease (hazard ratio = 4.5), female gender (hazard ratio = 2.4), fistula development (hazard ratio = 3), and body mass index (hazard ratio = 2.4 per 5 unit increase) were independent predictors of pouch failure. Quality-of-life (QOL) measurements for patients with a continent ileostomy were higher on all scales in comparison with patients who had the Kock reservoir and then reverted to a Brooke ileostomy. A recent review of outcomes for patients undergoing conversion of IPAA to continent ileostomy at this institution reported that despite the associated morbidity, the majority of this select group of highly motivated patients retain their continent ileostomy long-term, are highly satisfied with their choice of continent ileostomy, and enjoy a good QOL [26].

Conclusion

In conclusion, the quest for fecal continence after total proctocolectomy has evolved over the past 15 years. Currently, the preferred surgical option for ulcerative colitis is that of restorative proctocolectomy with ileoanal pouch, but that may be unsuitable for some patients. In such circumstances, for motivated patients who are fully informed of the pros and cons, a continent ileostomy is a valuable addition to the surgical alternatives.

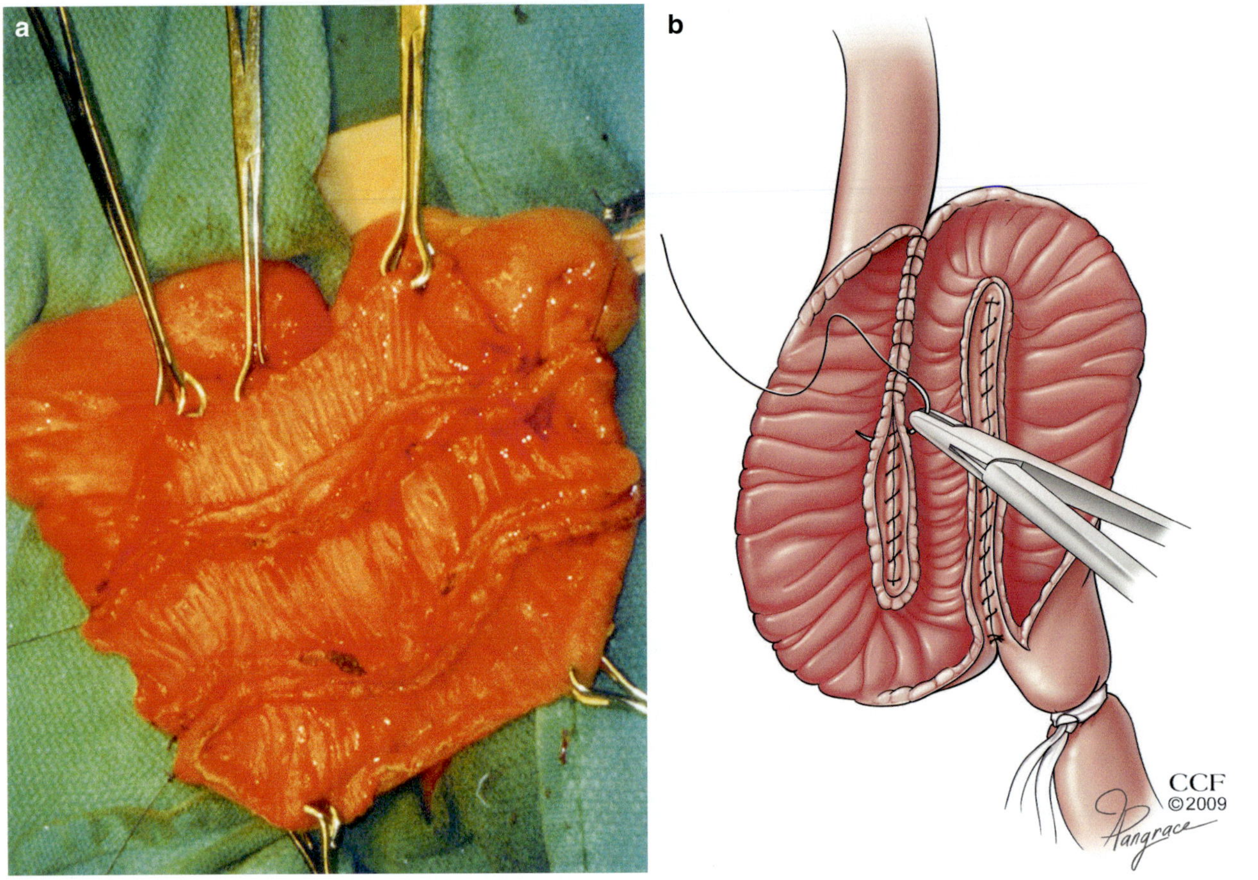

Fig. 10.9 Operative photograph (**a**) and illustration (**b**). Approximation of the mucosa of the back wall of the pouch (Illustration © CCF)

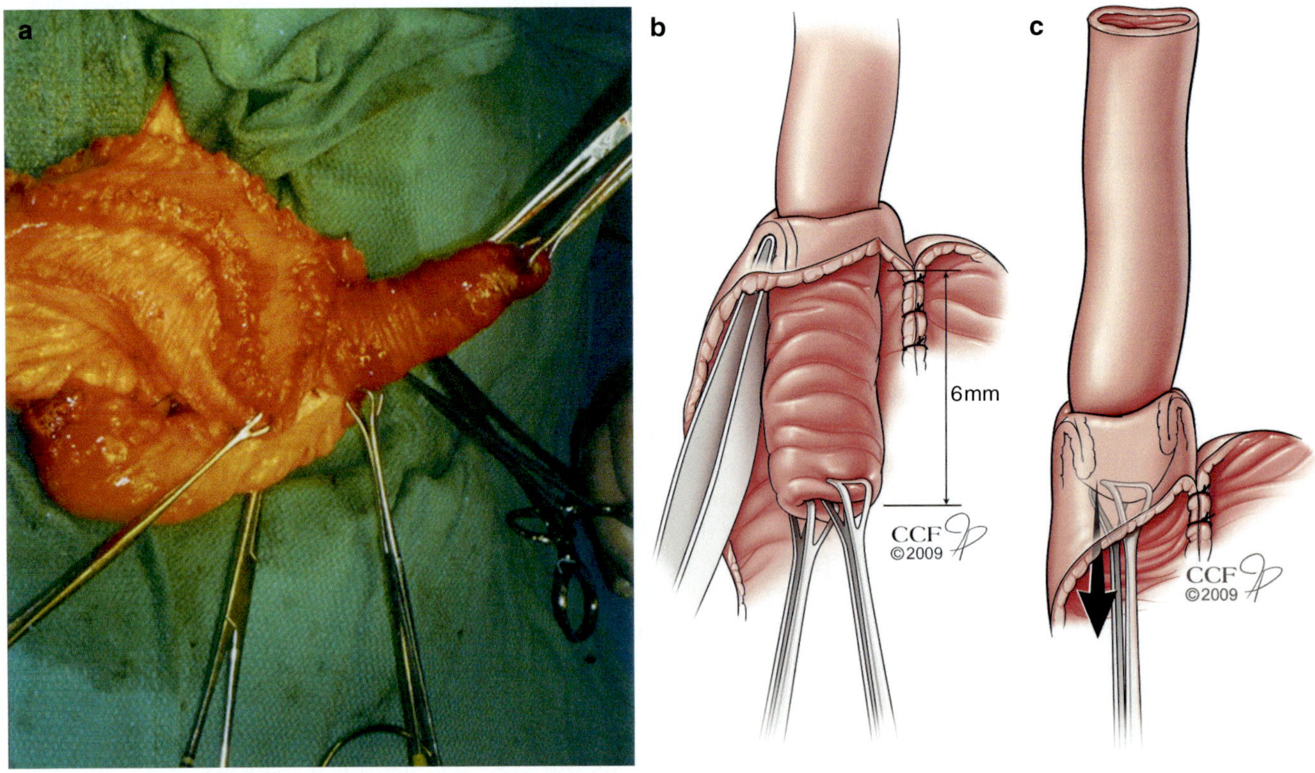

Fig. 10.10 Operative photograph (**a**) and illustrations (**b** and **c**). A 12-cm segment of ileum adjacent to the pouch is intussuscepted on itself to form a nipple valve (Illustrations © CCF)

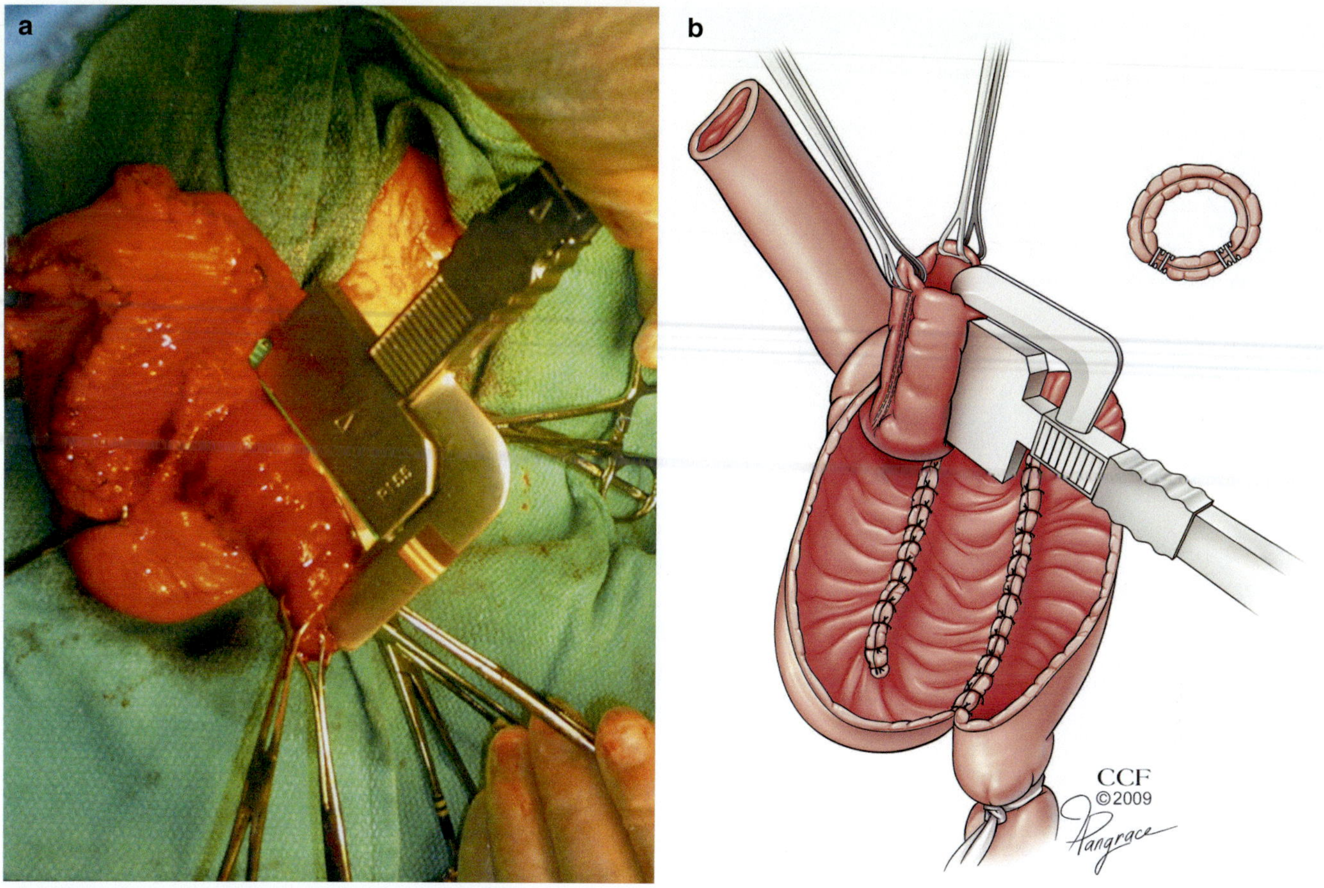

Fig. 10.11 Operative photograph (**a**) and illustration (**b**). The transverse stapler is used to place two parallel rows of staples on the inner aspect of the nipple valve on either side of the folded mesentery of the intussuscepted segment (Illustration © CCF)

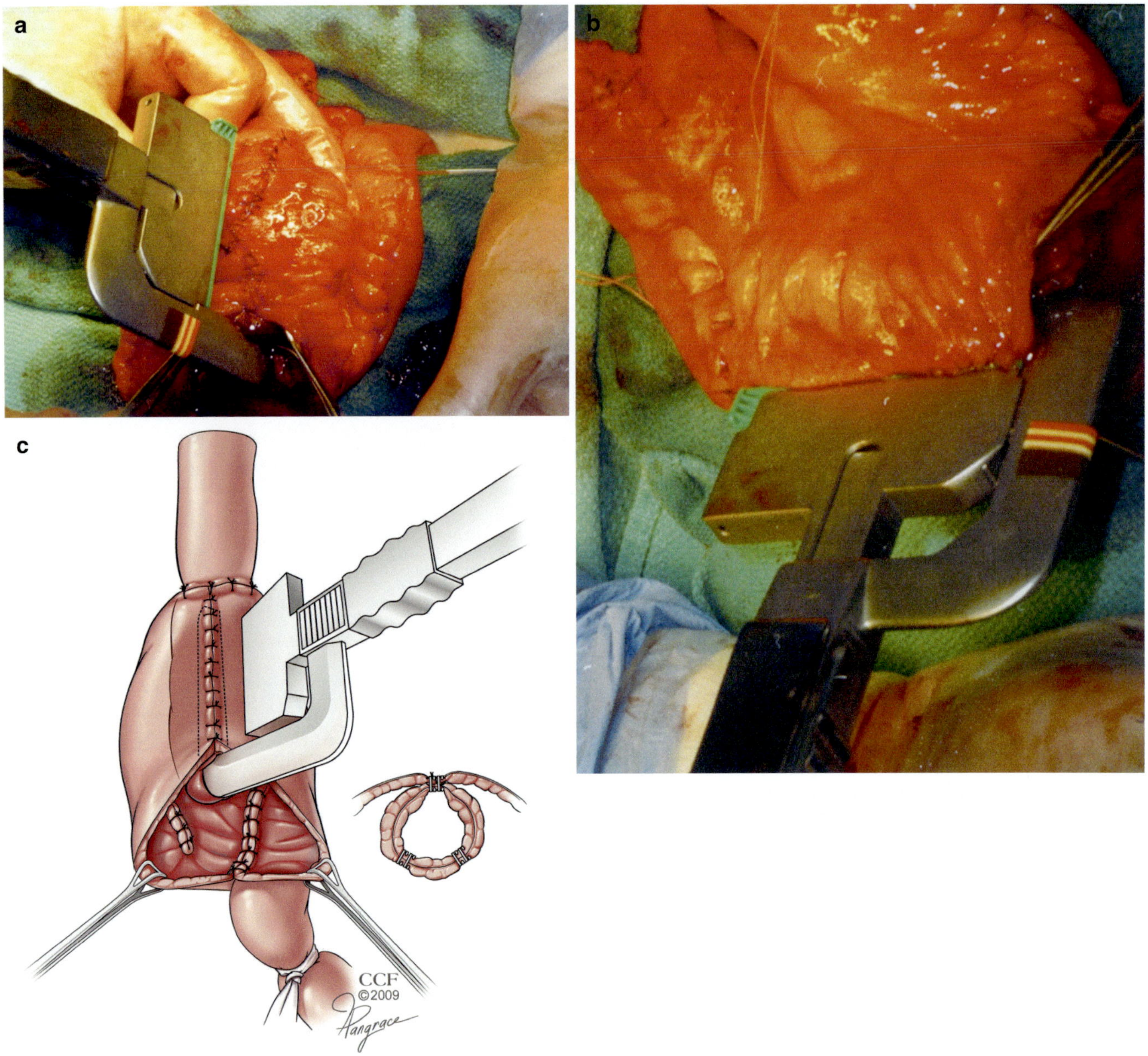

Fig. 10.12 Operative photographs (**a**, **b**) and illustration (**c**). The nipple valve is fixed to the pouch wall using the transverse stapler along the suture line previously placed to close the pouch wall (Illustration © CCF)

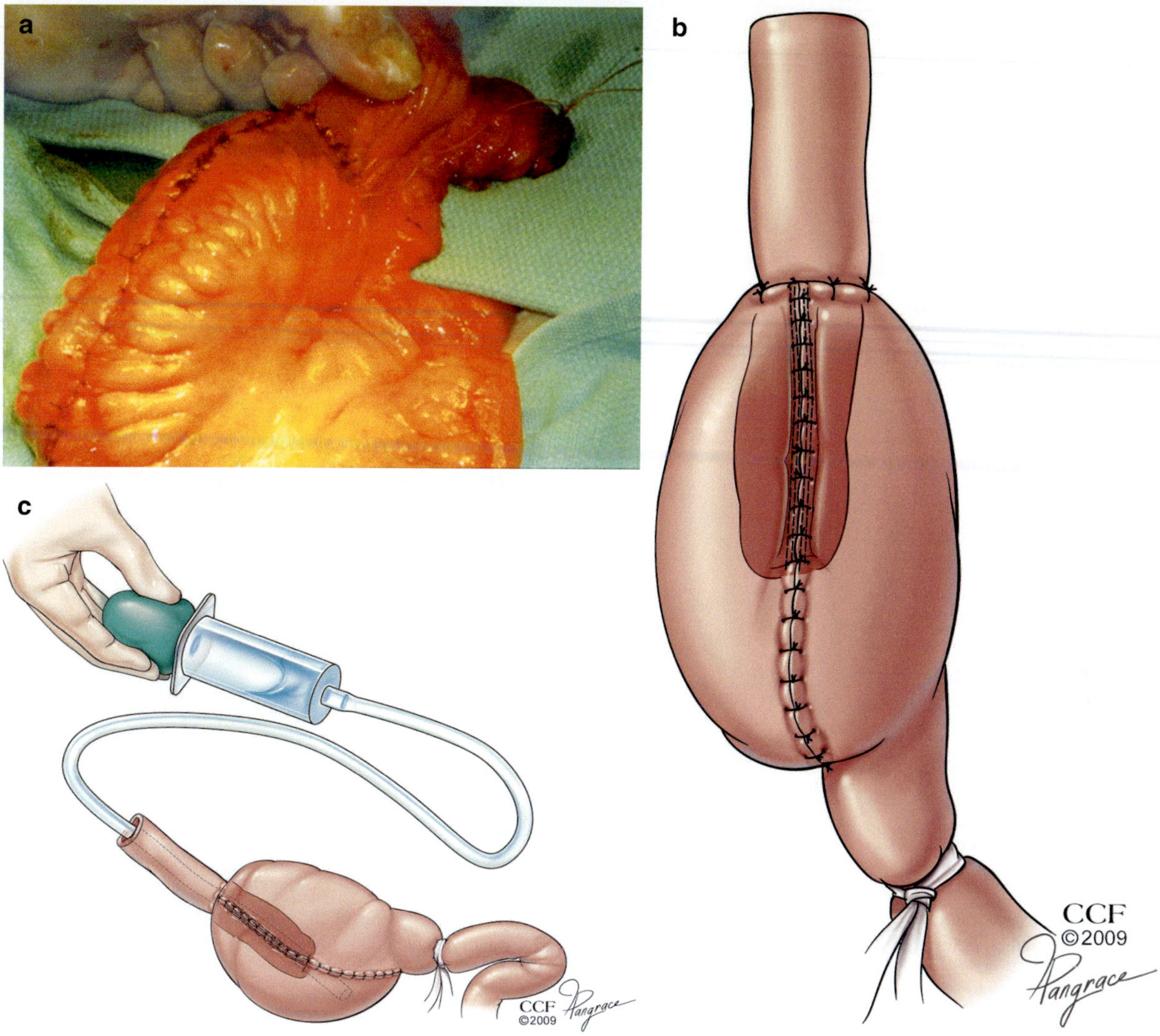

Fig. 10.13 Operative photograph (**a**) and illustration (**b**). The anterior wall of the pouch is then closed and (**c**) the pouch tested for integrity and continence (Illustrations © CCF)

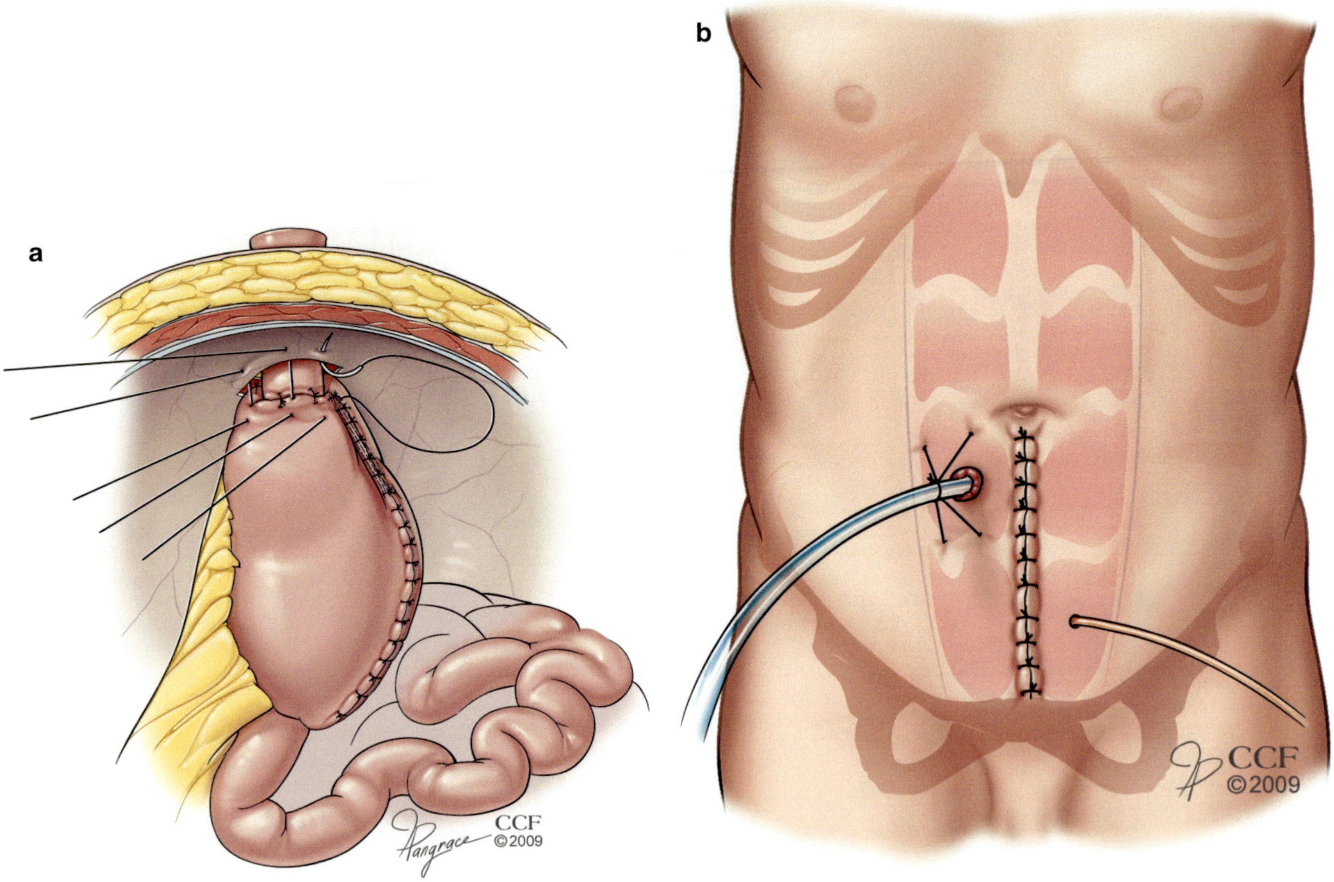

Fig. 10.14 (**a**) The exit conduit is brought through the abdominal wall, anchored to the inside of the abdominal wall and a drainage catheter secured safely in the pouch before (**b**) the abdomen is closed (Illustrations © CCF)

Table 10.2 Postoperative care protocol for patients with continent ileostomy

Day 1	Pouch irrigated every 2 h for the first 48 h.
Day 2	Pouch irrigated every 2 h for the first 48 h. Patient instruction begun: irrigation and dressing change.
Day 3	Pouch irrigated every 3–4 h unless thick effluent or clots. Catheter repositioning by daily shortening by 1 cm.
Day before discharge	Instruction regarding intubation and symptoms and signs of catheter blockage.
Day of discharge	Leg fitted with a bag.

Table 10.3 Intubation schedule for the continent ileostomy

First 3–4 weeks	Constant drainage of the catheter with irrigation 2–3 times a day and as needed with 30 cc of tap water
Next 3 weeks	Catheterization every 2–3 h during waking hours. Catheterization first thing in the morning and at bedtime. Catheter connected to constant drainage or emptied every 3–4 h at night. No eating or drinking within 2 h of bedtime.
Next 3 weeks	Catheterization every 3–4 h during waking hours. Catheterization first thing in the morning and at bedtime. No catheterization at night unless a full pouch is found on awakening. No eating or drinking within 2 h of bedtime.

References

1. Behrens DT, Paris M, Luttrell JN. Conversion of failed ileal pouch-anal anastomosis to continent ileostomy. Dis Colon Rectum. 1999;42(4):490–5; discussion 495–6.
2. Kusunoki M, Sakanoue Y, Shoji Y, et al. Conversion of malfunctioning J pouch to Kock's pouch. Case report. Acta Chir Scand. 1990;156(2):179–81.
3. Ecker KW, Haberer M, Feifel G. Conversion of the failing ileoanal pouch to reservoir-ileostomy rather than to ileostomy alone. Dis Colon Rectum. 1996;39(9):977–80.
4. Sjödahl R, Lemon E, Nyström PO, et al. Complications, surgical revision and quality of life with conventional and continent ileostomy. Acta Chir Scand. 1990;156(5):403–7.
5. Gerber A, Apt MK, Craig PH. The improved quality of life with the kock continent ileostomy. J Clin Gastroenterol. 1984;6(6):513–7.
6. Keltikangas-Järvinen L, Järvinen HJ. Psychosocial adaptation to ileostomy: a study after construction of conventional and continent stomies. Scand J Gastroenterol. 1987;22(2):202–6.
7. McLeod RS, Fazio VW. Quality of life with the continent ileostomy. World J Surg. 1984;8(1):90–5.
8. Ojerskog B, Hällström T, Kock NG, et al. Quality of life in ileostomy patients before and after conversion to the continent ileostomy. Int J Colorectal Dis. 1988;3(3):166–70.
9. Kock NG, Kock NG, Kock NG, Kock NG. Intra-abdominal "reservoir" in patients with permanent ileostomy. Preliminary observations on a procedure resulting in fecal "continence" in five ileostomy patients. Arch Surg. 1969;99(2):223–31.
10. Fazio VW, Church JM. Complications and function of the continent ileostomy at the Cleveland Clinic. World J Surg. 1988;12(2): 148–54.
11. McLeod RS, Fazio VW. The continent ileostomy. In: Jagelman DG, Jagelman DG, editors. Mucosal ulcerative colitis. Mount Kisco: Futura Publishing Co, Inc.; 1986. p. 241–75.
12. Okada Y, Arai Y, Oishi K, et al. Stable formation of the nipple valve in Kock pouch for diversion of the urinary tract. Surg Gynecol Obstet. 1989;169:315–8.
13. Goligher JC, Lintott D. Experience with 26 reservoir ileostomies. Br J Surg. 1975;62:893–900.
14. Kock NG, Brevinge H, Philipson BM, Ojerskog B. Continent ileostomy. The present technique and long term results. Ann Chir Gynaecol. 1986;75(2):63–70.
15. Olsson SA, Fredlund P, Pettersson U, Petersson BG. Continent ileostomy. A follow-up study of 60 patients. Acta Chir Scand. 1987; 153(2):119–22.
16. McLeod RS, Lavery IC, Leatherman JR, et al. Factors affecting quality of life with a conventional ileostomy. World J Surg. 1986;10(3):474–80.
17. Barnett WO. Current experiences with the continent intestinal reservoir. Surg Gynecol Obstet. 1989;168:1–5.
18. Fazio VW, Tjandra JJ. Technique for nipple valve fixation to prevent valve slippage in continent ileostomy. Dis Colon Rectum. 1992;35(12):1177–9.
19. Ecker KW, Hildebrandt U, Haberer M, et al. Biomechanical stabilization of the nipple valve in continent ileostomy. Br J Surg. 1996;83(11):1582–5.
20. Hultén L, Svaninger G. Facts about the Kock continent ileostomy. Dis Colon Rectum. 1984;27(8):553–7.
21. Vernava III AM, Goldberg SM. Is the kock pouch still a viable option? Int J Colorectal Dis. 1988;3(2):135–8.
22. Leijonmarck CE, Liljeqvist L, Poppen B, et al. Surgery after colectomy for ulcerative colitis. Dis Colon Rectum. 1992;35(5): 495–502.
23. Dozois RR, Kelly KA, Ilstrup D, et al. Factors affecting revision rate after continent ileostomy. Arch Surg. 1981;116(5):610–3.
24. Ojerskog B, Kock NG, Nilsson LO, et al. Long-term follow-up of patients with continent ileostomies. Dis Colon Rectum. 1990;33(3):184–9.
25. Nessar G, Fazio VW, Tekkis P, et al. Long-term outcome and quality of life after continent ileostomy. Dis Colon Rectum. 2006;49(3): 336–44.
26. Lian L, Fazio VW, Remzi FH, et al. Outcomes for patients undergoing continent ileostomy after a failed ileal pouch-anal anastomosis (IPAA). Dis Colon Rectum. 2009;52(8):1409–14.

Colostomy: Types, Indications, Formation, and Reversal

11

Thomas Garofalo

Introduction

The word ostomy is derived from the Latin word *ostium*, which is a small opening or orifice. A colostomy, therefore, is a procedure where the colon discharges stool through an artificial opening in the abdominal wall. There are five main indications for this procedure (Table 11.1) [1]; it can be performed either as a primary or secondary treatment (e.g., a diversion to "protect" a distal anastomosis or reconstruction).

Patient Education

The details and nuances of ostomy education will be discussed elsewhere, but some basics are worth mentioning here. Before surgery, the surgeon should hold a frank discussion with the patient regarding the possibility or certainty of a colostomy. To many patients, a *permanent* colostomy is initially unacceptable, but most understand when the lack of alternatives is explained to them.

When discussing a colostomy with the patient, it is important to explain how the colostomy will be made, the work needed to take care of it, and the potential long-term complications associated with it. Most importantly, the patient must understand that a colostomy is a change in his or her life and not the end of it. Further education in these matters will be discussed with the patient by an enterostomal nurse.

T. Garofalo
Department of Colorectal Surgery,
Digestive Disease Institute, Cleveland Clinic Foundation,
Cleveland, OH, USA
e-mail: garofat@ccf.org

Preparation

Marking the Site of a Colostomy

A few basic principles must be followed when marking the spot for a potential colostomy. Correct placement is important because it can make the colostomy easier to care for and possibly less obvious to others.

Table 11.1 Indications for colostomy

1. Obstruction
Congenital malformation
Neoplasm
Inflammation
Endometriosis
Ischemia
Radiation
2. Complications of inflammatory processes (diverticular disease, Crohn's disease, Ulcerative colitis)
Perforation
Fistula
Obstruction
3. Injury
Iatrogenic
Traumatic
4. Operations
Primary treatment
Secondary treatment (i.e., diversion)
5. Miscellaneous
Volvulus
Colonic dysmotility
Incontinence
Anal disease
Paralysis
Decubitus ulcers
Burns
Perineal infections

V.W. Fazio et al. (eds.), *Atlas of Intestinal Stomas*,
DOI 10.1007/978-0-387-78851-7_11, © Springer Science+Business Media, LLC 2012

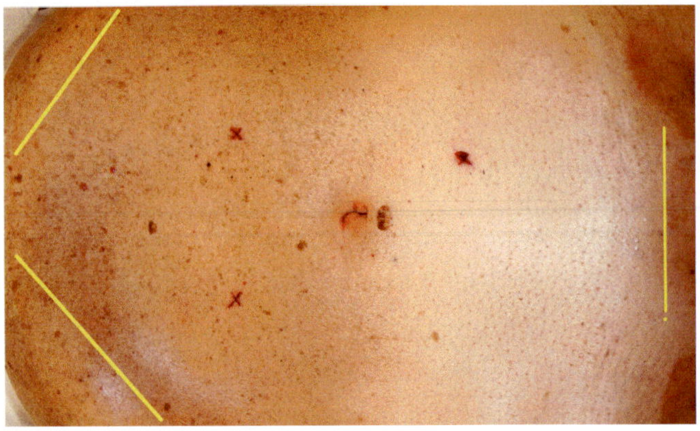

Fig. 11.1 Pre-operative abdomen with multiple potential colostomy sites marked. The *yellow lines* mark the costal margins and pubic tubercle

In the best of circumstances, an enterostomal nurse will have met with the patient preoperatively, conducted an education session, and marked the likely stoma site. However, the enterostomal nurse may not be available preoperatively and the surgeon may have to mark the patient. The surgeon may also be faced with performing an unexpected colostomy in the operating room with no previously marked site.

There are several factors to consider when marking a stoma site preoperatively. These include the patient's occupation, clothing style, belt line, flexibility, abdominal wall contour in the standing, sitting, and supine positions, any physical disabilities, location of previous abdominal scars, bony prominences, and abdominal girth [2]. The best site is on either side of the midline overlying the rectus muscle, 5 cm away from the umbilicus and any scars, bony prominences and, hopefully, the beltline. Additionally, the mark must be checked with the patient sitting to avoid any crevices and folds that may not be noted in the supine or standing positions [2] (Fig. 11.1).

Preoperative marking can be difficult in certain patients – e.g., a morbidly obese patient with a large pannus and those with multiple scars from previous abdominal procedures. In obese patients, it is always safer to place the ostomy in a supraumbilical position or else it may end up under the pannus where it will not be visible to the patient or allow for adequate appliance adhesion.

In patients with multiple scars and/or a compact torso, it may be necessary to choose several locations and ask them to wear the appliance for a day at a time in the different locations to see which one works best [2]. This, of course, only works in purely elective situations.

Intraoperative Stoma Marking

The need for a colostomy may become obvious intraoperatively, such as during trauma-related cases, in elective cases with unexpected and potentially life-threatening findings, or in unexpectedly complex cases with possible comorbidities that make a primary or unprotected anastomosis undesirable.

In these cases, it is important to remember that the stoma is likely to be temporary. However, a surgeon must always consider certain basic principles when planning a stoma, such as avoiding bony prominences, scars, and the umbilicus. Avoiding skin folds can be difficult if the patient is already lying flat. One way to check for folds is to first loosely approximate the midline skin with towel clamps, and then push on the abdominal wall skin from the proximal and distal ends of the incision. This may recreate skin folds that should be avoided. Finally, in obese patients, the lower abdomen should be avoided for the same reasons as noted in the previous section. Under these circumstances, it is best to try and place the stoma through the rectus muscle in either the left or right upper quadrant. Although not ideal, it will be easier for the patient to care for the stoma. If this placement is still difficult and there is no ideal location, the stoma can be brought out through the midline incision in the same way as a loop colostomy (see below).

Technique of End Colostomy

When creating a colostomy, the surgeon must follow these principles: (1) the bowel must be brought through the abdominal wall without tension, (2) stoma placement must be favorable so that the patient can easily apply a colostomy bag, (3) the bowel must be brought through the rectus muscle to lessen the risk of herniation, (4) the end of the bowel must be attached to the skin with primary suture to prevent stricture, and (5) the viability of the end of bowel must be demonstrated [3]. One premise that was stated in the first edition of this textbook – obliteration of the lateral gutter space to prevent volvulus and herniation of the small bowel – is now not usually performed.

It is with these basic principles in mind that we will describe the technique for colostomy formation. Laparoscopic colostomy formation is discussed in Chap. 12.

Preparation of the Abdominal Wall/Aperture

The previously marked site should be clearly identifiable (usually in the right lower quadrant). From here, it will be assumed that the abdomen is already open, and the resection portion of the procedure has already been completed.

A disc of skin is excised; the skin does not need to be elevated to do this. Four corners are marked using an electrocautery device, and they are connected in a circular fashion (Fig. 11.2a). For a standard colostomy, a disc of skin approximately 1.5–2 cm is removed (Fig. 11.2b). The dermis of the midline incision and the subjacent rectus fascia are held with Kocher clamps during construction of the stoma aperture, to keep the layers of the abdominal wall in alignment. A laparotomy pad is placed intraperitoneally under the stoma aperture and the abdominal wall is elevated with the surgeon's hand (Fig. 11.2c). The assistant now uses Army-Navy retractors to retract subcutaneous fat in a medial-to-lateral direction, and the electrocautery is used to divide the tissue vertically (Fig. 11.2d). Anterior rectus fascia is opened vertically; a cruciate incision is not necessary and may weaken the fascial layer and increase the risk for parastomal hernia. While the rectus muscle is exposed with the retractors, a large curved clamp is used to bluntly open the muscle fibers and expose the posterior rectus sheath. The posterior fascia is then opened to expose the intraperitoneal laparotomy pad (Fig. 11.2e). Care must be taken here as the inferior epigastric vessels can be injured.

The aperture is gently dilated using the surgeon's fingers. Generally speaking, the aperture should be dilated to two fingerbreadths (Fig. 11.2f). This is variable depending on the thickness of the abdominal wall and the amount of fatty tissue around the colon. If the fascial layer is dilated too much at this time, the risk of subsequent hernia increases. The layer can be at least partially closed once the colon has been delivered through the aperture.

Another laparotomy pad is now inserted into the aperture and around the midline wound and secured with a large curved clamp. This will allow the surgeon to control the opening and stem bleeding from the capillaries.

Preparation of the Bowel

Previous generations of colorectal surgeons were advised to avoid using the sigmoid colon when creating an end colostomy, especially a permanent one, due to the possibility that the blood supply to the sigmoid colon could be compromised during resection. That, in turn, could lead to ischemia and subsequent stricture or retraction of the stoma. The sigmoid colon may also be hypertrophied from the presence of diverticular disease and may be difficult to work with. In reality, it is often difficult to exactly determine where the descending

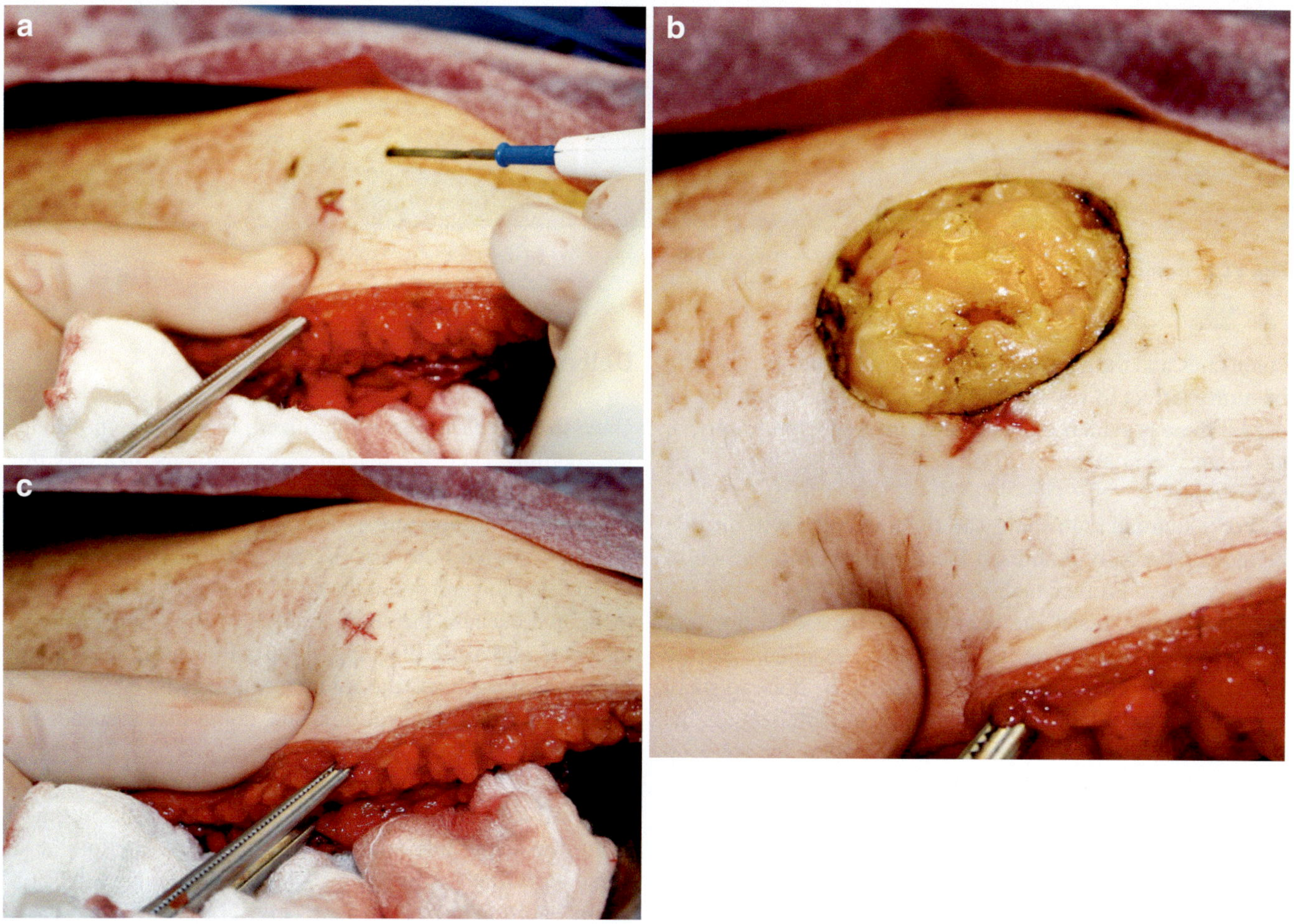

Fig. 11.2 (**a**) Marking the edges of the planned aperture with electrocautery. (**b**) Skin disk has been removed. (**c**) Fascial edge and skin edge are grasped and elevated. A laparotomy pad is placed to assist in elevation of fascia and protect underlying structures. (**d**) Exposing the anterior fascial layer. (**e**) Opening of the posterior fascia. Illustration © CCF. (**f**) Dilation of the aperture to the width of two fingers

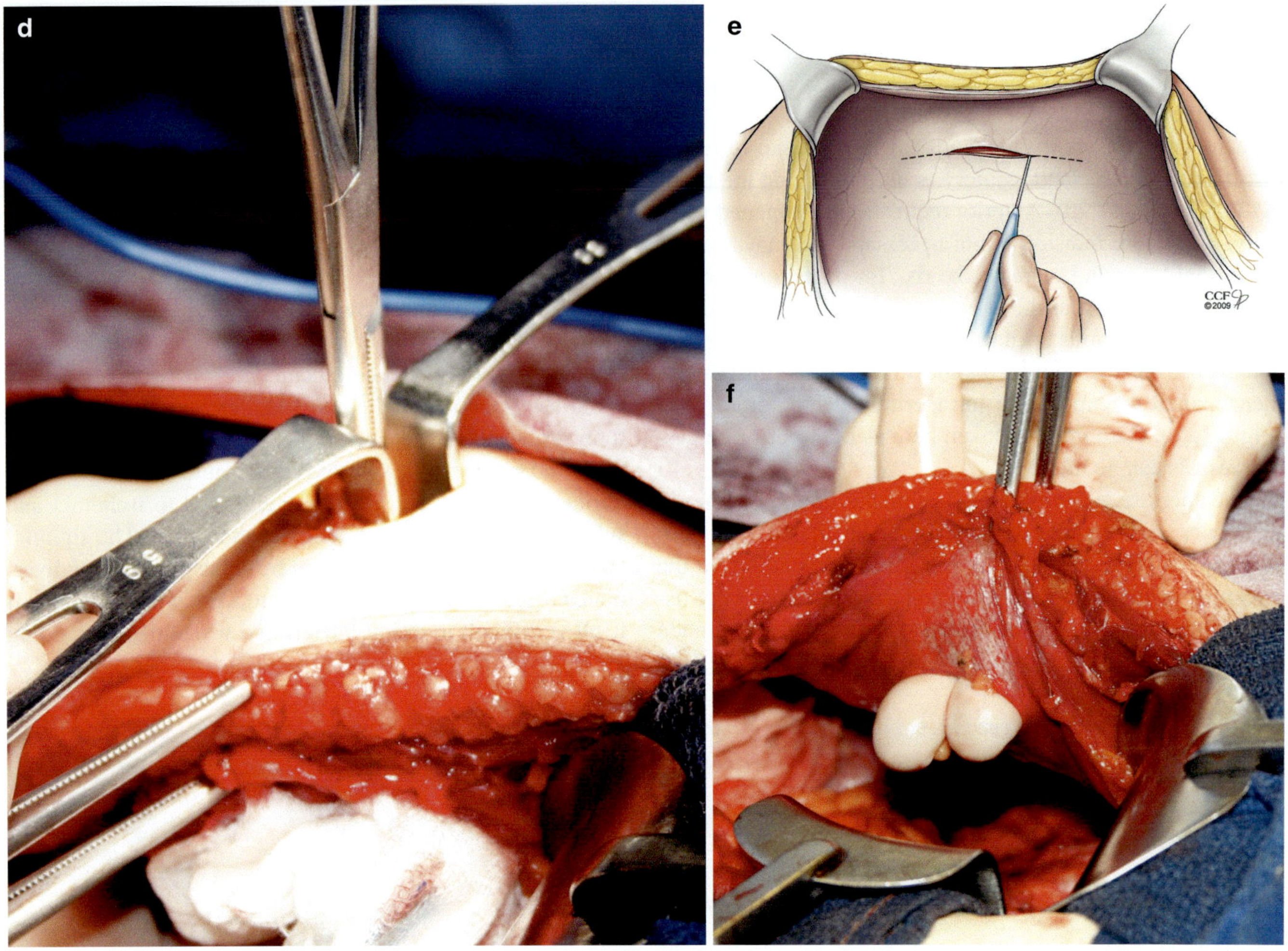

Fig. 11.2 (continued)

colon ends and the sigmoid colon begins. Therefore, it would be more correct to say that the sigmoid colon should not be used if there is evidence of ischemia, marked hypertrophy, or an extensive number of diverticuli in the segment to be exteriorized.

For a sigmoid colostomy, the sigmoid colon will already be at least partially mobilized from the resection portion of the procedure. Further mobilization may not be needed but the stoma must reach the skin around the stoma aperture without tension. Only in rare cases does the splenic flexure need to be mobilized. Mobilization should be done in small increments, and after each small amount of mobilization, the reach of the stoma should be checked by pulling the colon up through the midline incision adjacent to the fascia in the area of the aperture. Once the colon reaches 4–5 cm beyond the skin level, mobilization is complete. Most of the mobilization can be achieved solely by dividing the line of Toldt and dividing the retroperitoneal attachments of the colon. Only a minor amount of medial mobilization of the mesentery should be needed (Figs. 11.3 and 11.4).

Delivery of the Bowel

Once the bowel has been mobilized, it is delivered through the aperture. There are several ways to do this. In a very thin patient with a thin mesentery, it is possible to place two fingers through the aperture, grasp the colon and pull it through. Another method is to use two Babcock or Allis clamps to grasp the colon and pull it through. I generally do not use this technique because the sharper edges of the clamps can tear the colon and cause bleeding, devascularization, or contamination. This trauma to the colon may also cause enough damage that further mobilization of the colon may be needed to compensate for the colon that will need to be excised if it is devascularized. It is generally more preferable to insert a large curved clamp through the aperture, grasp the bowel along the staple line and pull it through the aperture at an angle such that the mesentery (with the vascular supply) is the last portion to be pulled out (Fig. 11.5).

The technique of tunneling the bowel under the peritoneum and out through the aperture was described in the first

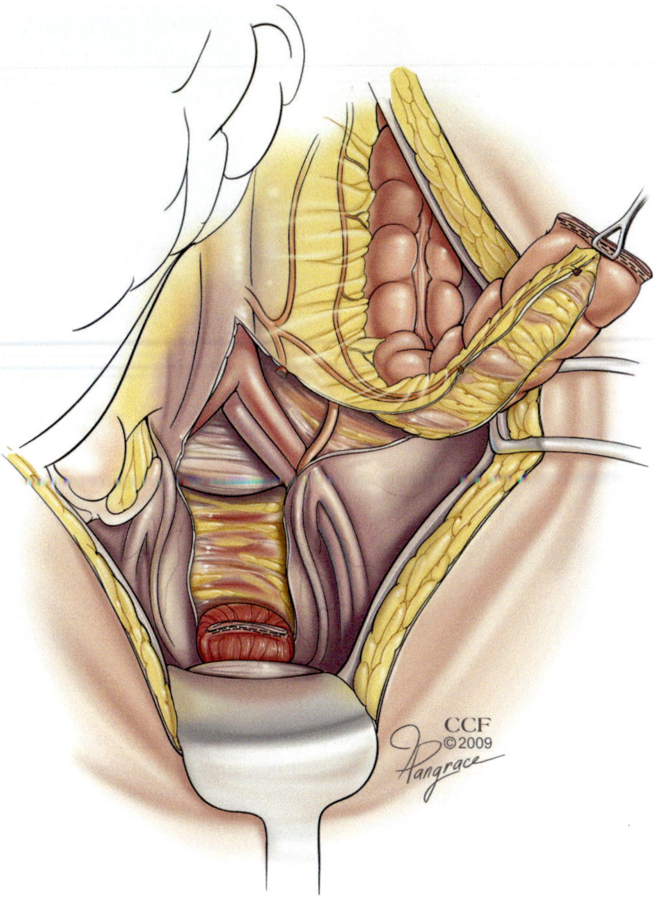

Fig. 11.3 Mobilization of colon. Illustration © CCF

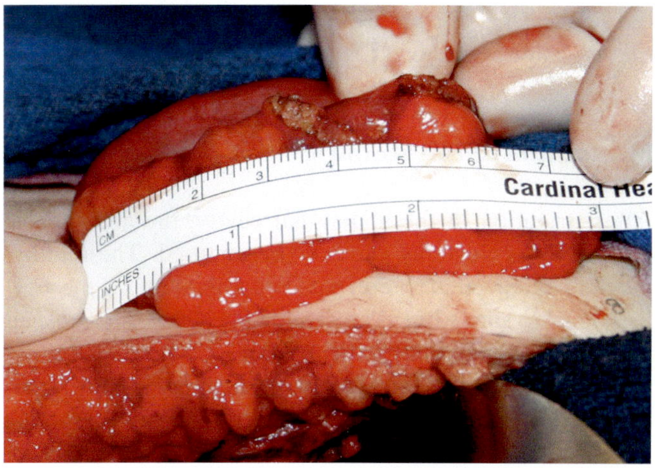

Fig. 11.4 Assuring adequate length of the mobilized colon. Note: The bowel has already been delivered through aperture

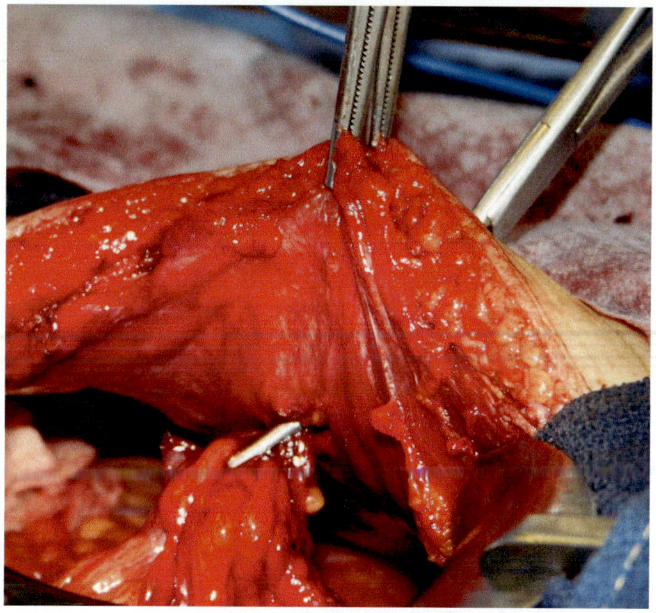

Fig. 11.5 Delivery of the bowel through the aperture. The staple line is grasped with a curved clamp and withdrawn through the aperture. The vascular supply should be the last portion of the bowel that is delivered

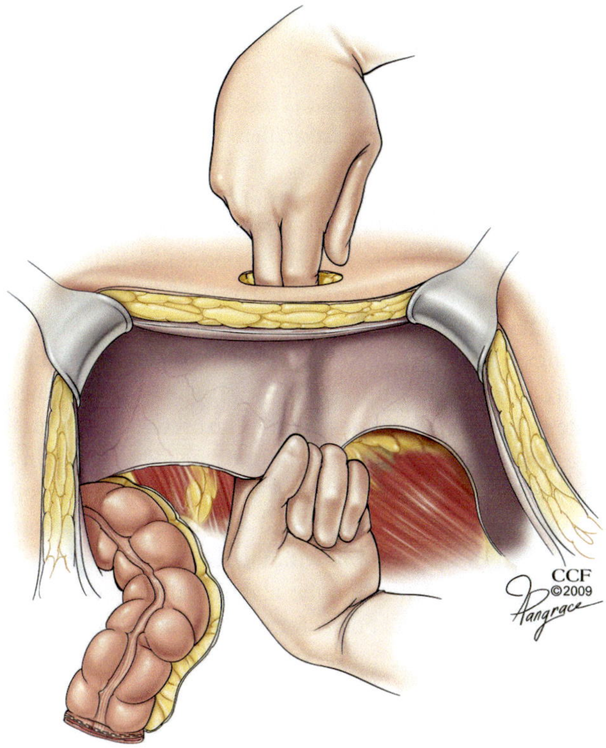

Fig. 11.6 Tunneling of the bowel to prevent herniation. Illustration © CCF

edition of this textbook (Fig. 11.6). This was described as a way of preventing herniation of the bowel. This technique is no longer routinely performed but is a good way of treating or preventing colostomy prolapse. Likewise, sutures between the internal fascial layer and the serosa of the bowel are unnecessary (Fig. 11.7). This technique will not provide any significant amount of fixation or prevent herniation. Additionally, if these sutures are placed improperly, a fistula can form.

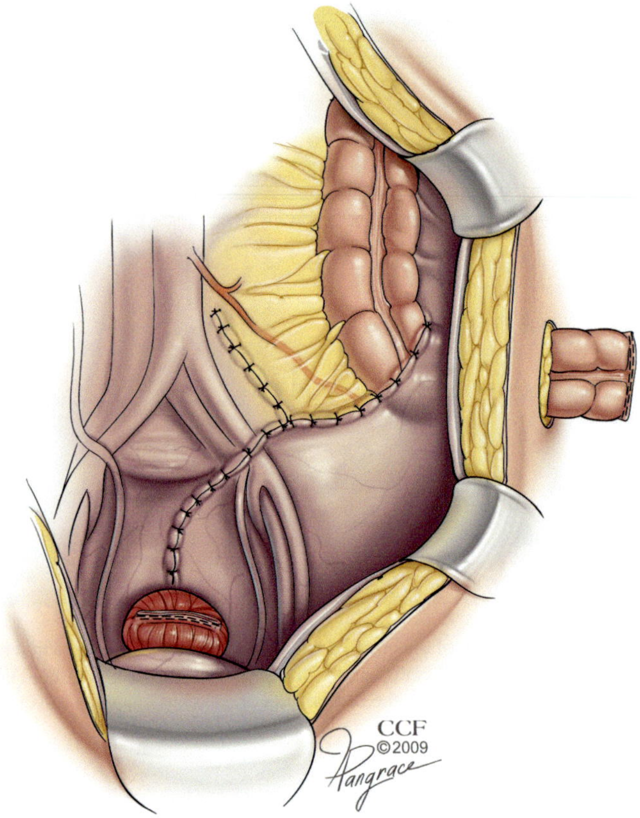

Fig. 11.7 Closure of peritoneum to assist in fixation of bowel and to help prevent prolapse and herniation. Illustration © CCF

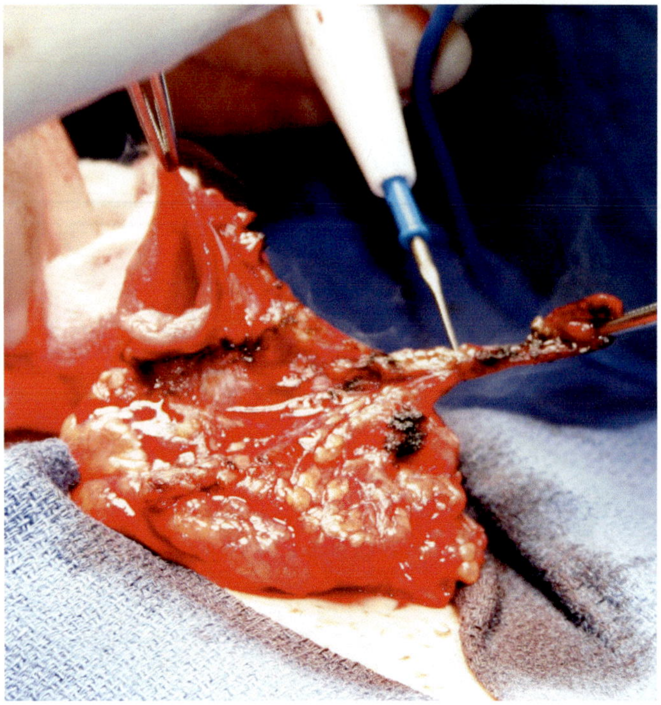

Fig. 11.8 Removal of excess fatty tissue and epiploica. Note in this photo that the bowel has already been delivered and is already open. This step can be performed before or after opening the bowel

In many cases, there is a large amount of fatty tissue on the colon and attached epiploica. The mesentery may also be quite thick. There are essentially two methods to address this problem. The first is to further dilate the aperture so that the colon can easily pass through the wall. The fascia can then be tightened as previously described. The other option is to trim the epiploica and thin out the fatty tissue (Fig. 11.8). In certain cases, this is feasible. The epiploica can be carefully removed with electrocautery and the mesenteric fat can be thinned out or even shrunk with the cautery to facilitate passage of the bowel through the abdominal wall. This is also helpful in everting the bowel for maturation. When removing this tissue, great care must be taken to avoid compromising the mesenteric blood supply. If the blood supply to the end of the bowel is compromised, further resection and mobilization will be needed.

If, after delivery of the bowel, the colostomy aperture is loose, it may require partial closure or occlusion. The internal fascia can be closed with interrupted absorbable monofilament sutures. These sutures are placed one at a time until the fascial defect is adequately closed (Fig. 11.9). At this point, the surgeon should be able to comfortably insert only his/her little finger between the bowel wall and the fascial layer. Defects larger than this can predispose to hernia formation. This area can then be "reinforced" with a bolster using adjacent adipose tissue or appendices epiploica and suturing it loosely to the facial layer on the peritoneal side of the defect. This step, however, is usually performed solely at the surgeon's discretion.

Maturation of the Stoma

After irrigation of the abdominal cavity, the abdomen is closed. The colostomy can now be matured. The midline incision is covered to prevent contamination of the new incision. If a staple line is present on the bowel, it is grasped and elevated and sharply excised (Fig. 11.10). Bleeding from the cut edge of the bowel is cauterized. At this point, bleeding should be brisk. Lack of bleeding or slow venous bleeding suggests that either devascularization of the bowel has occurred or that the vasculature is being impinged upon as it passes through the abdominal wall. In either case, the abdomen should be re-opened, the bowel should be returned to the abdominal cavity, and the blood supply of the stoma checked. If brisk bleeding is noted once the bowel is returned to the abdomen, this indicates impingement from the fascia. Either the aperture will need to be dilated further or the colon may need further mobilization to allow for a smoother turn into the aperture.

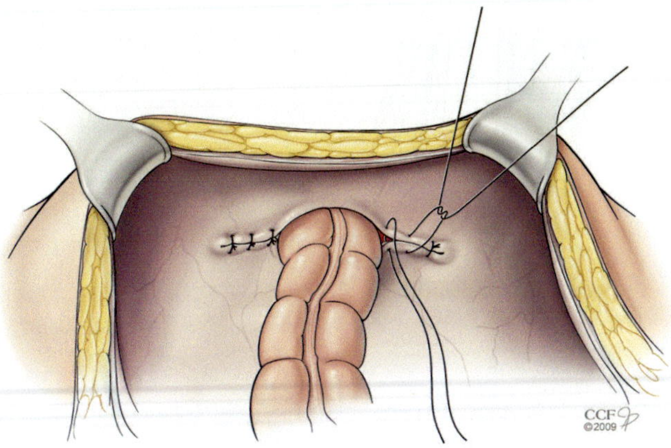

Fig. 11.9 Closure of internal fascial layer. Sutures should be interrupted so that a gradual closure takes place and can be easily adjusted. Illustration © CCF

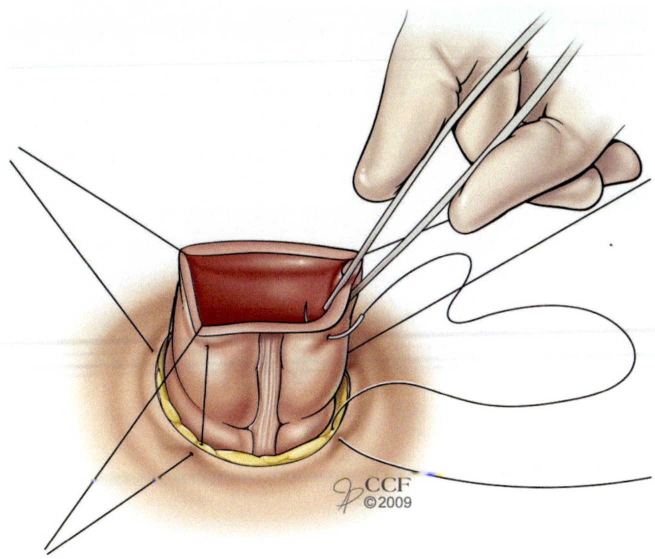

Fig. 11.11 Sutures are place in four quadrants and held with hemostats. Illustration © CCF

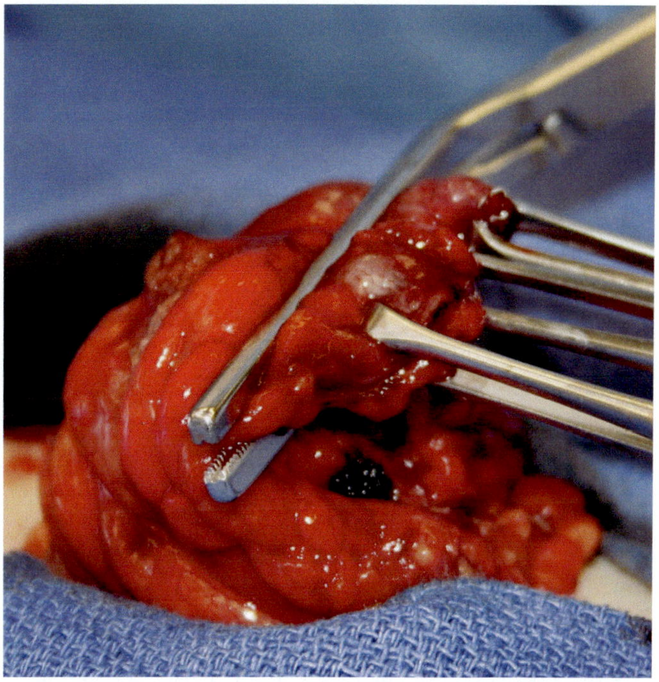

Fig. 11.10 The staple line is excised. The bowel is grasped with an atraumatic bowel clamp to prevent contamination. Bleeding from the cut edge should be brisk

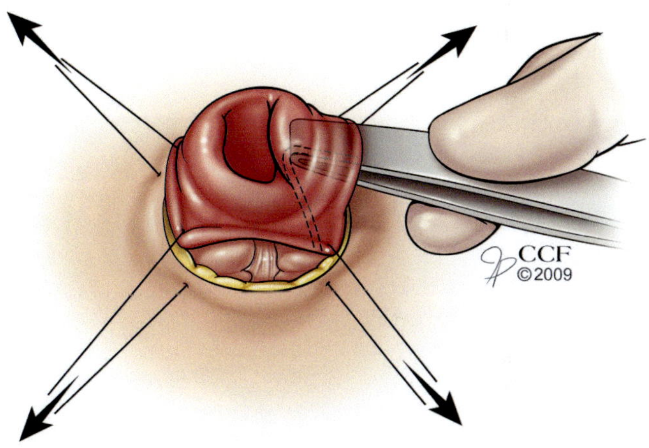

Fig. 11.12 Tension is placed on the quadrant sutures using eh hemostats. The blunt end of a forceps is used to evert the bowel wall. Illustration © CCF

The bowel edge is then everted using 3.0 chromic sutures (3.0 Vicryl suture can also be used). Four quadrant sutures are placed – typically beginning at the 2:00, 4:00, 8:00, and 10:00 o'clock positions (Fig. 11.11). The sutures are placed full thickness through the bowel wall and then through the dermal layer of the skin. The sutures are not passed through the serosal layer of the bowel at skin level. An Adson's forceps is used to assist the eversion as tension is placed on the sutures (Fig. 11.12). The sutures are then tied, and additional sutures are placed circumferentially as needed (Fig. 11.13). An ostomy appliance is cut to the appropriate size and placed (Fig. 11.14).

Closure of End Colostomy

Typically, closure of an end colostomy requires a laparotomy. Laparoscopic techniques can be used in certain circumstances and that will be discussed elsewhere.

Once the peritoneal cavity is open, any adhesions are lysed. The stump of the rectum or distal sigmoid colon must be identified and mobilized. The stump may have been previously marked with nonabsorbable sutures to facilitate identification. This step should be performed first because failure to identify and mobilize the rectal stump can, prevent safe closure of the colostomy. If the rectum cannot be identified and adequately mobilized, a permanent colostomy may be

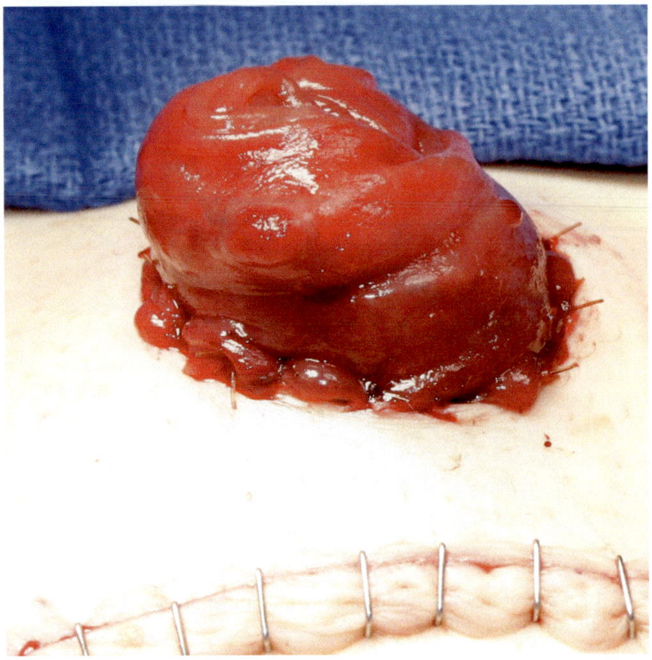

Fig. 11.13 After the bowel wall has been everted, additional sutures are placed at the mucocutaneous junction to complete the maturation of the colostomy

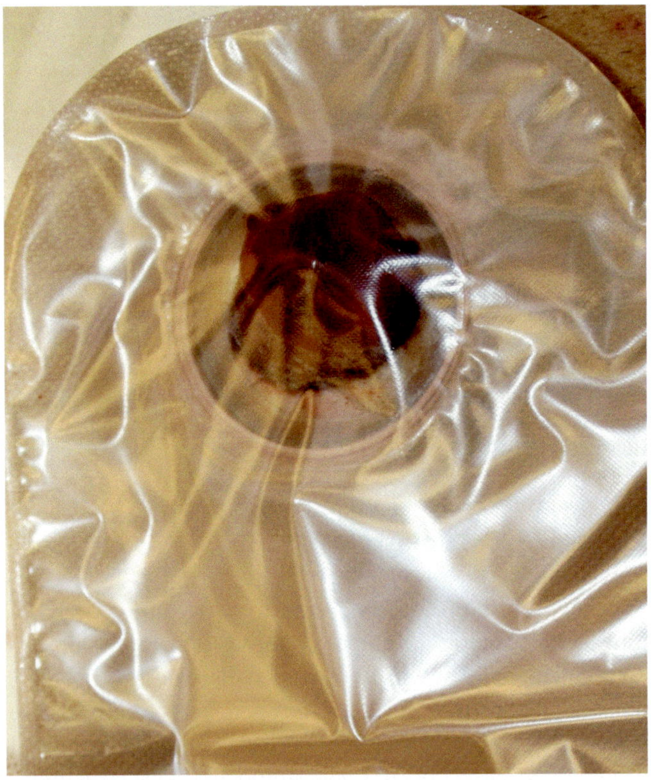

Fig. 11.14 An ostomy appliance is cut to allow easy passage of the colostomy

needed. If the reconnection is attempted in cases where mobilization is difficult, a temporary diverting ileostomy may be created to allow for healing. Additionally, if the stump cannot be mobilized at this point, there has been no manipulation of the colostomy and, therefore, no opportunity for injury to the colostomy and the development of subsequent complications.

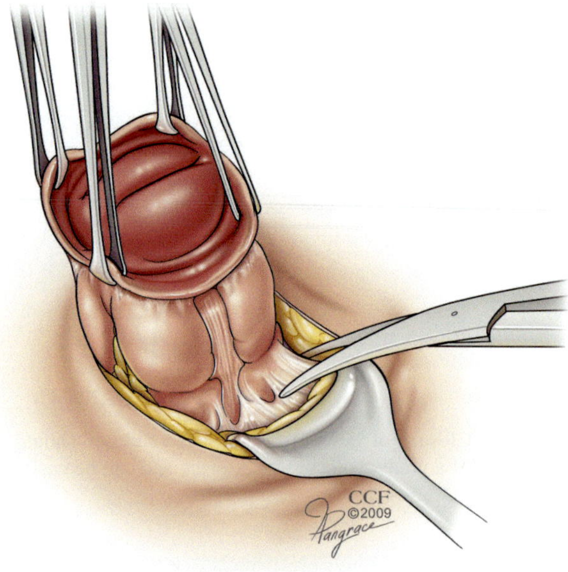

Fig. 11.15 A circumferential incision is made around the colostomy and the skin edges are grasped and elevated with clamps. The subcutaneous adhesions are divided to mobilize the bowel. Illustration © CCF

Once the stump has been mobilized, the bowel should be closely examined, and any residual sigmoid colon should be resected. The technique that is used for the anastomosis – end-to-end, side-to-end, stapled, or hand-sewn – is at the surgeon's discretion. However, a diverted rectum often atrophies and becomes fragile, so that safe insertion of a stapler transanally is difficult.

Once it has been deemed possible to proceed with reconstruction, the colostomy can be mobilized. A circumferential incision is made on the skin 2–3 mm around the mucocutaneous junction. The skin edges are grasped and elevated, and the subcutaneous adhesions divided (Fig. 11.15). This can be done using whatever instrument the surgeon feels most comfortable working with. I typically use sharp dissection with a #15-blade knife. Metzembaum scissors and even electrocautery can be used depending on the difficulty of the procedure. There is a subtle difference in color and texture between mesenteric fat and subcutaneous fat. Recognizing this difference is a key to easier mobilization. Near the fascial layer, one or two fingers can be placed from the inside surface to guide entry into the peritoneum. Care must be taken on the side of the bowel that contains the mesentery and blood supply. If the blood supply is compromised during mobilization, there will be resultant ischemia of a variable length of the distal part of the colon and resection of this ischemic portion of the bowel will be required. If there is no concern about the length or "reach" of the bowel (i.e., if it will be long enough to reach the distal rectal stump), it can

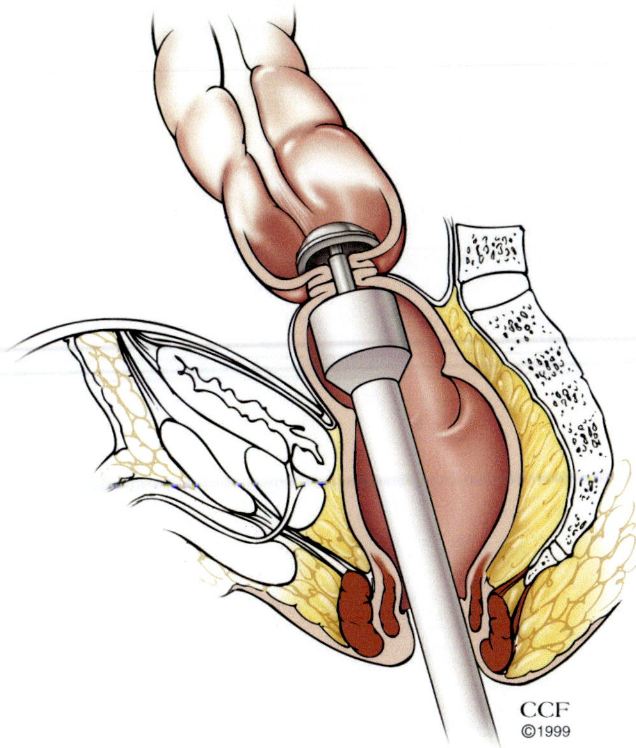

Fig. 11.16 Completion of colostomy reversal. End-to-end anastomosis using stapling device. Illustration © CCF

be divided on the peritoneal side using a GIA stapler in order to expedite the procedure. The remnant stump of colon in the abdominal wall can be excised later.

Once the colostomy mobilization is completed, the bowel is checked to ensure that the "reach" is adequate for a tension-free anastomosis. If there is redundancy, no further mobilization may be needed and the anastomosis is performed. If a significant amount of bowel has already been resected during a previous surgery, the splenic flexure will most likely need to be mobilized in order to achieve a tension-free anastomosis. Of course, care must be taken to avoid injuring the blood supply during mobilization, especially in areas containing adhesions and areas that may have been manipulated during previous surgeries. Anastomosis is performed in either a hand-sewn fashion or with an end-to-end stapling device (Fig. 11.16).

Once the anastomosis is completed, the colostomy aperture is closed. The fascial layer may need to be mobilized from the subcutaneous fat before it is closed with nonabsorbable sutures in an interrupted figure-of-eight fashion. Normally, 3–4 sutures are required. The subcutaneous tissue is irrigated and a pursestring suture (3.0 absorbable) is placed in the dermal layer. This is done in order to minimize the size of the resultant skin defect. The wound is then packed with a betadine-soaked Telfa pad. The skin can be closed primarily, but obliteration of the underlying dead space can be difficult and a seroma, hematoma, or abscess can form. Leaving the skin open to heal by secondary intention is safe and carries a smaller risk of infection and possibly a smaller chance of hernia formation. The resultant scar is not significantly larger or more disfiguring than those resulting from primary closure.

Technique of Loop End Colostomy

Indications

An end colostomy can be technically difficult to create in obese patients and in those who have a shortened, thick or friable mesentery and retraction. Stoma necrosis may be seen in 1–13% of these patients [4]. Under such circumstances, an end loop colostomy may be a better choice.

Prasad (1984) and Hebert (1988) described the end-loop stoma. It protects the blood supply to the end of the bowel and helps prevent complications of retraction and necrosis. Originally, the bowel was opened on the mesenteric border just proximal to the staple line at the divided end of the bowel. The staple line does not need to be buried in the subcutaneous tissue [4, 5].

Preparation of the Abdominal Wall

The technique of abdominal wall aperture creation is the same as for an end colostomy.

Delivery of the Bowel

The bowel is delivered in a fashion similar to that of a standard loop colostomy. The staple line can be reinforced prior to delivery. A penrose drain is passed though the mesentery 3–4 cm proximal to the cut edge. The drain is grasped with a large curved clamp that was previously placed through the aperture. The bowel is then carefully drawn through the aperture (Fig. 11.17). The drain is exchanged for a supportive rod (Fig. 11.18). The staple line is pushed into the subcutaneous tissue in order to create the typical loop.

Maturation of the Stoma

The bowel is then opened on the antimesenteric border 3–4 cm proximal to the divided end of the bowel (Fig. 11.19a). The proximal limb is everted and sutured to the skin with absorbable suture in the same fashion as for an end colostomy (see Fig. 11.12). The short, nonfunctional distal limb is buried within the subcutaneous tissue or just below the fascial layer (Fig. 11.19b). A *karaya ring* is placed, followed by an ostomy appliance.

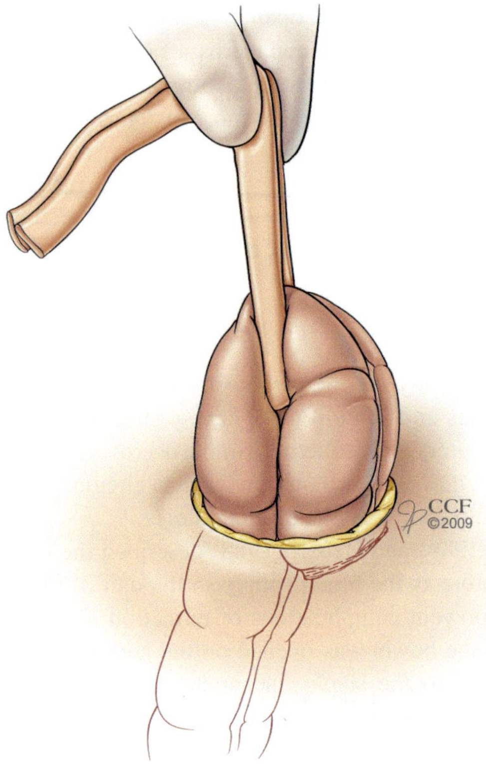

Fig. 11.17 Delivery of a loop (end) colostomy using a Penrose drain. Illustration © CCF

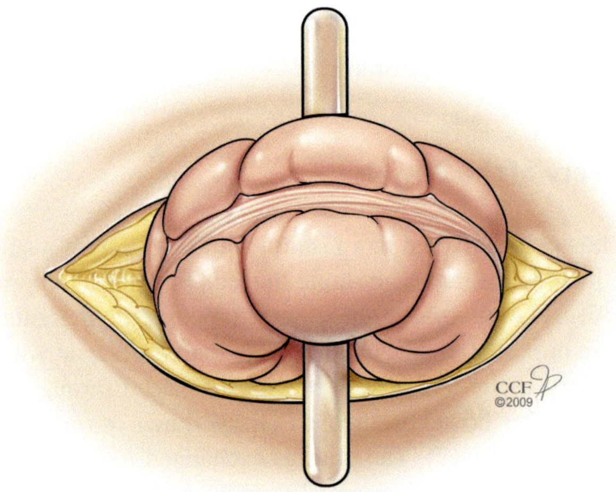

Fig. 11.18 Replacement of Penrose drain with a plastic supportive rod. Illustration © CCF

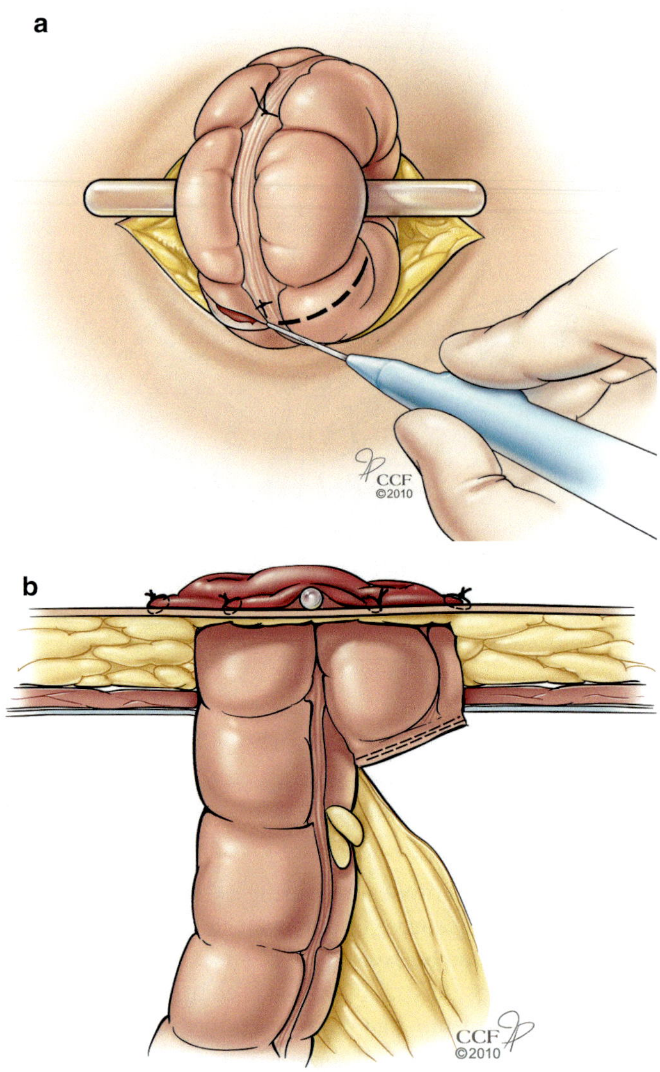

Fig. 11.19 (**a**) Opening of distal limb of loop. Illustration © CCF. (**b**) Suture placement for maturation of proximal limb and eversion of proximal limb of loop colostomy. Illustration © CCF

Closure of Loop End Colostomy

In cases where closure of this type of colostomy is indicated and possible, the technique is similar to that used for an end colostomy. After the abdomen is opened and the distal portion of the bowel is identified and prepared, the colostomy is mobilized and the loop returned to the abdominal cavity. The bowel is then mobilized as previously described, in order to achieve a tension-free anastomosis. It is better to resect the diverted portion of the colostomy and perform the anastomosis because the stoma site and the distal bowel, than to try to preserve the diverted loop by making two anastomoses in close proximity. However, if the reach for the anastomosis is an issue and if the distal limb is long enough (i.e. >3 cm), then closure of the colostomy with preservation of the distal loop will help. The anastomosis should be air tested for leaks.

Technique of Loop Colostomy

Use of the loop colostomy has declined over the past 20–25 years because loop ileostomy is generally considered a better form of fecal diversion [2]. However, loop colostomy

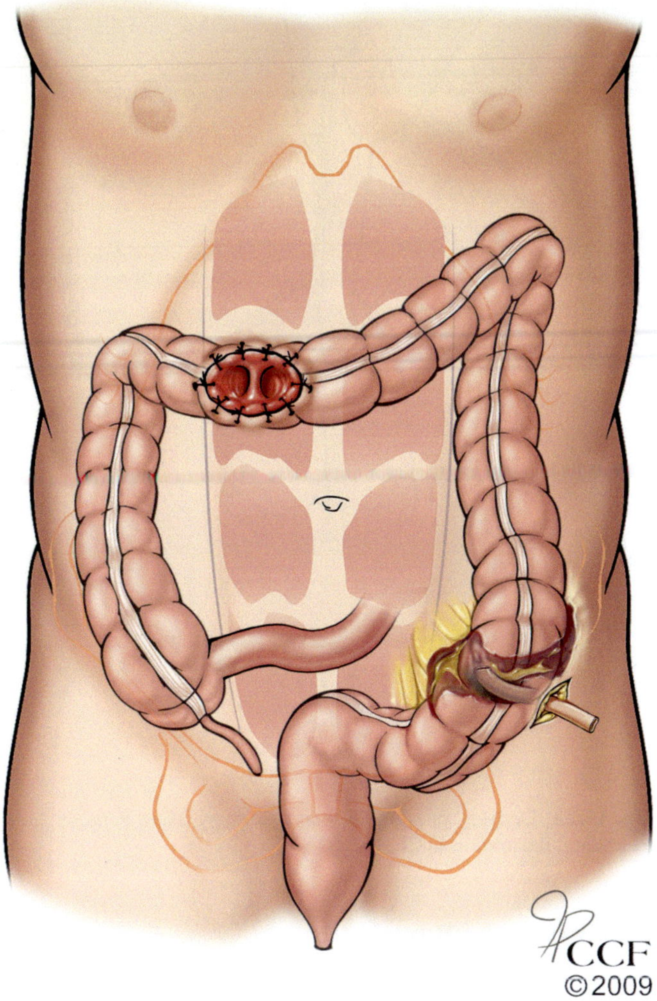

Fig. 11.20 Loop transverse colostomy. Illustration © CCF

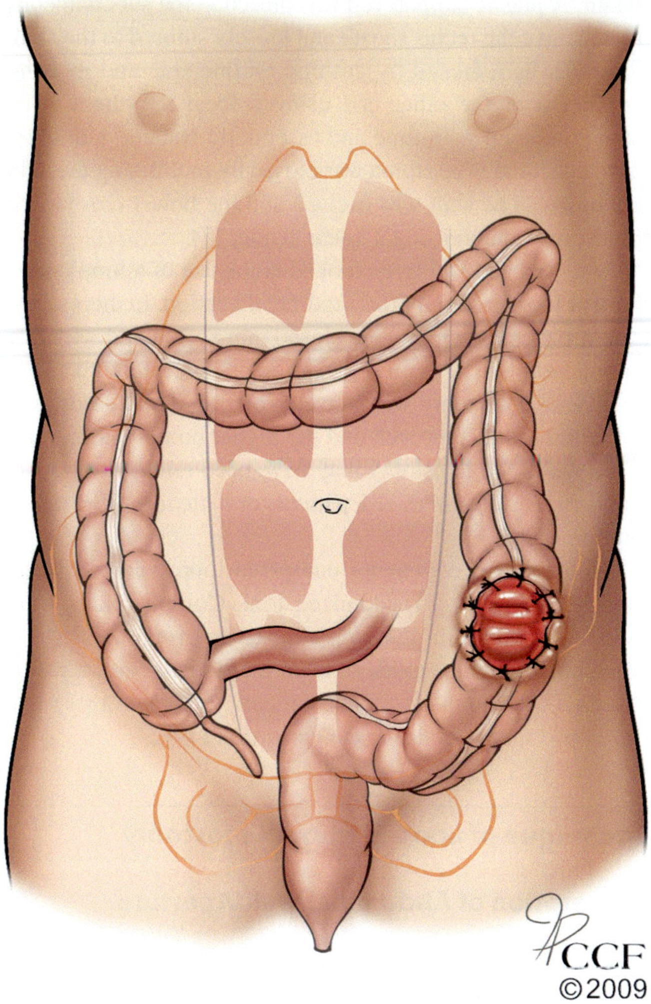

Fig. 11.21 Loop sigmoid colostomy. Illustration © CCF

still may have an important role in the management of acute large bowel obstruction [6].

Loop transverse colostomy (Fig. 11.20) or loop sigmoid colostomy (Fig. 11.21) is used to divert the fecal stream in extreme situations such as obliterative peritonitis, distal volvulus, or an obstructing distal cancer that is not resectable. It is also a useful technique in a sick patient with diverticulitis where the sigmoid colon will not easily reach the anterior abdominal wall and where mobilization of the splenic flexure is too much dissection. Here the end of the sigmoid can be stapled across, and a transverse loop colostomy made. Finally, a loop transverse colostomy is the easiest form of diversion in massively obese patients as the transverse colon is the most superficial part of the intestine in a patient lying supine, and so requires the least amount of mobilization to exteriorize.

Loop colostomies have a higher incidence of prolapse and parastomal hernia than end colostomy. A loop ileostomy is a better option in patients who have an obstructing distal tumor that potentially could be resected in the future (after neoadjuvant therapy, for example), and in cases of abdominopelvic sepsis from a distal perforation simply because it helps preserve the colon for future resection/reconstruction without injuring the blood supply. Additionally, ileostomies tend to be easier to manage, are odorless, and easier to close [6].

In strictly palliative cases, the transverse colon or the sigmoid colon can be passed though the rectus muscle via a muscle-splitting incision. This minimizes the invasiveness of the procedure and may decrease the risk for parastomal hernia. Of course, if the abdomen is already open, a loop transverse colostomy can easily be placed in the midline at the upper portion of the incision.

Loop colostomies are relatively easier to close than end colostomies. However, the mesentery of the colon – and in the case of a transverse colostomy, the omentum – can be injured and lead to bleeding that can be difficult to control.

Guivarc'h and colleagues described a slight variation in the loop colostomy technique. In their study, the colostomy was brought out through the lateral aspect of the rectus sheath. A plastic support rod was placed in the subcutaneous tissue above the rectus sheath and loosely sutured to the skin. The rod was removed by pushing on one side and incising the skin over the other end using a local anesthetic. The stoma retracted with time and essentially became a double-barreled stoma. The stoma was closed by mobilizing the skin and bowel. The skin was excised and the bowel closed in a transverse fashion using a linear stapler [7].

Rutegard and Dahlgren looked at the use of a loop colostomy or loop ileostomy for proximal diversion. In their study, transverse colostomies were closed more often and with few complications. The main complication associated with a loop transverse colostomy was bowel prolapse. Their study was not randomized, however, and the higher complication rates noted with loop ileostomy may have been related to the fact that they recruited high-risk patients or patients with a terminal disease [8].

Williams and colleagues compared loop colostomy and loop ileostomy in a randomized trial. Complications were twice as common in the loop colostomy group. Also, loop colostomy patients tended to need more visits with a stoma therapist than loop ileostomy patients (58% vs. 18%) and developed more hernias at the closure site [9].

Technique of Loop Sigmoid Colostomy

Preparation of Abdominal Wall/Aperture

The process used to prepare the abdominal wall is the same as that used for an end colostomy. However, because two limbs of bowel will pass through the abdominal wall, the aperture must be much larger (easily up to three fingers in diameter) [6]. In certain cases where the bowel is edematous due to inflammation, the aperture will need to be even wider. Of course, this increases the risk for parastomal hernia, but in all likelihood, this particular type of colostomy will be temporary.

Preparation/Mobilization of the Bowel

In a few cases where there is marked redundancy of the sigmoid colon, mobilization may not be needed because a loop of intestine will easily reach through the wall of the abdomen. This is more likely to be the case in a patient with nonresectable cancer. The reach should be determined in a fashion similar to that used with an end colostomy.

In most cases, some mobilization will be required. I start at the line of Toldt as it crosses the pelvic brim and work up toward the splenic flexure. The mesentery is carefully mobilized off the retroperitoneum. Again, it is important to mobilize only as much colon as will be needed to reach through the abdominal wall.

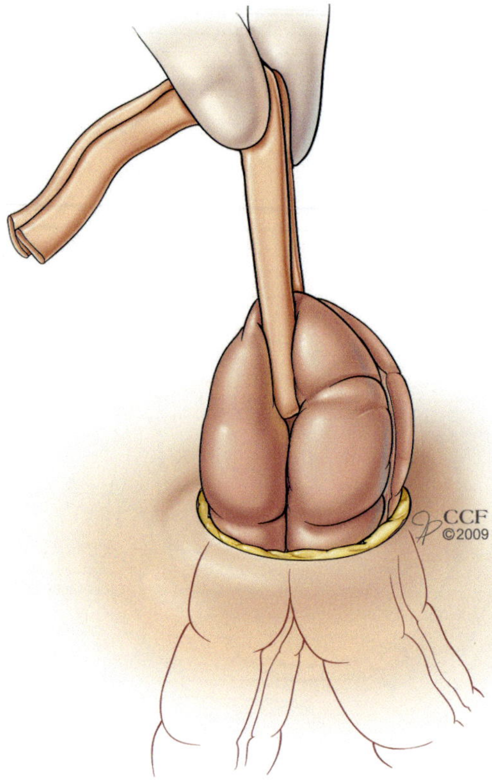

Fig. 11.22 Delivery of sigmoid loop colostomy using Penrose drain technique. Illustration © CCF

Delivery of the Bowel

The bowel is now delivered through the aperture. My preference is to create a small window through the mesentery and pass a penrose drain (either ½″ or 1″) around the bowel (Fig. 11.22). A large curved clamp is passed through the aperture, and the penrose is grasped. Even though there will always be some degree of bowel fixation present, it is still possible to inadvertently twist the loop of bowel as it is delivered through the abdominal wall. Therefore, I mark the proximal and distal limbs with different colored sutures in order to maintain orientation. At this point, the surgeon will need to decide whether the colostomy will be temporary or permanent. If temporary, I wrap the loops of bowel with an adhesion barrier in order to facilitate takedown at a later date. If permanent, I do not place the adhesive barrier. The drain is then carefully withdrawn. To expedite this process, I push the bowel through from the peritoneal side until the loop has fully threaded through the aperture. The drain is then clamped on one end and pulled through the mesentery so that the clamp is now under the bowel wall. The clamp is used to grasp a colostomy rod, which is then withdrawn through the mesenteric defect in order to support the loop (see Fig. 11.18). The surgeon generally decides which type of colostomy rod or support to use. I typically use a 3″ plastic rod with loops on either side. This is low profile and also allows for suture fixation if necessary. I do not suture the peritoneum to the bowel wall and I do not attempt to narrow the fascial opening. If the skin opening is too wide, I will place interrupted dermal sutures to close the skin defect around the bowel wall.

Maturation of the Stoma

Once the abdominal cavity is closed, the stoma is matured. The distal limb is marked with electrocautery in a curvilinear line along where it will be opened. The marking sutures can now be removed. The bowel is then opened. The distal limb is matured with absorbable sutures (full thickness in the bowel wall and through the dermal layer along the lower ½ of the aperture). Sutures are then placed full thickness through the bowel wall and to the dermal layer at the 12:00, 3:00, and 9:00 o'clock positions. Tension is placed on the sutures, and a small forceps is used to evert the proximal limb. The sutures are tied and additional sutures are placed as needed.

An ostomy appliance is applied. With the rod in place, it is often difficult to maintain a good seal. A *karaya ring* can be molded around the rod; the appliance can be placed on top of this. The rod is typically removed in 3–5 days. Ostomy care is generally easier after the rod is removed.

Closure of a Loop Sigmoid Colostomy

In some cases, it becomes possible to reverse a loop sigmoid colostomy. Closure of the loop colostomy begins again with a circumferential incision on the skin surrounding the colostomy. After the subcutaneous fat is entered, the edges of the skin are grasped with hemostats and elevated. The subcutaneous adhesions are taken down with sharp dissection. Care must be taken on the lateral surface of the mesentery. Due to the previous dissection needed to mobilize the sigmoid colon, there can be dense adhesions, and the mesentery can be easily damaged, leading to bleeding. Attempts to control this bleeding can lead to devascularization of the bowel that may require resection and subsequently make the closure more complicated.

Once the colon is mobilized, the colostomy is closed. Any adhesions on the proximal limb are divided in order to "unroof" it. The skin and mucocutaneous junction is excised sharply. Hemostasis is achieved with electrocautery along the bowel wall.

This type of colostomy can be closed with a stapling device in a side-to-side, functional end-to-end manner. Because of the relative fixation of the colon, this may be difficult. Therefore, a handsewn closure is recommended. This is performed in an interrupted, full-thickness fashion with absorbable suture (3.0 absorbable) (Fig. 11.23). A second seromuscular layer can be performed using either absorbable or nonabsorbable suture. The bowel is irrigated and returned carefully to the abdominal cavity. The fascial layer is mobilized as previously described and closed with nonabsorbable suture. The wound is partially closed with a pursestring suture and packed with a betadine-soaked, nonadhesive pad.

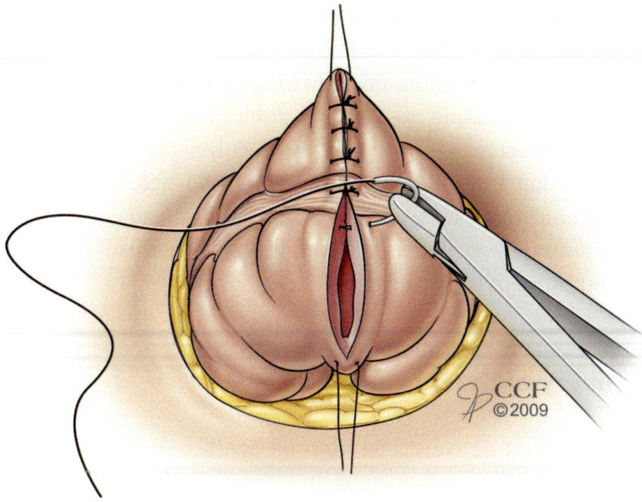

Fig. 11.23 Closure of loop colostomy. This can be done in 1 or 2 layers depending on bowel caliber and surgeon preference. Illustration © CCF

Technique for Loop Transverse Colostomy

As stated previously, a loop transverse colostomy can be used for diversion in patients with an unresectable distal obstruction or in cases of distal perforation and contamination. In the first scenario, the diversion will be permanent, and in the second one, temporary. Typically, in the latter case, the colostomy will be brought out through the upper portion of the midline incision.

Preparation of the Abdominal Wall/Aperture

When a colostomy is deemed "permanent," it can be brought out thought the rectus muscle in a fashion similar to that described for the loop sigmoid colostomy and end colostomy. Otherwise, the colostomy will be brought through the fascial layer at the superior aspect of a midline incision. Therefore, no special preparation is needed in this case.

Preparation of the Bowel

The usually loose and redundant transverse colon needs little preparation. The omentum is detached from the transverse colon in the area to be exteriorized. Otherwise, no other mobilization is necessary. The mesentery should not be manipulated any further as this may cause devascularization (and compromise future takedown) or compromise collateral blood flow, leading to distal colonic ischemia that may require resection. If the transverse colon does not easily reach so that a loop can be created, it is advisable to abandon a loop colostomy and proceed with a loop ileostomy instead. As previously explained, a single 1-in. penrose drain is placed through the mesentery.

Delivery of the Bowel

The bowel is delivered through an aperture made in either the right or left upper quadrant (through the rectus muscle as previously described). An alternative to this is to place the colostomy in the upper part of the midline incision as the abdominal fascia is closed. The bowel loop is positioned and secured with a single nonabsorbable suture (#1 nonabsorbable) in a figure-of-eight fashion placed to tighten the fascia around the bowel loop. Additionally, I prefer to turn the bowel so that the proximal limb is in an inferior position. The midline fascia can now be closed in the usual manner. The subcutaneous tissue is irrigated and the skin closed. The skin adjacent to the colostomy should be closed in a subcutaneous manner, which will provide a better fit for the ostomy appliance. The remaining portion of the skin is closed with skin clips. The Penrose drain is replaced with a 3-in ostomy rod that is oriented in a transverse position (see previous figures for details).

Maturation of the Colostomy

The colostomy is then matured in the same manner as described for the loop sigmoid colostomy. An ostomy appliance is applied. The opening in the appliance is cut so that the bowel is easily admitted, but an excessive amount of skin is not exposed.

Notes on Loop Colostomy

Although loop colostomies are used to divert the fecal stream, they are not always 100% efficient. Some solid and particularly liquid stool can pass into the distal limb and travel downstream. If there is a need to completely divert the fecal stream, a divided loop colostomy can be created. This is done by using the same techniques as described previously. After the bowel is secured with a rod and the abdomen closed, the distal limb of the loop is occluded. A linear or GIA stapler is inserted into the space created by the rod and fired so as to close the distal limb (Fig. 11.24). The distal limb should be secured to the fascial layer in this case to prevent it from retracting into the abdominal cavity. The staple line can then be buried into the subcutaneous tissue. The proximal limb is then matured in the same fashion as used for an end stoma.

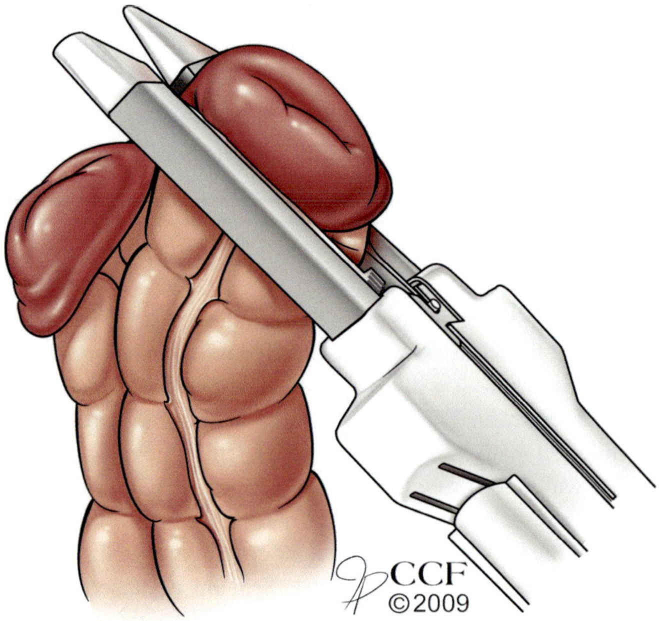

Fig. 11.24 Division of loop colostomy with stapled closure of distal limb. The distal limb can then be buried in the subcutaneous tissue. This should not be done in cases where there is a distal obstruction. Illustration © CCF

Obviously, this technique should not be used if the original reason for the stoma was diversion due to distal obstruction. This would lead to a closed loop obstruction with possible blow out of the distal limb, creating a fistula to the skin under the ostomy appliance. This in turn, would make it difficult or impossible for the appliance to adhere to the stoma. Likewise, if the distal limb retracts, the bowel contents could leak into the peritoneum and cause peritonitis. In these cases, the distal limb can be matured into a mucus fistula to allow for decompression (Fig. 11.25).

The process used to close this type of colostomy is more complex than that used for a standard loop colostomy. To completely mobilize the distal limb, the incision may need to be extended. Once both limbs are completely mobilized, the staple line will need to be excised from the distal limb. Although the choice of closure is dictated by surgeon preference, it may also depend on the amount of laxity in the limbs. A stapled side-to-side anastomosis, stapled end-to-side anastomosis, or handsewn end-to-end anastomosis can be performed. The bowel is returned to the abdominal cavity, and the resultant facial defect and wound are closed.

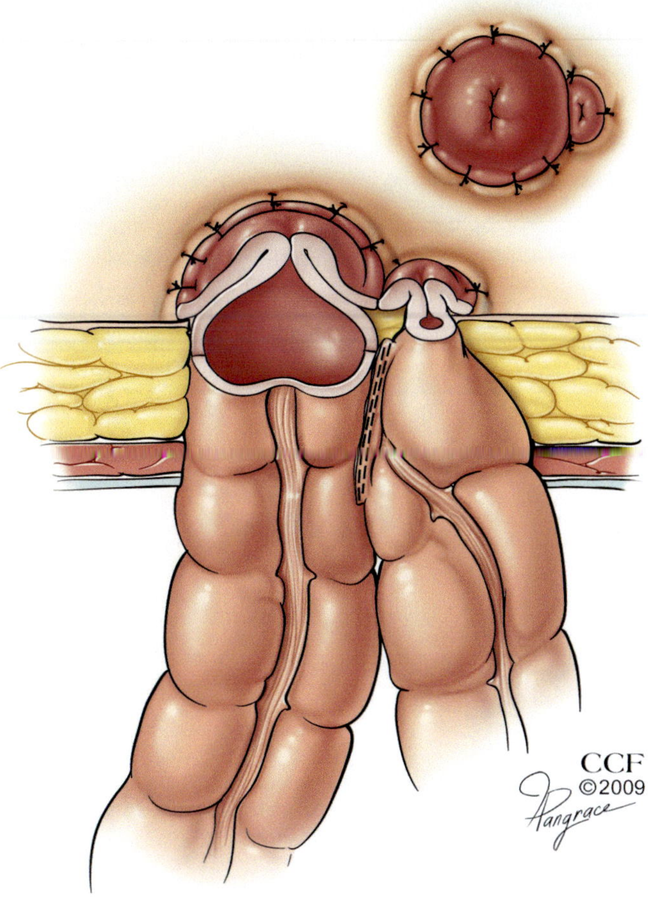

Fig. 11.25 Closed distal limb partially matured distal limb as a distal mucus fistula. The opening of the mucus fistula is incorporated into the ostomy appliance opening. Illustration © CCF

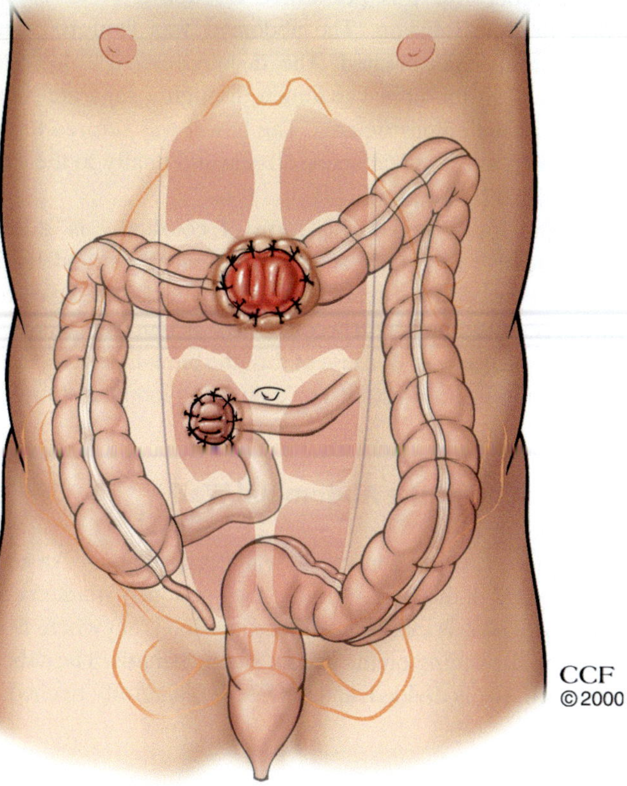

Fig. 11.26 Turnbull Blowhole colostomy. A decompressive colostomy created with a diverting loop ileostomy. Illustration © CCF

Technique of the "Blow-Hole" Colostomy

The use of a decompressive colostomy is useful in situations where there is severe distal obstruction or pseudo-obstruction. It is also particularly useful as a treatment for toxic megacolon as it can help improve or resolve symptoms with minimal intrusion on the abdomen and minimal physiologic stress on the patient.

Turnbull described the technique of an ileostomy in combination with a decompressive colostomy in 1971 [10] (Fig. 11.26). The dilated colon can often be seen bulging under the abdominal wall; this is the area (either midline or over the rectus muscle) where the ostomy should be located. If the area of dilated colon is not obvious, the most dilated portion of the transverse colon can be noted and marked using simple abdominal radiography. A metal marker is placed over the site, and an X-ray is taken to help gauge the location of the stoma. The skin is then marked.

Remzi and colleagues reviewed the current indications for this procedure. Because of improvements in medical care, the use of this technique has become rare. Seventeen patients at Cleveland Clinic underwent this procedure over an 18-year period. The indications included toxic megacolon associated with inflammatory bowel disease (6 patients); toxic megacolon associated with inflammatory bowel disease and pregnancy (2 patients); severe *Clostridium difficile* colitis (3 patients); adult Hirschsprung's disease (1 patient); pancreatitis with obstructing pseudocyst (1 patient); and malignant distal obstruction with metastases (4 patients) [11] (Table 11.2).

Table 11.2 Indications for "blow-hole" colostomy

1. Toxic Megacolon
2. Toxic Megacolon during pregnancy
3. Severe *Clostridium difficile*-associated colitis
4. Adult Hirschsprung's disease
5. Malignant distal colonic obstruction with metastases

Ooi and colleagues described in detail the two cases in which the Turnbull blowhole colostomy/ileostomy was used. Both patients had toxic megacolon associated with inflammatory bowel disease in the midst of their pregnancies. Both patients underwent the procedure without complications and both mothers and their babies did well. Both patients later underwent restorative proctocolectomy [12].

The procedure was performed through a 7- to 10-cm lower midline incision. The abdomen was explored, and an ileostomy was created. The decompressive colostomy was placed in the upper abdomen through a separate 5-cm incision in the epigastric area. The bowel was sutured to the fascia, then to the subcutaneous tissue and finally to the skin as described by Turnbull [12].

As previously noted, this form of colostomy is strictly decompressive in nature. A large amount of gas and liquid stool will initially pass out of the newly made hole in the colon. However, over time, it will become a low-output fistula and can spontaneously close. Because of this, the blow-hole colostomy must always be accompanied by a diverting loop ileostomy.

Preparation of the Abdominal Wall

There is no specific abdominal wall "preparation". An incision is made in the skin overlying the previously marked area where the colon is most dilated. The incision is anywhere from 2 to 4 in. depending on the patient's body habitus. The subcutaneous tissue is divided, and the fascia is carefully opened.

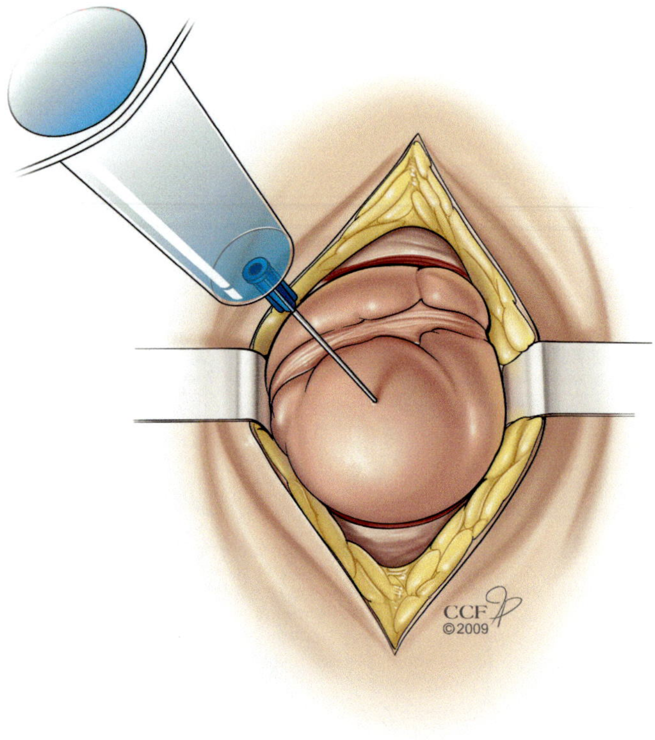

Fig. 11.27 Exposure of dilated colon. Note bulging appearance. Needle decompression may relieve some pressure to allow easier manipulation of bowel. Illustration © CCF

Delivery of the Bowel

In most instances, the colon will immediately bulge into the wound. Any manipulation or pulling on the colon should be minimized as it may easily rupture or bleed. The goal is to attach the seromuscular layer of the colon to the peritoneum and fascia without contaminating the peritoneal cavity [10] (Figs. 11.27 and 11.28).

Maturation of the Colostomy

The bowel wall is sutured to the peritoneum and the fascia using absorbable suture. A second layer of the bowel wall can be sutured to Scarpa's fascia [10]. Although this layer will not provide any strength, it will help prevent contamination. The colon is then incised in the midline; there will be a rush of gas and, likely, liquid stool (Fig. 11.29). This can be a very messy part of the case, and care should be taken to prevent contamination of the wound. The incision should be small at first and a pool-tip suction can be used to decompress the colon. The mucosa is then sutured to the skin (Fig. 11.30). An ostomy appliance is applied.

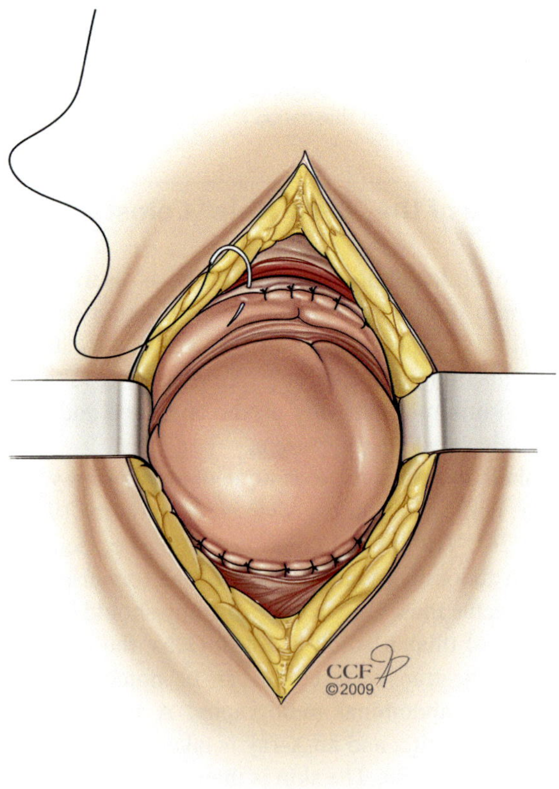

Fig. 11.28 The colon is first secured to fascial layer to prevent retraction and contamination. Sutures should be absorbable. Illustration © CCF

Technique of Cecostomy

There are three uses for a tube cecostomy: (1) cecal volvulus that has been reduced but is at risk for recurrence, (2) pseudo-obstruction, and (3) perforation of the cecum when resection

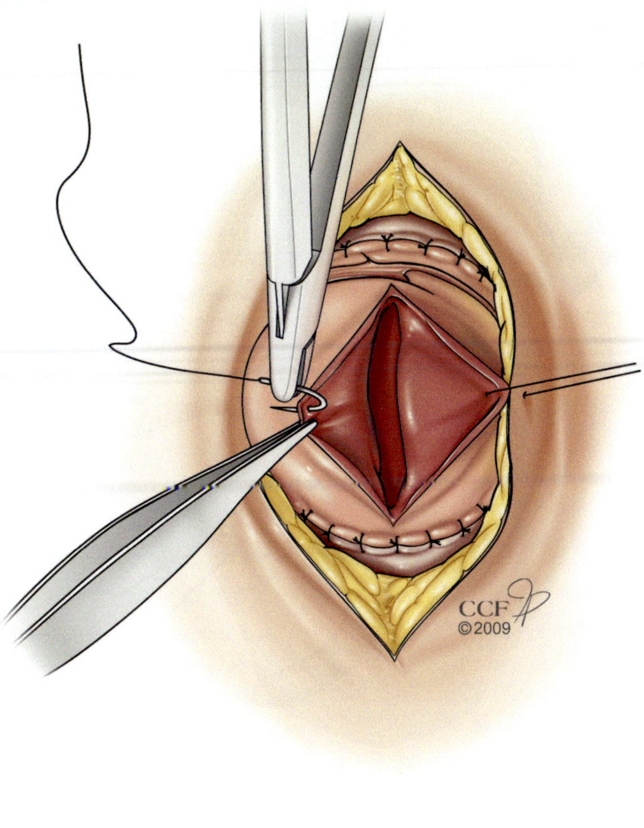

Fig. 11.29 Colon is opened. Laparotomy pads should be placed around wound edges and there is likely to be rush of gas and liquid stool. Illustration © CCF

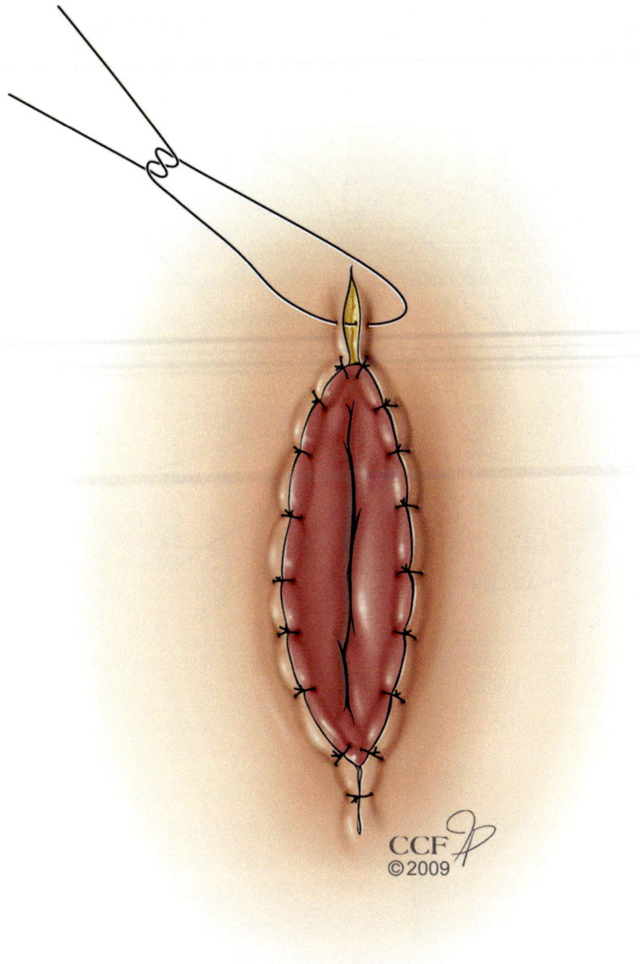

Fig. 11.30 Colostomy is matured. Edge of bowel is sewn to skin edge with absorbable suture. Illustration © CCF

is not possible [1]. Over time, improvements in surgical techniques have been made, and some conditions can now be managed medically. This has relegated cecostomy to a historical footnote. We will review the technique briefly here.

It is assumed the abdomen is already open. The cecum is isolated with laparotomy pads. A pursestring suture is placed, and a large mushroom-tip (32 French or larger) is inserted. The pursestring suture is tied (Fig. 11.31a, b). A second pursestring is placed and tied to imbricate the first one. The tube is then brought out through the abdominal wall via a stab incision in the right lower quadrant. After the cecum is brought into approximation to the abdominal wall, the cecum is secured to the abdominal wall with absorbable suture, and the tube is secured to the skin with a nonabsorbable suture that will be removed later [1] (Fig. 11.31c).

The tube should be irrigated regularly (3 times daily) and suctioned. Later, when the need for decompression has resolved, the tube can be removed, and the resultant low-output fistula will close spontaneously. Formal closure is rarely needed [1].

As previously stated, cecostomy is almost mentioned only in a historical footnote. Tube cecostomy is difficult to manage. The tube often leaks, becomes clogged, and is labor intensive for the nursing staff. Only in very rare circumstances will a cecostomy be a better option than either decompressive colostomy or ileostomy.

The Continent Colostomy

Prager described a two-piece device that acted as a continent colostomy. It consisted of a ring made of silicone and Dacron mesh that was sewn to the underside of the abdominal wall in the planned location of the new ostomy. The ring could also be cut and placed around an existing stoma. The bowel was brought through the ring and then the abdominal wall and matured in standard fashion. Additionally, it was thought that the ring would preclude hernia formation and, therefore, the stoma did not have to be placed through the rectus muscle. The second part of the device was a silicone balloon that acted as an obturator and occluded the bowel. The balloon was placed for gradually increasing periods of time over the next 5 postoperative days and then as tolerated. Some patients left the balloon in place for up to 10 h at a time. Patients complained of occasional mucus discharge. The study initially involved five patients who were followed for 6 months. There were no reports of infection, bowel necrosis, or ostomy

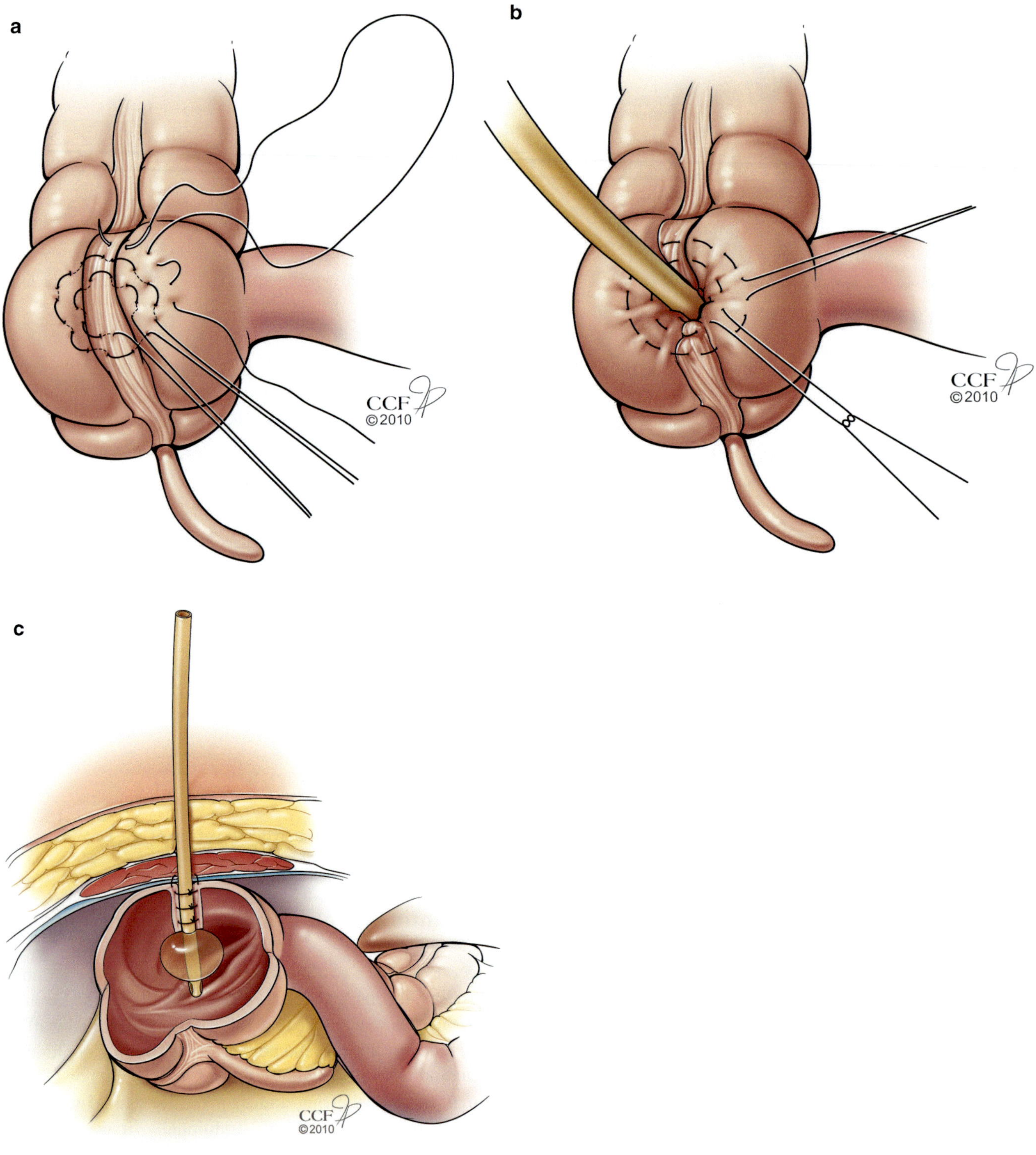

Fig. 11.31 (**a**) A purse-string suture in placed in the dilated cecum. Illustration © CCF. (**b**) A large bore tube in placed into the cecum (32 Fr or larger). Illustration © CCF. (**c**) The tube is brought through a stab incision in the skin and the cecum is secured to the anterior abdominal wall. Illustration © CCF

pain [13]. Despite this initial success, interest in the technique faded.

In 1981, Schmidt and colleagues began working with a continent perineal colostomy. They initially studied the use of a seromuscular tube that was fashioned from a segment of colon. It was wrapped around the segment of colon that would be sutured to the perineum. Animal models were initially used, and it was found that there was smooth muscle hypertrophy that mimicked the musculature of the anal sphincters and provided adequate continence [14].

In 1982, Schmidt and colleagues reported their experience with 509 patients who had undergone this procedure. Patients ranged in age from 7 to 84 years. Continence was achieved in 80%. Five patients subsequently underwent repeat resection and permanent colostomy for a variety of reasons. Manometric studies of this continent colostomy revealed resting pressures of 36 mmHg. There was an overall patient satisfaction level of 85%, and no deaths were reported [15].

Torres reported his experience with one patient using Schmidt's technique. Manometric studies revealed a resting pressure of 20 mmHg. Defecography revealed the ability to retain contrast up to 24 h. The patient was continent of solid and semisolid stool [16].

Santoro reported his experience with continent colostomies in 1994. He reported the results of 15 patients who had undergone standard abdominoperineal resection for cancer. There was either immediate or delayed reconstruction. The authors recommended waiting 6 months to 2 years before attempting reconstruction. They performed a perineal colostomy (handsewn anastomosis to the perineal skin) and a bilateral gracilis flap reconstruction of the perineal musculature. The right gracilis was placed posteriorly to act as the puborectal sling. The left gracilis was used to encircle the colon to act as the sphincter. An 8-cm colonic pouch was also used to increase the reservoir [17].

Patients were followed for 2–40 months. Satisfactory results were noted in 9 of the 15 patients. These patients passed 2–3 stools per day and none at night. However, there was some nocturnal leakage requiring pad usage. Manometric studies revealed a resting pressure of 15–20 mmHg and an anal canal length of 3–4 cm [17].

Summary

Over the years, continual improvements have been made in colostomy care and surgical techniques to improve the quality of life for patients with permanent colostomies. Despite these advances, ostomy patients still suffer from episodic leakage around the appliance and peristomal skin irritation. Irrigating the ostomy decreases some of these problems but this can be time-consuming for the patient [13].

References

1. Aldrete J. Diverting and venting colostomy techniques and colostomy closure. Mastery of surgery. 2nd ed., Volume II. Little, Brown, Inc: 1992. p. 1201–17.
2. Orkin BA, Cataldo PA. Intestinal stomas in the ASCRS textbook of colon and rectal surgery. 1st ed. Springer Science and Business Media; 2007. p. 622–42.
3. Turnbull RB, Weakley F. End sigmoid colostomy. Atlas of intestinal stomas. 1st ed. The C.V. Mosby Company; 1967. p 145–51.
4. Hebert J. A simple method for preventing retraction of and end colostomy. Dis Colon Rectum. 1988;31(4):328–9.
5. Prasad ML, Pearl RK, Abcarian H. End loop colostomy. Surg Gynecol Obstet. 1984;158(4):380–2.
6. Keighley MRB. Stomas. Atlas of colorectal surgery. Churchill Livingstone, Inc: 1996. p. 61–92.
7. Guivarc'h M, Mosnier H, Roullet-Audy JC. Protective transverse loop colostomy associated with low colo-rectal anastomoses. Int J Colorectal Dis. 1997;12:340–1.
8. Rutegard J, Dahlgren S. Transverse colostomy or loop ileostomy as diverting stoma in colorectal surgery. Acta Chir Scand. 1987;153: 229–32.
9. Williams NS, Nasmyth DG, Jones D, Smith AH. De-functioning stomas: a prospective controlled trial comparing loop ileostomy with loop transverse colostomy. Br J Surg. 1986;73(7):566–70.
10. Turnbull RB, Hawk WA, Weakley FL. Surgical treatment of toxic megacolon: ileostomy and colostomy to prepare patients for colectomy. Am J Surg. 1971;122:25–31.
11. Remzi FH, Oncel M, Hull TL, Strong SA, Lavery IC, Fazio VW. Current indications for blow-hole colostomy:ileostomy procedure. A single center experience. Int J Colorectal Dis. 2003;18:361–4.
12. Ooi BS, Remzi FH, Fazio VW. Turnbull blowhole colostomy for toxic ulcerative colitis in pregnancy. Dis Colon Rectum. 2003;46(1):111–5.
13. Prager E. The continent colostomy. Dis Colon Rectum. 1984;27: 235–7.
14. Schmidt E, Bruch HP, Romen W, Rothhammer A. Experimental and clinical studies on continent colostomy. Eur Surg Res. 1981;13: 202–12.
15. Schmidt E. The continent colostomy. World J Surg. 1982;6:805–9.
16. Torres RA, Gonzalez MA. Perineal continent colostomy: report of a case. Dis Colon Rectum. 1988;31:957–60.
17. Santoro E, Santoro R, Santoro E. Perineal reconstruction with continent colostomy after the miles operation. Semin Surg Oncol. 1994;10:208–16.

Laparoscopic Ostomy Surgery

12

Daniel P. Geisler and Hermann Kessler

Introduction

Construction of a stoma, either an ileostomy or a colostomy, is an ideal indication for laparoscopy because only minimal dissection is required, almost no mesenteric manipulation is necessary, and the procedure is generally simple. The benefits of a laparoscopic approach for stoma formation include minimal pain, quick recovery, and a low complication rate. Additionally, a laparoscopic approach allows for a very thorough exploration of the entire abdominal cavity, an advantage that normally cannot be achieved by a "blind" or a "limited open" approach despite successful reports in the literature. Biopsy specimens may be obtained quickly and the small and large bowel may be easily examined in a hand-to-hand or hand-over-hand technique as is often necessary for Crohn's disease or partial bowel obstruction. Also, the portion of the intestine chosen for the stoma may be assessed accurately. Laparoscopy also permits one to see that the intestinal loop is properly oriented as it is brought through the stoma site. The indications for a laparoscopic stoma formation are identical to those for open surgery. The techniques for stoma maturation are also the same as those for an open procedure. The importance of a carefully selected stoma site should be emphasized and is best determined in conjunction with a stoma nurse. This premarked site is an ideal place to gain initial access to the abdominal cavity, with the pneumoperitoneum being maintained by use of an extra small wound protector device. This device also assists in delivering the stoma through the abdominal wall.

D.P. Geisler (✉)
West Penn Allegheny Health System, Pittsburgh, PA, USA
e-mail: dgeisle1@wpahs.org

H. Kessler
Department of Surgery, University of Erlangen, Erlangen, Germany

Patient Positioning and Port Placement

The most common types of enteric stoma are ileostomy, transverse colostomy, and sigmoid colostomy. The proposed ostomy site is chosen and marked based on a preoperative assessment of the abdominal wall with the patient in the sitting, standing, and lying positions. For the procedure itself, the patient may be placed in the supine or lithotomy (split-leg) position with the latter more desirable as it allows for greater mobility around the patient as well as access to the perineum. General anesthetic is used and an orogastric tube and Foley catheter are placed. A full bowel prep is preferred if a colostomy is being performed but is usually not necessary for creation of a loop ileostomy. The procedure begins at the proposed stoma site. For an ileostomy, this is usually in the right lower quadrant over the rectus sheath; for a transverse colostomy it is the right upper quadrant, and for a sigmoid colostomy it is the left lower abdomen. For the creation of a loop ileostomy, the surgeon and camera operator are on the patient's left side with the scrub nurse between the legs. For loop colostomy, the surgeon and camera operator are on the patient's right side with the scrub nurse between the legs (Fig. 12.1). The patient is placed in the modified lithotomy position (yellow fins or split-leg bed) with the arms tucked at the side.

With the initial port placed in the right lower quadrant, the position of a second port is then determined. Additional ports are usually only needed if there are adhesions that need to be addressed. A mirror image of this set-up is used for creation of an end colostomy with the need for additional ports determined by the laxity of the sigmoid colon and need for an endoscopic stapling device.

The number of trocars needed and their positioning is largely determined by the extent of dissection needed to allow for a tension-free stoma. Patients undergoing creation of a loop ileostomy frequently only need a 5 mm trocar in addition to the port at the stoma site if there are no intra-abdominal adhesions (Fig. 12.2). Additional ports may be added to assist with dissection. A more traditional

V.W. Fazio et al. (eds.), *Atlas of Intestinal Stomas*,
DOI 10.1007/978-0-387-78851-7_12, © Springer Science+Business Media, LLC 2012

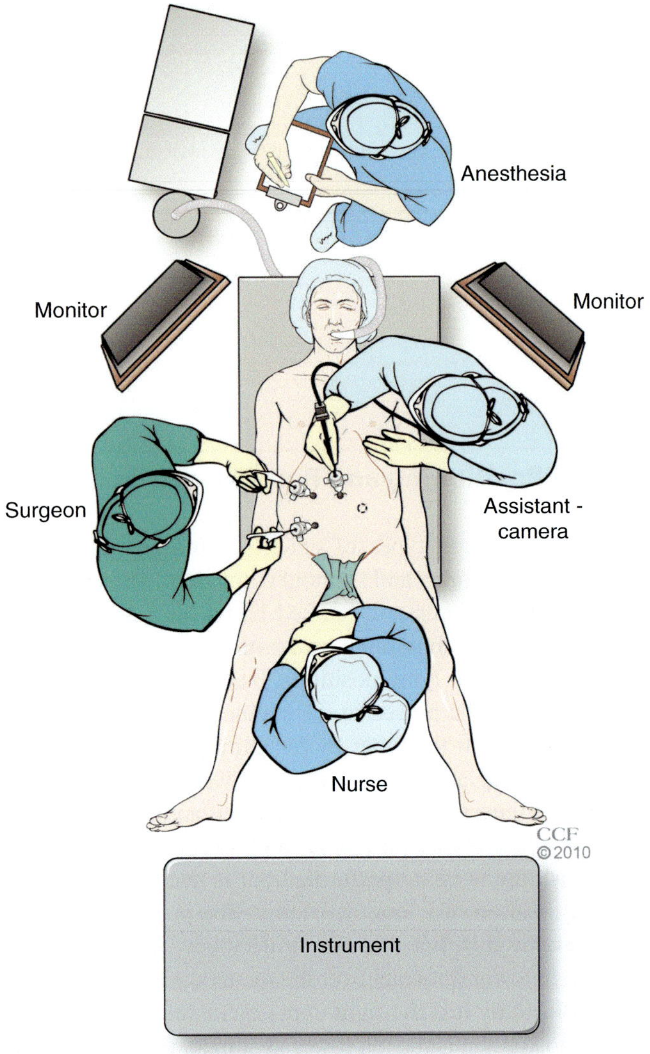

Fig. 12.1 Room set-up for loop colostomy. The surgeon is positioned on the patient's right. Illustration © CCF

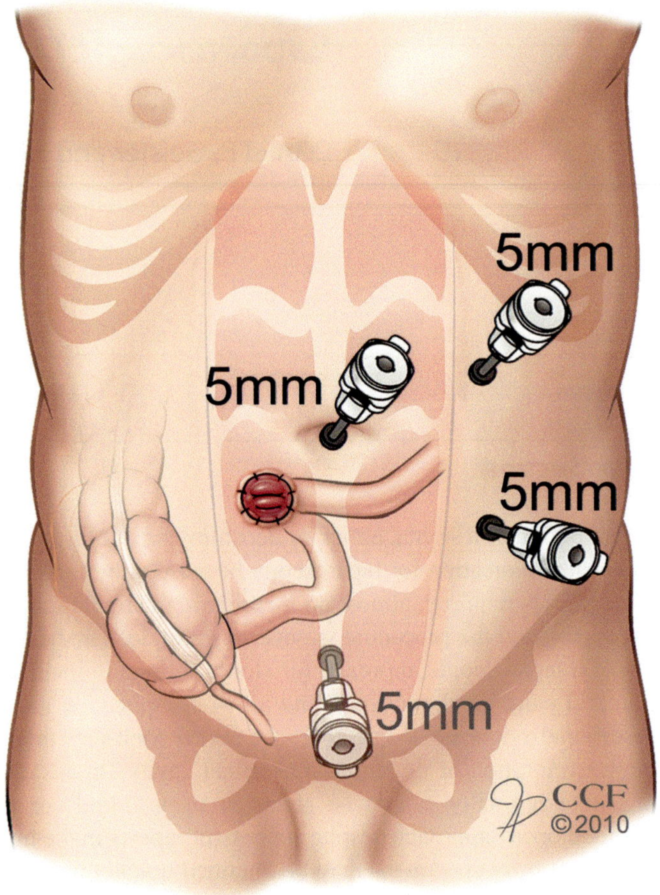

Fig. 12.2 Port-placement for loop ileostomy. Illustration © CCF

port-placement is typically employed when performing an end sigmoid colostomy (Fig. 12.3). This helps facilitate both the lateral dissection and the transection of the bowel.

For a loop ileostomy, the patient is placed in the Trendelenburg, left-side down position. The surgeon and camera operator are on the patient's left side. A 2–3 cm ellipse of skin is excised and the subcutaneous tissue is incised in a vertical fashion. The fascia is then identified and incised in a vertical fashion. The peritoneum is opened with sharp dissection in an open fashion. An extra small wound protector can be placed with a 10–12 mm trocar secured with a Penrose around it. Alternatively, as a first cannula, a Hassan trocar may be inserted using an open technique. Carbon dioxide (CO_2) is used to establish pneumoperitoneum. A 30-degree laparoscope is routinely used. A 10-mm cannula is then inserted lateral to the rectus sheath in the midabdomen or lower quadrant of the opposite side of the stoma site. Any exploration or biopsy should be carried out now and mobilization of the bowel, especially the colon, should be performed if necessary. One to two additional 5-mm cannulas may have to be inserted on the opposite side of the stoma site trocars for this purpose. At the terminal ileum, an intestinal site for ileostomy should be chosen 10–20 cm upstream of the ileocecal valve to avoid any tension on the bowel. After this, the surgeon should place the laparoscope in the cannula opposite the stoma site and an endoscopic Babcock-type instrument through the stoma site cannula. After a thorough examination and inspection of the abdominal cavity and identification of the ileocecal region, an appropriate segment of terminal ileum is selected for deliverance through the fascial defect. The entire width of the intestine is grasped firmly and the grasper is locked. Care should be taken to assure that there are no twists of the bowel, that there is no proximal small bowel lateral to the stoma, and that the mesentery of the ileostomy is not under tension. The bowel may be oriented to the stoma with the afferent loop either in a medial or inferior position. Releasing pneumoperitoneum somewhat may be necessary to fully evaluate the amount of tension needed to bring the loop comfortably

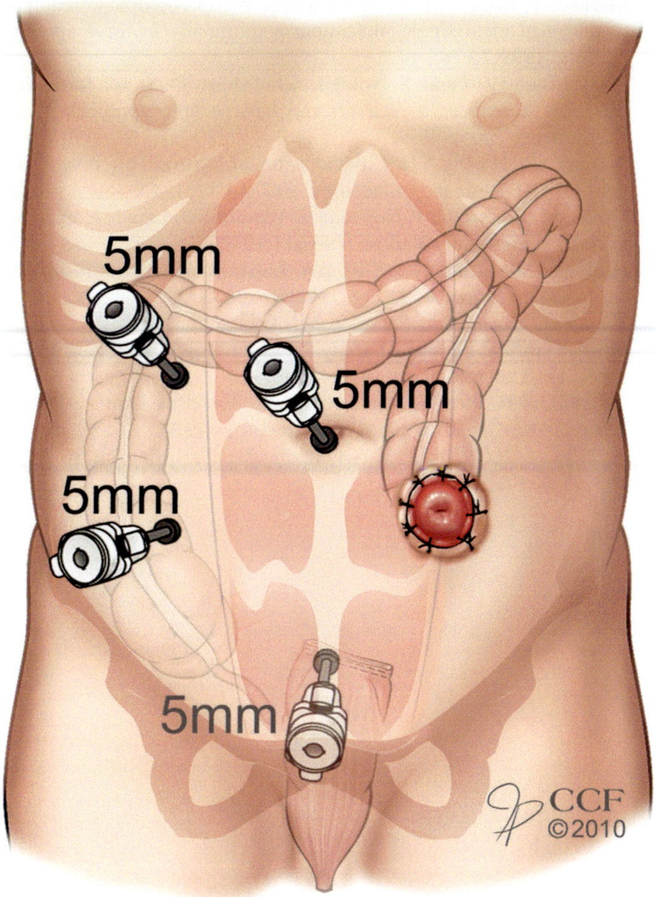

Fig. 12.3 Port-placement for loop sigmoid colostomy. Illustration © CCF

up to the skin. After this, any rotation on the shaft of the Babcock clamp must be prevented. The laparoscope is removed, pneumoperitoneum is fully released, and the endoscopic Babcock instrument is left with its tip positioned just below the fascia. The stoma site cannula is pulled out. The posterior sheath incision may need to be enlarged. The stoma is then matured as in an open operation.

For an end colostomy, the patient is placed in the Trendelenburg position. A 3 cm ellipse of skin is excised and the subcutaneous tissue is incised in a vertical fashion. The fascia is then identified and incised in a vertical fashion. The peritoneum is opened with sharp dissection in an open fashion. An extra-small wound protector can be placed with a 10–12 mm trocar secured with a Penrose around it. The surgeon and the camera operator are on the patient's right side. A 30° laparoscope is routinely used. After a thorough examination of the abdominal cavity, it may also be necessary to place the patient in the right-side down position to deliver the small bowel out of the pelvis. A third trocar of the 10–12 mm variety is frequently needed both for mobilization of the sigmoid colon as well as for transection of the sigmoid colon if an end colostomy is being made. It should be noted that a loop stoma is recommended if there is any concern about distal obstruction.

Discussion

For decades, stoma construction has been performed by laparotomy. In contrast, laparoscopic stoma formation has been an option only for about the past 15 years and has found rapid acceptance.

In the early 1990s, single cases were published, with later-on results and experiences in laparoscopic stoma creation becoming more comprehensive [1–3]. Without exception, all studies concluded that the laparoscopic approach is reliable, technically feasible, and effective [1, 2, 4].

In particular, with the stoma being applied as the sole abdominal intervention, the laparoscopic approach appears to be an excellent option [1, 3, 5–7].

Hardly any studies comparing laparoscopic and open stoma construction have been published so far. Young et al. compared a small group of 19 laparoscopic patients with a historical group of 23 conventional stoma patients. However, surgery was indicated almost exclusively for benign diseases, and a number of patients underwent additional anal or perianal procedures in the same session. Despite these restrictions, the authors concluded that the laparoscopic stoma construction may be associated with less postoperative pain, earlier postoperative return to a normal diet and recovery of peristalsis, as well as a shorter hospital stay [8]. Scheidbach et al. compared the results of two prospective multicenter studies and found similar favorable results [9].

In almost all analyses, significant advantages were found to be associated with the laparoscopic approach in terms of general and specific postoperative morbidity. In studies comparing open and laparoscopic approach, postoperative mortality was significantly higher in the laparotomy groups. On the other hand, conventional laparotomy may be superior to laparoscopy if exploration of a region within the abdominal cavity is necessary which cannot be easily accessed by means of minimally invasive techniques.

Summary

The laparoscopic approach to stoma creation allows for the minimally invasive creation of a stoma while also affording the surgeon and patient a very thorough examination of the abdominal cavity. While this approach has not been thoroughly studied by means of a prospective randomized trial, several retrospective studies have shown that this approach is safe and effective. Most published studies have reported decreased morbidity while achieving the same expected advantages associated with a minimally invasive approach.

Conclusion

A laparoscopic approach to stoma formation should be considered for most patients needing proximal diversion. While the procedure is safe and effective, its true benefits lie in the minimally invasive approach associated with such a procedure while maintaining the same desired outcome and assuring minimal surgical trauma.

References

1. Oliveira L. Laparoscopic stoma creation and closure. Semin Laparosc Surg. 2003;10:191–6.
2. Schwandner O, Schiedeck THK, Bruch HP. Stoma creation for fecal diversion: Is the laparoscopic technique appropriate? Int J Colorectal Dis. 1998;13:251–5.
3. Marusch F, Koch A, Kube R, Gastinger I. Laparoscopic creation of stomas—an ideal single indication in minimally invasive surgery. Chirurg. 1999;70:785–8.
4. Liu J, Bruch HP, Farke S, Nolde J, Schwandner O. Stoma formation for fecal diversion: a plea for the laparoscopic approach. Tech Coloproctol. 2005;9:9–14.
5. Wexner SD, Hwang YH. Clinical status of laparoscopic bowel surgery for GI malignancy. Oncology. 2000;14:1131–43.
6. Oliveira L, Reissman P, Nogueras J, Wexner SD. Laparoscopic creation of stomas. Surg Endosc. 1997;11:19–23.
7. Hollyoak MA, Lumley J, Stitz RW. Laparoscopic stoma formation for faecal diversion. Br J Surg. 1998;85:226–8.
8. Young CJ, Eyers AA, Salomon MJ. Defunctioning of the anorectum—historical controlled study of laparoscopic vs. Open procedures. Dis Colon Rectum. 1998;41:190–4.
9. Scheidbach H, Ptok H, Schubert D, et al. Palliative stoma creation: comparison of laparoscopic vs conventional procedures. Langenbecks Arch Surg. 2007;394(2):371–4. Epub ahead of print doi 10.2007/s00423-007-0220-3

Ostomies in Trauma

13

Matthew C. Byrnes and Greg J. Beilman

Introduction

Injuries to the colon represent a challenging and controversial facet of trauma surgery. Colonic trauma can be treated with primary repair, diversion, resection and anastomosis or resection and diversion, depending upon the extent of the injury. These are the standard options for treating all types of colon pathology; however, traumatic injuries to the colon represent a fundamentally different form of colon pathology compared to elective or other emergent colon procedures. The injured colon often has vascular compromise. Additionally, there is a likelihood of postoperative shock that may lead to further malperfusion of the remaining colon segment. Trauma patients tend to be younger and healthier than other populations requiring colon surgery, so they may be more resistant to such insults. These divergent components of colonic injuries have generated much of the controversy that has surrounded the treatment of these injuries over the past two decades.

Each avenue of the treatment algorithm has benefits and pitfalls. The ultimate goal in treating colonic injuries is to restore physiologic stability and avoid postoperative complications. Diversion has been historically considered to be the safest option [1–5]; however, the abdomen must frequently be left open after completing a trauma laparotomy due to concerns for intra-abdominal compartment syndrome. An ostomy adjacent to an open abdomen may yield increased infectious complications. Additionally, there are more psychological components to consider when creating ostomies in trauma patients [3, 4]. These patients tend to be younger than patients undergoing elective colon resections and are never prepared for an ostomy prior to their injury. There are also pitfalls to colonic repair without diversion. Trauma patients may be multiply injured and have severe organ derangement. Each insult could be life threatening, so an anastomotic leak could be a fatal complication.

Herein, we review the indications for colostomies in trauma patients. We then review the techniques that can be employed to create a manageable colostomy.

History

The first serious attempts at performing laparotomy for trauma took place in the late 1800s. Prior to this time, abdominal gunshot wounds were nearly universally fatal. Mortality rates of abdominal gunshot wounds were well over 50% in the first half of World War II. Dr. Ogilvie in Great Britain and the office of the Surgeon General in the United States issued separate decrees that colon trauma should be treated with diversion [2, 3]. The mortality rates of colon injuries decreased in the second half of WWII. This military dictum was translated into civilian practice, and diversion became the primary mode of treatment for several decades. In 1979, Stone et al. performed a randomized, prospective trial designed to evaluate diversion versus primary repair in a highly selected population of injured patients (no fecal spillage, hemodynamically stable, and no delay to operation) [6]. They found decreased abdominal infections in the group undergoing primary repair (15% versus 29%). This marked a transition point favoring primary repair over ostomies in trauma.

Indications for Colostomy – by Type of Injury

Colonic trauma can be categorized by the amount of damage to the colon wall [3, 7]. Nondestructive injuries encompass less than 50% of the circumference of the colon wall, do not involve devascularization, and have minimal injury of the surrounding tissue (Fig. 13.1). These lesions are most commonly caused by stab wounds or low velocity gunshot wounds. Destructive injuries to the colon wall encompass

M.C. Byrnes (✉) • G.J. Beilman
Department of Surgery, University of Minnesota,
Minneapolis, MN, USA
e-mail: byrne147@umn.edu

V.W. Fazio et al. (eds.), *Atlas of Intestinal Stomas*,
DOI 10.1007/978-0-387-78851-7_13,

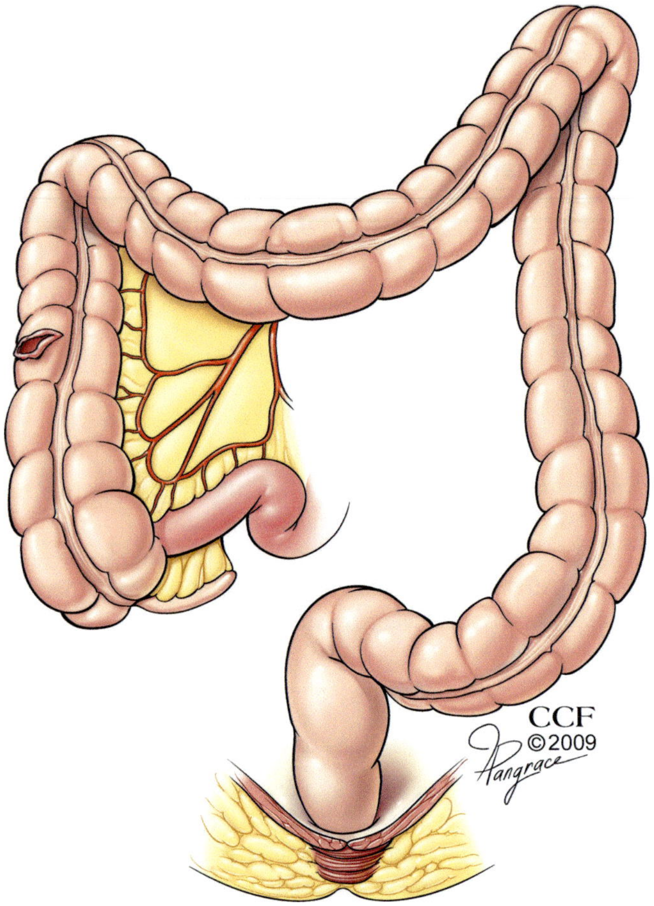

Fig. 13.1 Nondestructive colonic injury. Illustration © CCF

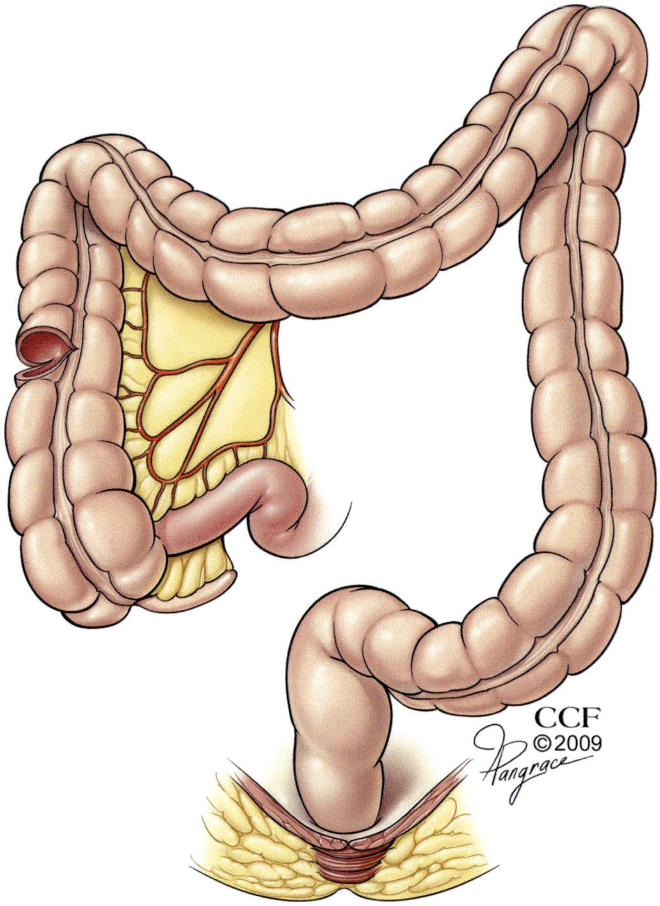

Fig. 13.2 Simple destructive injury to right colon. Illustration © CCF

greater than 50% of the colon circumference or involve devascularization (Figs. 13.2–13.4). These injuries are typically caused by blunt trauma or higher velocity gunshot wounds. There is significant variability in the presentation of destructive lesions, with the spectrum ranging from simple transection of the colon to complete obliteration of large segments of bowel in major blast injuries.

Numerous studies, review articles, and meta-analyses have indicated that most nondestructive injuries can safely be repaired primarily without diversion. There is a large volume of retrospective data that indicate that primary repair is preferable to diversion [8–13]. Maxwell et al. summarized these studies and found an increased risk of complications among patients who were diverted compared with patients who were treated with repair without diversion (31% versus 14%) [1]. However, mortality rates in these studies were less than 1%, which suggests that they represented a low-risk patient population. Initial prospective studies were criticized because they either excluded high-risk patients or were nonrandomized [6, 14, 15]. As such, it was generally agreed that low-risk patients (no hypotension, no fecal spillage, no delay to operation) could be treated without diversion, but there was significant debate about treating patients with a risk factor for anastomotic failure. There are now several randomized prospective studies that evaluated a mixture of nondestructive and destructive injuries among all patients regardless of risk factors [16–19]. Complication rates ranged between 20% and 30% and were similar between the groups. Sasaki et al. reported an additional 7% complication rate among patients undergoing colostomy reversal [18]. The complication rate of colostomy reversal has been reported by other authors and has been cited as an additional reason to perform repair without diversion [20–22]. A recent Cochrane meta-analysis evaluated six randomized prospective trials comparing primary repair to diversion [23]. Mortality was similar between the groups, but overall complications were higher among the patients undergoing diversion (OR = 0.54).

The aforementioned studies included a mixture of nondestructive injuries amenable to primary repair and destructive injuries requiring resection; however, few studies focused specifically on destructive wounds. Accordingly, it is difficult to extrapolate these results to patients with higher grade, destructive injuries. The largest prospective study to date was published by Demetriades et al. in 2001 [24]. Nineteen trauma centers participated in the study. All patients in the study had a destructive injury that required resection. The

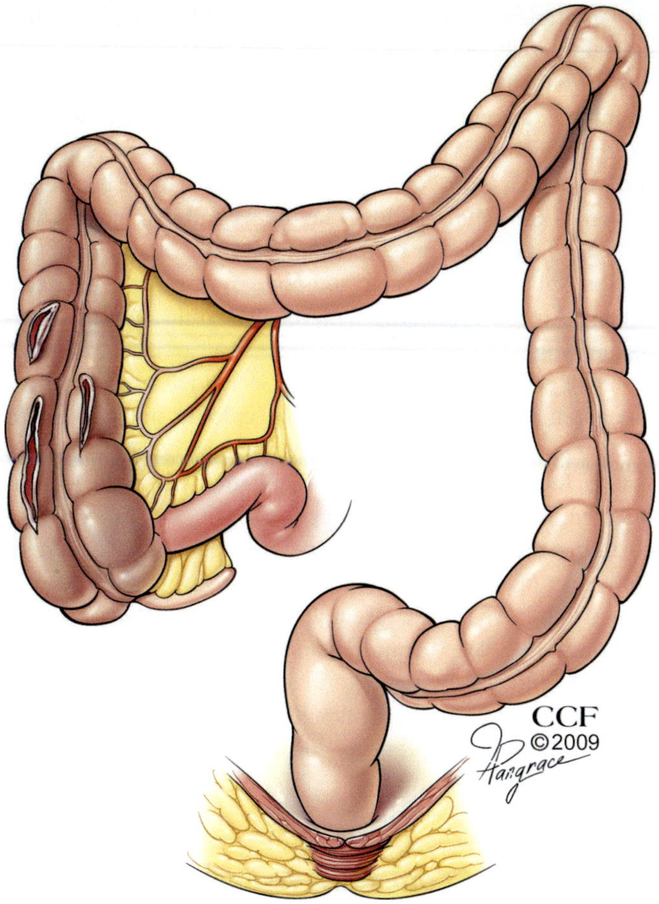

Fig. 13.3 Devascularization. Illustration © CCF

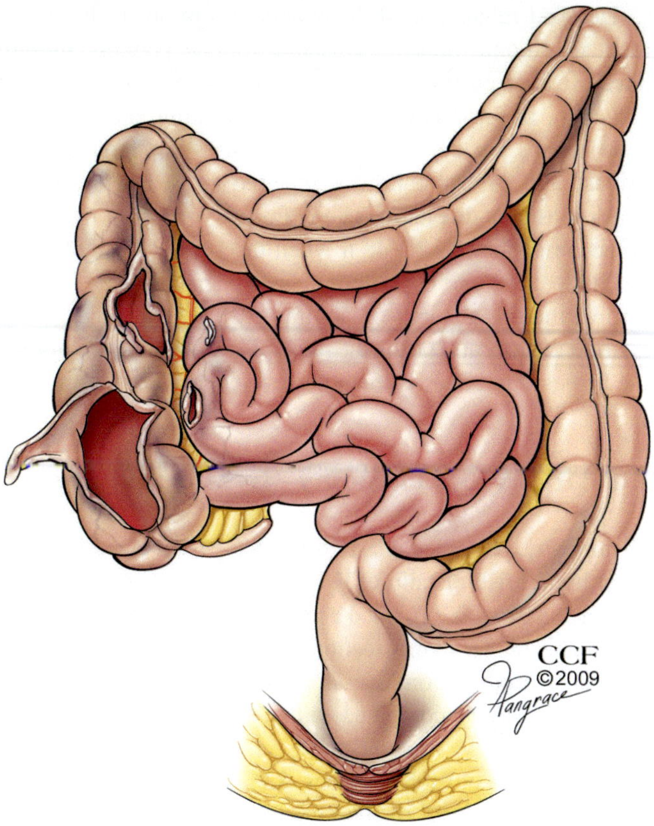

Fig. 13.4 Major blast injury. Illustration © CCF

decision to divert the patient was left to the discretion of the trauma surgeon. Mortality related to colon pathology was 1% in the diverted group and 0% in the nondiverted group. There was a 6.6% anastomotic leak rate. Patients were categorized as high risk or low risk. High-risk patients were defined as patients with hypotension, severe fecal spillage, a penetrating abdominal trauma index of ≥25, or the requirement of six or more units of packed red blood cells. This group of patients had historically been considered to have the highest risk of anastomotic complications. Complications were similar between the high-risk patients who underwent diversion or repair without diversion. The mortality rate among high-risk diverted patients was higher than high-risk patients who underwent repair without diversion (4.5% versus 0%). This led the authors to conclude that all patients should be treated with anastomosis without diversion regardless of risk factors.

Historically, delayed time to operation has been considered an absolute indication for diversion. Kamwendo et al. randomized patients with colonic injury to receive either primary repair or diversion [25]. Patients who underwent laparotomy within 12 h were compared to patients with delayed treatment. There was not an increased risk of complications among the patients who underwent primary repair after an operative delay. The authors concluded that operative delay is not an indication for colostomy.

Although the preponderance of the literature supports repair of colonic injuries without diversion, there are certain high-risk populations that have been poorly studied. These groups include patients who have multiple risk factors (hypotension, fecal spillage, and delayed operation), patients with severe edema of the bowel wall, or patients with high velocity (military type) gunshot wounds or severe blast injuries with a significant amount of devitalized tissue. Previous studies have indicated that repair without diversion is appropriate in patients with a single high-risk factor; however, no studies have evaluated the select group of patients with multiple high-risk factors for anastomotic failure. Accordingly, we recommend proceeding with diversion in these groups of patients. Severe edema of the bowel wall increases the likelihood of anastomotic failure, as the tissue is not as amenable to healing. Groups of patients suffering high-velocity gunshot wounds or severe blast injuries have never been evaluated prospectively. Nonetheless, the general wisdom among surgeons is that diversion is safer in this population. We also recommend proceeding with colostomy in patients on high-dose vasopressor medications, as perfusion to the anastomotic segment may be compromised.

Delayed repair (24–48 h) is another option in the treatment of colonic injuries. Unstable trauma patients should have a truncated operation that is completed with an open abdomen. In this "damage control" procedure, hemorrhagic solid organs are packed, vascular injuries are rapidly controlled, and enterotomies are repaired or resected without anastomosis or diversion. The definitive operation can then be accomplished in 24–48 h when the patient is stable and coagulopathies and hypothermia have been corrected. In this setting, there is generally a significant amount of fluid resuscitation that occurs during the interval between operations, so the bowel may be too edematous to support an anastomosis.

Indications for Colostomy – by Site of Injury

Historically, left-sided anastomoses have been considered to be at higher risk of failure. There is also a higher theoretical risk of sepsis with left-sided anastomotic leaks, as the bacterial load is higher in this section of the colon. The largest retrospective study reported an increased risk of complications of colocolostomy compared with ileocolostomy [26]. The largest prospective trial to date reported a 4.2% complication rate with ileocolostomy versus 8.9% with colocolostomy [24]. Considering all of the aforementioned data, diversion should be seriously considered for patients with a left-sided colonic injury and a high risk factor for anastomotic failure.

Rectal injuries differ from colonic injuries in terms of blood supply and difficulty of operation. Rectal injuries can be difficult to expose and repair, especially in patients with a narrow pelvis. Intraperitoneal rectal injuries that can easily be visualized can be repaired without diversion in the lowest-risk patients [27, 28]. However, if the injury is difficult to visualize, requires a resection, or there is a high-risk factor (extensive spillage, hypotension, or delayed time to operation), the patient should be diverted [29].

Special Situations

One of the most vexing problems faced by trauma surgeons is the presence of an ostomy and an open abdomen. This group of patients is at a very high risk of subsequent intra-abdominal infection. There is no class I or class II data to direct the care of these patients. As such, experience should dictate the treatment of individual patients. We recommend placing the ostomy more laterally in this situation (through the most lateral portion of the rectus muscle) in order to divert the fecal stream further away from the open wound. We recommend placing a suction-assisted dressing in the midline wound to prevent stool from leaking into the wound (Fig. 13.5a–d). This will control the peritoneal drainage and will protect the wound from fecal contamination. There are also multiple commercial products available that accomplish the same goals (KCI Wound Vac, San Antonio, TX or Blue Sky, Carlsbad, CA).

Injured patients may have significant perineal wounds with significant tissue loss. This can be the result of a gunshot wound or, more commonly, blunt trauma to the perineum. If there is enough tissue loss that the wound will have to heal by secondary intent or be repaired with a tissue flap, consideration should be given to temporarily diverting the fecal stream. An end colostomy with mucus fistula should be performed (Fig. 13.6).

Open pelvic fractures represent a unique indication for diversion, in that there may be no colonic injury present. A laceration overlying a pelvic fracture can be contaminated with a fecal stream. Such contamination can lead to life-threatening osteomyelitis and pelvic sepsis. Because of these concerns, fecal diversion has generally been the procedure of choice for open pelvic fractures. Recently, reports have suggested that there is little research supporting such a treatment algorithm [30]. We recommend proceeding with diversion in patients with a pelvic fracture overlying large lacerations near the fecal stream. Patients with small lacerations that can be easily closed or anteriorly located open fractures do not require diversion.

Techniques of Colostomy Formation in Trauma Patients

A destructive lesion that requires diversion should first be evaluated for the extent of injury. The colon should be resected to healthy tissue with good vascularity. A standard end colostomy should be brought up and matured (Fig. 13.7).

There are anatomic considerations that must be taken into account when choosing the type of diversion technique. The ascending colon is attached to the retroperitoneum laterally. Even with complete mobilization of the right colon, there is usually not enough length to bring up an end colostomy. Injuries to the ascending colon can be treated in three different ways. The right colon can be resected and an ileocolostomy can be performed. Alternatively, the right colon can be repaired primarily. Both of these repairs can be protected with a loop ileostomy. This allows preservation of the ileocecal valve. If the injury is near the cecum, we perform a cecal resection and an end ileostomy (Fig. 13.8).

The remainder of the colonic injuries can be treated with resection and colonic diversion. There is almost always enough length in the transverse colon to bring up an end colostomy with a long Hartmann's pouch. Injuries to the descending colon should be treated with resection to the transverse colon with formation of an end transverse colostomy. Injuries to the sigmoid colon should be treated with a standard Hartmann's pouch and end colostomy.

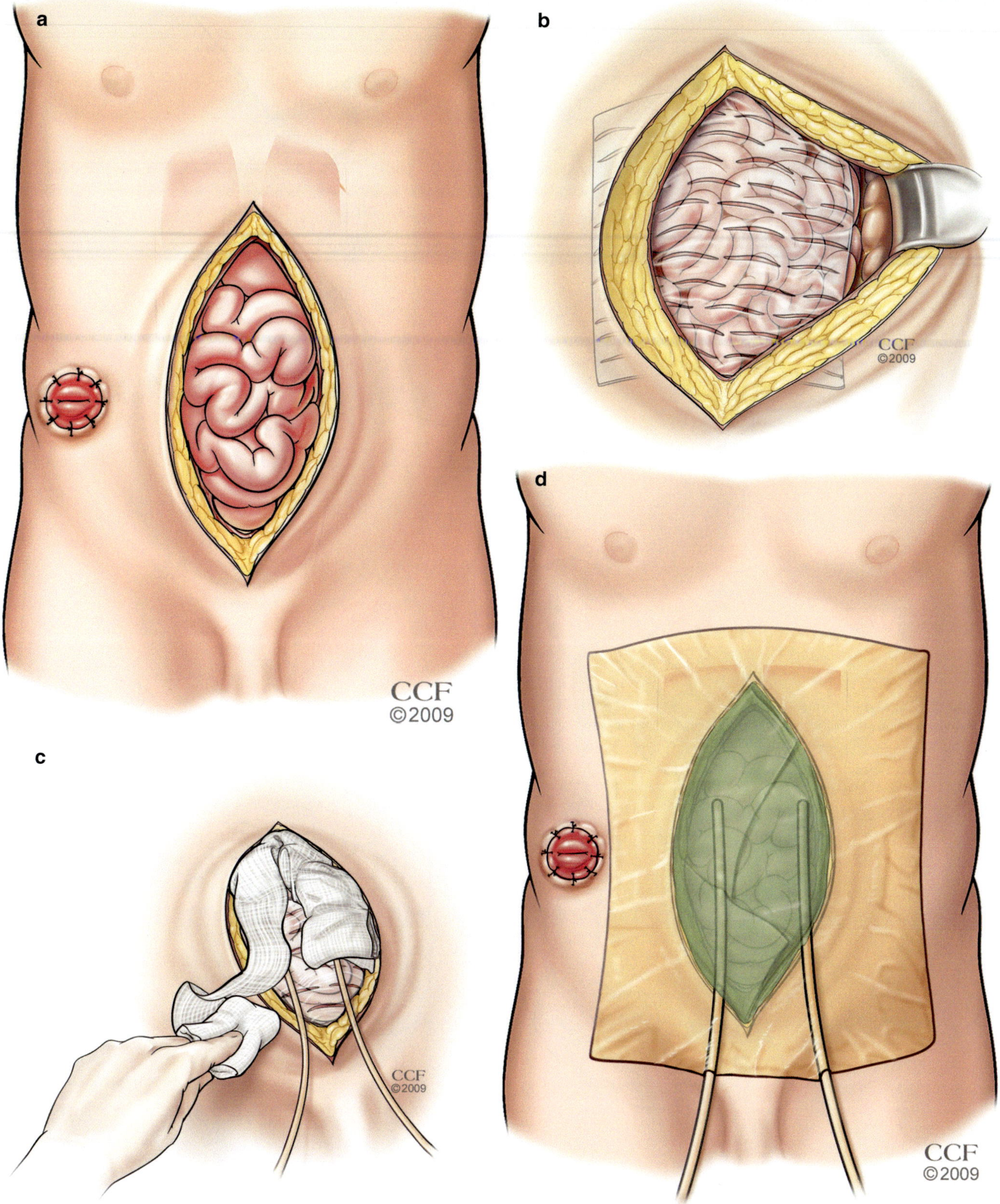

Fig. 13.5 (**a**) Open abdomen with extreme lateral ostomy. (**b**) Open abdomen covered with vacuum-assisted dressing. (**c**) Abdominal wound packed with gauze and drain. (**d**) Complete wound cover with Ioban™. Illustrations © CCF

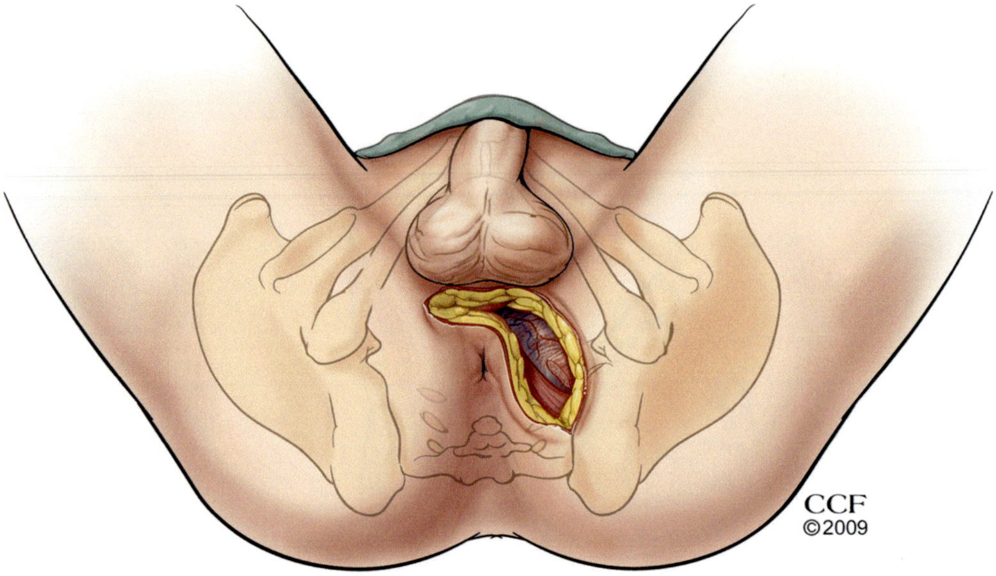

Fig. 13.6 Large perineal wound. Illustration © CCF

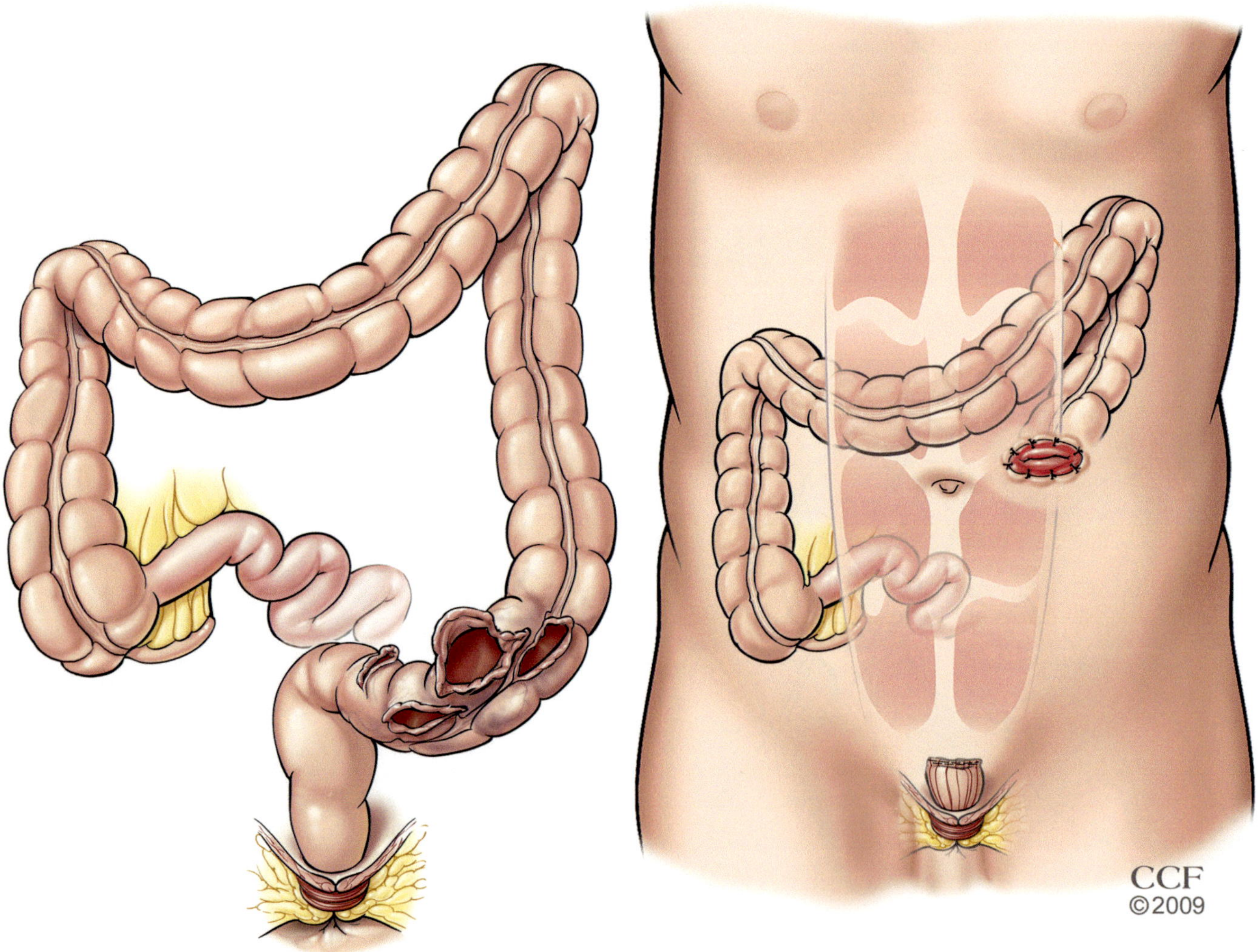

Fig. 13.7 Blast injury with left hemicolectomy. Illustration © CCF

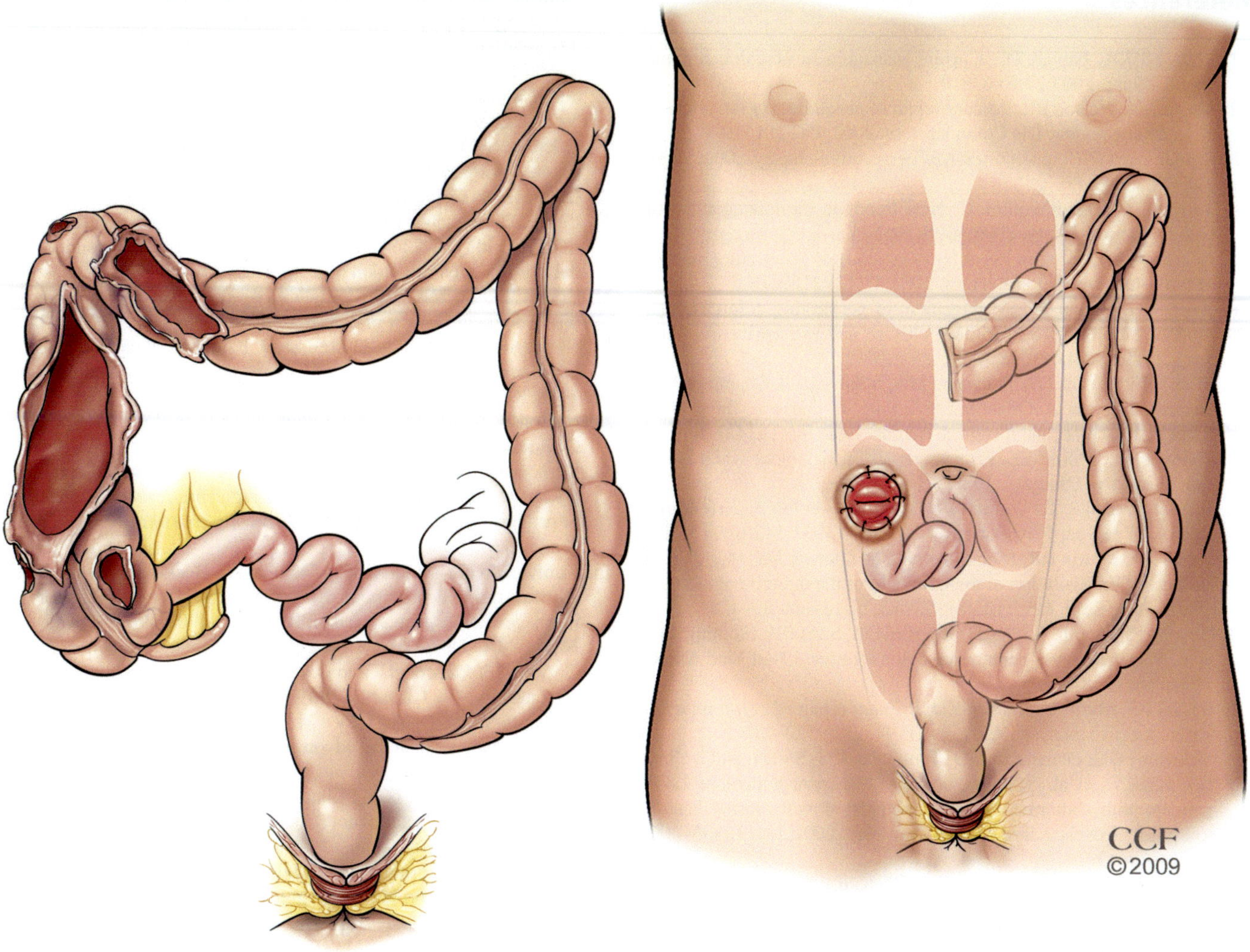

Fig. 13.8 Blast injury with right hemicolectomy. Illustration © CCF

A previously used technique was exteriorization of repair. The injured colonic segment was repaired primarily and was brought up into the wound or through another skin incision. This was fraught with complications of bowel desiccation and necrosis, so it has fallen out of favor and is not suggested by the authors.

Indications for Small Bowel Diversion

The bulk of this chapter focuses on colon injuries. Nearly all of the literature on bowel diversion distal to the ligament of Treitz focuses on colon injuries. Nearly all small bowel injuries should be treated with primary repair or resection and anastomosis. Small bowel diversion for a small bowel injury should only be undertaken in certain disastrous injuries such as a destructive small bowel injury coupled with an injury to the portal vein. In this situation, a standard end ileostomy or jejunostomy can be created. The primary use of ileostomy in the trauma setting is to divert enteric contents away from a colonic injury. Either a loop ileostomy or an end ileostomy will suffice as described elsewhere in this chapter.

Conclusion

The treatment of colonic injuries is complex and requires consideration of the patient's physiologic condition, their premorbid status, the extent of the injury, and the vascular supply. Although there has been a significant trend toward repair without diversion in recent years, there still is a role for colostomy in high-risk patients. Surgeons should be familiar with the techniques for performance of colostomy in the injured colon.

References

1. Maxwell RA, Fabian TC. Current management of colon trauma. World J Surg. 2003;27(6):632–9.
2. Singer MA, Nelson RL. Primary repair of penetrating colon injuries: a systematic review. Dis Colon Rectum. 2002;45(12):1579–87.
3. Demetriades D. Colon injuries: new perspectives. Injury. 2004;35(3): 217–22.
4. Tzovaras G, Hatzitheofilou C. New trends in the management of colonic trauma. Injury. 2005;36(9):1011–5.
5. Adesanya AA, Ekanem EE. A ten-year study of penetrating injuries of the colon. Dis Colon Rectum. 2004;47(12):2169–77.
6. Stone HH, Fabian TC. Management of perforating colon trauma: randomization between primary closure and exteriorization. Ann Surg. 1979;190(4):430–6.
7. Moore EE, Cogbill TH, Malangoni MA, Jurkovich GJ, Champion HR, Gennarelli TA, et al. Organ injury scaling, II: pancreas, duodenum, small bowel, colon, and rectum. J Trauma. 1990;30(11):1427–9.
8. Shannon FL, Moore EE. Primary repair of the colon: when is it a safe alternative? Surgery. 1985;98(4):851–60.
9. Wiener I, Rojas P, Wolma FJ. Traumatic colonic perforation. Review of 16 years' experience. Am J Surg. 1981;142(6):717–20.
10. Burch JM, Martin RR, Richardson RJ, Muldowny DS, Mattox KL, Jordan Jr GL. Evolution of the treatment of the injured colon in the 1980s. Arch Surg. 1991;126(8):979–83; discussion 83–4.
11. Bostick PJ, Heard JS, Islas JT, Johnson DA, Sims EH, Fleming AW, et al. Management of penetrating colon injuries. J Natl Med Assoc. 1994;86(5):378–82.
12. Sasaki LS, Mittal V, Allaben RD. Primary repair of colon injuries: a retrospective analysis. Am Surg. 1994;60(7):522–7.
13. Velmahos GC, Demetriades D, Toutouzas KG, Sarkisyan G, Chan LS, Ishak R, et al. Selective nonoperative management in 1,856 patients with abdominal gunshot wounds: should routine laparotomy still be the standard of care? Ann Surg. 2001;234(3):395–402; discussion –3.
14. George Jr SM, Fabian TC, Voeller GR, Kudsk KA, Mangiante EC, Britt LG. Primary repair of colon wounds. A prospective trial in nonselected patients. Ann Surg. 1989;209(6):728–33; 33–4.
15. Demetriades D, Charalambides D, Pantanowitz D. Gunshot wounds of the colon: role of primary repair. Ann R Coll Surg Engl. 1992;74(6):381–4.
16. Chappuis CW, Frey DJ, Dietzen CD, Panetta TP, Buechter KJ, Cohn Jr I. Management of penetrating colon injuries. A prospective randomized trial. Ann Surg. 1991;213(5):492–7; discussion 7–8.
17. Gonzalez RP, Falimirski ME, Holevar MR. Further evaluation of colostomy in penetrating colon injury. Am Surg. 2000;66(4):342–6; discussion 6–7.
18. Sasaki LS, Allaben RD, Golwala R, Mittal VK. Primary repair of colon injuries: a prospective randomized study. J Trauma. 1995; 39(5):895–901.
19. Falcone RE, Wanamaker SR, Santanello SA, Carey LC. Colorectal trauma: primary repair or anastomosis with intracolonic bypass vs. Ostomy. Dis Colon Rectum. 1992;35(10):957–63.
20. Berne JD, Velmahos GC, Chan LS, Asensio JA, Demetriades D. The high morbidity of colostomy closure after trauma: further support for the primary repair of colon injuries. Surgery. 1998;123(2):157–64.
21. Curran TJ, Borzotta AP. Complications of primary repair of colon injury: literature review of 2,964 cases. Am J Surg. 1999;177(1):42–7.
22. Demetriades D, Pezikis A, Melissas J, Parekh D, Pickles G. Factors influencing the morbidity of colostomy closure. Am J Surg. 1988;155(4):594–6.
23. Nelson R, Singer M. Primary repair for penetrating colon injuries. Cochrane Database Syst Rev. 2003;3:CD002247 Review.
24. Demetriades D, Murray JA, Chan L, Ordonez C, Bowley D, Nagy KK, et al. Penetrating colon injuries requiring resection: diversion or primary anastomosis? An AAST prospective multicenter study. J Trauma. 2001;50(5):765–75.
25. Kamwendo NY, Modiba MC, Matlala NS, Becker PJ. Randomized clinical trial to determine if delay from time of penetrating colonic injury precludes primary repair. Br J Surg. 2002;89(8):993–8.
26. Murray JA, Demetriades D, Colson M, Song Z, Velmahos GC, Cornwell 3rd EE, et al. Colonic resection in trauma: colostomy versus anastomosis. J Trauma. 1999;46(2):250–4.
27. McGrath V, Fabian TC, Croce MA, Minard G, Pritchard FE. Rectal trauma: management based on anatomic distinctions. Am Surg. 1998;64(12):1136–41.
28. Weinberg JA, Fabian TC, Magnotti LJ, Minard G, Bee TK, Edwards N, et al. Penetrating rectal trauma: management by anatomic distinction improves outcome. J Trauma. 2006;60(3):508–13; discussion 13–14.
29. Velmahos GC, Gomez H, Falabella A, Demetriades D. Operative management of civilian rectal gunshot wounds: simpler is better. World J Surg. 2000;24(1):114–8.
30. Lunsjo K, Abu-Zidan FM. Does colostomy prevent infection in open blunt pelvic fractures? A systematic review. J Trauma. 2006; 60(5):1145–8.

CCF Color Photo Gallery

14

Victor W. Fazio, Paula Erwin-Toth, James M. Church, and James S. Wu

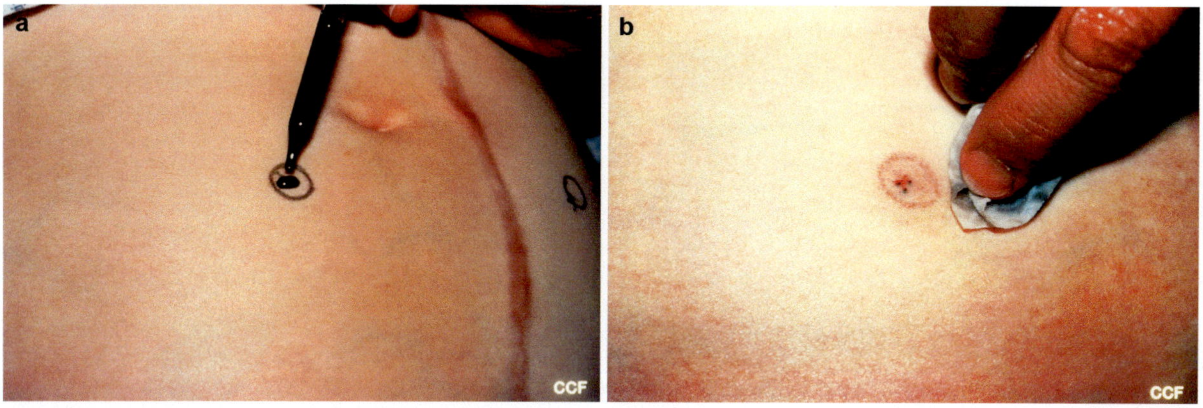

Fig. 14.1 (**a**, **b**) Stoma site-tattoo with India ink

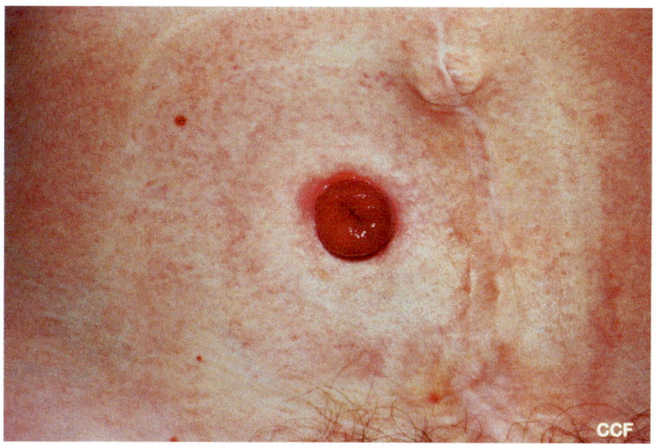

Fig. 14.2 End ileostomy, conventional Brooke construction

V.W. Fazio (✉)
Department of Colorectal Surgery, Digestive Diseases Institute, Cleveland Clinic Lerner College of Medicine of Case Western Reserve University, Cleveland Clinic Foundation, Cleveland, OH, USA
e-mail: faziov@ccf.org

P. Erwin-Toth
The Rupert B. Turnbull School of WOC/ET, Cleveland Clinic/ET, Cleveland, OH, USA

J.M. Church • J.S. Wu
Department of Colorectal Surgery, Digestive Diseases Institute, Cleveland Clinic Foundation, Cleveland, OH, USA

V.W. Fazio et al. (eds.), *Atlas of Intestinal Stomas*,
DOI 10.1007/978-0-387-78851-7_14, © Springer Science+Business Media, LLC 2012

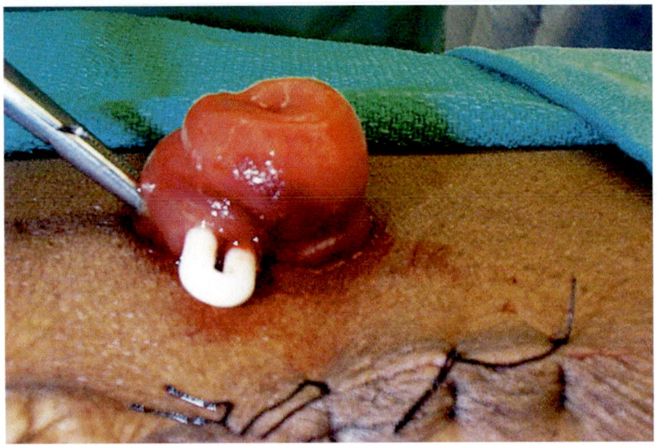

Fig. 14.3 Loop Ileostomy. The diminutive inactive lumen is identified with the instrument

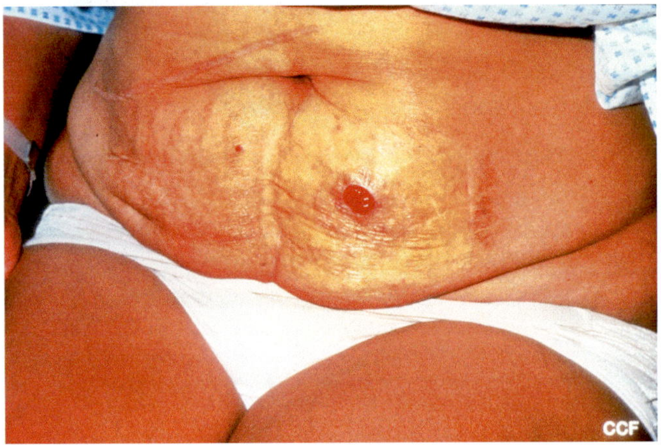

Fig. 14.4 End descending colostomy

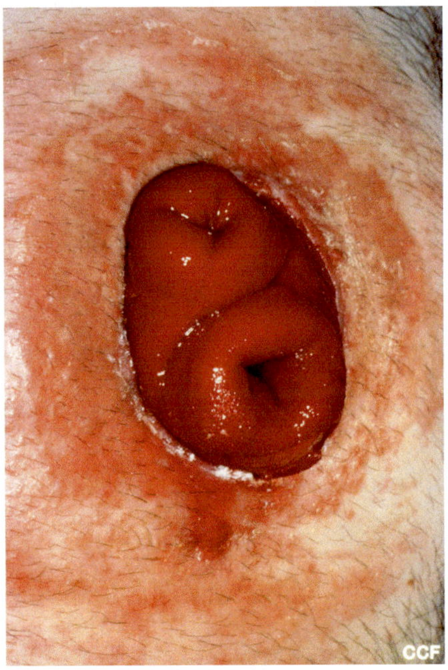

Fig. 14.5 Transverse loop colostomy

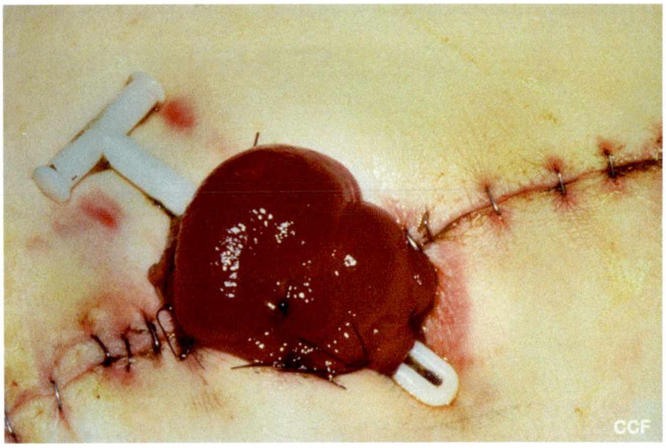

Fig. 14.6 Transverse loop colostomy through incision (not usually recommended)

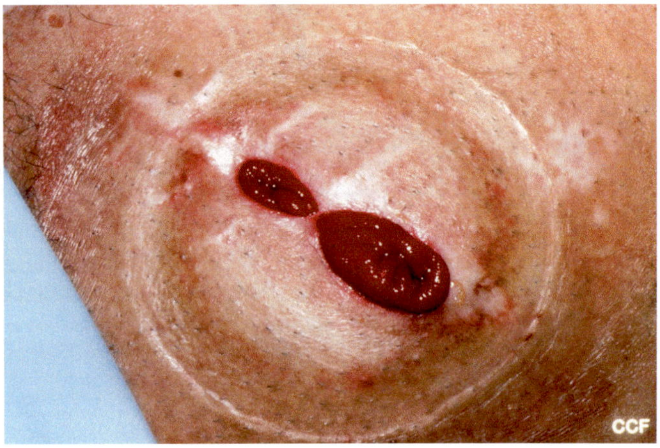

Fig. 14.7 Divided sigmoid colostomy and mucous fistula

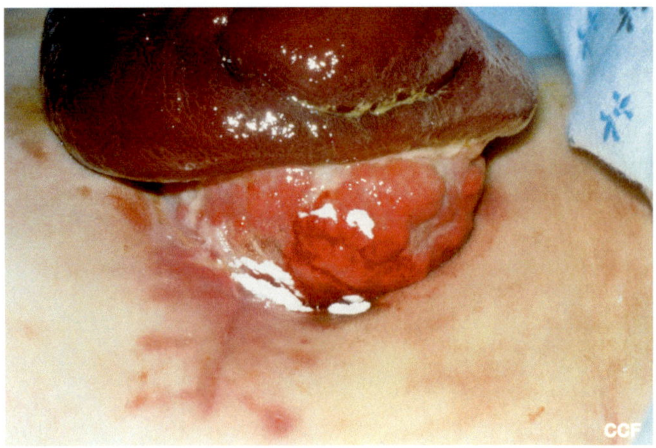

Fig. 14.8 Loop colostomy, incomplete stoma maturation

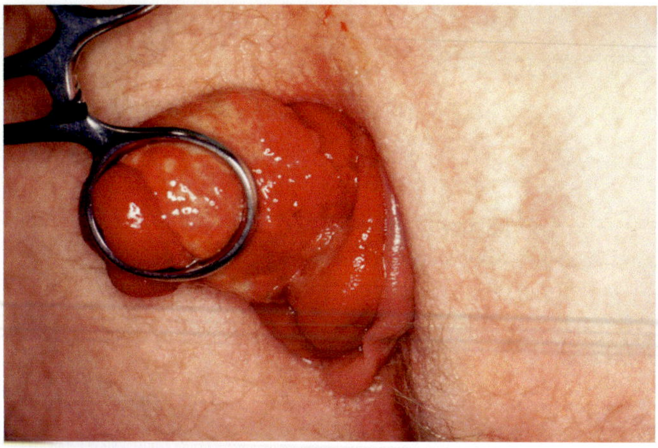

Fig. 14.9 Unmatured ileostomy-serosal granulation tissue

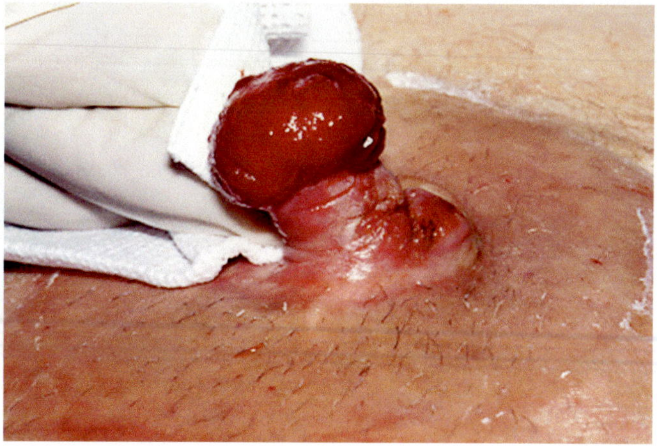

Fig. 14.11 Skin-grafted ileostomy

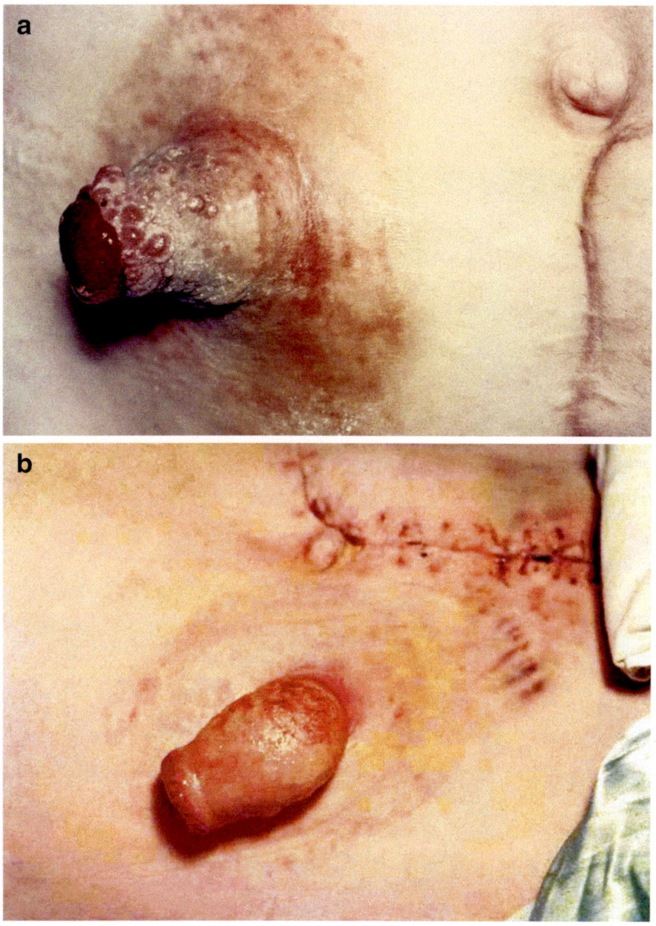

Fig. 14.10 Skin-grafted ileostomy. (**a**) Courtesy Frank L. Weakley, MD. (**b**) Courtesy Victor Fazio, MD

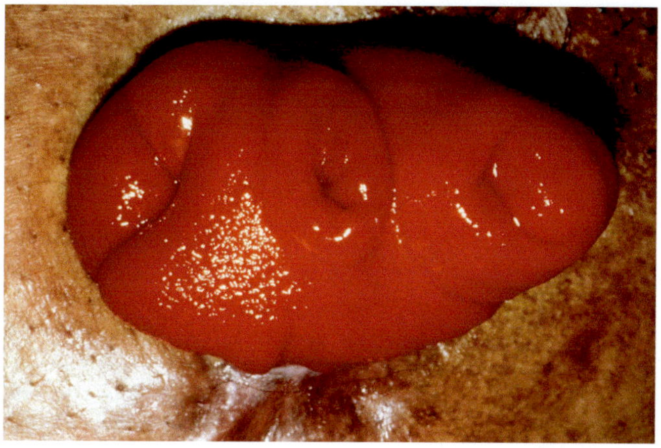

Fig. 14.12 Loop cecoileostomy. The third orifice is the appendix

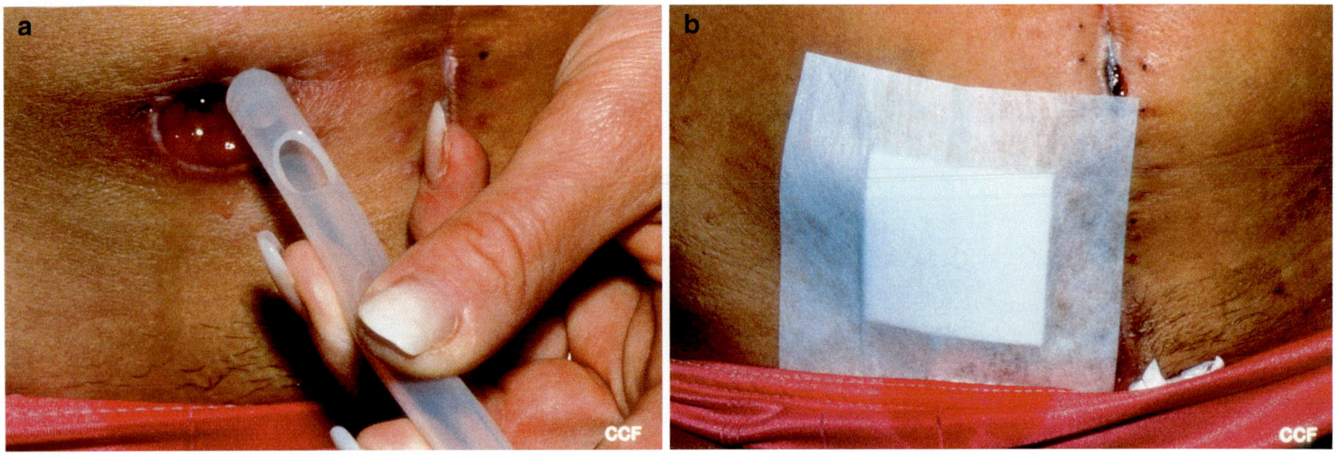

Fig. 14.13 (**a**) Continent ileostomy and intubation tube managed by patient. (**b**) Continent ileostomy with dressing

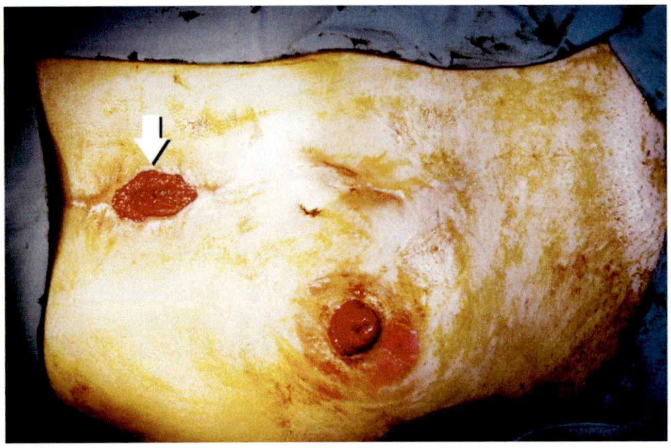

Fig. 14.14 Blowhole colostomy (*arrow*), loop ileostomy in a patient with toxic megacolon

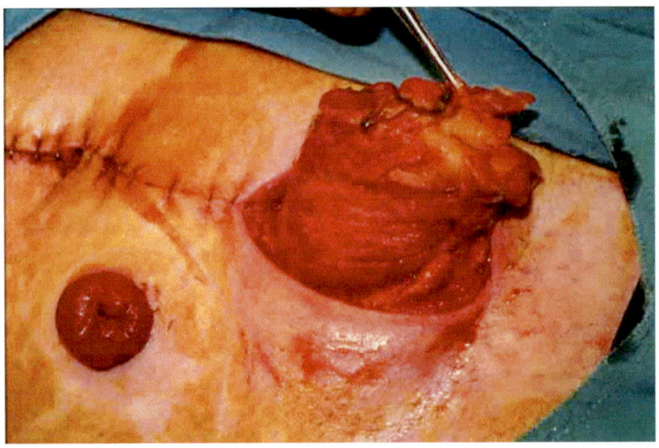

Fig. 14.15 End ileostomy and exteriorized rectosigmoid after subtotal colectomy for toxic colitis. The rectosigmoid is secured above the skin with gauze to prevent retraction back into the abdomen; maturation to a mucous fistula is delayed

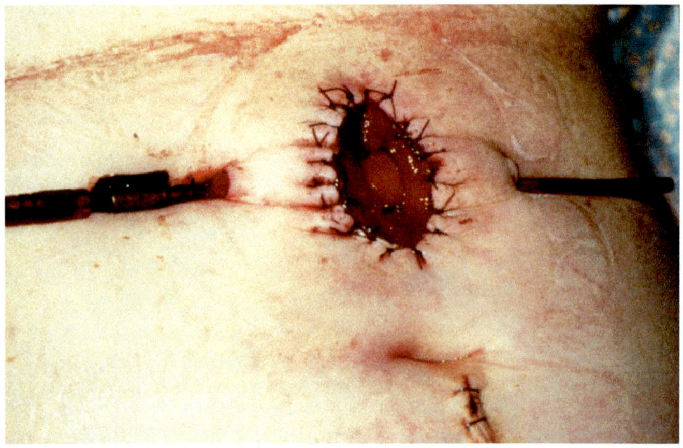

Fig. 14.16 Subcutaneous stoma support rod (courtesy Rupert B. Turnbull, Jr., MD)

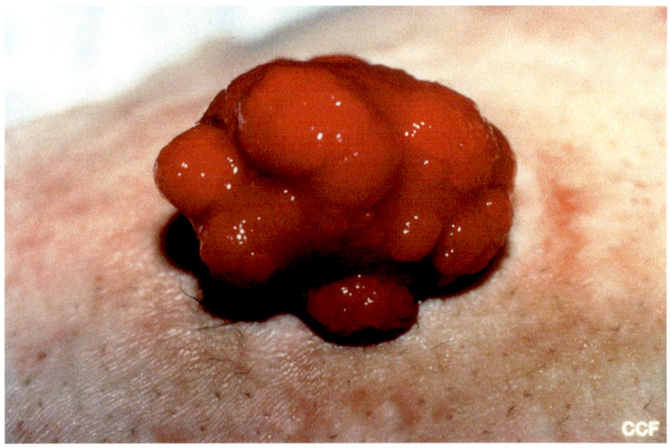

Fig. 14.17 Ileostomy, profuse granulomatous tissue

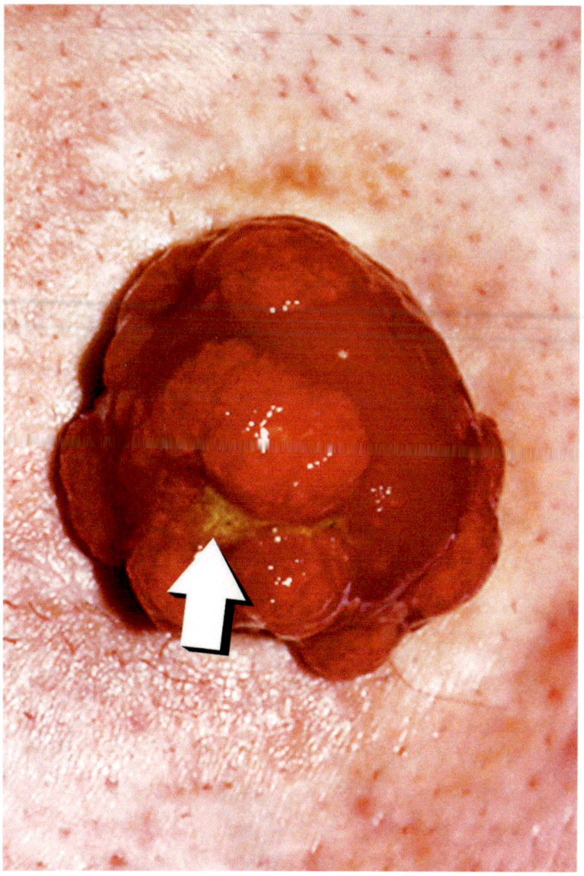

Fig. 14.18 Crohn's ileitis. Note ulceration (*arrow*)

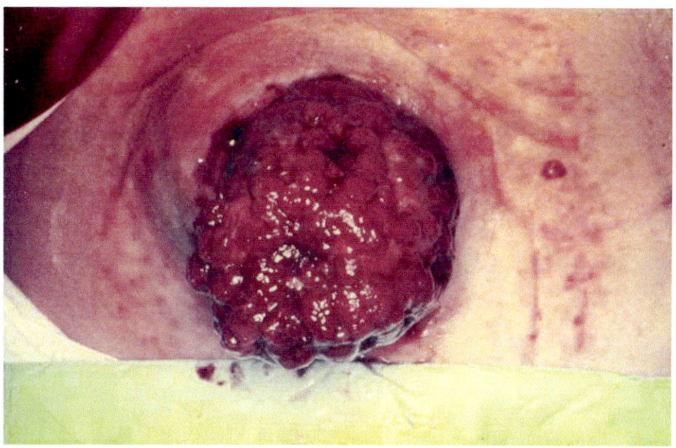

Fig. 14.19 Colostomy affected by Crohn's disease; patient underwent completion proctocolectomy and ileostomy

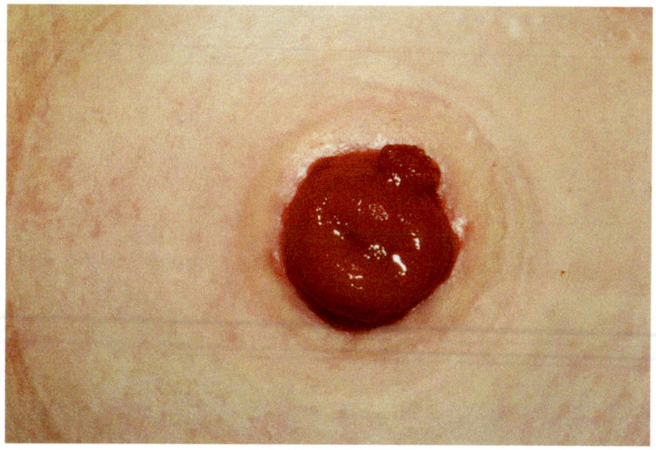

Fig. 14.20 Ileostomy polyp in a patient with familial adenomatous polyposis

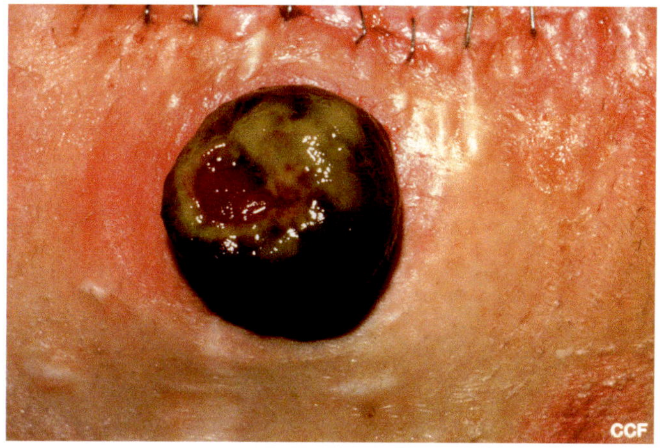

Fig. 14.21 Pseudomembranes on ileostomy in a patient with *Clostridium difficile* enteritis

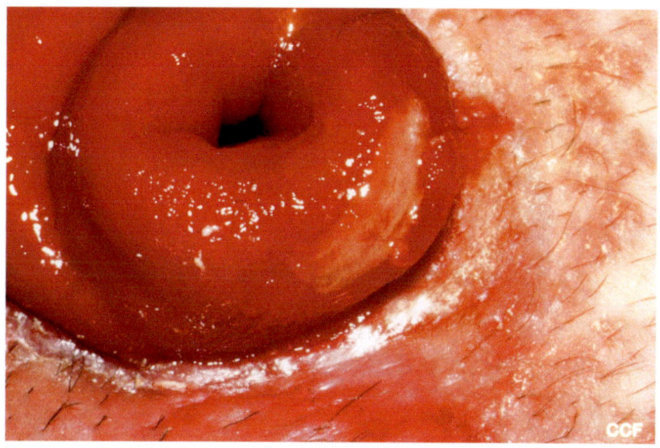

Fig. 14.22 Ileostomy, mucosal trauma from pressure

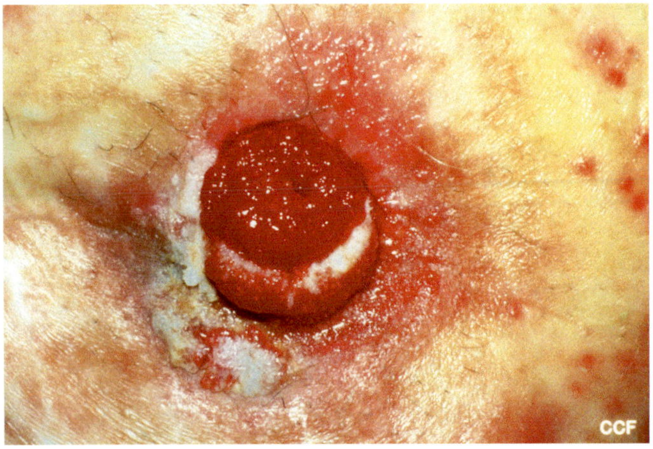

Fig. 14.23 Ileostomy, mucosal trauma-appliance aperture too small

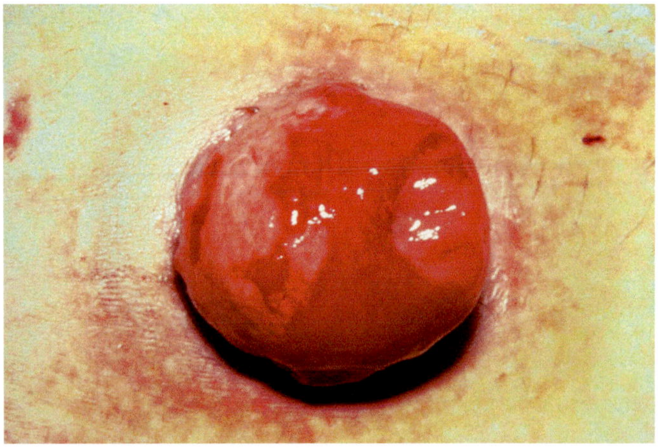

Fig. 14.24 Mucosal ischemia

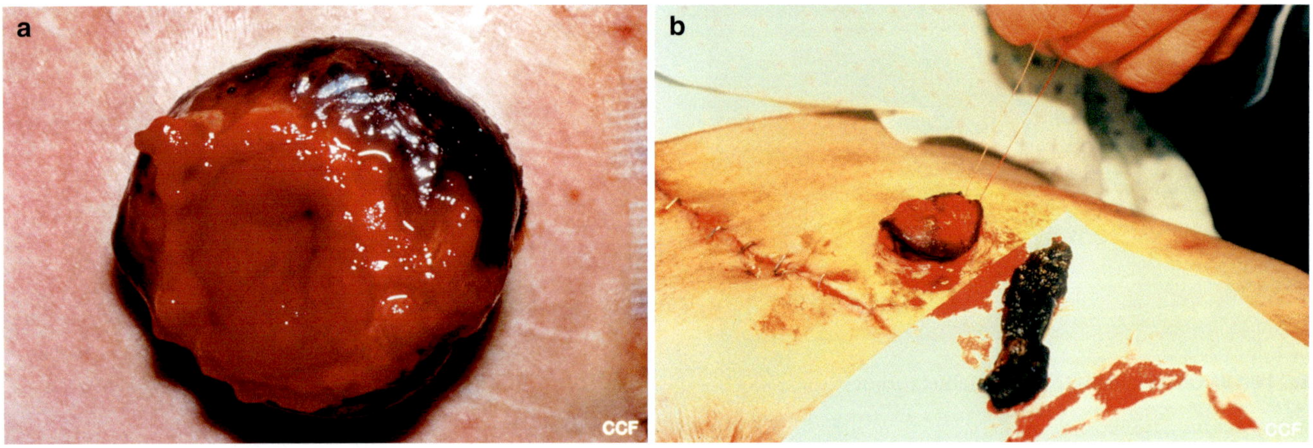

Fig. 14.25 (**a**) Ileostomy, marginal ischemia. (**b**) Ileostomy, local revision, excision of devitalized tissue

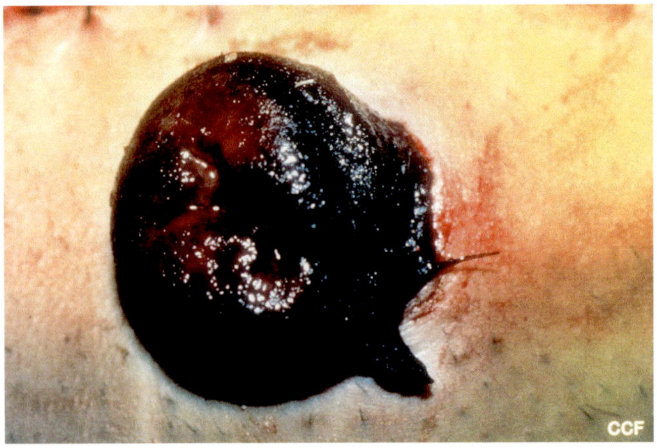

Fig. 14.26 Ileostomy, ischemia

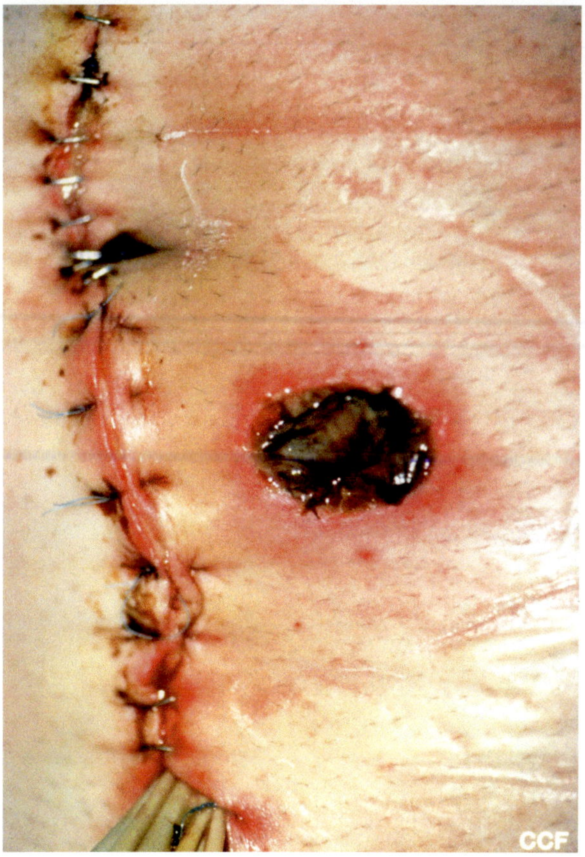

Fig. 14.27 Gangrenous end sigmoid colostomy

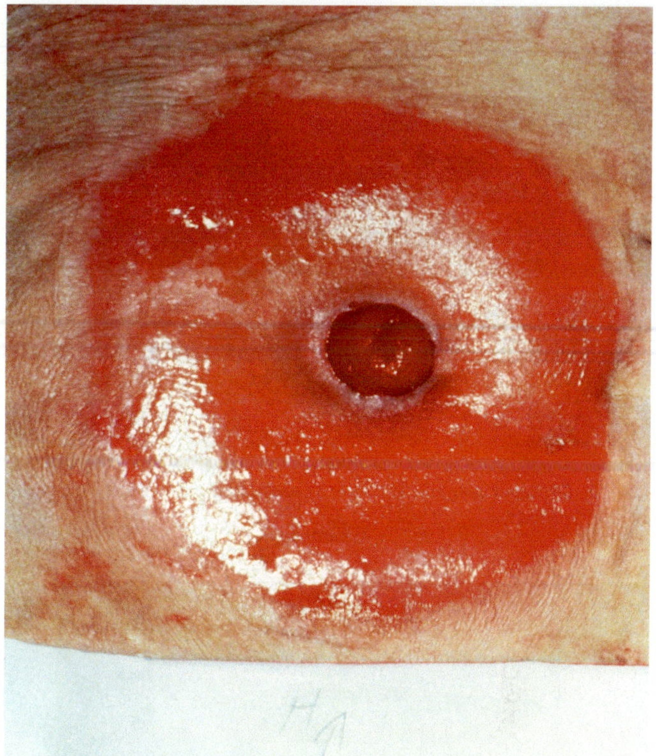

Fig. 14.29 Ileal conduit, acute contact dermatitis due to urine leak

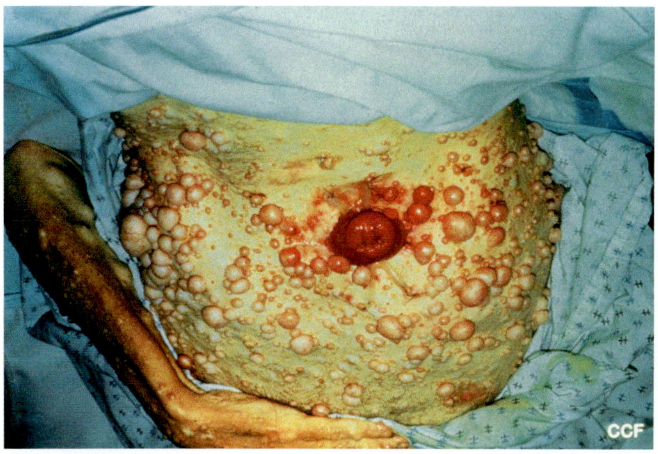

Fig. 14.28 End ileostomy, neurofibromatosis (von Recklinghausen's disease)

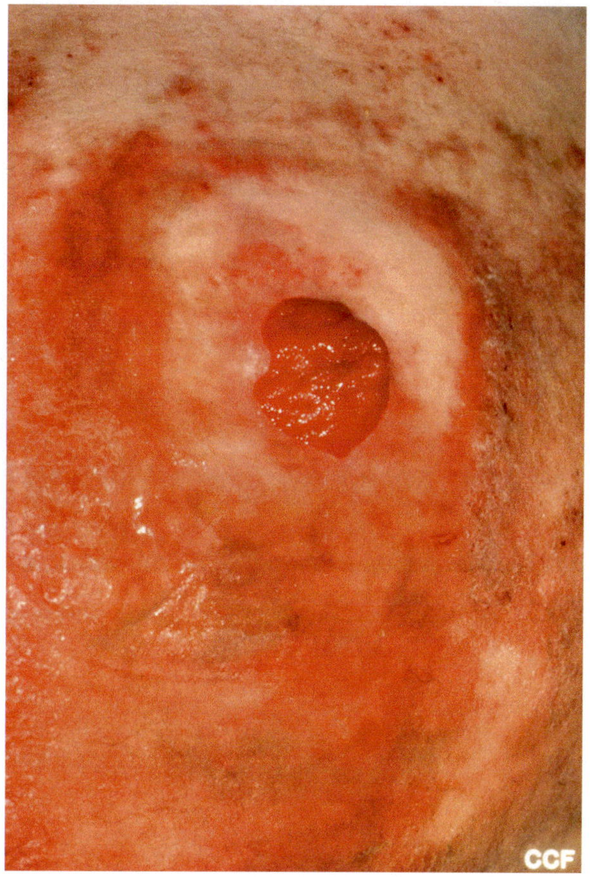

Fig. 14.30 Chronic reactive dermatitis to stoma bag

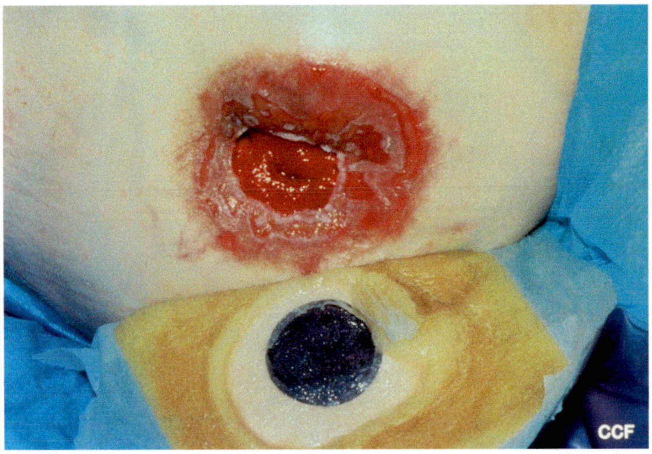

Fig. 14.31 Ileal conduit, leakage, skin destruction caused by contact of skin with urine

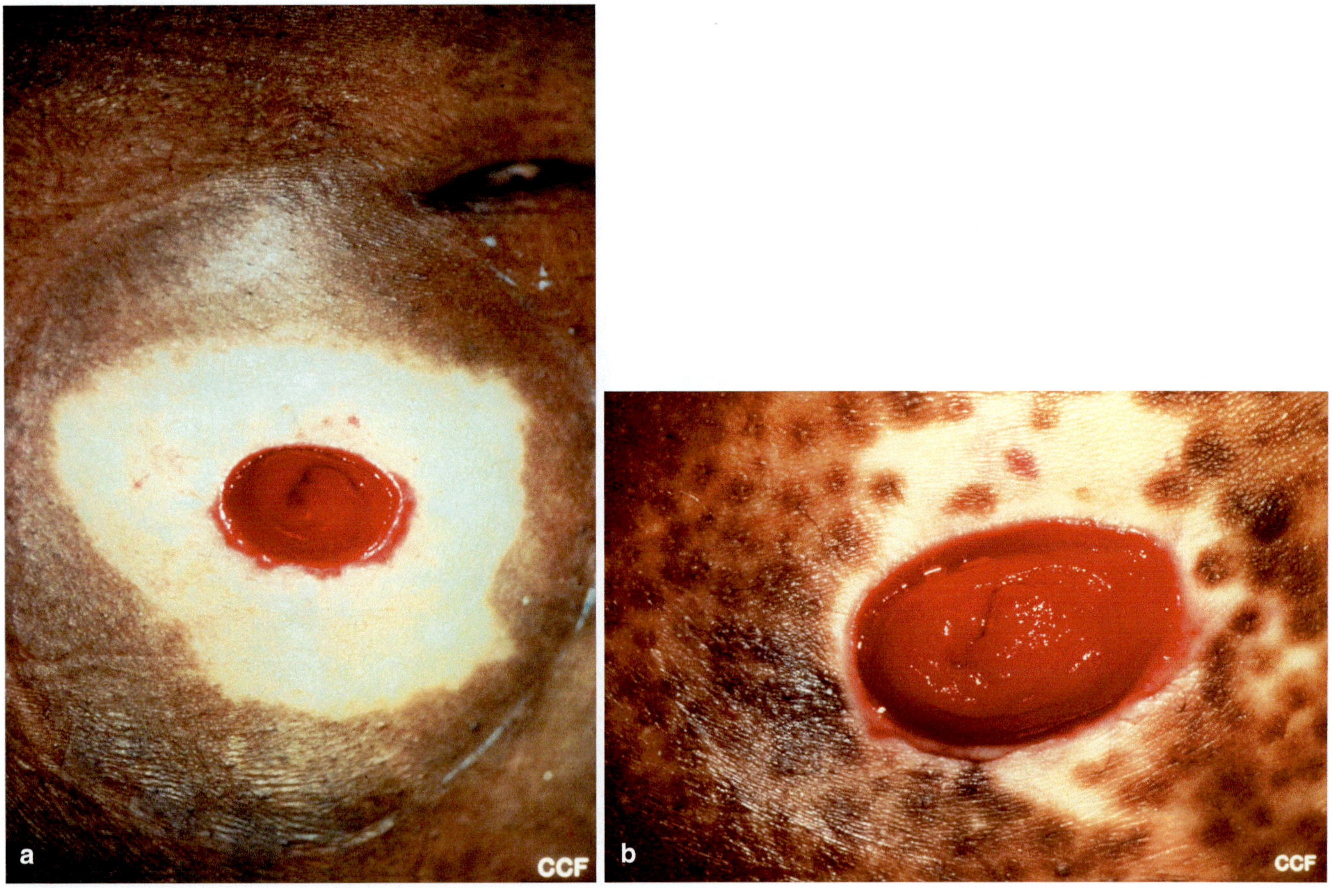

Fig. 14.32 (**a**) Ileal conduit, vitiligo. (**b**) Ileal conduit, vitiligo, melanin returning

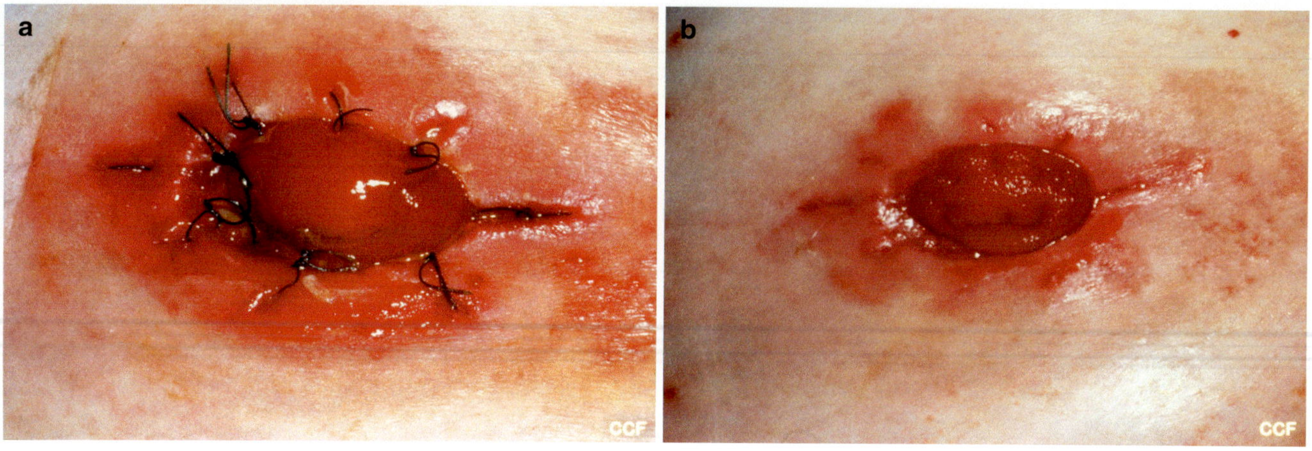

Fig. 14.33 (**a**) End ileostomy. Mechanical trauma from sutures. (**b**) End ileostomy after suture removal

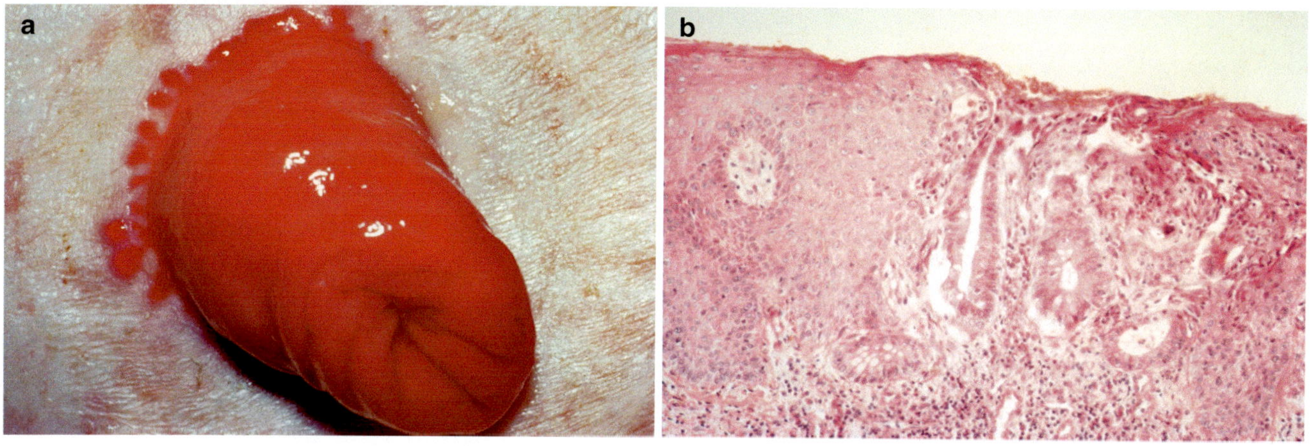

Fig. 14.34 (**a**) Intestinal mucosal implants along parastomal needle tracks (macroscopic). (**b**) Intestinal mucosa implants along parastomal needles tracts (microscopic)

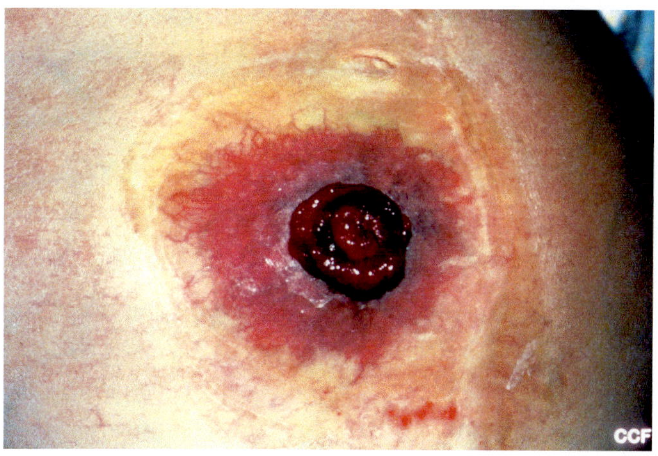

Fig. 14.35 Ileostomy, caput medusae

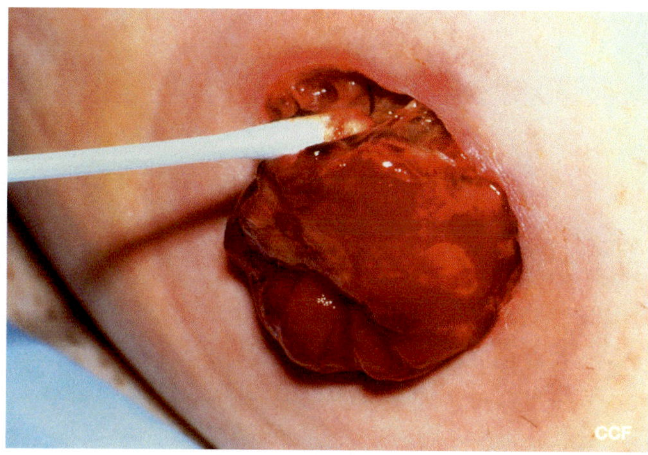

Fig. 14.36 Ileostomy, partial mucosal separation

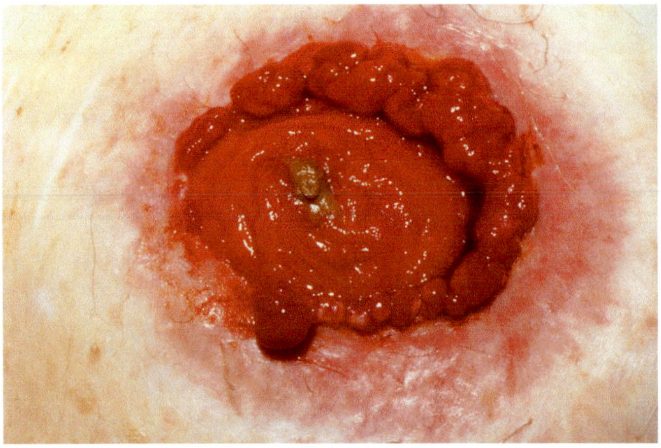

Fig. 14.37 Transverse colostomy, peristomal granulation tissue

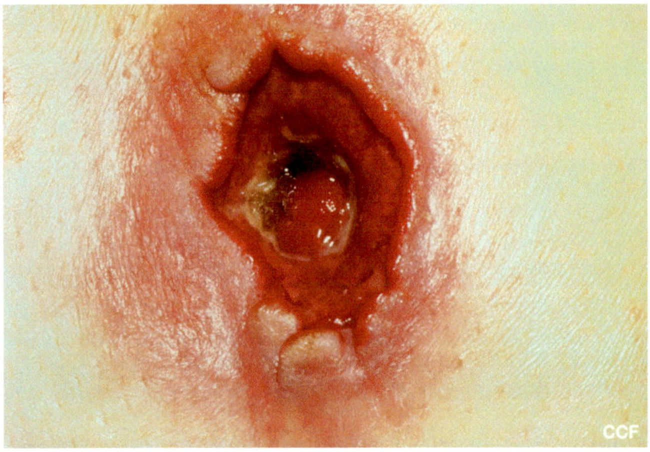

Fig. 14.38 End descending colostomy, total mucosal separation

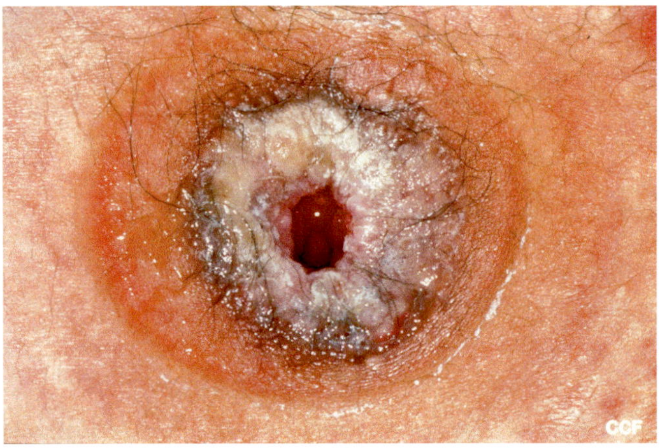

Fig. 14.39 Pseudoverrucous lesion due to chronic hydration of the peristomal skin

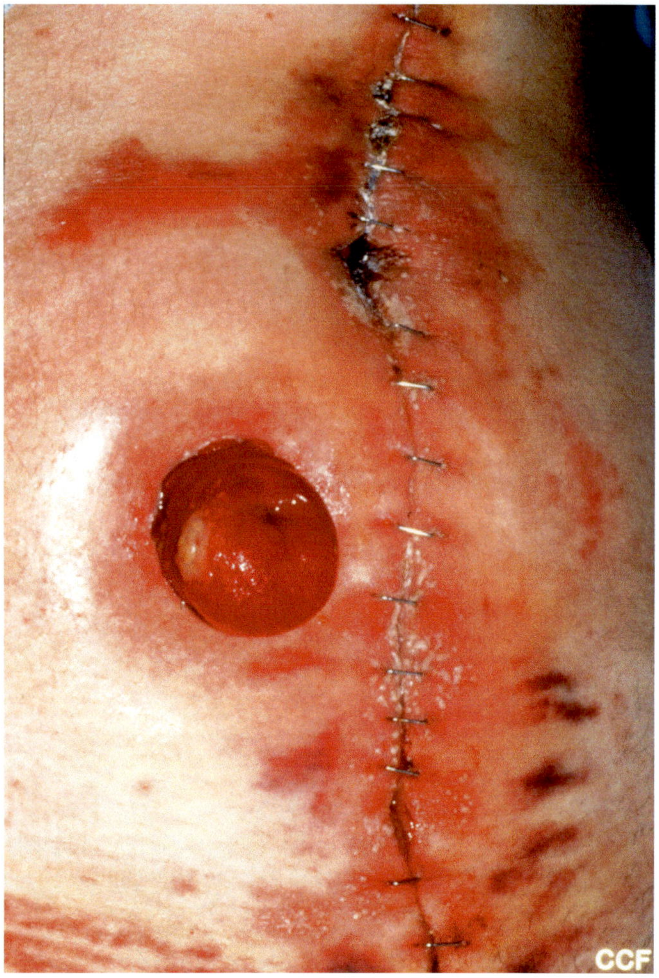

Fig. 14.40 Stoma too close to midline incision. This situation increases the risk of leakage and wound infection. A fungal rash is seen around the incision

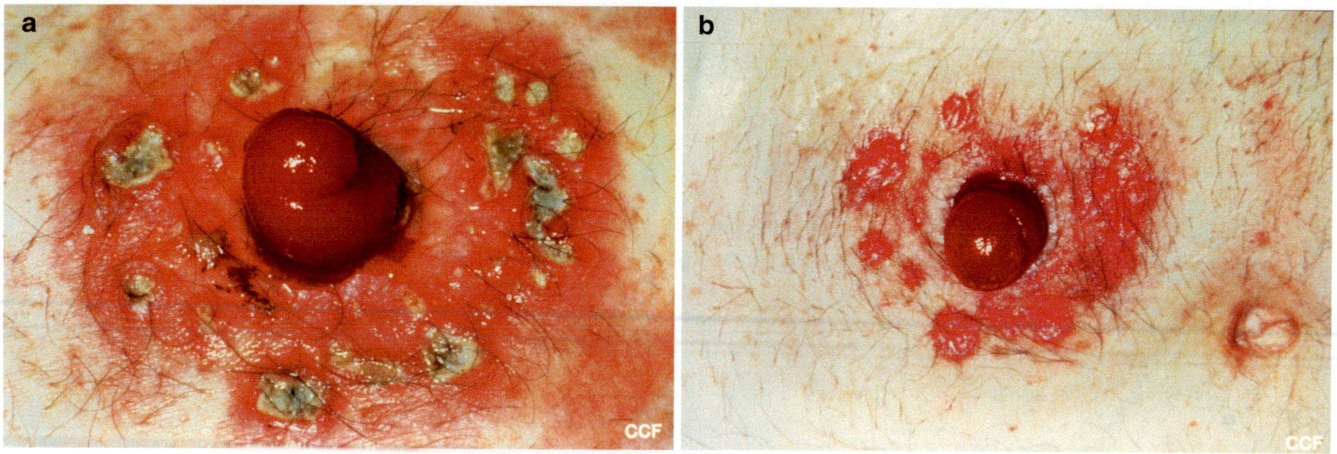

Fig. 14.41 (**a**) Ileal conduit, folliculitis due to depilation from traumatic removal of skin barrier. (**b**) Ileal conduit, folliculitis resolving with correct pouching and antibiotic treatment

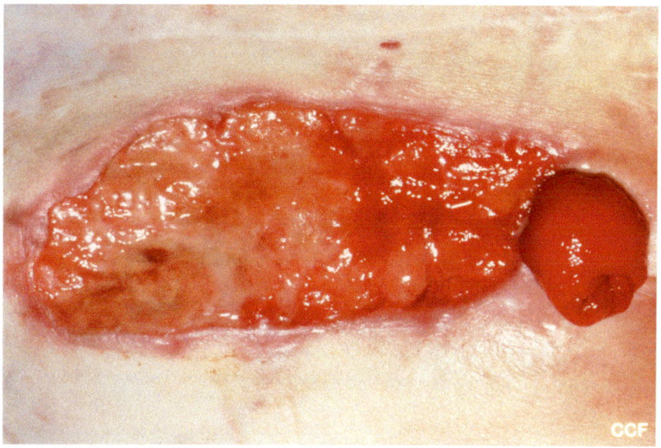

Fig. 14.42 Peristomal ulcer extending laterally from stoma. The base is granulating; the edges are shelved with a tendency to undermine

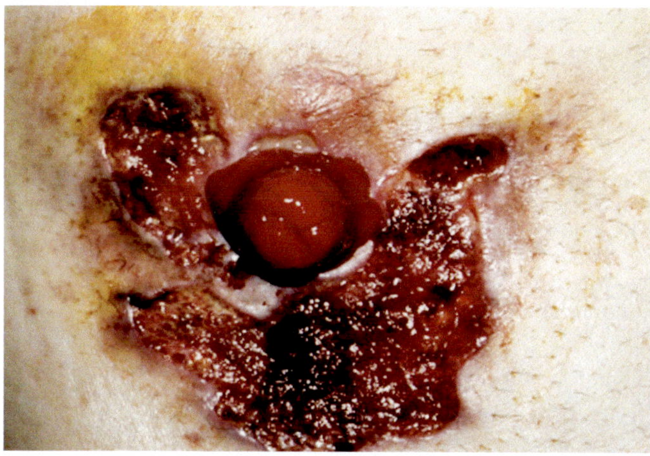

Fig. 14.43 Pyoderma gangrenosum adjacent to an ileostomy in a patient with inflammatory bowel disease. The base of the ulcer shows the typical black ulcer reflective of necrosis

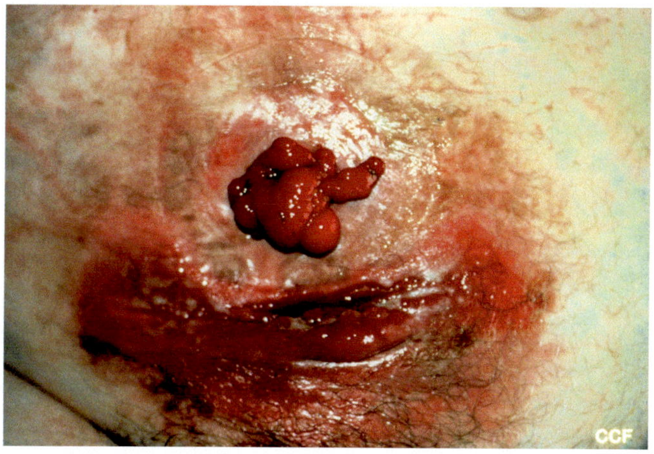

Fig. 14.44 Mechanical trauma from stoma plate

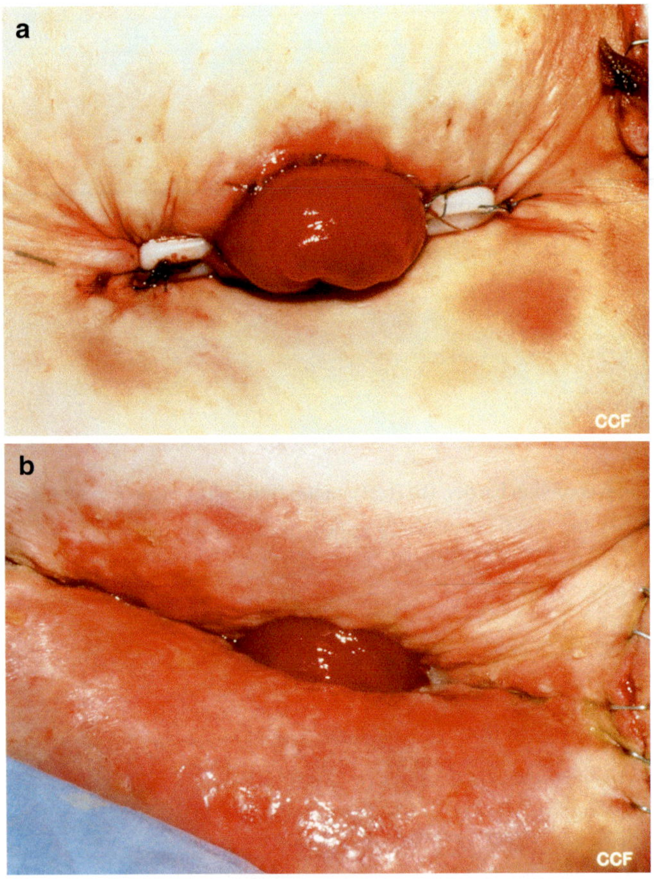

Fig. 14.45 (**a**) Tension on ileostomy exacerbating skin crease. (**b**) Loop ileostomy, recessed stoma after removal of support rod

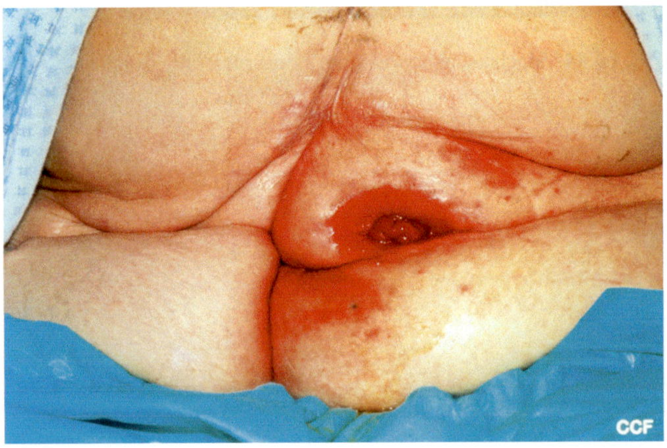

Fig. 14.46 Loop jejunostomy, location in skin crease resulting in leakage and skin destruction

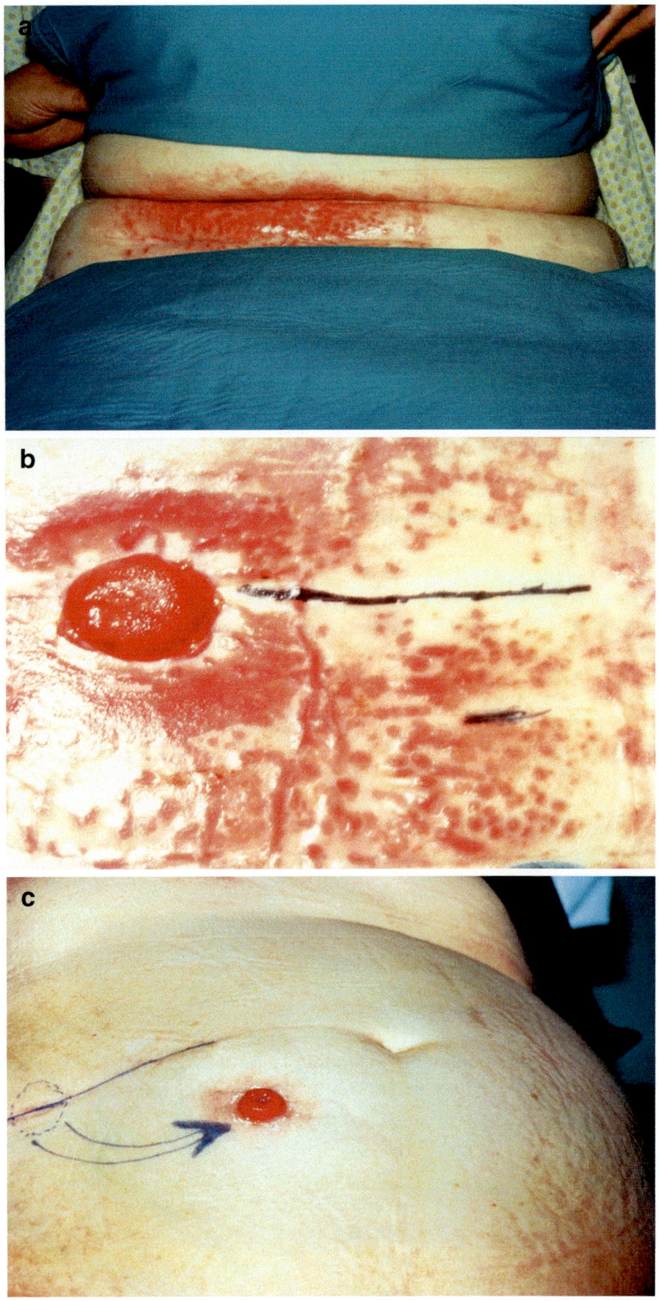

Fig. 14.47 (**a**) Ileostomy in a skin crease, sitting. (**b**) Ileostomy in a skin crease, supine. (**c**) Ileostomy in a skin crease, corrected by stoma relocation

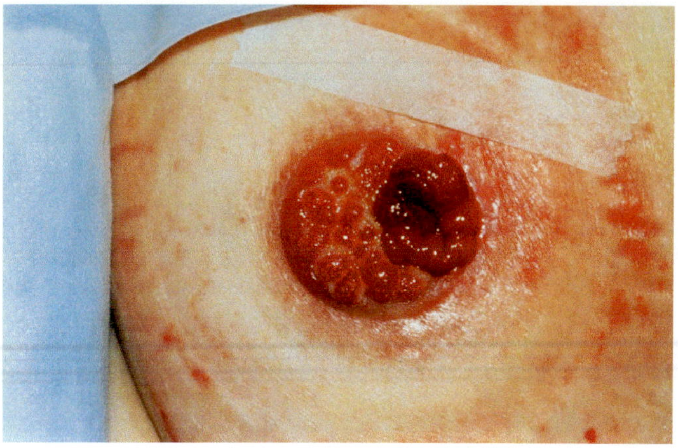

Fig. 14.48 Dermatitis, pouch opening too large

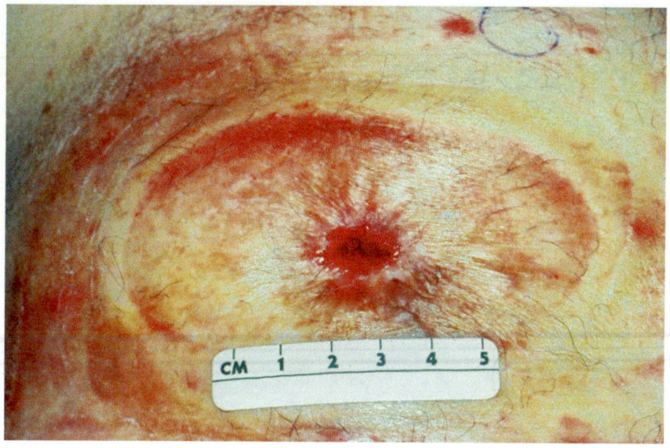

Fig. 14.51 Stoma stricture

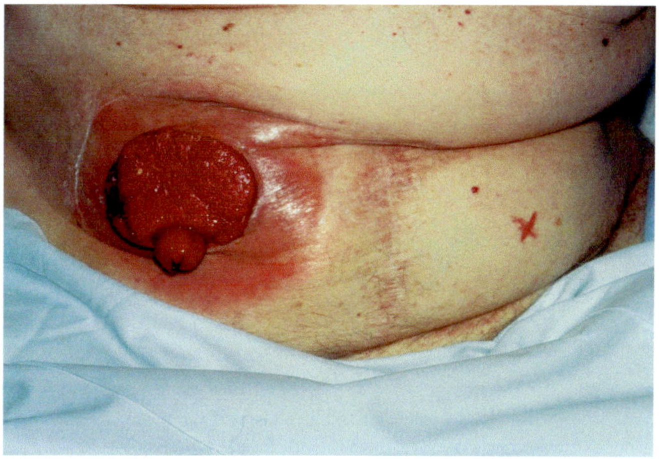

Fig. 14.49 Ileostomy, parastomal squamous cell carcinoma from chronic chemical irritation

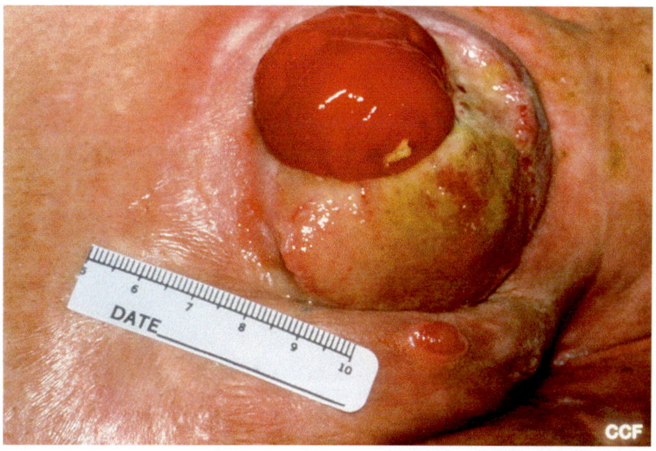

Fig. 14.50 Ileostomy, parastomal cancer with island metastasis

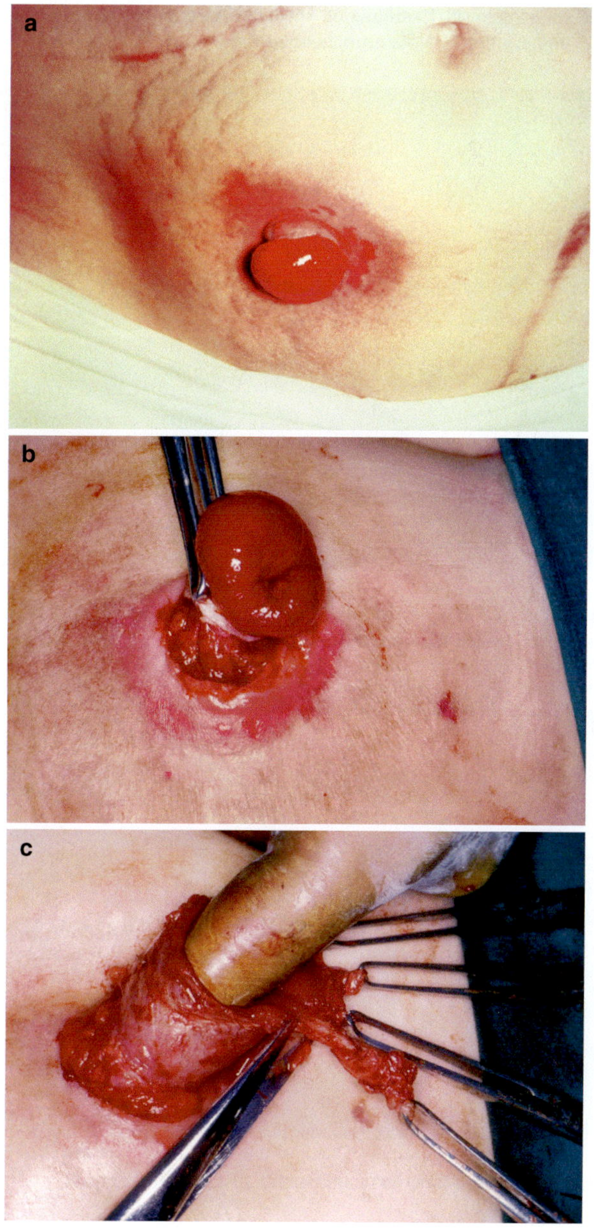

Fig. 14.52 (**a**) Ileostomy stricture: "Bishop's Collar" due to delayed stoma maturation. (**b**) Ileostomy stricture revision. Stoma mobilization. (**c**) Ileostomy stricture revision. Excising the constricting scar tissue

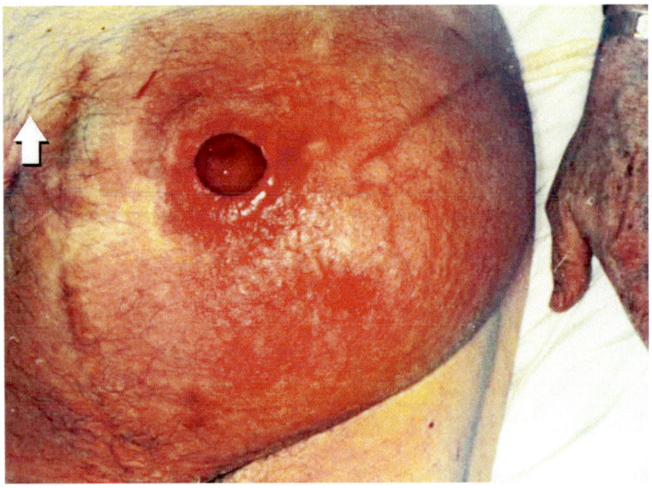

Fig. 14.53 Parastomal abscess due to perforation caused by catheter used for irrigation. Examination revealed marked tenderness, fluctuance, and erythema. Note normal area (*arrow*)

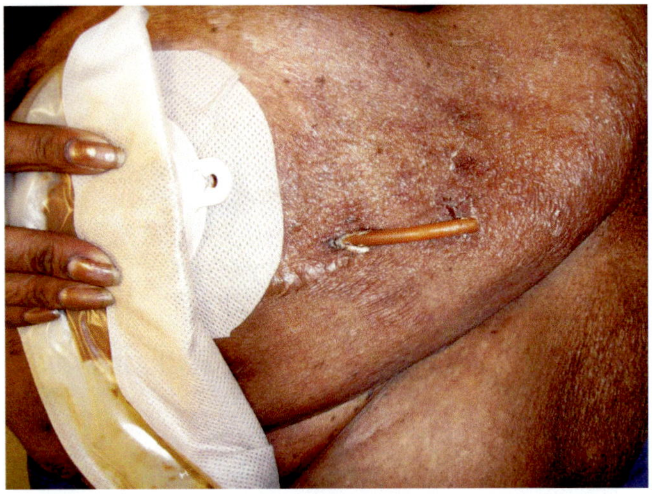

Fig. 14.54 Paracolostomy abscess drained lateral to the appliance to avoid interference with pouching by the drain

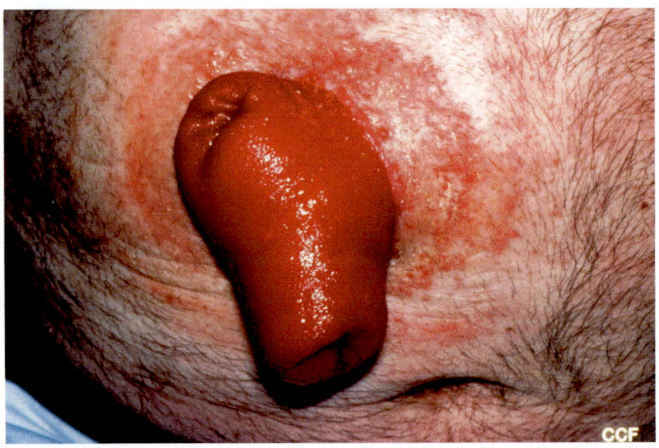

Fig. 14.55 Loop transverse colostomy, distal limb prolapse

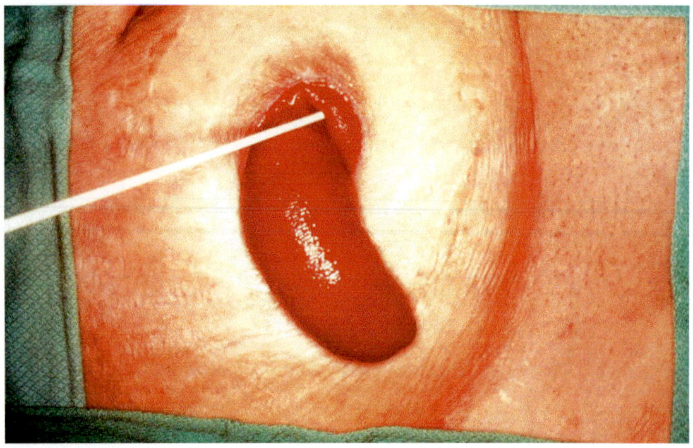

Fig. 14.56 Loop ileostomy prolapse. The pointer identifies the second lumen

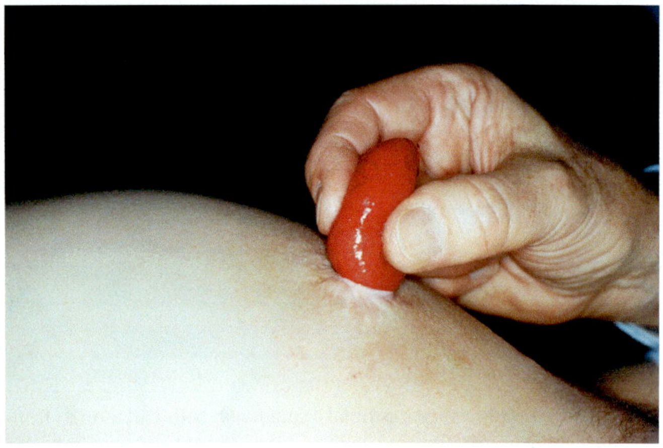

Fig. 14.57 Ileostomy prolapse in pregnancy. The prolapse reverts to normal after delivery (pre-glove era, courtesy Rupert B. Turnbull, Jr., MD)

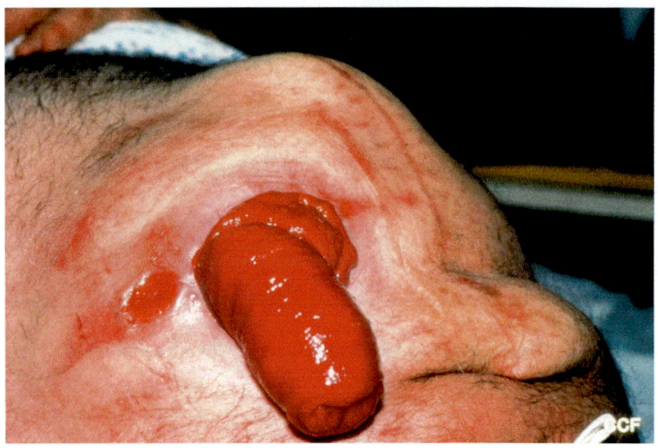

Fig. 14.58 Loop transverse colostomy prolapse, parastomal pressure ulcer due to ostomy belt, incisional hernia

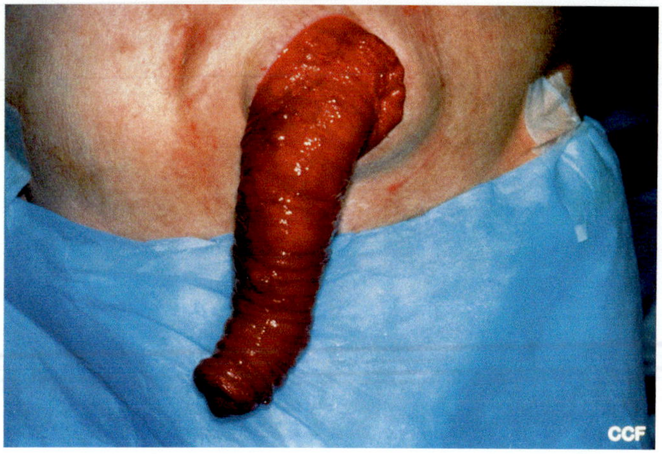

Fig. 14.59 Loop transverse colostomy, prolapse. The tip of the prolapse is becoming ischemic

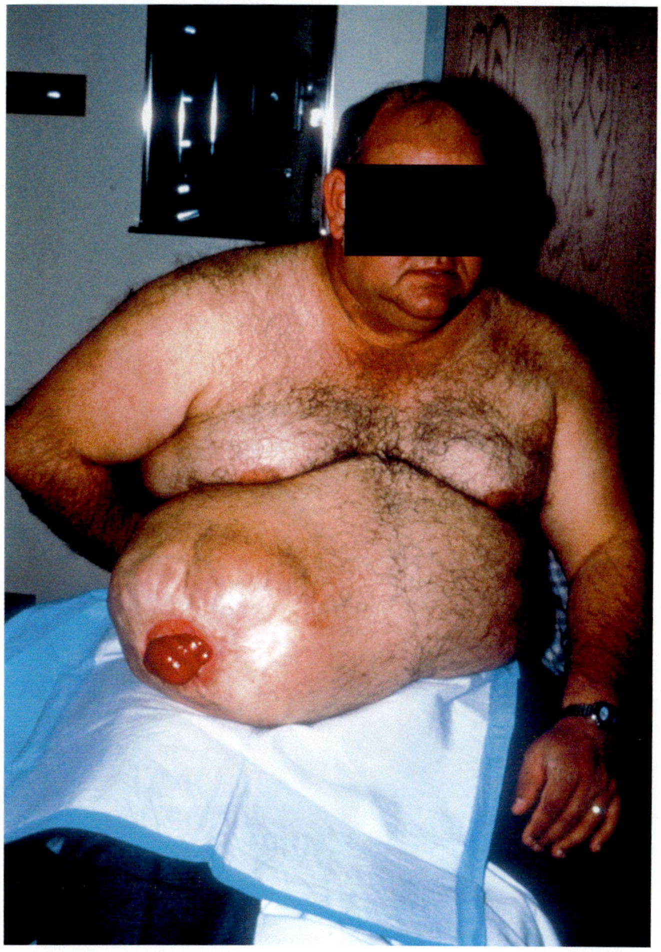

Fig. 14.60 Paracolostomy hernia. Ectopic stoma site outside of the rectus sheath

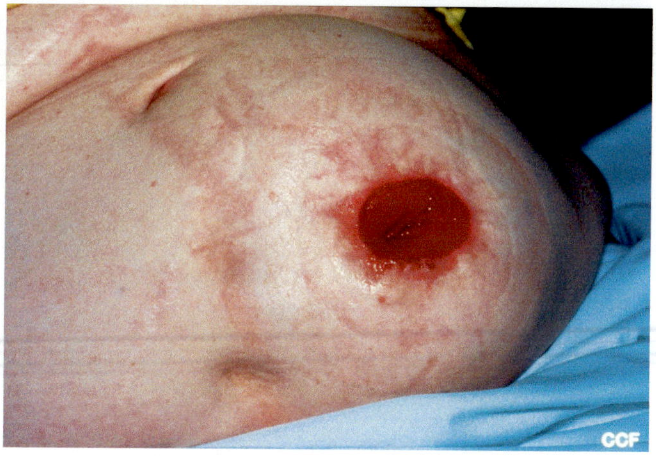

Fig. 14.61 Paracolostomy hernia

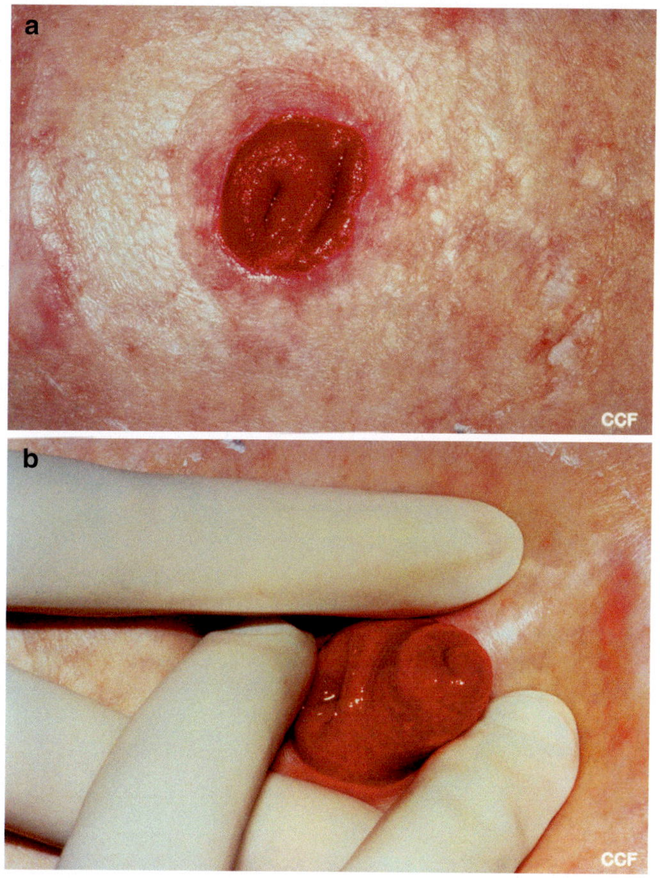

Fig. 14.62 Flush stoma (**a**), everted with pressure (**b**)

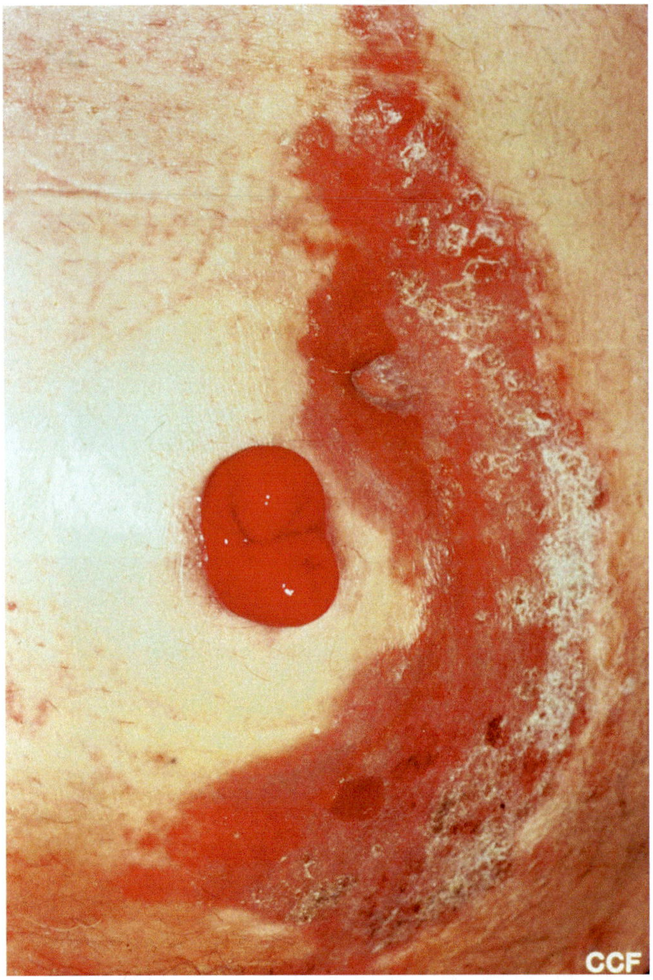

Fig. 14.63 Psoriasis

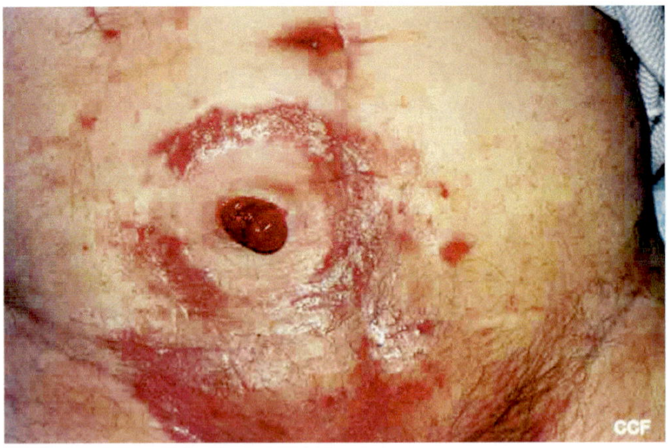

Fig. 14.64 Candidiasis

Fig. 14.66 (**a**) Parastomal necrotizing fasciitis. (**b**) Necrotizing fasciitis debridement to viable tissue. (**c**) Parastomal necrotizing fasciitis. Split-thickness skin graft needed

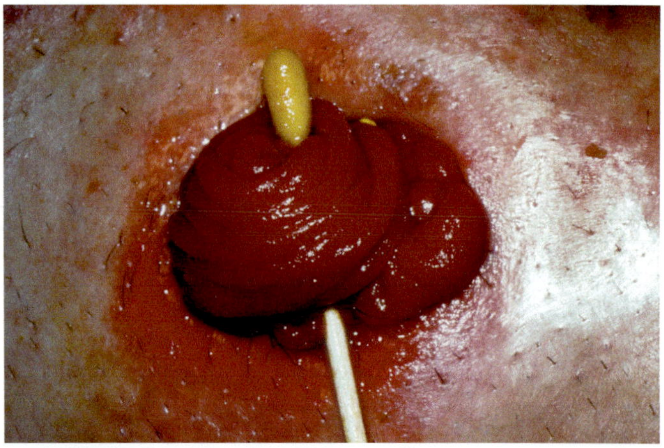

Fig. 14.65 Ileostomy fistula

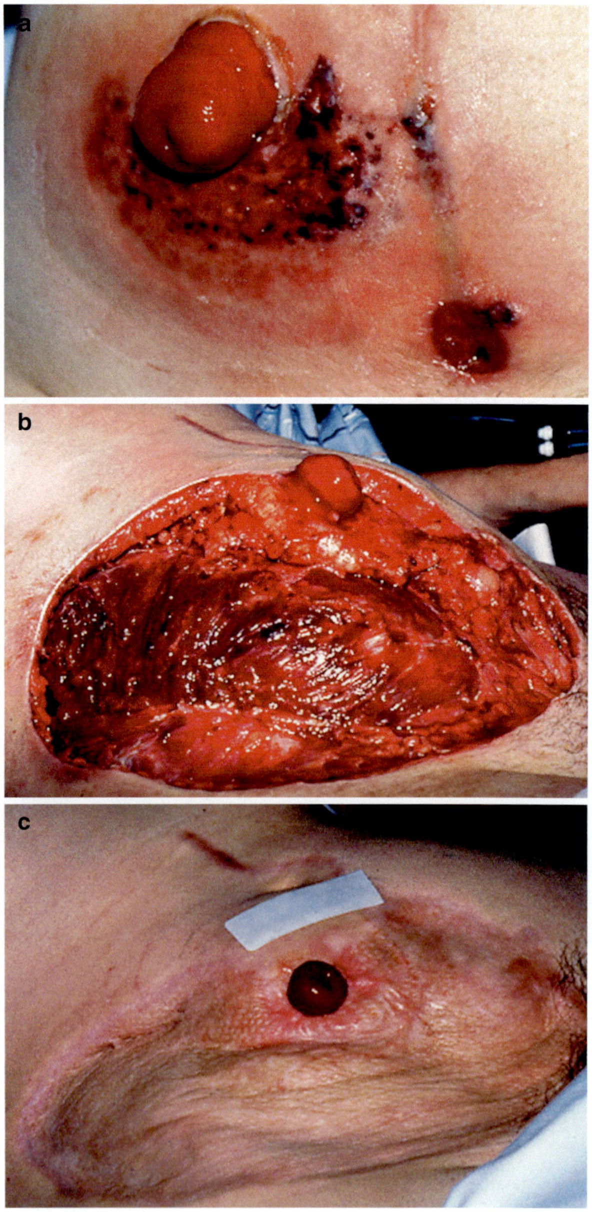

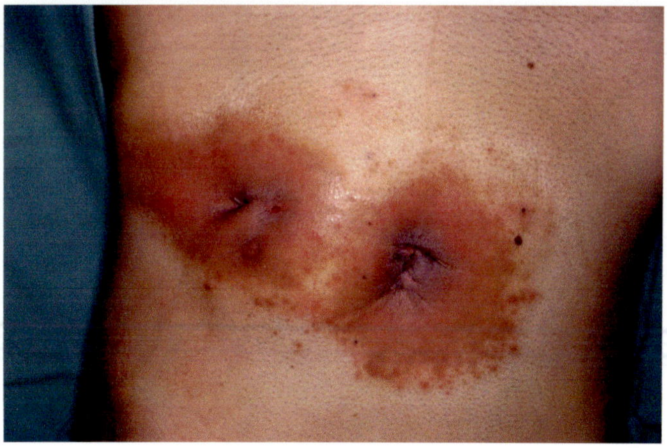

Fig. 14.67 Enterocutaneous fistula

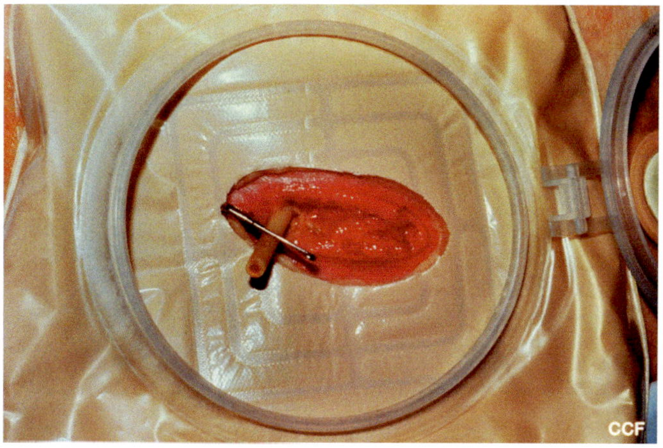

Fig. 14.68 Enterocutaneous fistula managed using pouch with window

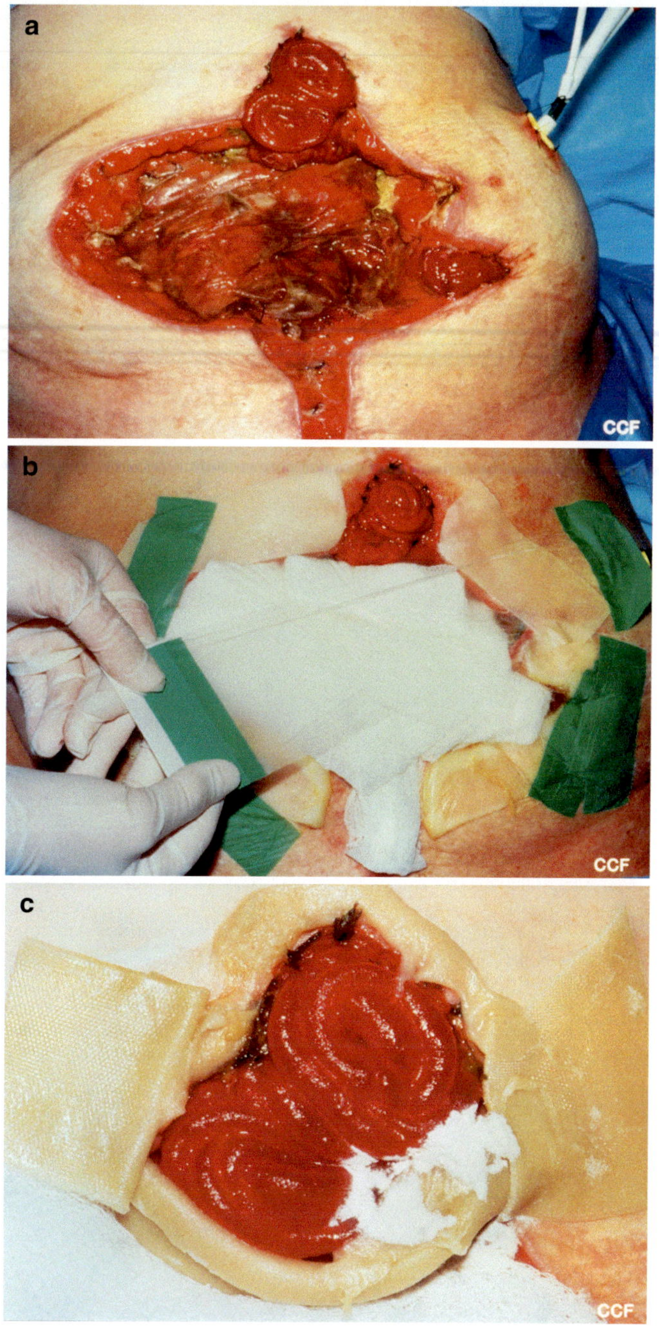

Fig. 14.69 (**a**) Loop ileostomy and wound dehiscence. (**b**) Open wound packed with saline gauze dressing and covered with clear adhesive film dressing. (**c**) Loop ileostomy surrounded with pectin paste, powder, and wedges before pouch is applied

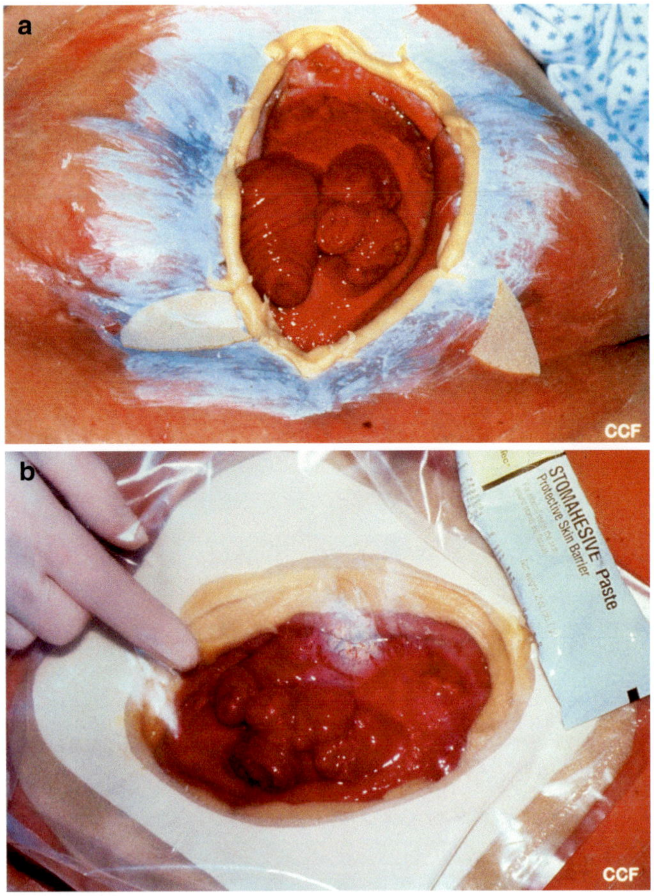

Fig. 14.70 (**a**) Enterocutaneous fistula: setting the stage for pouching with cement, pectin paste, and wafer wedges. (**b**) Enterocutaneous fistula: custom-fitted fistula appliance

Acknowledgements Stoma images courtesy of Dr. Rupert B. Turnbull, Jr., M.D.; Frank L. Weakley, M.D.; Victor W. Fazio, M.D.; Paula Erwin-Toth, RN; James M. Church, M.D.; and James S. Wu, M.D.

Stomas Via Percutaneous Endoscopy

15

Michelle D. Inkster and John J. Vargo II

I cannot see why the indications should not be as great to open the intestinal canal to put nourishment in, as to open it to take a foreign body out.

– Egeberg (a Norwegian Army surgeon) 1837 [1]

Introduction

Although nutritional assessment has been an important part of surgical training for many years, discussion about enteral feeding was not included in the first edition of this atlas, which was devoted to elegant descriptions of the surgical placement of stomas. The delivery of nutrition was changed dramatically in 1979 with the introduction of endoscopic methods of enteral tube placement by Gauderer and colleagues [2]. The concept, however, of creating a fistula into the stomach to feed patients enterally was first proposed by Egeberg in 1837 [3]. In the gut, protein malnutrition causes gastric and intestinal mucosal atrophy, decrease in villus height and crypt depth, changes in water and electrolyte balance, and changes in the production of fat-soluble vitamins [4]. Delivery of nutrients to the gastrointestinal tract does not provide any benefit unless there is going to be adequate absorption, therefore the decision to place a feeding tube must be based on whether this intervention will actually benefit the patient.

Enteral nutrients provide improved motility – the nutrients in a meal determine the motility response that dictates efficacy of digestion and absorption [5], improved blood flow in the superior mesenteric artery [6], decreased permeability, and increased immunoglobulin A (IgA) secretion [7], decreased bacterial translocation [8], improved mucosal immunity and an improved mucous layer [9, 10]. All of these help to maintain the integrity of the gastrointestinal tract. With enteral feeding, wound healing is improved in burn patients [11, 12]. In patients with renal failure, enteral nutrition is the preferred route for nutritional support [13]. Finally, patients who are malnourished and who receive enteral feeding recover more quickly from surgery. For example, De Gennaro reported that, for patients with colorectal cancer, when the albumin level was less than 2.8 g/dL the postoperative complication rate rose to 70% with a mortality rate of 4% [14]. Many critically ill patients, however, are either too ill or have too short a life expectancy to institute enteral feeding. For patients who have adequate nutritional status there is no difference in outcome whether or not they receive enteral nutrition [15].

The development of nutritional concepts and devices that can deliver that nutrition started many years ago. The first enteral feedings have been attributed to Herodotus Euterpe in ancient Egypt [16]. He noted that the Egyptians, next to the Libyans, were the healthiest people in the world: "for three successive days each month they purge the body by means of emetics and clysters." Hippocrates is also credited with enteral feeding; in his treatise "On Ancient Medicine" he expounds on different diets for different situations so that those who are ill will suffer less because of the wrong diet [17]. US President Garfield, on the other hand, was given nutrient enemas every 4 h for 79 days before his death [18]. This added nutrition did not prevent him from dying from wound contamination.

The development of feeding tubes could be thought to have started with the Romans who would induce vomiting during and after a banquet in order to make room for more food and also to settle the stomach. Feathers and fingers were used with good effect [19]. Tubes for feeding into the stomach developed from bougies or sounds that were used for blind extraction of foreign bodies. These tubes were designed to clasp fish bones and extract them and were made from

M.D. Inkster (✉)
Digestive Disease Institute, Cleveland Clinic Foundation, Cleveland, OH, USA
e-mail: inkstem@ccf.org

J.J. Vargo II
Department of Gastroenterology and Hepatology, Digestive Disease Institute, Cleveland Clinic Foundation, Cleveland, OH, USA

V.W. Fazio et al. (eds.), *Atlas of Intestinal Stomas*,
DOI 10.1007/978-0-387-78851-7_15,

perforated metallic tubes [20], whale bone, lead, and silver [21]. When the patient could not swallow, Capivaceus and Fabricious ab Aquapendente tried to find solutions to this problem. In 1568, Capivaceus [22] utilized a tube that was introduced through the mouth into the esophagus. The upper end was attached to an animal bladder into which the nutrient fluid was inserted prior to expression [23, 24]. In 1617, Aquapendente devised a thin silver tube that he threaded through the nostril to feed patients who had tetanus [25]. In 1790, John Hunter, the famous surgeon, is reported to have given one of the first orogastric feeds by using a syringe with a hollow or flexible tube made by a watchmaker of whale bone and eel skin and that was long enough to extend into the stomach so that the lungs would not be affected in persons who had drowned [25]. Later he proposed that a feeding tube could be passed into the stomach for patients who had suffered a stroke and who were unable to swallow [26].

It is generally agreed that the first gastroscope was designed and used by Kussmaul in 1868. It was rigid and stated to be "one of the most lethal instruments in the surgeon's kit." The first fiber-optic gastroscope was designed by Heinrich Lamm in 1930, but his work languished during the Second World War [27]. Visual acuity remained a significant problem even though the endoscope was now more flexible. Van Heel was asked by the Dutch government to work on periscopes for submarines in the 1940s and realized that light leaked between the bare fibers when they touched each other. He solved the problem of poor image resolution by coating the fibers with plastic. He was then able to transmit images through a 400 fiber bundle up to a distance of half a meter [27]. Basil Hirschowitz, a South African gastroenterologist, then at the University of Michigan, used this concept to "evaluate peering into the body" [27]. Techniques for delivering nutrition into the stomach were greatly advanced from early attempts when, in 1937, an interpretable photograph was taken with an external camera and, in cooperation with the Eastman Kodak Company, a better light source was developed that allowed increased light to operate in conjunction with the camera shutter [28]. Further development of fiber-optic endoscopes not only allowed visualization of the stomach but also possibilities for advances in therapy, as the endoscopist could now see into not only the stomach but also the duodenum [29].

Successful surgical gastrostomy tube placement was first performed by Verneuil in France in 1876 [30]. For many years though, the enteral feeding method of choice was a Stamm Gastrostomy tube, which was introduced in 1894 [31]. This surgical technique requires an incision through the abdominal wall as far away from the pylorus as possible, lifting the stomach up past the omentum and using two purse-string sutures to anchor it to the abdominal wall. Leaking and hemorrhage if the sutures are not tight enough are major potential complications. This technique has persisted since its introduction with only slight modification to allow for jejunostomy. It was not until 1980 that the feeding tubes that are now widely used were unveiled by Gauderer, Ponsky, and Izant who had all been working in children's hospitals and who had devised a method to insert a feeding tube into the pediatric stomach using endoscopy [32]. This procedure was a safe way to introduce nutrition for children who had brain damage and who had severe musculoskeletal deformities. The concept was simple and possible because of the development of fiber-optic endoscopes, an appropriate light source, and advances in the design and availability of equipment that was now readily available in any operating room. This technique has had some modifications since its introduction, but the principles remain the same whether the tube is placed in the stomach or the jejunum.

General Indications for a Feeding Tube

Delivery of nutrients can be via gastrostomy, cervical pharyngostomy, duodenostomy, and jejunostomy. The route chosen depends on whether there will be a need for short-term or long-term access. Then the decision must be made as to whether there are any contraindications to placement of a feeding tube. Mechanical obstruction and dysmotility, for example, can preclude using the gastrointestinal tract. During times of critical illness, there is often a decrease in gastric emptying and colonic motility but early use of the gastrointestinal tract can prevent dysmotility [5]. There is limited long-term application for a tube that passes through the esophagogastric junction as it can lead to aspiration with a mechanically induced laxness of the lower esophageal sphincter. Cervical pharyngotomy has limited usefulness as well. Patients can be unwilling to have the latter placed because they are not cosmetically acceptable, although there are indications for this technique for selected patients.

Gastrostomy tubes are indicated when patients cannot maintain adequate nutrition with oral intake and where there is an expectation that the patient will survive to achieve long-term clinical benefit from the intervention [33]. For example, patients with head and neck cancer are candidates for long-term nutritional support, especially when surgery is expected to be extensive and chemotherapy and radiation therapy are planned. Benefits include improved tolerance compared with nasogastric tubes, ease of use, patient and caregiver satisfaction, reduction in aspiration pneumonia, and cost-effectiveness. Gastrostomy tubes are also placed for long-term decompression, for example, when the patient has a mechanical obstruction due to a malignancy or intractable gastroparesis. The percutaneous endoscopic gastrostomy (PEG) tube is placed to suction and can improve the quality of life for the patient. Because a chronic nasogastric tube does not need to be placed, care of the patient is also simplified.

Table 15.1 Indications and contraindications for a feeding tube

Indications	Contraindications
Amyotrophic lateral sclerosis	*Absolute*
Burns	Coagulopathy
Crohn's disease	Intestinal dysmotility
Decompression	Marked hepatomegaly
Delivery of medication	Portal hypertension
Hypoxic encephalopathy	Sepsis
Long-term enteral feeding	*Relative*
Macroglossia secondary to amyloidosis	Ascites
Respiratory failure	Esophageal obstruction
Tracheoesophageal fistula	Intestinal obstruction (feeding)
	Morbid obesity
	Peritoneal dialysis
	Peritoneal metastases
	Previous gastrectomy

Comorbid conditions may delay placement of a percutaneous endoscopic gastrostomy (PEG) or percutaneous endoscopic jejunostomy (PEJ) tube. For example, severe malnutrition where the albumin level is below 2.8 g/dL may lead to failure of the site to heal and wound infection may occur [34]. The presence of severe gastric ulceration may lead to significant bleeding after the procedure. Appropriate patient selection is part of the preoperative evaluation and is an important part of the process (see Table 15.1).

Indications for a Jejunostomy Tube

For individuals in whom there is significant risk of regurgitation of stomach contents into the cervical esophagus or ineffective gastric emptying or gastroparesis, jejunostomy tube placement may be a good alternative. Jejunostomy tubes were initially placed surgically, requiring laparotomy and general anesthesia. Shike described direct PEJ placement in 1987 in patients who had undergone gastrectomy [35]. Mellert in Germany described direct PEJ in 39 patients in 1994 who had undergone either partial or total gastrectomy for cancer, esophageal perforation, severe trauma, or who had esophageal fistulae [36]. His group showed that endoscopic placement was not only feasible but also exposed the patient to less procedural risk.

Techniques

PEG Tube Placement

There are two techniques that are commonly used for PEG tube placement: the "push" technique of Ponksy [37] and the "pull" technique of Sacks-Vine [38]. The patient's abdomen must first be examined to evaluate for an appropriate area for the gastrostomy site. Extensive scars from prior surgery may make it difficult to place the tube in the best site within the stomach. Feeding is usually withheld for 8 h prior to the procedure to ensure an empty stomach. A prophylactic antibiotic that will cover gram-negative organisms is given intravenously just before the procedure.

The patient is placed in reverse Trendelenburg position at about 45°: this allows the stomach to be in a dependent position within the abdomen. One operator is at the head of the patient to perform the gastroscopy while the second performs the actual tube placement. An esophagogastroduodenoscopy (EGD) is performed and the best site for tube placement is selected by the second operator palpating the abdomen with gentle pressure while the first operator illuminates the stomach with the gastroscope (Fig. 15.1). The stomach is fully insufflated to appose the stomach with the anterior abdominal wall. The safety of the site is verified [39, 40] by using the safetrack technique. The abdomen is draped and prepared in the usual sterile fashion. A syringe containing several milliliters of local anesthesia is introduced just beyond the skin at the selected point. Under constant view by the endoscopist, the needle of the syringe is advanced while negative pressure is maintained within the syringe. The endoscopist should see the end of the needle enter the lumen at the same time as his/her partner sees air bubbles in the barrel of the syringe. If air bubbles are seen before the needle enters the stomach, the needle has passed through another air-containing structure such as the colon or small bowel. In this event, the needle is withdrawn and another site is selected.

Once the correct site has been identified and confirmed, the skin is infiltrated with local anesthetic. A transverse incision is made through the abdominal wall. The introducer needle is pushed through the incision into the gastric cavity (Fig. 15.2) and a guidewire is threaded through the needle, grasped with the endoscopic snare, and pulled out through the patient's mouth. The PEG tube is looped through the thread – "blue through," lubricated well, and the PEG tube is pulled back through the patient's mouth into the stomach. The tube is then pulled out through the skin incision by the second operator (Fig. 15.3) until the button is snug against the gastric wall. It is anchored on the outside with a bumper (Fig. 15.4). The mushroom button decreases the likelihood of tube migration and keeps gastric contents from leaking onto the skin because of the antireflux valve [41].

The stomach and small bowel should not be overdistended, as overfilling of the stomach and small bowel may "lift" the transverse colon and increase the probability of colon injury [42]. Colonic injury usually presents with peritonitis. Gastrocolic fistula results from interposition of the colon between the anterior abdominal wall and the stomach. Patients are often asymptomatic except for transient fever or ileus. The problem is usually discovered months after PEG

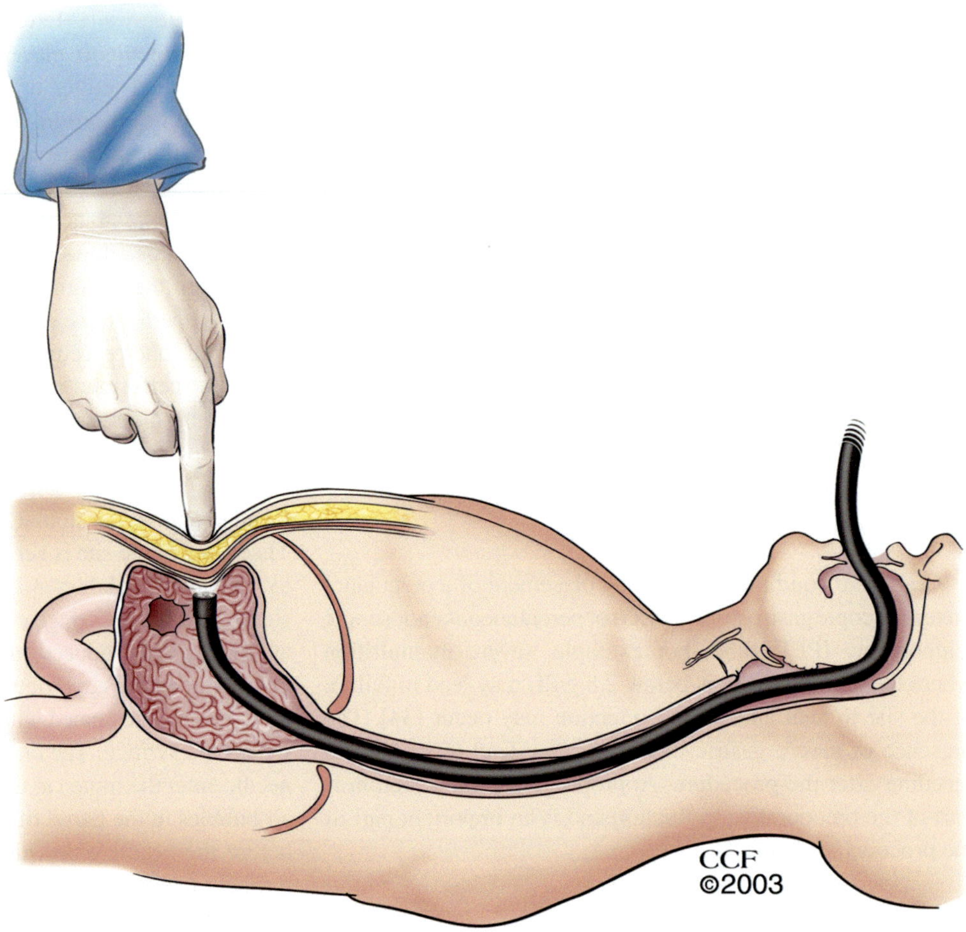

Fig. 15.1 The first operator illuminates the gastric wall from the inside with the endoscope. The second operator places a finger on the outside of the abdomen and palpates gently to produce a bulge in the stomach wall that is visible on the inside. Illustration © CCF

tube placement when the original tube is removed or manipulated [43]. Extensive tension of the external bolster against the abdominal skin should be avoided to prevent buried bumper syndrome (see Fig. 15.5f) [44]. Epithelialization can cover the internal stoma with gastric mucosa and result in complete closing of the orifice. Fatal cases have been reported. A buried bumper should be removed even if the patient is asymptomatic because of the risks of tube impaction in the abdominal wall and gastric perforation. The PEG tube should not migrate if the external bumper is properly positioned. The PEG tube can be dislodged into the pylorus and cause gastric outlet dysfunction. If the PEG tube is a Foley catheter type, deflating the balloon and withdrawing the tube should provide relief.

In obese patients, placement of a PEG feeding tube is often considered impossible because of an inability to transilluminate the abdominal wall. Inadvertent puncture of the transverse colon, or even puncture of the left lobe of the liver, can occur. Kirby [45], however, was able to place PEG tubes endoscopically in obese patients with a body mass index up to 63 kg/m^2. Gastrostomy tubes were placed successfully in 130 of 134 obese patients with a 0% procedure-related mortality. Of 355 patients evaluated, 14 did not receive a PEG tube. Four procedures were aborted because of paucity of anatomical landmarks and failure to illuminate the abdominal wall.

Peristomal infections are the most common complications of PEG tube placement; although in patients who are compromised neurologically, aspiration pneumonia is more common [46]. Because systemic infections can occur and are often underinvestigated, antibiotics are given prior to the procedure. One gram of cefazolin administered intravenously prior to the procedure reduces the rate of infection, although the reduction is variable depending on the study reported. Pneumoperitoneum is common after placement of a PEG tube and can persist for several weeks [47]. This is a benign condition but can result in diagnosis of a perforated viscus when those involved are unaware of this association. See Table 15.2 and Fig. 15.5a–g for common complications of PEG tube placement.

Pharyngostomy

Klopp described cervical pharyngostomy in 1951 in a patient who had cancer of the cervical esophagus with complete obstruction [48]. The tube was placed through an open neck

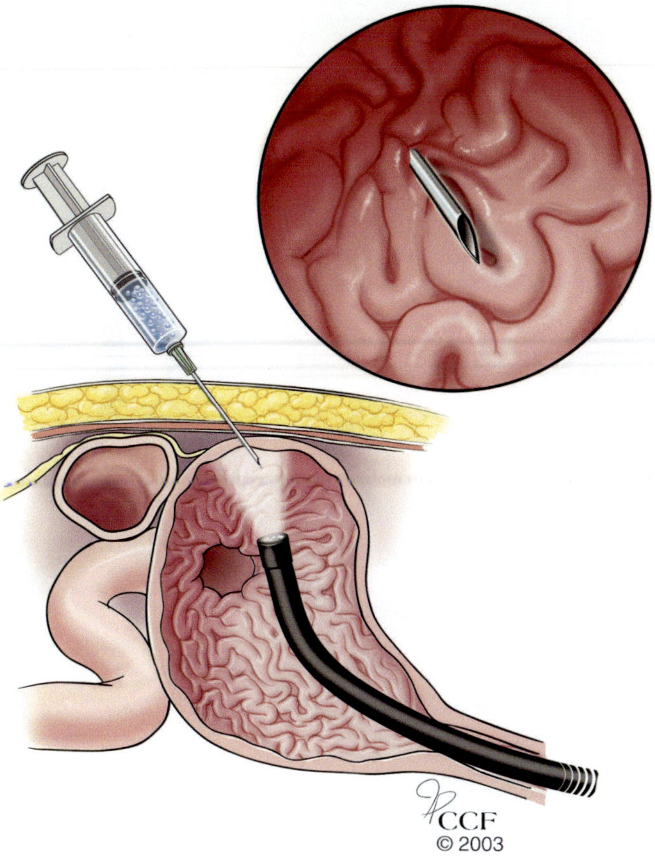

Fig. 15.2 The SafeTack technique is used to place the finder needle. The second operator inserts a syringe containing fluid through the abdominal wall from the outside. Traction is applied to the syringe. Bubbles should be observed by the second operator at the same time that the first operator sees the needle enter the stomach. If bubbles are noted before this, the needle is withdrawn and a new site selected as the needle may have entered the colon. Illustration © CCF

dissection procedure and was used successfully for many years in a simplified fashion for patients with neurologic disease and those with extensive facial trauma. Bucklin and Gilsdorf developed a feeding pharyngostomy tube that could be performed at the bedside with the patient awake [49]. The main indication for this approach was for patients who constantly removed nasogastric tubes or who had aphagopraxia (Table 15.3). It is a technique that can be used successfully for head and neck patients who require prolonged tube feeding. This type of tube is also appropriate for patients with advanced intra-abdominal malignancy who would benefit from palliative decompression but who are not candidates for conventional PEG tube placement [50, 51]. This technique was used at the Cleveland Clinic by Mackey and Ponsky and found to be safe and effective for decompression in malignant gastrointestinal obstruction [52].

The tube can be hidden under a high collar and the patients can care for this tube themselves at home by using a mirror to look at the site. It is better then using an NG tube as it avoids sinusitis and interference with speech or swallowing for this very select group of patients.

Direct Percutaneous Jejunostomy (DPEJ)

Direct percutaneous jejunostomy (DPEJ) is a modification of PEG placement. The original description of a PEG/PEJ was a one-piece apparatus that consisted of a gastrostomy tube and a smaller jejunostomy tube that was drawn through the pylorus into the duodenum (JET/PEG). This technique was complicated by the jejunostomy tube falling back into the stomach as the endoscope was withdrawn. It also did not prevent aspiration as the pylorus was made incompetent with the placement of the jejunostomy tube. The first PEJ tube was placed by Ponsky and Aszodi in 1984 [53]. Shike (1987) later placed PEJ tubes in cancer patients with prior gastric resection [54].

DPEJ tubes should be placed beyond the ligament of Treitz, or at least in the third or fourth portion of the duodenum. These tubes may be more difficult to replace if dislodged and they may need more nursing care. PEJ tubes that are anchored by balloon are more likely to have long-term problems with balloon rupture and difficulty with replacement of the balloon. Mushroom catheter placement is preferred. Jejunostomy tubes may be placed over a wire or a pediatric endoscope may be used instead of a gastroscope. The lumen of the jejunum is much smaller than the lumen of the stomach so that placement has to be more precise. The most important part of the procedure is using the impression made by a finger applying pressure to the abdomen from the outside to mark the point of insertion of the PEJ tube because the light from a forward viewing endoscope places the point of insertion a little further forward than the actual end of the instrument. Using the light as a reference point can therefore result in placement of the tube in a nonoptimal position. Peristalsis can also change the location of the loop in relation to the abdominal wall. It is therefore important to ascertain the appropriate puncture point very close to the time of actual puncture of the skin [55].

A safetrack is verified by using a 19–21 gauge needle. The needle is secured with an endoscopic snare to stabilize the segment of jejunum. The larger trochar needle can then be inserted adjacent to the finder needle. It is important to maintain fixation of the finder needle so that the jejunum does not fall away from the abdominal wall. After the stylet is removed from the trochar, a guidewire is inserted and the procedure completed as for a standard pull-type PEG. It is not known what length of time is required for this track to mature. It is prudent to allow 6 weeks before removing the DPEJ and perhaps longer in malnourished patients. Feeding can begin within 24 h.

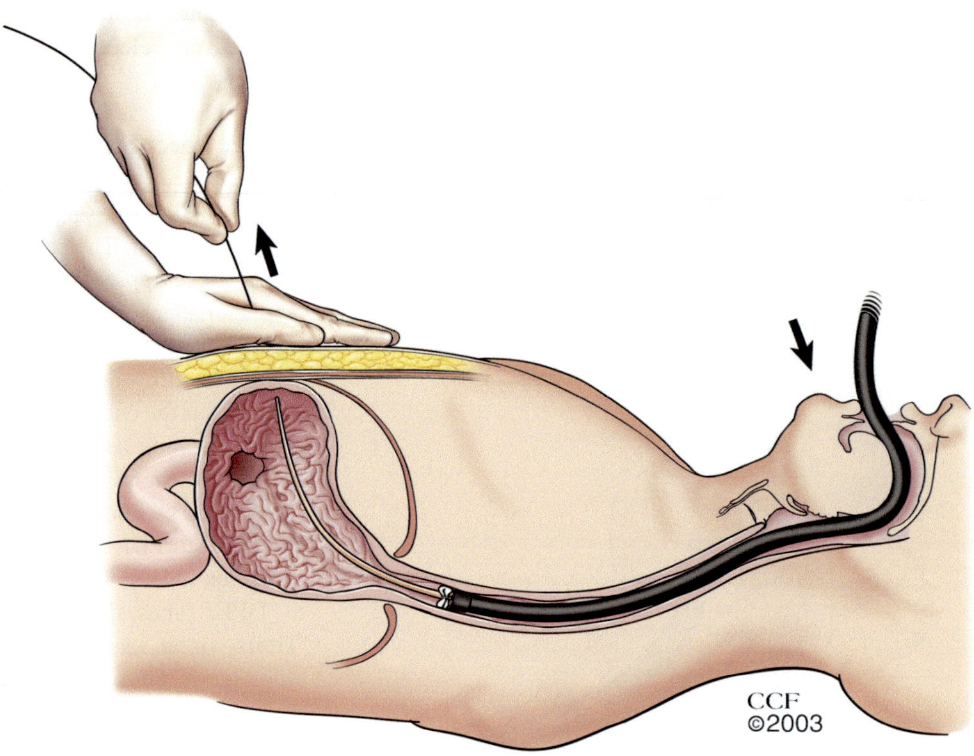

Fig. 15.3 The endoscope has been removed from the stomach, the snare has been pulled through the patient's mouth, and the PEG tube has been attached. The endoscope is then reinserted into the stomach, and force applied to pull the snare attached to the bumper through the abdominal wall. Illustration © CCF

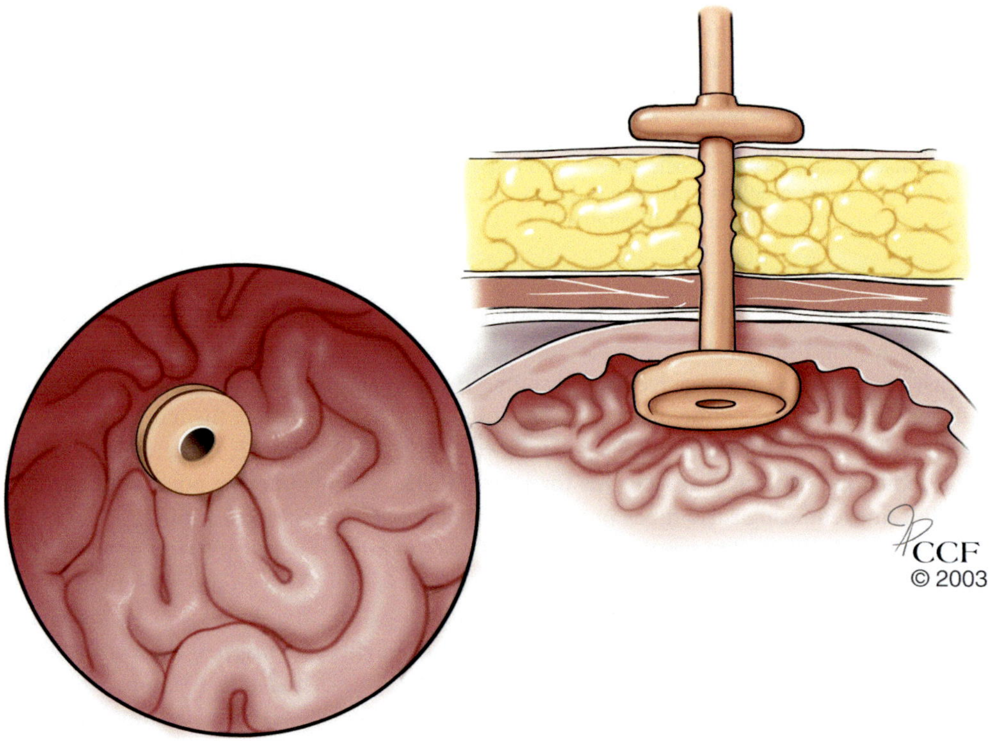

Fig. 15.4 The mushroom catheter in place on the inside of the stomach while the external bumper is placed loosely against the abdominal wall. The external bumper will be adjusted the day after the procedure. Illustration © CCF

The question of successful PEG placement in obese patients was addressed by Kirby as detailed previously. The question of successful DPEJ placement in obese patients was addressed by Mackenzie and colleagues [56] who found that, of 80 DPEJ placed in 75 patients, DPEJ placement was feasible whether the patients were obese or not but that adverse events were more common in patients with a body mass index (BMI) greater than 25. These were jejunal

Table 15.2 Complications of PEG tube placement

Major	Minor
Aspiration pneumonia	External leakage
Buried bumper syndrome	Peristomal infection
Dehiscence of the wound	Tube blockage
Gastrocolic fistula	Tube dislodgement
Gastric perforation	
Perforation of the transverse colon	
Peritonitis	
Seeding of the abdominal skin with metastases	
Subcutaneous abscess	

obstruction, jejunal volvulus, necrotizing fasciitis/death, and sepsis in a total of five patients. Success rate was 96% for underweight, 81% for normal weight, and 73% for overweight patients. Maple used computed tomography (CT) scans to try to predict the success of DPEJ placement [57]. There was poor sensitivity and specificity in this study, but an abdominal wall thickness of greater that 3 cm was associated with a greater likelihood of placement failure. See Table 15.4 for common complications of DPEJ placement and Fig. 15.5a–g.

Radiological Placement of Gastrostomy Tubes

When a feeding tube cannot be placed by an endoscopist, the procedure may be deferred to a radiologist. One method that has been used by radiologists is to place an NG tube the night before the procedure and to administer a dilute barium solution into the gut so that on the day of the procedure the contrast should be in the colon and the operator can avoid puncturing the colon. The NG tube is then placed to suction 2–3 h prior to the procedure. Fluoroscopy is used to evaluate the abdomen before selecting a skin site. Glucagon may be given to decrease gastric peristalsis and emptying. Air is then insufflated through the nasogastric tube and distention monitored by fluoroscopy. In selecting an appropriate puncture site, some radiologists also use ultrasound examination of the abdomen so that the liver can be visualized as well as the superior epigastric artery, thereby minimizing the risk of bleeding. When the initial catheter is placed, a peel-away sheath is often necessary. The feeding tube is pushed through the abdominal wall into the stomach and secured after the location in the lumen of the stomach has been confirmed. The use of gastropexy anchors may or may not be used; both methods have been described. Proper tube placement can be confirmed with water-soluble contrast injection if desired. Placement of direct gastrostomy tubes is technically less difficult than placement of direct jejunostomy tubes. Because there can be more complications with primary DPEJ placement, some radiologists will only replace them [58].

Percutaneous Cecostomy (PEC) and Percutaneous Sigmoid Colostomy

Tube cecostomy had been used successfully in the 1960s for patients who had colorectal cancer and in emergencies such as post-traumatic fractures or for patients with ileus [59]. In 1985, Ponksy introduced the percutaneous cecostomy (PEC) for colonic decompression for two patients who had Ogilve's syndrome [60]. The mushroom catheter was placed in the cecum with immediate decompression. The first patient died a week later from progressive respiratory and renal failure but the second patient was discharged a week later without surgical intervention and with resolution of his sepsis. More recently, Holm and Baron used cecostomy tubes for palliation for patients who had decreased colonic transit time secondary to narcotic use, tumor obstruction, or progressive neuromuscular disease [61]. PEC tubes are not used to meet nutritional needs in adults, rather they are used for decompression and to prevent pain from abdominal bloating, antegrade washout for chronic constipation, and to alleviate obstruction for patients with neoplasms.

In 1996, Chait in Canada published his series of PEC tubes in children [62]. Between June 1995 and September 1996 he placed 42 PEC tubes in children who had fecal incontinence and troublesome soiling, unresponsiveness to rectal enemas, requirement for diapers, and anorectal malformations. Twenty-nine patients had spina bifida, nine had imperforate anus, three had cloacal anomalies, and one had Hirschprung's disease. Ten patients were ambulatory and the rest used wheelchairs. The development of the Trapdoor device (Cook Medical, Bloomington, Indiana) allowed all patients to have a low-profile device, irrespective of their size or weight. These are now known as the Chait Trapdoor™ Cecostomy Catheters and are used for antegrade irrigation of the bowel. They appear to be a standard of care both in Canada and in the United Kingdom. For indications and contraindications for this procedure in children see Table 15.5 and in adults, Table 15.6. Common complications are detailed in Table 15.7.

Technique

Placement of the Chait Trapdoor Cecostomy™ tube is a two-step procedure. These patients are given a bowel preparation, if possible, via nasogastric tube until rectal drainage is clear. Fluoroscopy is used for visualization and glucagon is used to paralyze the bowel. A balloon catheter is placed into the rectum and air instilled until the cecum is sufficiently insufflated. Then the rectal balloon is inflated to keep the balloon in place and to keep the air in the colon. Insufflation is monitored by ultrasound. A temporary loop retention drainage catheter (for example, a Dawson-Mueller drainage catheter)

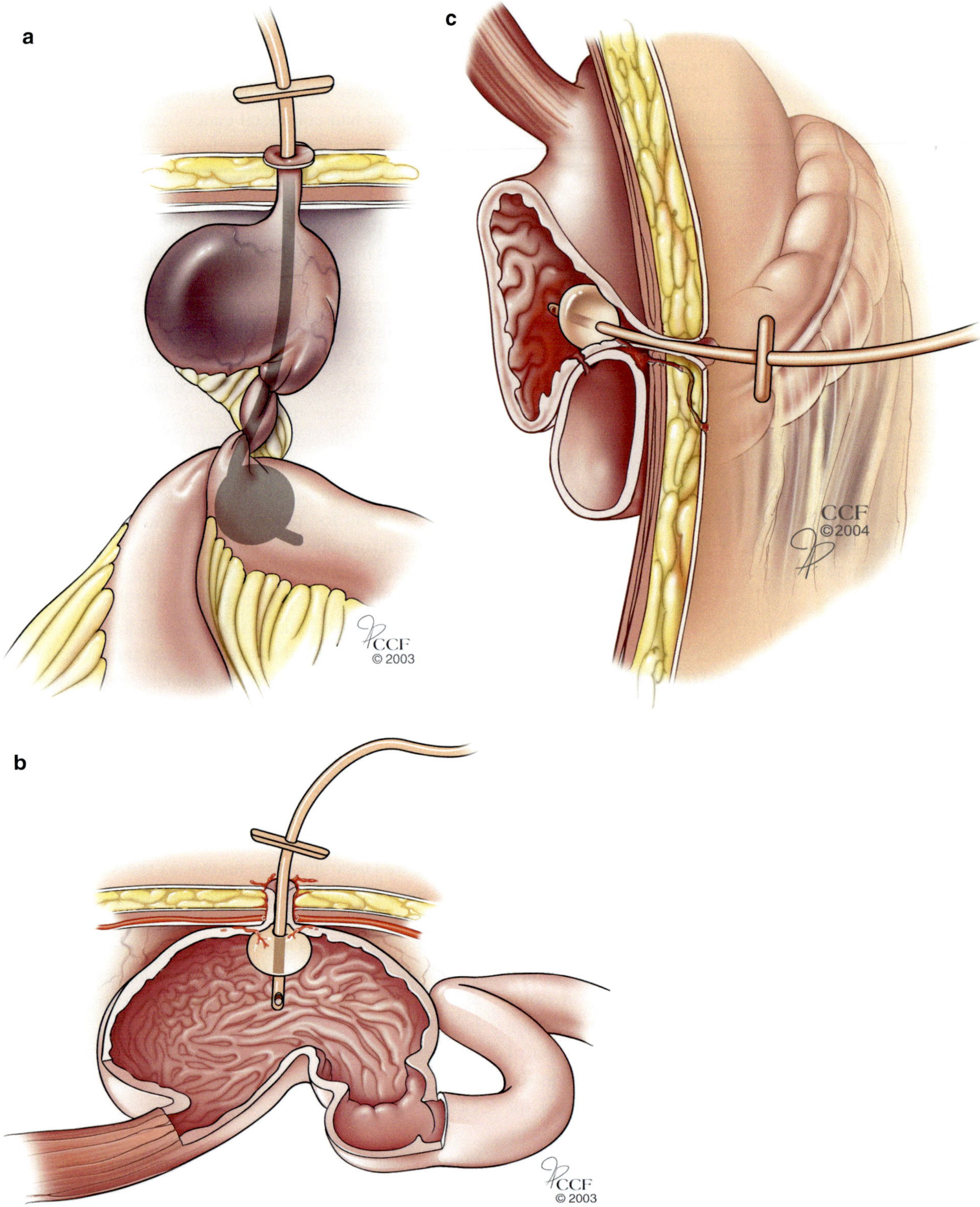

Fig. 15.5 Complications that can occur with placement of PEG and DPEJ tubes. (**a**) Torsion of the stomach around the insertion site. (**b**) Leakage around the insertion site. (**c**) Gastrocolic fistula. (**d**) Migration of the tube within the stomach and insertion into the opposing wall. A balloon catheter was used and an external bumper was not used. (**e**) Migration of the tube within the stomach so that it is coiled and not flush with the abdominal wall. (**f**) Buried bumper syndrome. (**g**) Intussusception of the catheter within the small bowel lumen. Illustrations © CCF

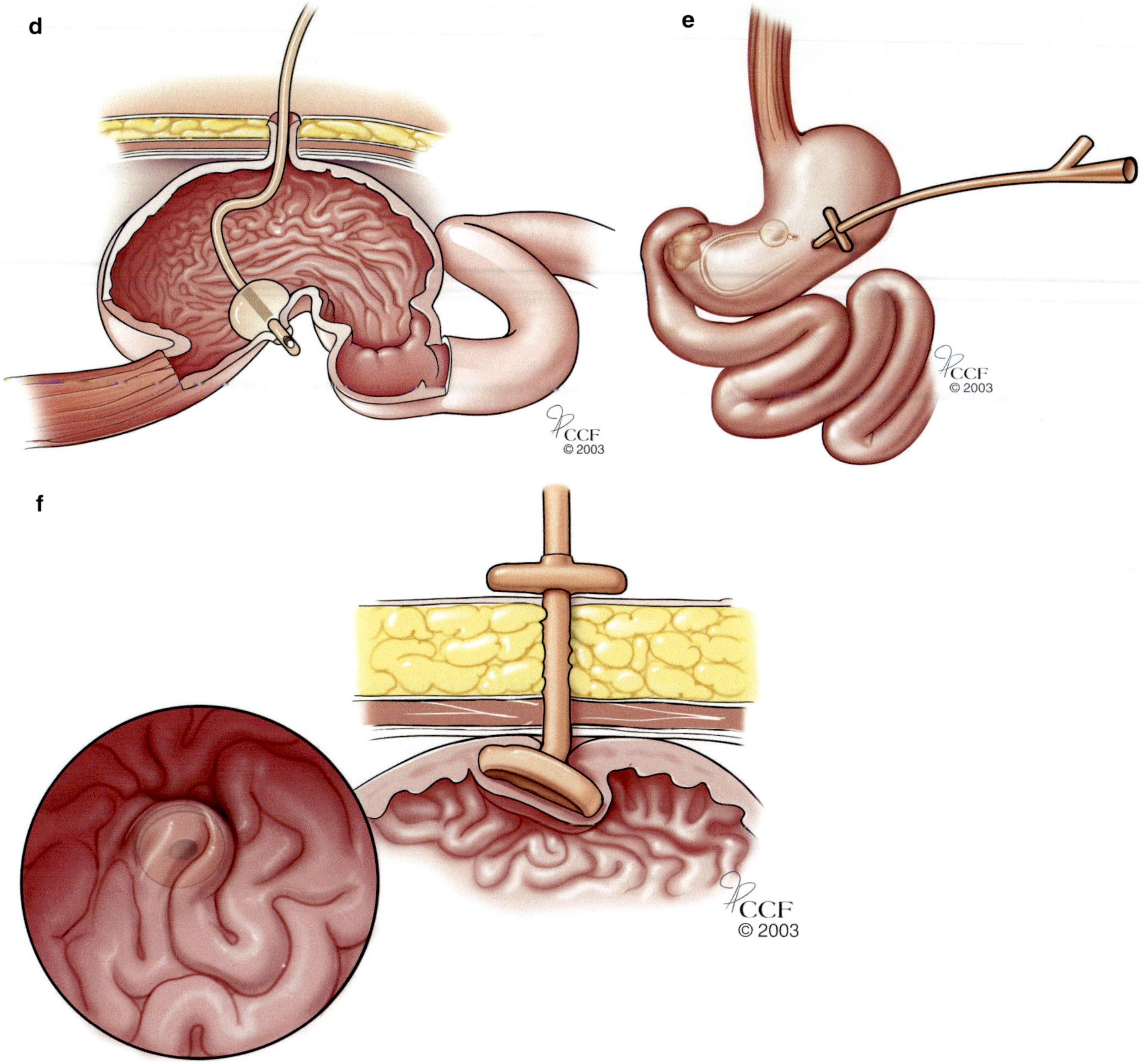

Fig. 15.5 (continued)

g

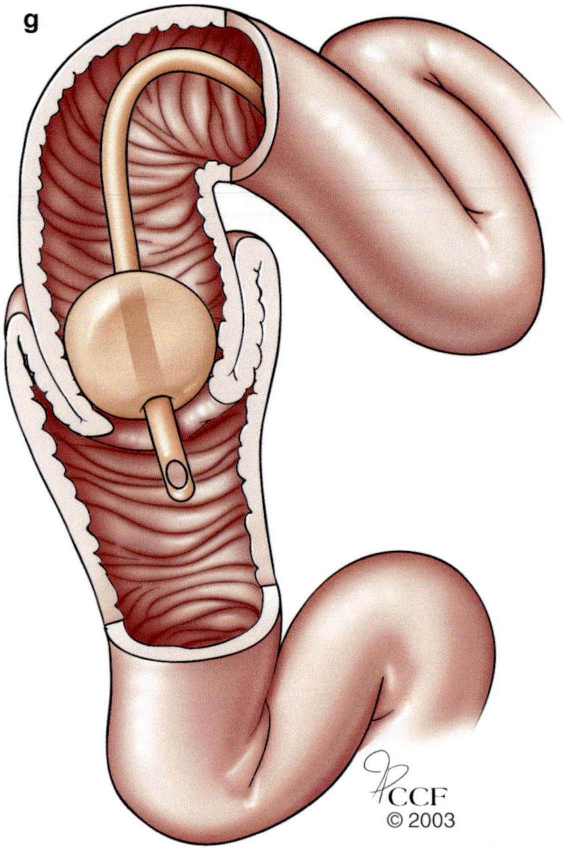

Fig. 15.5 (continued)

Table 15.3 Complications of pharyngostomy tube placement

Accidental removal
Exuberant granulation tissue around the exit wound
Hemorrhage
Hyperemia around the stoma
Kinking of the tube
Persistent cervical fistula

Table 15.4 Complications of DPEJ placement

Abdominal cramping
Abdominal distention
Constipation
Displacement of the tube
Focally thickened jejunal folds
Jejunal hematomas
Jejunal volvulus
Migration of the tube
Nausea
Occlusion of the tube
Retrograde flow of feeding material
Small bowel intussusceptions
Small bowel obstruction

Table 15.5 Indications and contraindications for pediatric cecostomy tube placement

Indications	Contraindications
Cloacal anomalies	Previous abdominal surgical procedures
Imperforate anus	Coagulopathies
Klippell Fell Syndrome	Known medical problems that put them at risk
Myelomeningocele	
Paraplegia	
Sacral agenesis	
Spina bifida	

Table 15.6 Indications for adults for percutaneous cecostomy [60]

I. Antegrade irrigation
II. Decompression
A. Malignant colonic obstruction
Colon cancer
Pelvic malignancies
B. Benign colonic obstruction
Colonic pseudo-obstruction (Ogilvie syndrome)
Neurogenic bowel
C. Fecal incontinence

Table 15.7 Complications of percutaneous cecostomy

Peristomal infection
Peritonitis – leakage of fecal contents during placement of device
Granulation tissue around insertion site
Placement into the terminal ileum
Self-removal of catheter

is placed percutaneously into the cecum and the track allowed to mature. Suture anchors are recommended to assist the introduction of the temporary drainage catheter. The patient flushes the temporary catheter twice every day with 10 mL of water. This is continued for 1 week in conjunction with a normal rectal enema regimen. Then antegrade enemas can begin. After maturation (approximately 6 weeks) the temporary catheter is removed and the Chait Trapdoor catheter is placed (Fig. 15.6a–d). A metal stiffener is inserted into the catheter to straighten the coils and to push the catheter through the tract over a prepositioned wire guide. Once the catheter is inserted, the guide wire is removed until the Trapdoor is flush against the access site. The catheter coils reform in the cecum once the guidewire has been removed. Contrast injection is used to confirm placement and patency in the cecum. The patient inserts a metal cannula tip into the opening of the Trapdoor and administers a phosphate enema, followed 15 min later by a saline enema via gravity until drainage is clear – usual volume is 200–500 mL.

This technique is now an accepted method for the previously mentioned conditions in a number of countries. In the United Kingdom it is also approved for sigmoid colostomy

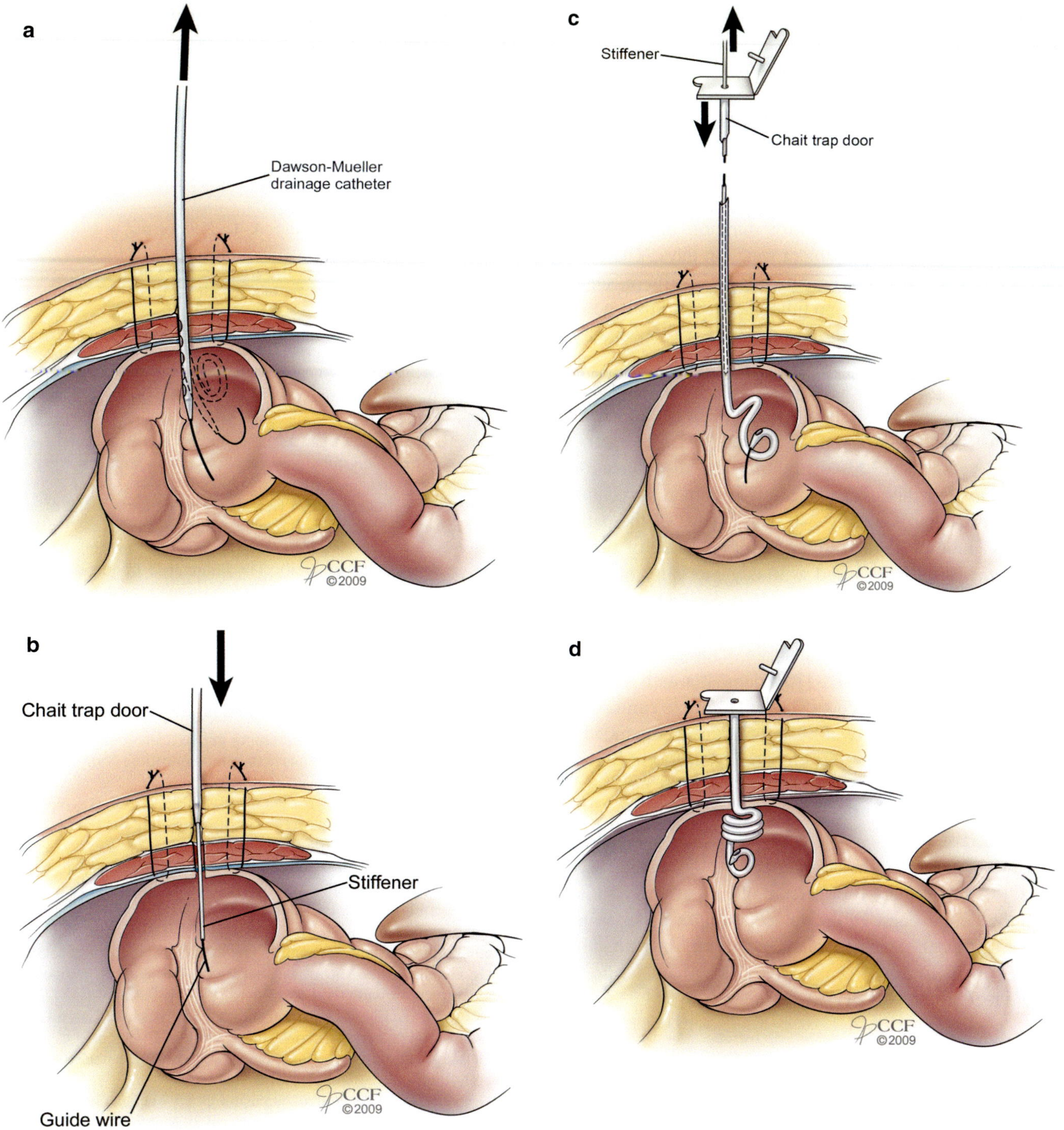

Fig. 15.6 Placement of the Chait Trapdoor Cecostomy tube™. (**a**) The Dawson Mueller tube in place in the cecum. (**b**) Placement of the Chait Trapdoor with a metal stiffener. (**c**) The stiffener has been removed allowing the distal end to coil in the cecum. (**d**) The Chait Trapdoor in place. Illustrations © CCF

in patients who have sigmoid volvulus, fecal impaction, constipation, incontinence, and for the delivery of anti-inflammatory agents for patients with colitis. Baraza confirmed the utility of this technique in adults with colonic pseudo-obstruction, and slow transit constipation [63]. Van den Berg in the United States, however, performed colonic manometry in children with defecation disorders prior to insertion and determined that, for patients without high amplitude propagating contractions, the placement of a cecostomy tube was less likely to be beneficial [64].

Outcomes

Anis reported that of 191 patients 76% would have a PEG tube placed again, 84% felt that feeding was easier, 63% that the tube was cosmetically acceptable, and 60% that the tube increased survival [65]. Data from the Scottish MND Register was evaluated for 142 patients who had PEG tubes placed between 1989 and 1998 [66]. Mean age at insertion was 66.8 years with a mean disease duration of 24 months. Median survival after placement was 146 days. The 30-day mortality was 25%. Placement did not confer a survival advantage compared with no tube placement, but it was felt that the unexpectedly high mortality rate was secondary to lack of selection bias.

Rabeneck published a study of long-term outcomes in 1996 in which 7,369 patients who received a PEG tube between 1990 and 1992 were evaluated [67]. The mean age was 68.1 years and 23.5% died during the hospitalization in which the PEG tube was placed. The median survival was 7.5 months (approximately 240 days). Most of the patients had PEG tube placement in the terminal phase of their illness. Other studies reported a 30-day mortality of 22% at 30 days [68], and 67% at 30 days [69]. Several studies have looked at poor prognostic factors for PEG placement. These include hypoalbuminemia (albumin <2.8 g/dL) in which 6-month mortality was 44% [70], dementia with a 6-month mortality of 81%, and in patients with multiple comorbid illness a 6-month mortality of 50% [65]. Kirby concluded that it is important to concentrate on patient selection and reducing complications [71]. The role of jejunostomy tube feeding in long-term enteral feeding has not yet been clearly established.

Outcomes for the Chait Trapdoor PEC tube are detailed in Refs. [62, 63]. Ninety-four percent of patients were satisfied with the effectiveness of the device, rating it better than the irrigation/bowel cleansing routine that they had previously used. Ninety-seven percent of the 124 patients said they would recommend the device to others.

Conclusion

Gauderer reflected on the development of endoscopic placement of gastrostomy tubes in 1999 [72]. His original intentions were to provide a technique to simplify catheter placement and he and his colleagues clearly accomplished that goal. There are now multiple kits available to insert these tubes and multiple indications for the use of the procedure. Most of the problems associated with actual tube placement are minor and can be treated fairly easily. The major complications, however, such as transverse colon through-and-through perforation can lead to death. Most of the patients are debilitated medically and malnourished and care must be exercised in selection of patients who undergo this procedure. The person who performs the procedure needs to critically assess each patient for suitability prior to performing the procedure.

References

1. Tam W, Schoeman M, Oliver I. To PEG or not to PEG? IMVS Newsl. 1999;37:12–3.
2. Gauderer MWL, Ponsky JL, Izant Jr RJ. Gastrostomy without laparotomy: a percutaneous endoscopic technique. J Pediatr Sur. 1980;15:872–5.
3. Chernoff R. History of tube feeding. An overview of tube feeding: from ancient time to the future. Nutr Clin Pract. 2006;21:408–10.
4. DeWitt RC, Kudsk KA. The gut's role in metabolism, mucosal barrier function and gut immunology. Infect Dis Clin North Am. 1999;13(2):465–81.
5. Ono H, Azuma T, Miyaji H, et al. Effects of percutaneous endoscopic gastrostomy tube placement on gastric antral motility and gastric emptying. J Gastroenterol. 2003;38:930–6.
6. Sieber C, Beglinger C, Jager K, Stalder GA. Intestinal phase of superior mesenteric artery blood flow in man. Gut. 1992;33:497–501.
7. Alverdy J, Chi HS, Sheldon GF. The effect of parenteral nutrition on gastrointestinal immunity. The importance of enteral stimulation. Ann Surg. 1985;202(6):681–4.
8. MacFie J. Enteral versus parenteral nutrition: the significance of bacterial translocation and gut-barrier function. Nutrition. 2000; 16(7/8):606–11.
9. Shikora SA, George B. Nutrition for the critically ill patient. In: Shikora SA, George B, editors. Nutrition support. Theory and therapeutics. New York: Jones and Bartlett; 1997. p. 464–85.
10. Sacks GS, Kudsk KA. Maintaining mucosal immunity during parenteral feeding with surrogates to enteral nutrition. Nutr Clin Pract. 2003;18(6):483–8.
11. Patton ML, Haith Jr LR, Germain TJ, Goldman WT, Raymond JT. Use of percutaneous endoscopic gastrostomy tubes in burn patients. Surg Endosc. 1994;8:1067–71.
12. Yowler CJ, Pruitt Jr BA. Enteral nutrition in burns. Ch 19. In: Rombeau JL, Rolandelli RH, editors. Clinical nutrition. Enteral and tube feeding. 3rd ed. Philadelphia: WB Saunders; 1984. p. 333–48.
13. Cano N, Fiaccadori E, Tesinsky P, et al. ESPEN guidelines on enteral nutrition: adult renal failure. Clin Nutr. 2006;25:295–310.
14. De Gennaro VA. Nutritional assessment and role of preoperative assessment of parenteral nutrition. JPEN. 1980;4:314–6.
15. Rombeau JL. Enteral nutrition and critical illness. In: Enteral nutrition, Ronnie Chernoff, series editor, 1994. p. 25–36; ch 3.
16. Herodotus, Euterpe, p. 19, Ancient Greek library, www.greektexts.com/library. Accessed 28 Mar 2010.
17. Hippocrates, On ancient medicine, pp. 1–11, Ancient Greek Library, www.greektexts.com/library. Accessed 28 Mar 2010.
18. Rutkow I, Schlesinger Jr AM, editors. James A. Garfield: The American Presidents Series: The 20th President 1881. New York: Macmillan; 2006. p. 119–27.
19. Friedenwald J, Morrison S. The history of the stomach tube with some notes on the duodenal tube. Am J Dig Dis. 1938;5(3):165–70.
20. Modlin IM. A brief history of endoscopy. Milano: MultiMed; 2000. p. 11.
21. Kravetz RE. Stomach (Ewald) tube. Am J Gastroenterol. 2005; 100(7):1444–5.
22. Modlin I. A brief history of endoscopy. Milano: MultiMed; 2000. p. 12.
23. Allison SP. History of nutritional support in Europe pre-ESPEN. Clin Nutr. 2003;22 Suppl 2:S3–5.

24. Lennard-Jones JE. Historical overview. Ch 1. In: Jeremy Nightingale, editor. Intestinal failure. Cambridge: Cambridge University Press; 2001. p. 3–15.
25. McCamish MA, Bounos G, Geraghty ME. History of enteral feeding: past and present perspectives. Ch 1. In: Rombeau JL, Rolandelli RH, editors. Clinical nutrition. Enteral and tube feeding. 3rd ed. Philadelphia: WB Saunders; 1997.
26. Gorman RC, Mchael H. Torosian, Marcel Dekker, Inc New York 1995 Nance ML. Morris JB. Enteral feeding technique. Ch 17. In: Nutrition for the hospitalized patient: basic science and principles of practice
27. Woodward B, Husson EB. Ch 1. History of fiber optics. In: Fiber optics installer and technician guide., John Wiley and Sons; 2005. p. 1–12.
28. Modlin I. A brief history of endoscopy. Milano: MultiMed; 2000. p. 89.
29. Given MF, Lyon SM, Lee MJ. The role of the interventional radiologist in enteral alimentation. Eur Radiol. 2004;14:38–47.
30. Verneuil M. Communique une Observation de gastro-stomie pratique'e avec success pour un retrecissement cicatriciel infranchissable de l'oesophage. Bulletin de l'Academie de medicine. 1876;2(5):1023–38.
31. Stamm M. Gastrostomy by a new method. Med News. 1894;65: 324–6.
32. Gauderer MW, Ponsky JL, Izant Jr RJ. Gastrostomy without laparotomy. J Pediatr Surg. 1980;15(6):872–5.
33. Doyle FM, Kennedy NP. Nutritional support via percutaneous endoscopic gastrostomy. Proc Nutr Soc. 1994;53:473–82.
34. Gibbs J, Cull W, Henderson W, Daley J, Khuri SF. Preoperative serum albumin level as a predictor of operative mortality and morbidity: results from the National VA Surgical risk study. Arch Surg. 1999;134(1):36–42.
35. Shike M, Schroy P, Ritchie MA, Lightdale CJ, Morse R. Percutaneous endoscopic jejunostomy in cancer patients with previous gastric resection. Gastrointest Endosc. 1987;33(5):372–4.
36. Mellert J, Naruhn MB, Grund KE, Becker HD. Direct endoscopic percutaneous jejunostomy (EPJ). Clinical results. Surg Endosc. 1994;8:867–70.
37. Ponsky JL. How I do it: percutaneous endoscopic gastrostomy. J Gastrointest Surg. 2004;8(7):901–4.
38. Sacks BA, Vine HS, Palestrant AM, et al. A non-operative technique for establishment of a gastrostomy tube on the dog. Invest Radiol. 1983;18:485–7.
39. Foutch PG, Talbert RN, Waring JP and Sanowski RA. Percutaneous endoscopic Gastrostomy in patients with prior abdominal surgery: virtues of the safe tract. Am J Gastroenterol. 1988;83:147–50.
40. Foutch PG, Talbert GA, Gaine JA, Sanowski RA. The gastrostomy button, a prospective assessment of safety, success and spectrum of use. Gastrointest Endosc. 1989;35(1):41–4.
41. Funaka B, Zaleshi GX, Lorenz J, et al. Radiologic gastrostomy placement: pigtail versus mushroom retained catheters. Am J Radiol. 2000;175:375–9.
42. Kinoshita Y, Udagawa H, Kajiyama Y, et al. Cologastric fistula and colonic perforation as a complication of percutaneous endoscopic gastrostomy. Surg Laparosc Endosc Percutan Tech. 1999;9:220–2.
43. Shrag SP, Sharma R, Jaik NP, et al. Complications related to Percutaneous Endoscopic Gastrostomy (PEG) tubes, A comprehensive critical review. J Gastrointest Liver Dis. 2007;16(4):407–18.
44. Gencosmanoglu R, Koc D, Tozun N. The buried bumper syndrome: migration of internal bumper of percutaneous endoscopic gastrostomy tube into the abdominal wall. Case report. J Gastroenterol. 2003;38:1077–80.
45. McGarr SE, Kirby DF. Percutaneous endoscopic gastrostomy (PEG) placement in the overweight and obese patient. J Parenter Enteral Nutr. 2007;31(3):212–6.
46. Suzuki Y, Irashima K, Ishibashi Y, et al. Covering the percutaneous endoscopic gastrostomy (PEG) tube prevents peristomal infection. World J Surg. 2006;30:1450–8.
47. Wiesen AJ, Siderikis K, Fernandes A, et al. True incidence and clinical relevance of pneumoperitoneum after PEG placement: a prospective study. Gastrointest Endosc. 2006;64(6):886–9.
48. Klopp CT. Cervical pharyngostomy. J Thorac Surg. 1951;21(5): 490–1.
49. Bucklin DL, Gilsdorf RB. Percutaneous needle pharyngostomy. J Parenter Enteral Nutr. 1985;9(1):68–70.
50. Kendrick ML, Sarr MG. Prolonged gastrointestinal decompression of the inoperable abdomen: the forgotten tube pharyngostomy. J Am Coll Surg. 2000;191(2):221–3.
51. Higaki F, Oishi M, Higaki T, Hayata Y. Old-fashioned but modern tube cervical esophagotomy. Am J Surg. 2006;192(3):385–7.
52. Mackey R, Chand B, Oshi H, Kameoka S, Ponsky JL. Percutaneous transesophageal gastrostomy tube for decompression of malignant obstruction: report of the first case and our series in the US. J Am Coll Surg. 2005;201:695–700.
53. Ponsky JL, Aszodi A. Percutaneous endoscopic jejunostomy. Am J Gastroenterol. 1984;79(2):113–6.
54. Shike M, Schroy P, Ritchie MA, Lightdale CJ, Morse R. Percutaneous endoscopic jejunostomy in cancer patients with previous gastric resection. Gastrointest Endosc. 1987;33:372–4.
55. Shike M. Editorial. Predicting the success of percutaneous endoscopic jejunostomy placement: the endoscope light outshines the CT scan. Gastrointest Endosc. 2006;63:431–2.
56. MacKenzie SH, Haslem D, Hilden K, Thomas K, Fang J. Success rate of direct percutaneous endoscopic jejunostomy in patients who are obese. Gastrointest Endosc. 2008;67:265–9.
57. Maple JT. Editorial. Direct percutaneous endoscopic jejunostomy in the obese: proceed with caution. Gastrointest Endosc. 2008;67(2): 270–2.
58. Richard Duszak Jr. Percutaneous gastrostomy and jejunostomy. http://www.emedicine.medscape.com. Accessed 29 Jun 2010.
59. Gerber A, Thompson Jr RJ. Use of a tube cecostomy to lower the mortality in acute large intestinal obstruction due to carcinoma. Am J Surg. 1985;110:893–6.
60. Ponsky J, Aszodi A, Perse D. Percutaneous endoscopic cecostomy: a new approach to nonobstructive colonic dilation. Gastrointest Endosc. 1985;32(2):108–11.
61. Holm AN, Baron TH. Palliative use of percutaneous endoscopic gastrostomy and percutaneous endoscopic cecostomy tubes. Gastrointest Endosc Clin North Am. 2007;17:795–803.
62. Chait PG, Shandling B, Rochards HM, Connelly BL. Fecal incontinence in children: treatment with percutaneous cecostomy tube placement – a prospective study. Pediatr Radiol. 1997;203:621–4.
63. Baraza W, Brown S, McAlindon M, Hurlstone P. Prospective analysis of percutaneous endoscopic colostomy at a tertiary referral center. Br J Surg. 2007;94:1415–20.
64. van den Berg MM, Hogan M, Caniano DA, Di Lorenzo C, Benning MA, Mousa HM. Colonic manometry as predictor of cecostomy success in children with defecation disorders. J Pediatr Surg. 2006; 41:730–6.
65. Anis MK, Abid S, Jafri W, et al. Acceptability and outcomes of the percutaneous endoscopic gastrostomy (PEG) tube placement – patients' and caregivers' perspectives. BMC Gastroenterol. 2006;6:37.
66. Forbes RB, Colville S, Swingler RJ. Frequency, timing and outcome of gastrostomy tubes for amyotrophic lateral sclerosis/motor neurone disease. A record linkage study from the Scottish Motor Neurone Disease Register. J Neurol. 2004;251:813–7.
67. Rabeneck L, Wray NP, Petersen NJ. Long-term outcomes of patients receiving percutaneous endoscopic gastrostomy tubes. J Gen Intern Med. 1996;11:287–93.
68. Smith BM, Perring P, Engoren M, Sferra JJ. Hospital and long-term outcome after percutaneous endoscopic gastrostomy. Surg Endosc. 2008;22:74–80.
69. Taylor CA, Larsen DE, Balard DJ, Bergstrom LR, Silverstein MD, Zinsmeister AR, et al. Predictors of outcome after percutaneous

endoscopic gastrostomy: a community based study. Mayo Clin Proc. 1992;67:1042–9.
70. Nair S, Hertan H, Picthumoni CS. Hypoalbuminemia is a poor predictor of survival after percutaneous endoscopic gastrostomy in elderly patients with dementia. Am J Gastroenterol. 2000;95(1):133–6.
71. Kirby DF. Editorial. Surgical gastrostomies versus endoscopic gastrostomies. A tube by any other name. Mayo Clin Proc. 1995;70:914–6.
72. Gauderer MWL. Review. Percutaneous endoscopic gastrostomy and the evolution of contemporary long-term enteral access. Clin Nutr. 2002;21(2):103–10.

Gastrointestinal Stomas in Infants and Children

16

David K. Magnuson and Oliver S. Soldes

Introduction

Stomas of the gastrointestinal tract represent some of the most commonly performed surgical procedures, and most frequent management dilemmas, in the practice of pediatric surgery. The wide variety of congenital anomalies and functional disorders of the intestinal tract encountered by the pediatric surgeon has led to the development of a creative and sometimes unconventional repertoire of options for providing access and decompression of the GI tract at every level. Some of the first surviving patients of decompressive enterostomy operations were children with congenital intestinal obstructions, and over the long history of stomal development by general surgeons treating adults there has been a parallel development of stoma techniques directed at addressing pediatric diseases. Often, the techniques first developed in adults were adapted for children with good results. On occasion, a surgical problem unique to children required a solution that had no corollary in the adult surgical experience, requiring the development of an innovative approach for a rare disease process that did not present a large enough clinical volume to submit new ideas to objective analysis. Over the years, accumulated experience has played a large role in selecting and discarding these techniques. In this chapter, we present an overview of gastrointestinal stoma techniques that have proven to be useful over time and which have been widely adopted as standard options in the care of children with gastrointestinal problems. A number of selected references are also offered for further reading.

D.K. Magnuson (✉) • O.S. Soldes
Department of Pediatric Surgery,
Cleveland Clinic Foundation, Cleveland,
OH, USA
e-mail: magnusd@ccf.org

Gastrostomy in Children

Gastrostomy tubes are used in children for long-term feeding, medication administration, hydration, and gastric venting for a variety of medical and surgical conditions. They are also intermittently employed for gastric access for endoscopy and esophageal dilation for conditions such as chronic esophageal strictures due to caustic ingestions and esophageal atresia. They may provide access for transgastric jejunal feeding tubes as well.

There are several clinical considerations unique to the placement of a gastrostomy tube in a child. Gastrostomy in adults is often associated with clinical circumstances associated with end-of-life care (e.g. advanced malignancy), conditions causing permanent disability and immobility (e.g. stoke and traumatic brain injury), and institutionalization in long-term care facilities. Pediatric gastrostomy tubes are usually utilized for a period of months to years in patients who often thrive later. These children are often physically active with relatively mild disabilities. Patients with gastrostomy tubes are usually mobile and attend school. Participation in mainstream schooling and activities outside the home make the presence of conventional long gastrostomy tubes inconvenient.

Historically, the Stamm technique for open placement of gastrostomy tubes described for adults was also employed in children. The percutaneous placement of gastrostomy tubes in children was first reported in 1980, and represented a significant new development in the nutritional management of patients with feeding difficulties who had otherwise functional gastrointestinal tracts [1]. This technique is described elsewhere in this volume and is essentially the same in children as adults. The percutaneous endoscopic gastrostomy (PEG) procedure was rapidly adopted as the standard for placement of gastric feeding tubes in both children and adults who were not otherwise undergoing laparotomy. Two problems emerged, however, in children who underwent

V.W. Fazio et al. (eds.), *Atlas of Intestinal Stomas*,
DOI 10.1007/978-0-387-78851-7_16, © Springer Science+Business Media, LLC 2012

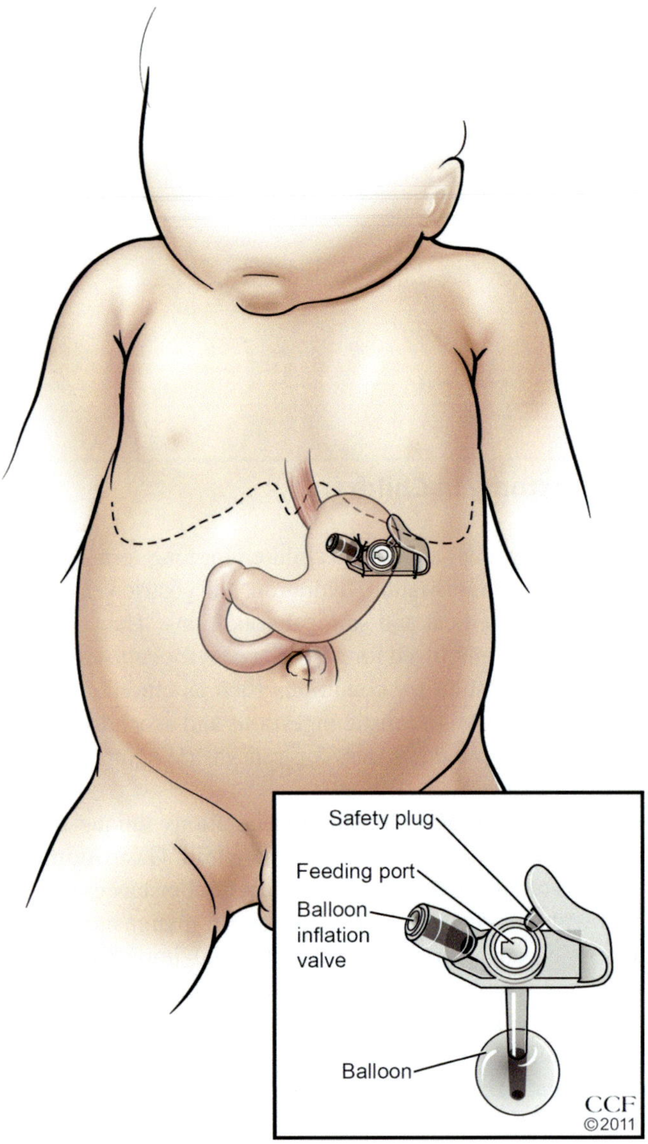

Fig. 16.1 Gastrostomy button

placement of a PEG tube: accidental dislodgment of the tube by children who grabbed at the strange device attached to their bodies, and leakage of gastric contents through tracts that had become progressively dilated by the constant movement and levering action of the tube against the thin abdominal wall of a child.

A major innovation occurred with the development of the skin-level silicone gastrostomy "button" with a feeding port that accommodates a detachable external catheter (Fig. 16.1) [2, 3]. These low-profile devices free the patient from a long protruding catheter, allow better concealment of the appliance and wearing of tight fitting clothes, and offer improved cosmesis. Furthermore, a short skin-level device reduces the mechanical forces exerted by the tube on the abdominal wall site. Reduction of the mechanical forces reduces erosion and enlargement of the gastrostomy site, formation of chronic granulation tissue, and leakage of gastric contents around the button. The internal balloon makes theses tubes much more difficult to displace than a soft mushroom catheter and obviates the need for suturing the tube to the skin to prevent accidental removal. These appliances are also used for jejunal feeding tubes, and for cecal access to perform antegrade colonic irrigation programs in children with intractable constipation or incontinence.

Variations of these silicone gastrostomy buttons, with inflatable internal balloons or rigid nonballoon internal bumpers, are in common use worldwide. The tubes with rigid nonballoon bumpers are more difficult to remove and more durable. They often require a brief general anesthesia in small children to replace because of the force required to pull the nondeflatable button through the tract. When nonballoon buttons and tubes are exchanged for balloon buttons, the external portion of the stem may be cut and the internal portion with the rigid "mushroom" retrieved endoscopically to avoid the soft-tissue damage caused by pulling the internal bumper forcefully through the tract. This extra step avoids tract enlargement and the potential consequences of granulation tissue formation and leakage.

Minimally Invasive Primary Placement of Gastrostomy Buttons

In the years since the PEG procedure and gastrostomy button revolutionized enteral access in children, the usual approach has been to place a PEG tube initially, and replace it with a button device after a 6 week interval to allow secure healing of the stomach to the abdominal wall before manipulating the tract. The clear preference for the eventual placement of a button, and the fact that tube complications occur with some regularity during the interval before conversion from tube to button, has led to the widespread application of a minimally invasive approach for the primary placement of gastrostomy buttons.

The endoscopic technique can be performed with any sized gastroscope, as it is used only for insufflation and visualization (Figs. 16.2–16.10). The main difference between the technique for primary button placement as compared to the PEG is the need to stabilize the stomach against the abdominal wall during button placement, as dilation of the tract and introduction of the button from the outside both involve forces that tend to push the two tissue planes apart. Although prefabricated "T-fasteners" may be used, we have found these unsatisfactory in children as the internal metallic toggling T-bar often becomes embedded in the gastric and abdominal walls, and may erode to the surface resulting in prolonged inflammation, swelling, pain, and drainage. We now use a pair of temporary transabdominal monofilament U-stitches that are less reactive and completely removable [4]. These stay sutures

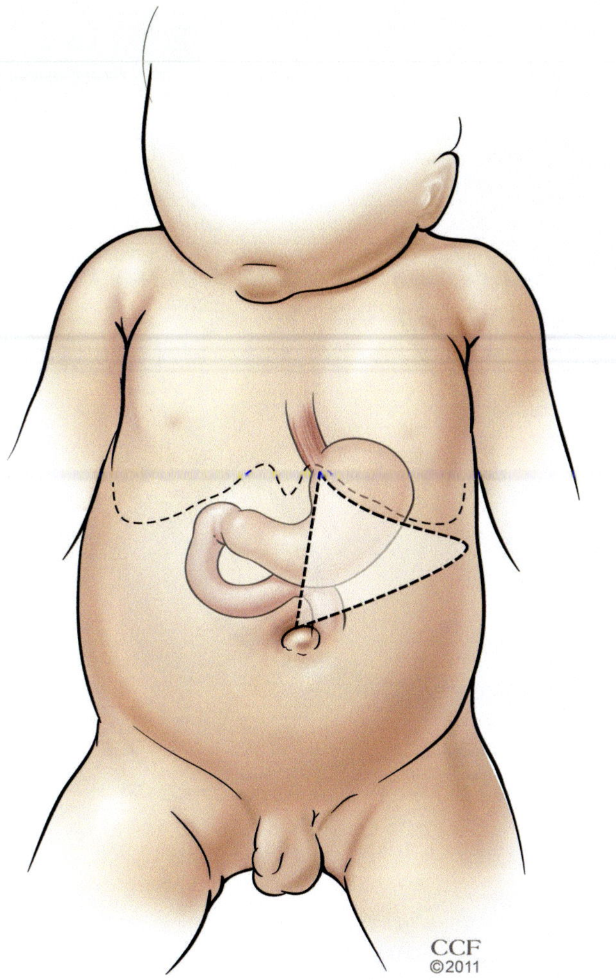

Fig. 16.2 Anatomic placement of gastrostomy tubes and buttons. Triangle. Avoid linea alba and costal margin

can be replaced by simple full-thickness suture technique in a small child, or, on a larger patient, by introducing a suture through one introducer needle, and retrieving it with either a laparoscopic port site closure device or a suture loop "snare" introduced through a second needle. The basic technique for endoscopic primary button placement can be easily adapted to the laparoscopic approach.

Roux-Y Button Jejunostomy for Feeding

Gastrostomy is generally the preferred method of long-term feeding access in children, allowing both bolus and continuous feeding with fewer complications than a jejunostomy. Jejunostomy tubes generally necessitate continuous feedings, which are cumbersome in active children. Continuous feedings tether patients to a feeding pump, limiting mobility and play. Jejunostomy tubes may be employed in cases of severe gastroparesis or failed surgical management of gastroesophageal reflux, or in cases where the stomach is unsuitable for gastrostomy tube placement, such as prior resection, altered body habitus in spastic quadriplegia, and congenital microgastria.

In cases where a long-term feeding jejunostomy is needed, the authors prefer a Roux-Y button jejunostomy over a simple loop jejunostomy for a number of reasons. The placement of a balloon button in a simple loop jejunostomy may obstruct the small bowel in a young child. The Roux-Y technique permits the placement of a button within the end of the defunctionalized Roux limb, avoiding the presence of an obstructing balloon within the intestinal stream [5]. Just as for a gastrostomy, the skin-level button tube has definite advantages. Infants and children with thin abdominal walls may develop an enterocutaneous fistula from localized skin breakdown and ulceration at the site of a conventional tube. The Roux-Y conduit quickly diverts the formula away from the jejunostomy site, reducing local skin irritation from leakage of succus and irritation at the tube site. The creation of a dedicated feeding conduit discourages the retrograde flow of formula that may occur in loop jejunostomies, particularly in patients with global motility disorders. The loop jejunostomy with a tunneled catheter is generally suitable for short-term feeding access and is infrequently used. In addition, in very small infants, a Witzel tunnel may compromise the lumen if too much jejunal wall is imbricated over the catheter.

Roux-Y button jejunostomies can be created by both laparoscopic and open technique (Figs. 16.11–16.14). In both procedures, a Roux limb is fashioned by standard techniques. The jejunum is divided approximately 15 cm distal to the ligament of Treitz with a linear stapler. A 20 cm Roux-Y limb is fashioned with an end-to-side anastomosis. The anastomosis is usually hand sewn in infants, but may be stapled in older children. Two purse-string sutures of 4–0 polyglycolic acid are placed in the antimesenteric border of the jejunum, just proximal to the terminal end of the Roux limb. A stab incision is made in the left upper quadrant of the abdominal wall. A small enterotomy is made inside of the purse-string sutures and a 12 Fr gastrostomy button of appropriate length is passed through the abdominal wall and into the jejunum. In difficult cases, a guidewire and dilators, identical to those used in gastrostomy placement, may be helpful. The balloon is inflated and the purse-strings tied. The jejunum around the tube placement site and along the Roux limb are tacked to abdominal wall.

Stomas in Necrotizing Enterocolitis

Necrotizing enterocolitis (NEC) is a disease unique to infants that is most often a complication of prematurity. Intestinal hypoperfusion and ischemia of unclear etiology produces intestinal injury of varying severity ranging from mild transient ischemia to isolated focal perforation and, on occasion,

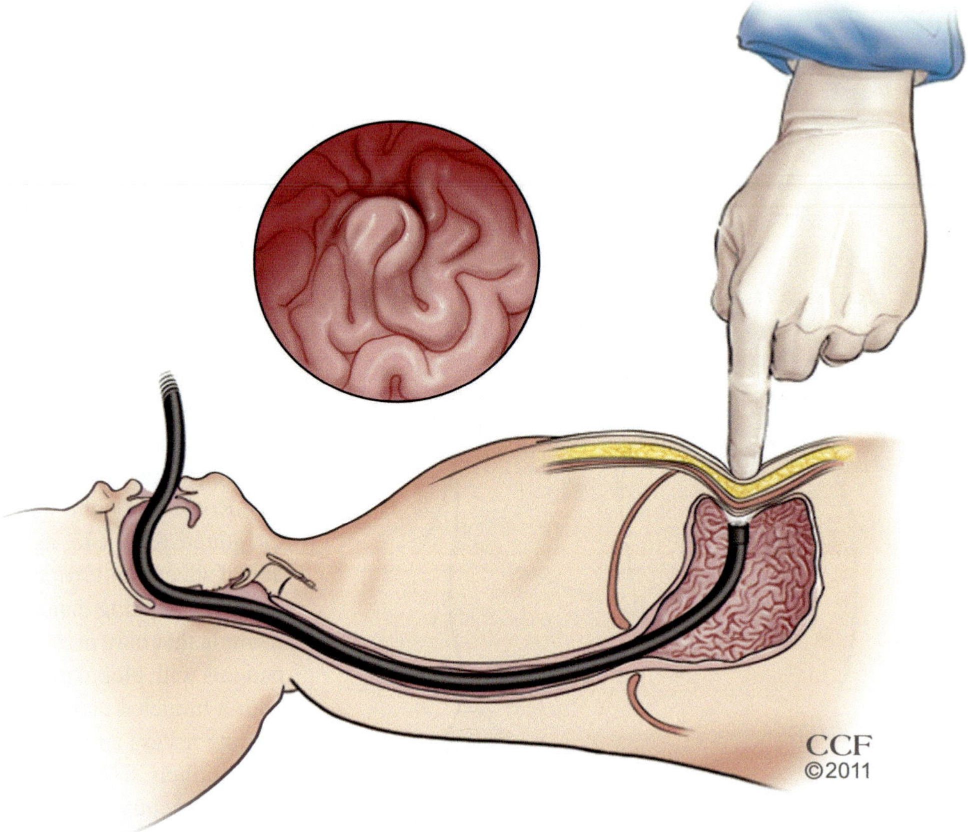

Fig. 16.3 Endoscopic insufflation of stomach and determination of gastrostomy site. Avoidance of liver and transverse colon

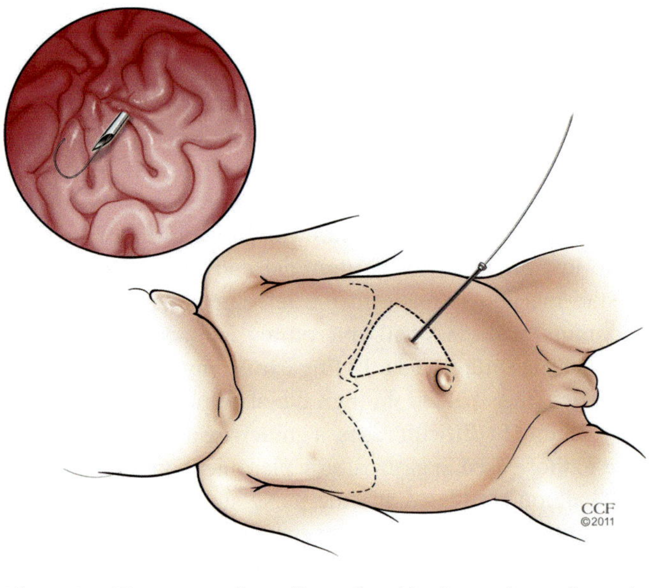

Fig. 16.4 Placement of needle and guidewire under endoscopic guidance

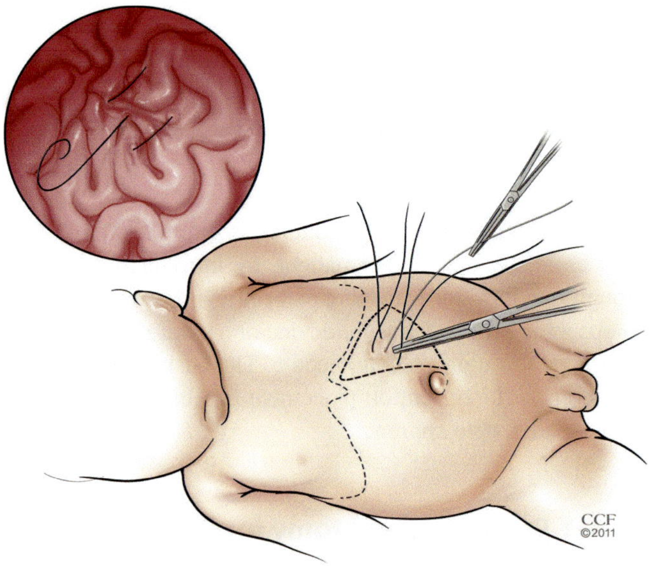

Fig. 16.5 Placement of two transabdominal U-stitches to provide four-point fixation

pan-intestinal necrosis. The areas of ischemia are often patchy with viable bowel segments separating areas of frank necrosis. In the event of significant intestinal loss, even short viable segments a few centimeters long must be preserved to mitigate against short-gut syndrome. In such cases, especially where hypoperfusion and generalized peritonitis is a concern, anastomosis is avoided and multiple stomas may be created. The foreshortened mesentery of the neonatal gut that has been exposed to peritoneal contamination often makes it impossible to create stoma sites distant from the exploratory incision without damaging the tenuous blood supply of the externalized bowel. Diverting stomas in infants

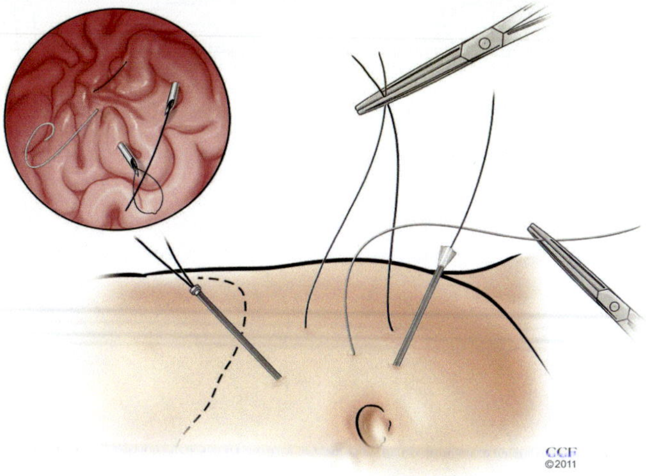

Fig. 16.6 Alternative approaches to U-stitch placement in larger patients. Introduction of monofilament suture through needle and retrieval by suture loop snare (depicted), or with laparoscopic port site closure device (Endo-Close, Covidien Surgical)

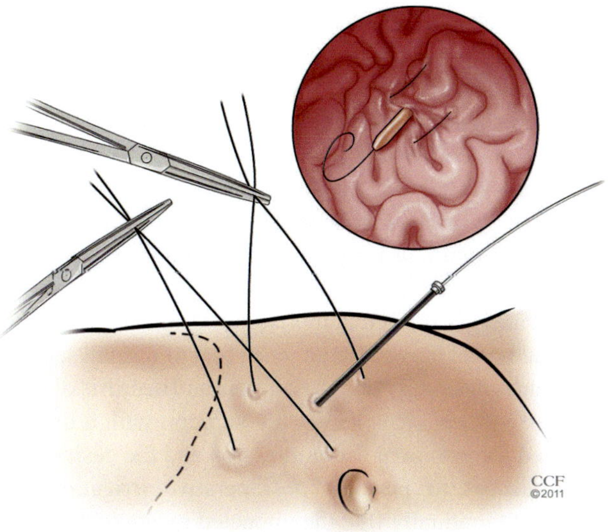

Fig. 16.7 Dilation of tract with U-stitch traction

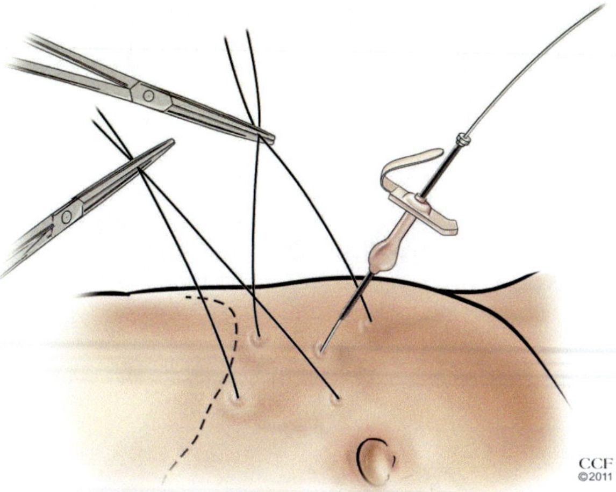

Fig. 16.8 Introduction of button with stent over wire

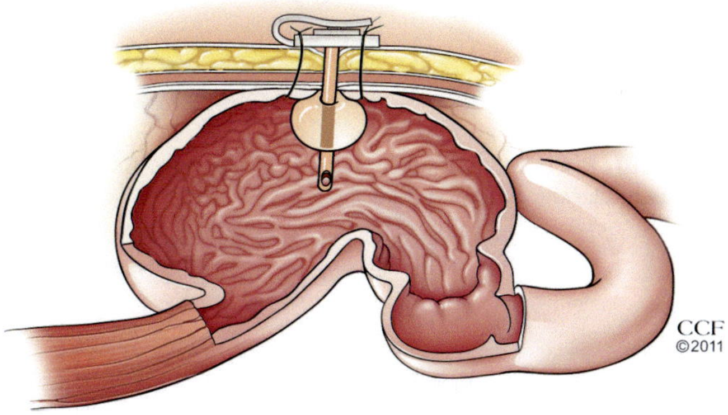

Fig. 16.9 Tying U-stitches over button as bolster

may be brought out directly through the abdominal incision, which is usually oriented transversely across the supraumbilical abdominal wall. Proximal and distal stomas may be placed at both poles of the incision, and intervening stomas may simply be lined-up within the middle of the incision itself (Fig. 16.15). Surprisingly, the risk of wound infection is low, probably owing to the lack of a significant adipose layer "dead-space" in premature neonates. The same lack of abdominal wall thickness makes stomal prolapse an eventual problem if the stomas are not reversed in an expeditious manner. The diminutive stomas created in premature infants do not need to be formally matured and attempts to do so may further damage the bowel ends. The segment of bowel to be brought out is simply tacked to the fascia with seromuscular stitches to the bowel wall. The mucosa at the end of the stoma will spontaneously roll over and mature within a few days (Fig. 16.16). The segments will grow with time and are later reconnected.

Stomas in Congenital Intestinal Obstruction

The unique needs of the neonate with a congenital bowel obstruction have led to the introduction of a variety of innovative stomas that provide proximal decompression while also addressing other germane surgical problems at the same time. The main surgical condition that provided the impetus for a novel approach to intestinal decompression was meconium ileus, an uncommon condition characterized by the endo-luminal obstruction of the fetal intestine by abnormal meconium. The condition is pathognomonic for cystic fibrosis and results from the abnormal chemical composition of gastrointestinal secretions resulting from a defective

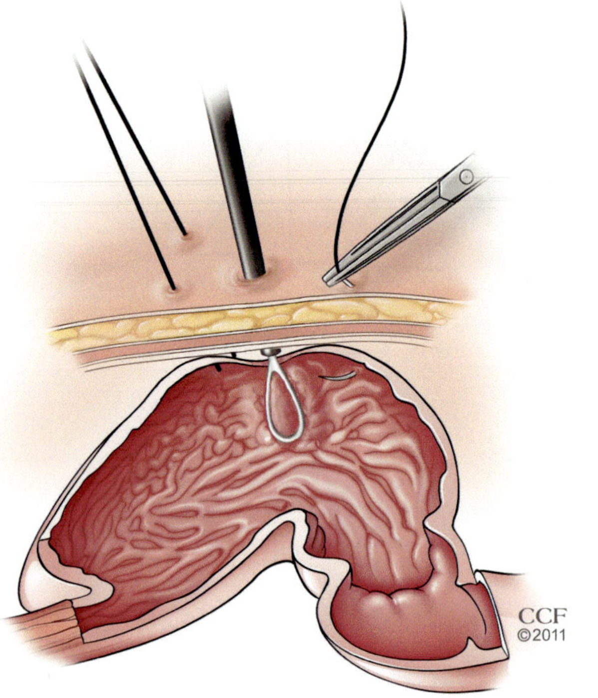

Fig. 16.10 Placement of U-stitches during laparoscopy. Advantage in selecting exact site on gastric wall

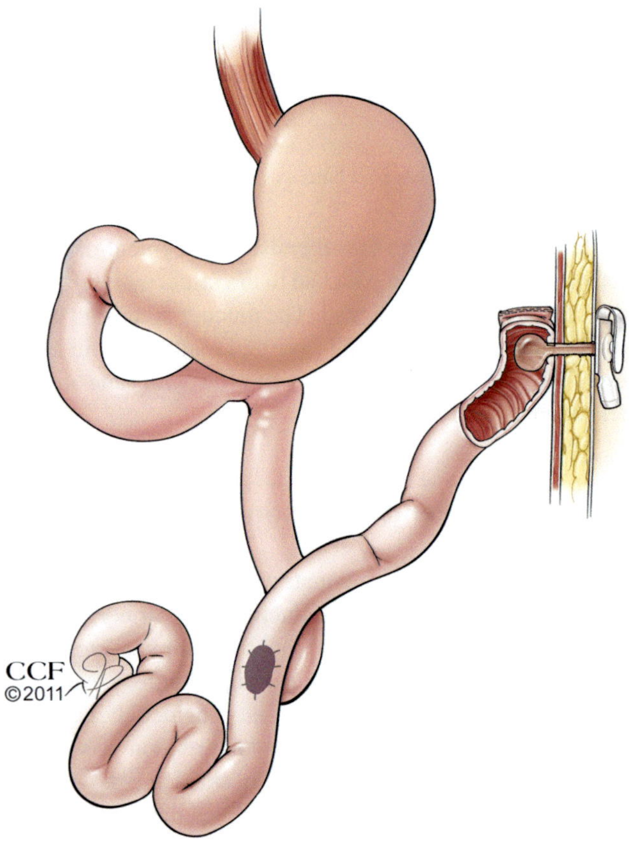

Fig. 16.11 Roux-Y button jejunostomy

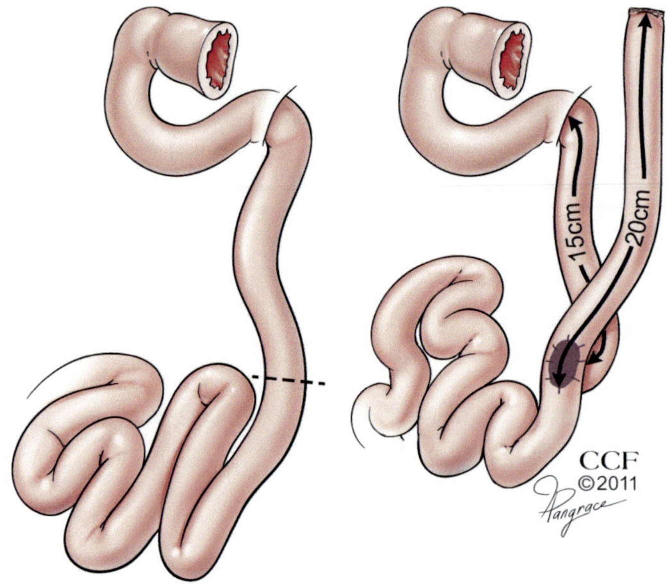

Fig. 16.12 Creation of Roux-Y limb

chloride-transport mechanism. Meconium produced under these conditions in the fetal gut becomes extraordinarily tenacious and inspissated, filling and blocking the lumen of the distal small intestine with an immovable caste.

Surgeons confronted with a neonate suffering from meconium ileus found that the inspissated meconium caste often could not be safely dislodged and removed at the time of initial surgery without irreparably damaging the bowel [6, 7]. Resection of the meconium-packed bowel is usually contraindicated, as it often comprises a significant proportion of the total bowel length. Often, resection of a small segment of intestine is necessary due to ischemia and necrosis of the most affected portion. This leaves the surgeon with a dilemma – the need for proximal decompression and the desirability for distal access to perform postoperative irrigations in an attempt to gradually free the impacted meconium.

Three basic approaches to stoma formation have gained acceptance, as well as many modifications to fit unique circumstances (Figs. 16.17a–c). Gross originally utilized the double-barrel Mikulicz stoma to create a proximal venting stoma adjacent to a distal access stoma. This procedure allowed for intestinal resection to be done after abdominal wall closure, a tangible benefit in an era of limited antibiotic options. He recommended the suturing together of the afferent and efferent stomal limbs so that a crushing clamp could later be placed, fusing and opening the adjacent intestinal walls and re-establishing intestinal continuity below the fascial level. The venting stoma could then be closed in a lesser operation at a later date; occasionally the venting portion of the stoma would atrophy and close by itself, obviating further surgery.

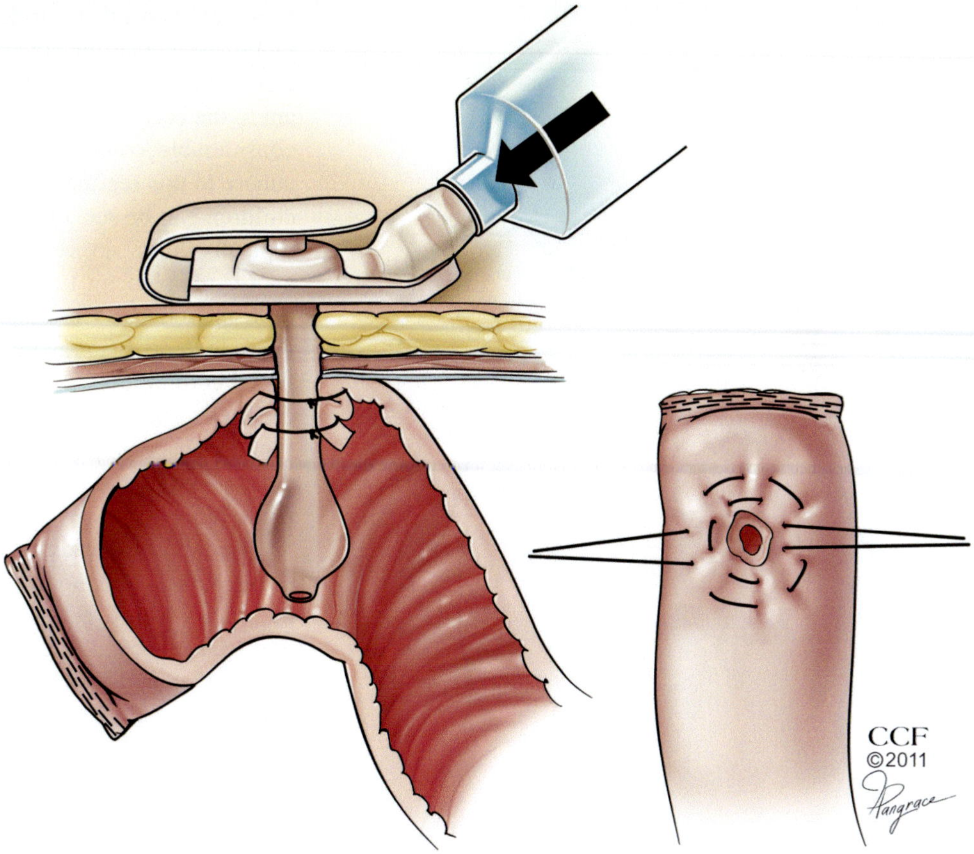

Fig. 16.13 Insertion of button into Roux-Y limb

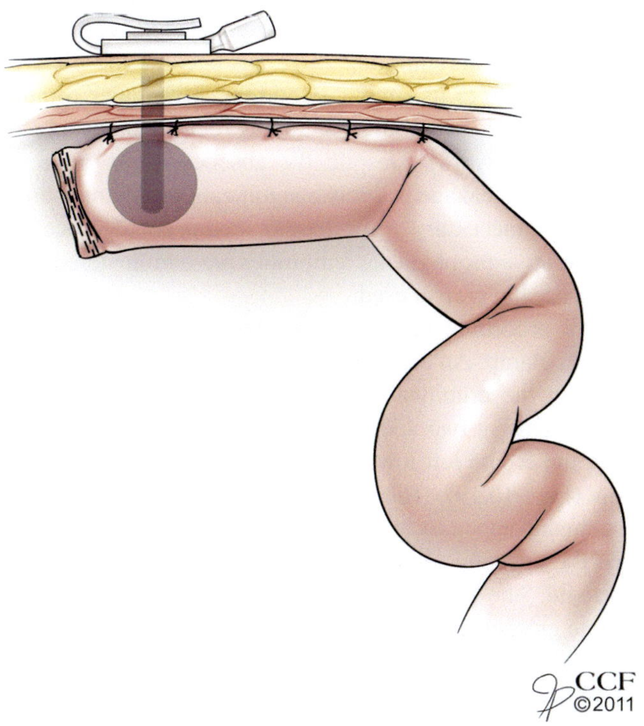

Fig. 16.14 Complete Roux-Y button jejunostomy

Bishop and Koop refined this approach, describing an anastomosis between the end of the proximal bowel with the antimesenteric side of the distal segment (essentially creating a Roux-Y limb), and bringing the end of the distal segment through the abdominal wall as an end-stoma. This allowed egress of intestinal effluent, easy access to the distal limb for irrigations, and the advantage of a smaller, more easily cared-for single stoma, which had a greater likelihood of spontaneous regression and closure than did the double barrel Mikulicz stoma. Santulli recommended the opposite configuration, creating a side-to-end anastomosis to provide better egress through a larger proximal limb. The Santulli stoma had the disadvantage of externalizing the dilated proximal limb, which proved harder to care for and more prone to prolapse when it decreased in size, while the benefits of better egress were never realized as the Bishop-Koop stoma proved to provide adequate output on a consistent basis. The contemporary management of meconium ileus in most cases involves the intraoperative irrigation of the intestinal lumen with surface-active agents, such as N-acetylcysteine, and removal of the inspissated meconium through enterotomies. This allows for immediate reconstruction and avoidance of stomas altogether in most patients. The traditional stoma options are still occasionally used in refractory patients and those whose physiologic condition will not allow for a lengthy laparotomy and creation of enterotomies.

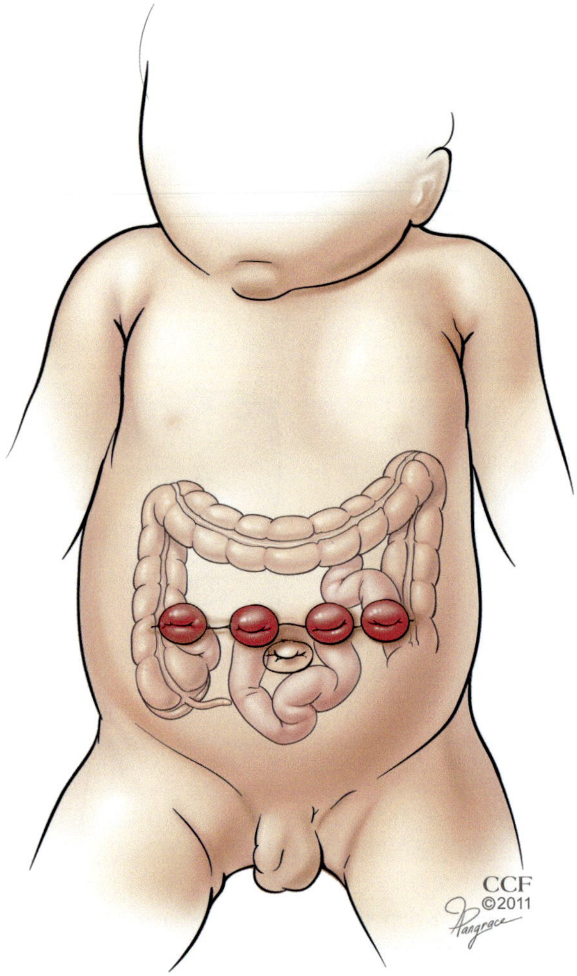

Fig. 16.15 Multiple intestinal stomas for necrotizing enterocolitis

The Santulli stoma has also been used in infants with jejunoileal atresia, as the marked sized discrepancy between the dilated proximal and atretic distal bowel often precludes end-to-end anastomosis. The Bishop-Koop stoma is also an effective means of connecting the disparate intestinal segments in patients with atresia. Although the distal segment caliber is often tiny, it grows and distends rapidly, and the small venting stoma derived from the distal bowel may be sufficient for the liquid effluent from the small intestine. Furthermore, the anastomosis between the dilated proximal bowel and the antimesenteric side of the distal bowel is more easily accomplished.

Appendicostomy for Antegrade Colonic Irrigation

Appendicostomy for antegrade enemas is a suitable treatment for severe constipation and overflow incontinence when all other medical management (dietary modification and laxatives) and other surgical reconstructive measures have failed and a diverting colostomy is not desired. Patients catheterize the appendicostomy stoma nightly and deliver irrigant to the cecum, completely emptying the colon. It requires considerable commitment from the patient and family to adhere to this regimen. However, with sufficient effort most children can be socially continent and clean. These patients typically have severe anorectal malformations with poor anorectal sphincter function, absent rectal evacuative function, and reduced sensation of rectal distention. Other indications include neurogenic constipation from spina bifida, spinal cord injuries, and delayed diagnosis of tethered spinal cord. Occasionally, they may be used for severe refractory functional constipation or patients with Hirschsprung's disease who have not responded to palliative pull-through procedures.

The appendicostomy stoma may be brought directly through the abdominal wall or hidden in the base of the umbilicus with excellent cosmesis. An extended preoperative trial of bowel management with large-volume nightly saline enemas is performed to assess the effectiveness of enemas in achieving continence, and to prepare the patient and family for the use of the appendicostomy. If the patient and family are unable to comply with the trial of enemas, they may be unwilling to catheterize the stoma and perform the antegrade irrigations postoperatively.

An appendicostomy may be performed by laparoscopic or open technique. With the open technique, an antireflux valve is usually created with a cecal submucosal tunnel or by cecal wrapping. More recently, laparoscopic appendicostomy without an antireflux valve has become the preferred technique due to its simplicity and the advantages common to laparoscopic procedures, including reduced pain and more rapid recovery [8]. Despite the absence of an antireflux mechanism, leakage is rarely a significant problem. A bowel prep is unnecessary prior to the laparoscopic procedure. Preoperative prophylactic antibiotics are administered and a standard skin prep is used.

The procedure begins by everting the umbilicus with a Kocher clamp. An inverted V-shaped incision (Fig. 16.18) is made in the umbilical skin. A 5 mm laparoscopic port is placed. One or two additional 5 mm ports are placed in the right upper and left lower quadrants to facilitate the dissection (Fig. 16.19). The retroperitoneal attachments of the cecum and appendix are divided and the cecum mobilized so that the appendix may be easily delivered via the umbilical port site. The tip of the appendix is grasped with a laparoscopic grasper. The port is removed and the tip of the appendix is delivered approximately 2 cm via the umbilicus. The tip of the appendix is opened with a needle point electrocautery and the incision extended 1 cm along the antimesenteric border to spatulate the opening. The appendix is catheterized with a 10 Fr balloon-tipped catheter and the catheter tip is

Fig. 16.16 Spontaneous maturation of and end stoma in premature infant

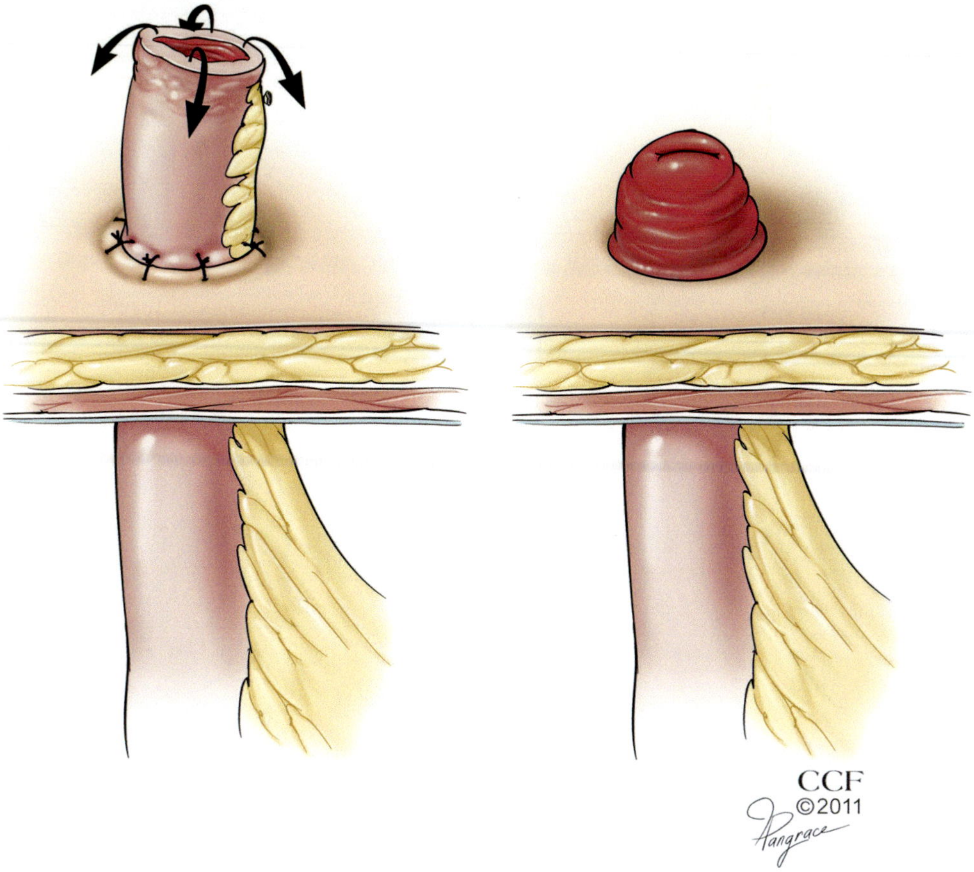

advanced well into the cecum. The balloon is inflated and brought back to the internal appendiceal orifice. The appendix is tacked to the umbilical fascia in four quadrants with 4–0 polyglycolic acid sutures to prevent retraction and prolapse. The inverted V-shaped umbilical skin flap is then sutured in a full-thickness fashion to the spatulated opening at the tip of the appendix, with the epidermal surface of the V-flap continuous with the mucosal surface of the appendiceal lumen. This arrangement creates a short subcutaneous tunnel that helps conceal the opening, and interposes a durable and distensible flap of skin into the appendicostomy orifice that might otherwise be prone to stricture (Fig. 16.20). The remainder of the circumference of the appendicostomy is sutured to the umbilical skin to complete the anastomosis.

The patient resumes a regular diet the next day and antegrade irrigations via the catheter may begin. If a preoperative enema trial has been successfully completed, the parents will already be experienced with the technique of enema administration and the patient may be discharged after the first irrigation. The standard regimen consists of homemade saline solution (1.5 tsp table salt in 1 L warm water). These are given nightly at a volume of 15–20 mL/kg, over 15 min, to achieve a daily bowel movement that empties the colon completely. Three weeks postoperatively, the catheter is removed in the clinic and the patient and family are instructed in intermittent catheterization with a lubricated 10 Fr red rubber catheter. The catheterizations are done twice daily for 1 month and then nightly thereafter.

Leveling Colostomy for Hirschsprung's Disease

The history of colostomy formation in infants with "congenital megacolon" is both interesting and instructive. Harald Hirschsprung, a Danish pediatrician and pathologist, first described the anatomic features of fatal congenital megacolon in infants in 1886: a dilated colon with muscular hypertrophy, transitioning to more normal-appearing distal colon and rectum (Fig. 16.21). Resection of the dilated bowel and formation of a proximal colostomy were occasionally life saving, but subsequent colostomy closure resulted in recurrent symptoms, enterocolitis, sepsis, and death. Although surgeons of the day speculated that the distal, normal-appearing bowel was in fact the pathological cause of a functional obstruction, it took 60 years before this hypothesis was proven and the histological hallmarks of Hirschsprung's disease (HD) were identified: absence of ganglion cells and neural hypertrophy in the normal-appearing distal segment.

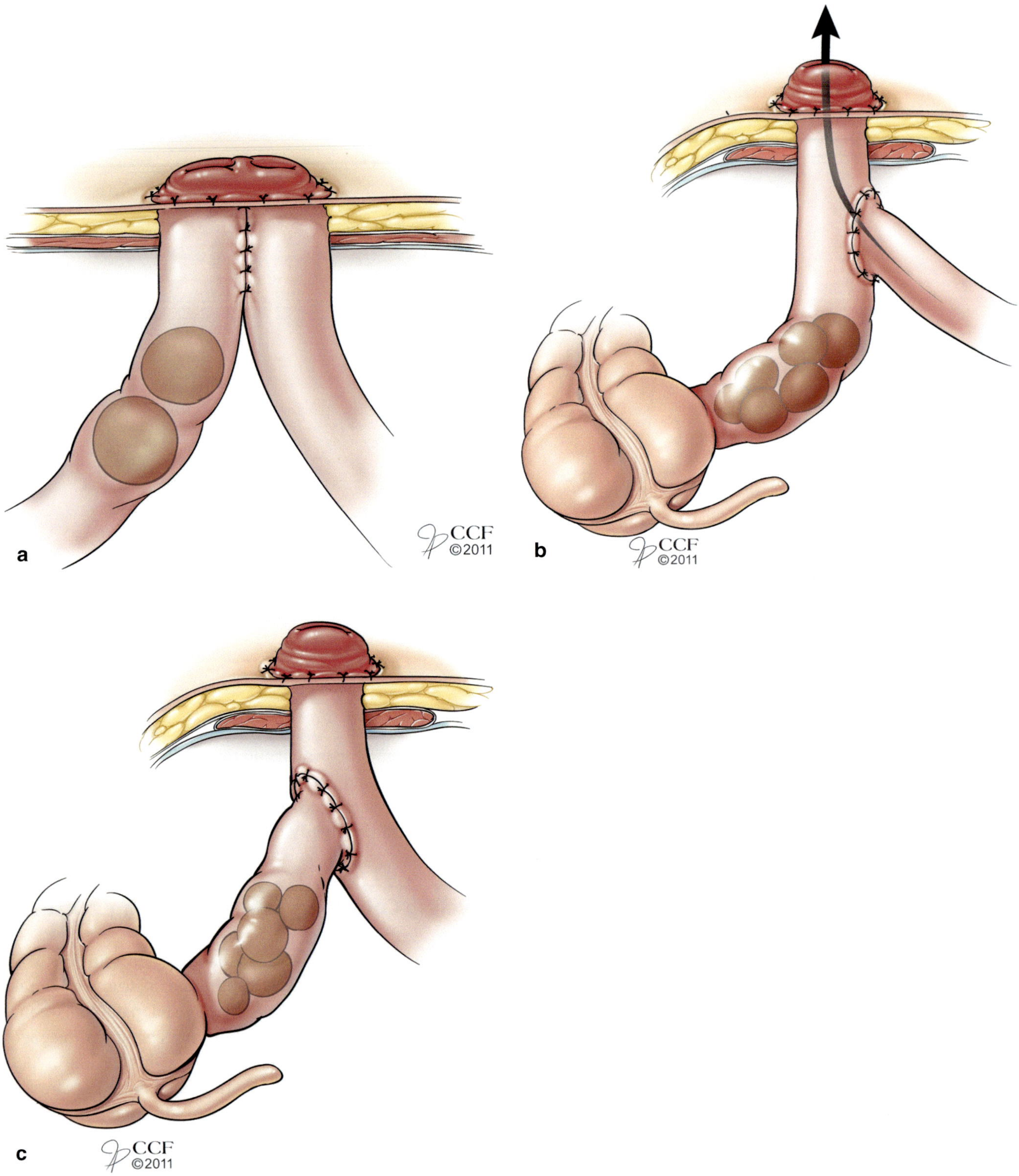

Fig. 16.17 Various stomas for congenital intestinal obstruction. (**a**) Mikulicz. (**b**) Bishop-Koop. (**c**) Santulli

The absence of intramural ganglion cells in both the submucosal and myenteric plexuses causes impairment of receptive relaxation and failure of peristalsis. This realization explained why colostomy closure resulted in recurrent disease. The first palliative pull-through procedure to "bypass" the aganglionic segment was reported by Swenson and Bill shortly after the pathologic features of HD become widely known [9].

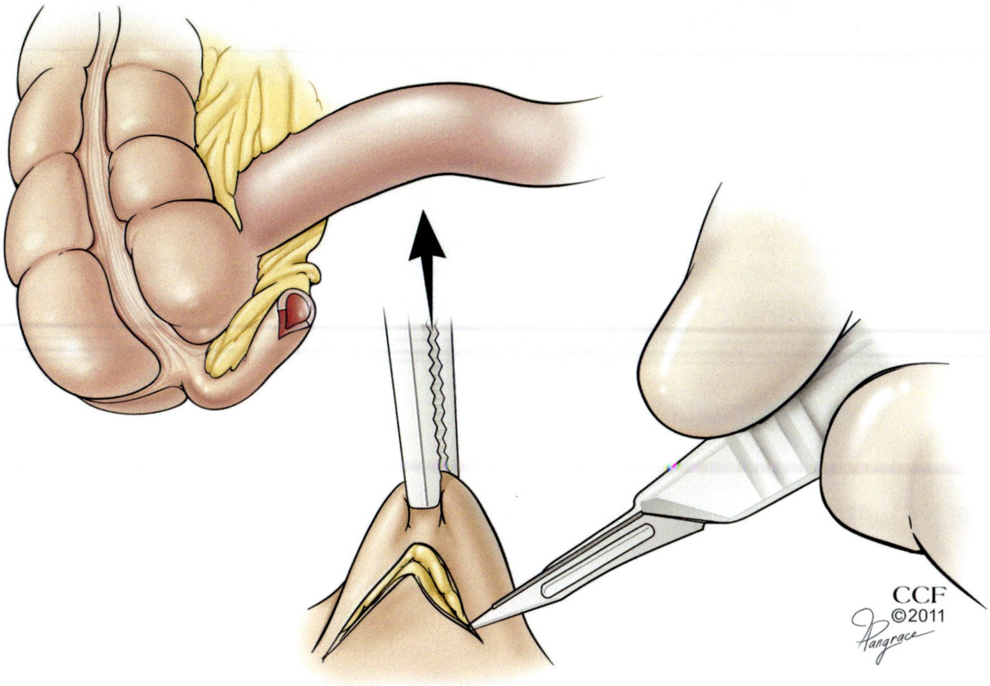

Fig. 16.18 Umbilical flap for appendicostomy

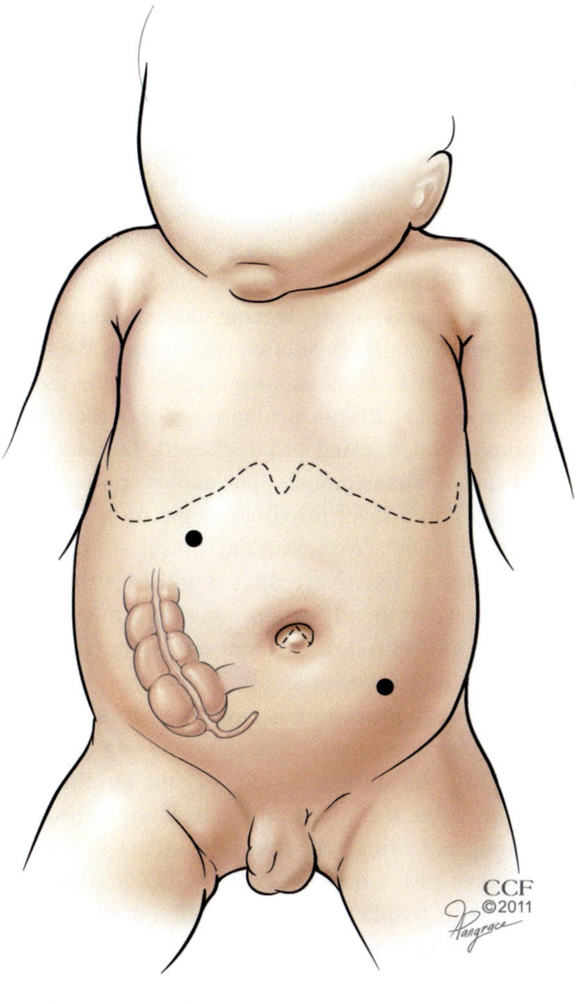

Fig. 16.19 Laparoscopic port placement for appendicostomy

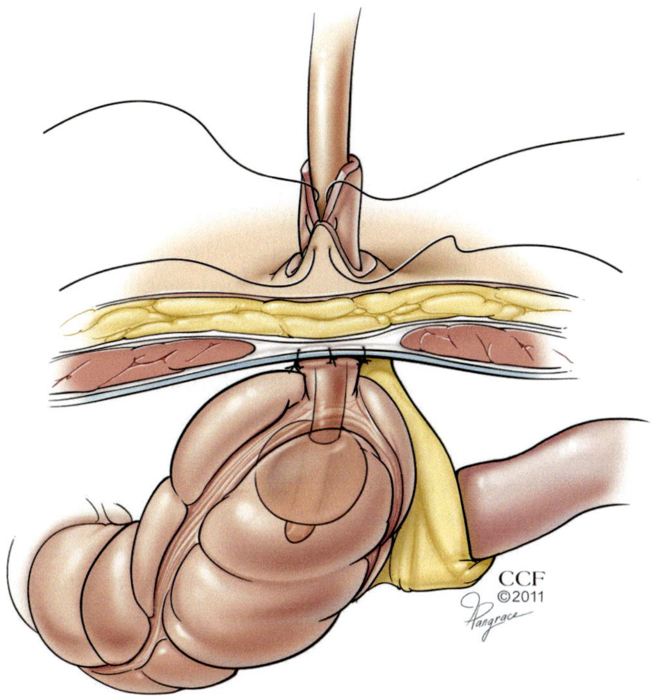

Fig. 16.20 Catheterized umbilical flap anastomosis in appendicostomy

There are now a number of palliative surgical options for Hirschsprung's disease, most of which can be performed without a protective colostomy in selected patients. Historically, however, the initial approach to a child suspected of having HD was to confirm the diagnosis by performing a transanal rectal wall biopsy, and then to perform a "leveling"

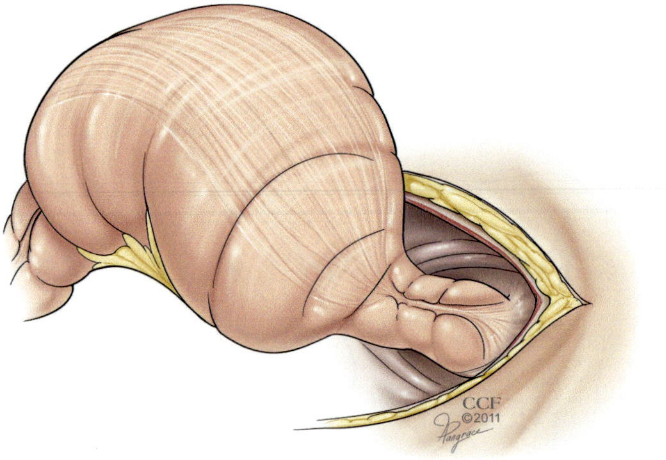

Fig. 16.21 Appearance of colon in typical Hirschsprung's disease

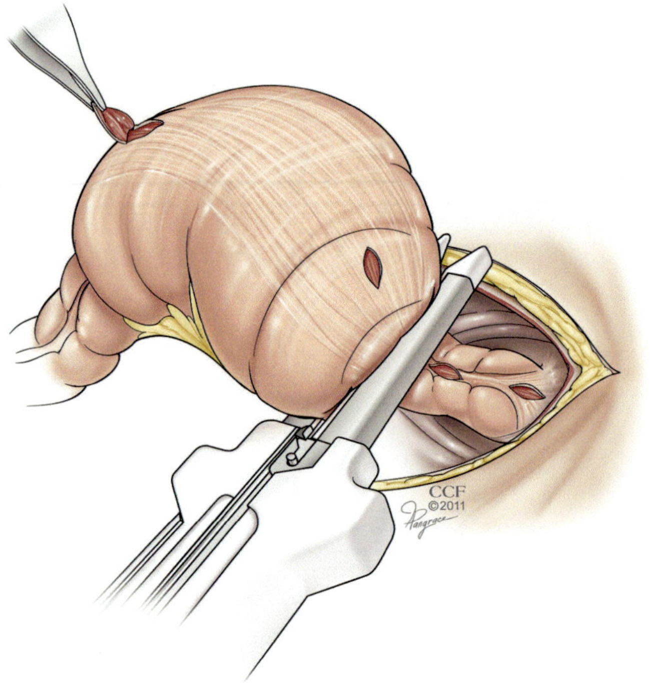

Fig. 16.22 Serial seromuscular biopsies to establish level of aganglionosis. Biopsies are performed through the antimesenteric *Tinea coli*, preserving mucosal layer intact. Limited resection of grossly abnormal colon segment

colostomy for temporary decompression. The modifier "leveling" was added to stress the importance of defining the zone of transition between normal ganglionic bowel and distal aganglionic bowel, and to perform a colostomy above that "level." Currently, leveling colostomies are still indicated in two groups of patients: those who present with acute stasis enterocolitis with significant physiologic compromise, and those with a delayed diagnosis in whom the proximal colon is chronically dilated and thick-walled – unsuitable for a pull-through procedure in its present state and in need of a longer period of decompression to regain a normal caliber.

Thus, a leveling colostomy is the combination of serial seromuscular colon wall biopsies for frozen section analysis, proceeding proximally from the peritoneal reflection, and the formation of a colostomy in the confirmed ganglionic bowel (Fig. 16.22). The transition zone is often characterized by a funnel-like reduction in caliber from proximal to distal. Although ganglion cells may be present histologically within this tapered segment, residual neural hypertrophy often persists and muscular relaxation is impaired. The "level" of aganglionosis is not circumferentially even; the leading edge of ganglion cell loss occurs around the bowel circumference in an undulating fashion over a length of several centimeters, resulting in adjacent zones that differ with respect to innervation. Therefore, the colostomy should be created at a level at least several centimeters proximal to the site of the most distal ganglionated biopsy specimen. The most dilated and hypertrophied segment of ganglionic bowel may be discarded as long as the remaining bowel will be of sufficient length to reach the anus. The transition zone occurs in the rectosigmoid region in roughly 75% of cases, in the more proximal colon in about 15% ("Long-segment HD"), at the ileocecal junction in about 10% ("Total-colon HD"), and rarely in the more proximal intestinal tract.

When the diagnosis is known from prior rectal biopsy and the typical recto-sigmoid transition zone is suspected radiologically, the procedure is usually done through an oblique left-lower quadrant incision. Some advocate performing a loop colostomy in the ganglionic proximal sigmoid colon, reasoning that a loop stoma does not interrupt the mesenteric blood supply, leaving more options when the definitive pull-through procedure is performed. We find that the propensity for loop stomas to prolapse make them less desirable, and that chronic prolapse renders the proximal limb chronically congested and thickened, and less suitable for a pull-through anastomosis. The authors prefer a simple end colostomy at a level proximal to the most dilated and hypertrophied bowel. We resect any bowel above the transition zone that is massively dilated and hypertrophied as we feel bowel chronically compromised in this fashion is an unreliable pull-through segment even after decompression. Preservation of bowel length in this area is irrelevant, and a pull-through procedure is easily performed using any point in the sigmoid or proximal left colon. In creating the end colostomy, the authors divide only the terminal vascular arcade to allow the colostomy to be straightened as it is externalized, and usually position the stoma in the lateral (superior) pole of the incision (Fig. 16.23). Some surgeons prefer a mucous fistula for decompression of the distal segment, but a closed distal pouch is well tolerated as long as no dilated bowel is left above the transition zone. If a mucous fistula is performed, it is usually placed in the lower

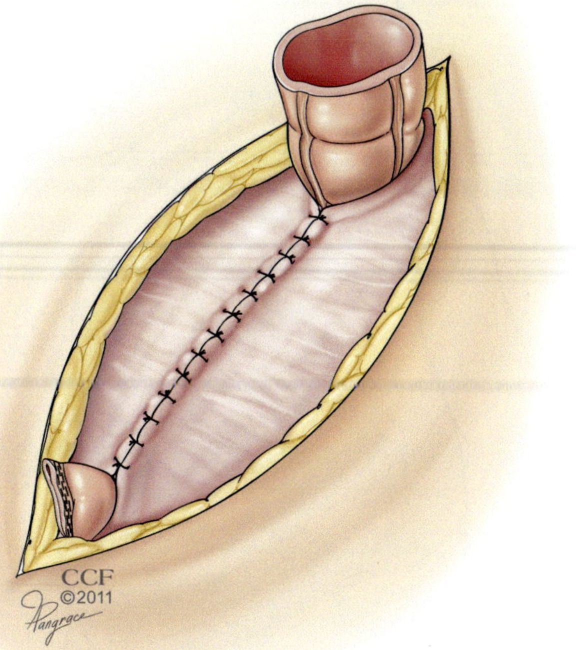

Fig. 16.23 End colostomy in upper pole of incision. Vented mucous fistula in lower pole

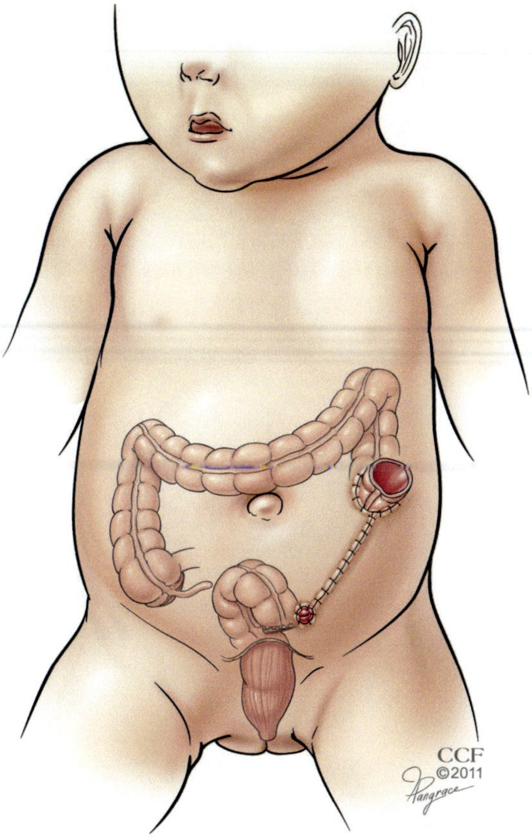

Fig. 16.24 Completed "leveling" colostomy and mucous fistula

pole of the incision, and may be performed at skin level, excising a corner of the staple line to provide a simple vent (Fig. 16.24).

If the transition zone is suspected of being more proximal than the rectosigmoid, then a vertical midline incision may be used and the stoma created where appropriate. If intraoperative frozen section biopsies are unobtainable, either because the operation is performed on an emergency basis or appropriate pathology expertise is unavailable, then a loop stoma may be created in the proximal transverse colon (Fig. 16.25). This option decompresses in both directions and will be above the transition zone in approximately 85% of cases, and close enough to it in the remainder to provide effective emergency decompression if required. Seromuscular biopsies are taken and processed for later examination. If the gross appearance of the bowel suggests total colon involvement, an end ileostomy should be performed.

Colostomy for Anorectal Malformations

Anorectal malformations are a heterogeneous group of congenital defects occurring in about 1 in 4,000 births. They are broadly classified according to the patient's sex, the distance from the end of the atretic rectum to perineum, and the presence or absence of fistulas in the perineum and genitourinary systems. Anorectal malformations are commonly associated with genitourinary, sacral, cardiac, tracheoesophageal, and other anomalies, which must be investigated. Their complexity and heterogeneity precludes an in-depth discussion of definitive management of anorectal malformations and the associated anomalies here. Detailed descriptions are found in many excellent chapters by Pena and other experts in standard pediatric surgery texts [10, 11]. Broadly speaking, colostomies are usually constructed for "high" defects prior to more complex reconstructions. "Low" defects are usually reconstructed primarily in the neonatal period. Decisions about "high" or "low" defects are made most of the time based on the perineal examination, cross-table lateral films, and urinalysis. These clinical decisions are generally delayed for 18–24 h after birth to allow time for meconium to appear on the perineum, as in the case of imperforate anus with perineal fistula, allowing identification of these "low" defects by visual inspection.

A colostomy is indicated in neonates with complex or "high" defects (females with a cloaca, a rectovestibular fistula, or no obvious perineal cutaneous fistula; males with a flat underdeveloped perineum and buttocks, genitourinary

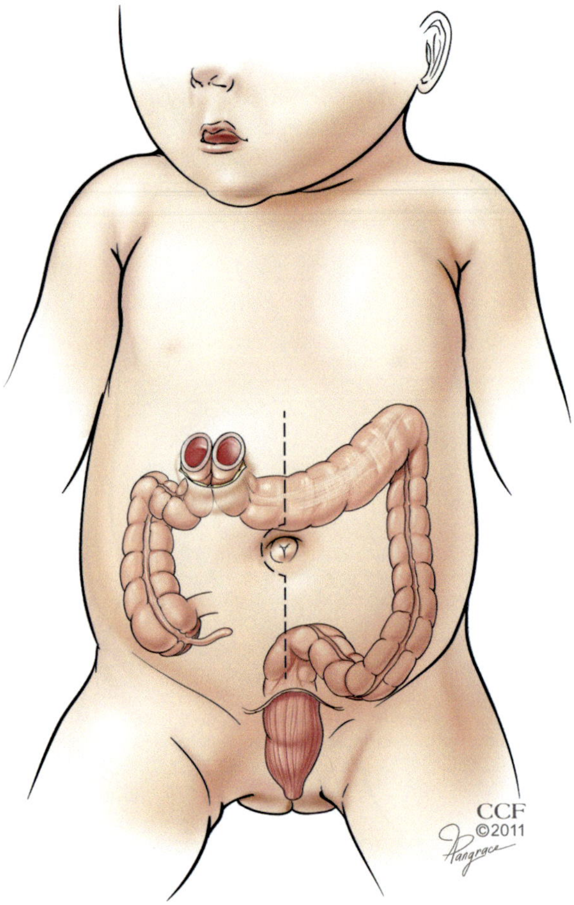

Fig. 16.25 Proximal transverse loop colostomy

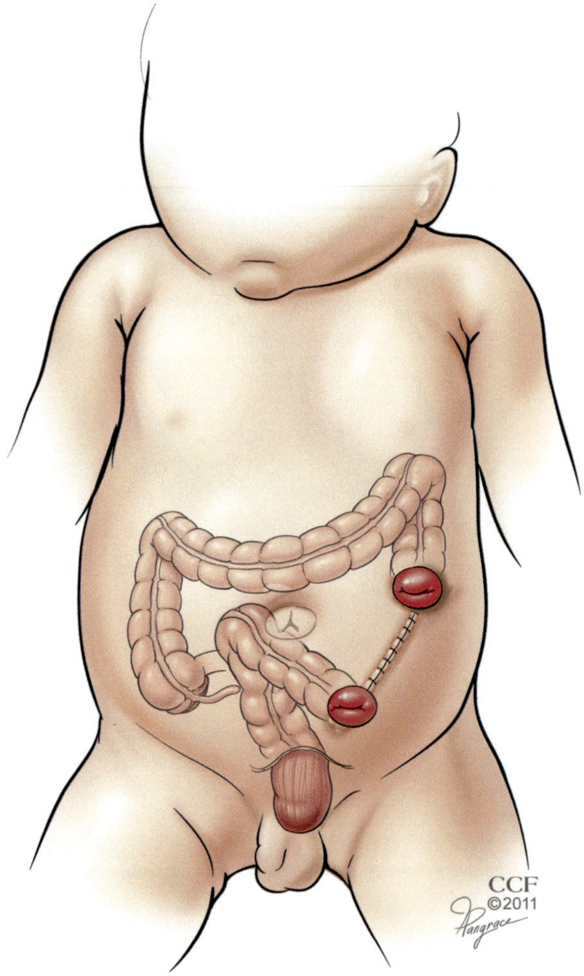

Fig. 16.26 Descending divided colostomy for anorectal malformations

fistula or without a perineal fistula). In environments of limited resources and expertise with anorectal malformations, when failure to relieve the distal obstruction will result in significant harm, a colostomy may be the wisest initial course of action. Girls with a rectoperineal cutaneous fistula may undergo dilations of the fistula, until an anoplasty can be performed.

A descending divided colostomy with a distal mucous fistula done via a left lower quadrant oblique incision is recommended (Fig. 16.26). The proximal colostomy and a small mucous fistula are brought out at the upper and lower ends of the wound and the fascia and skin are closed in between. The distal meconium is irrigated out. This configuration allows the proximal colostomy to be bagged separately from the mucous fistula to prevent urinary tract infection, in the case of genitourinary fistulas. The mucous fistula allows access to the distal colon for colostography to define rectourethral and bladder neck fistulas, passage of urine to reduce metabolic acidosis from absorption, and decompression of the distal segment to avoid megarectosigmoid. The divided descending colostomy reduces the risk of stomal prolapse, versus loop colostomies. The critical point in the construction of the descending colostomy is to open it just distal to the fixed portion of the descending colon and proximal to the more mobile sigmoid colon. This prevents prolapse of the proximal stoma and allows adequate distal length for the rectosigmoid colon to reach the perineum at the time of definitive reconstruction via a laparoscopic pull-through or posterior sagittal anorectoplasty.

References

1. Gauderer MW, Ponsky JL, Izant Jr RJ. Gastrostomy without laparotomy: a percutaneous endoscopic technique. J Pediatr Surg. 1980;15:872–5.
2. Gauderer MWL. Feeding gastrostomy button: experience and recommendations. J Pediatr Surg. 1988;23:24–8.
3. Gauderer MWL, Picha GJ, Izant RJ. The gastrostomy "button" – a simple, skin-level, nonrefluxing device for long-term enteral feedings. J Pediatr Surg. 1984;19:803–5.
4. Nixdorff N, Diluciano J, Ponsky T, et al. The endoscopic U-stitch technique for primary button placement: an institution's experience. Surg Endosc. 2010;24:1200–3.

5. Williams AR, Borsellino A, Sugarman ID, et al. Roux-en-Y feeding jejunostomy in infants and children. Eur J Pediatr Surg. 2007;17:29–33.
6. Bishop HS, Koop CE. Management of meconium ileus: resection, Roux-en-Y anastomosis and ileostomy irrigation with pancreatic enzymes. Ann Surg. 1957;145:410–4.
7. O'Neill JA, Grosfeld JR, Boles ET, et al. Surgical management of meconium ileus. Am J Surg. 1970;119:99–105.
8. Nanigian DK, Kurzrock EA. Intermediate-term outcome of the simplified laparoscopic antegrade continence enema procedure: less is better. J Urol. 2008;179:299–303.
9. Swenson O, Rheinlander H, Diamond I. Hirschsprung's disease: a new concept of the etiology – operative results in thirty-four patients. N Engl J Med. 1949;241:551–6.
10. Pena A. Atlas of surgical management of anorectal malformations. New York: Springer; 1990.
11. Shaul DB, Harrison EA. Classification of anorectal malformations – initial approach, diagnostic tests and colostomy. Semin Pediatr Surg. 1997;6:187–95.

Antegrade Colonic Enema (ACE) 17

Brooke Gurland, Crina V. Floruta, and Ian C. Lavery

Introduction

Retrograde rectal irrigation through various enema techniques is a well-accepted practice to empty the lower bowel and to relieve constipation and fecal soiling in patients with functional bowel disorders [1]. However, retrograde enemas can be technically challenging for elderly and disabled patients and may require caregiver assistance. For the patient with severe bowel dysfunction who is contemplating a permanent colostomy, the antegrade colonic enema (ACE) procedure may be a viable option. This procedure allows easy access to the colon through the abdominal wall with intermittent catheterization, irrigation of the colon, and rapid, controlled bowel purging (Fig. 17.1). The goal is to avoid wearing a stoma pouch while allowing the patient to independently manage his or her own bowel activities.

The ACE technique was first described by Malone in 1990 using the appendix as the conduit but since them the cecum, ileum, and left colon have been utilized as the continence mechanism [2–5]. Malone adapted this concept from the urology literature where a cutaneous appendicovesicostomy was introduced to maintain urinary continence [6]. These procedures have become increasingly popular for children with spinal dysraphism and anorectal malformations and are well reported in the pediatric literature [7]. The ACE procedure is gaining recognition in the adult population for patients with colonic neurologic dysfunction, colonic inertia, obstructed defecation, and fecal incontinence [8–15].

Variations to the traditional ACE procedure have also been reported with success. The results of laparoscopic ACE procedures using the technique of in situ appendix without cecoplication have promising results [16, 17]. Left-sided ACE procedures with irrigation of the descending colon for

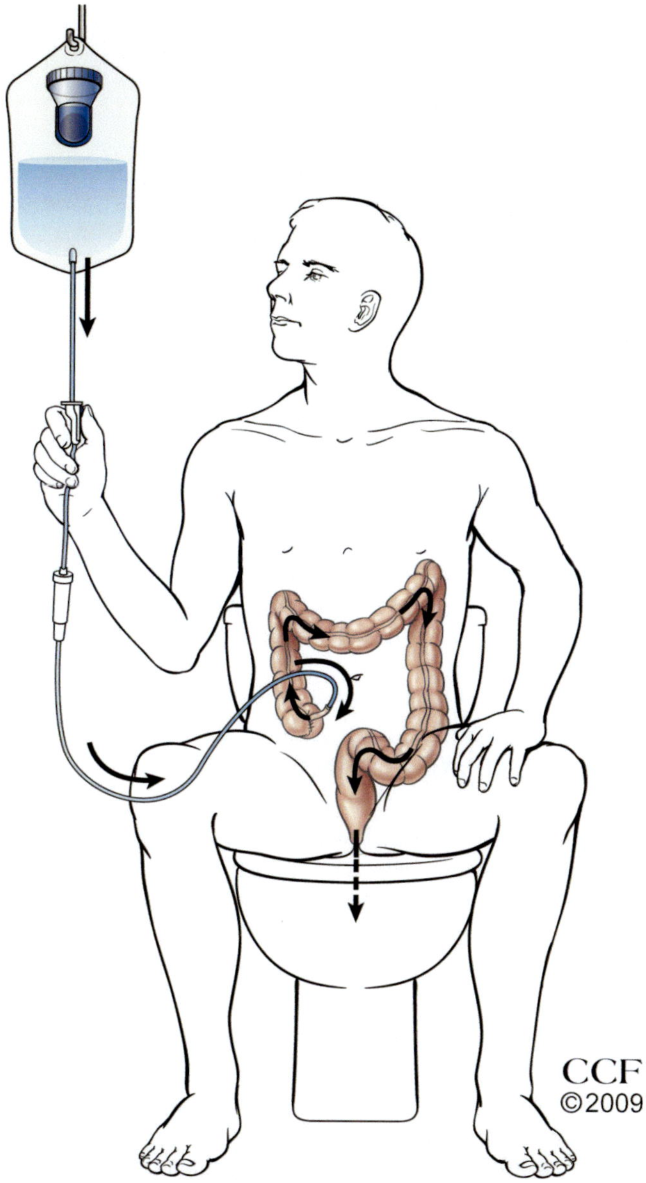

Fig. 17.1 The catheter is intermittently inserted into an orifice on the anterior abdominal wall and into the cecum for irrigation of the colon and rapid and controlled bowel purging. Illustration © CCF

B. Gurland (✉) • C.V. Floruta • I.C. Lavery
Department of Colorectal Surgery, Digestive Disease Institute, Cleveland Clinic Foundation, Cleveland, OH, USA
e-mail: gurlanb@ccf.org

V.W. Fazio et al. (eds.), *Atlas of Intestinal Stomas*,
DOI 10.1007/978-0-387-78851-7_17, © Springer Science+Business Media, LLC 2012

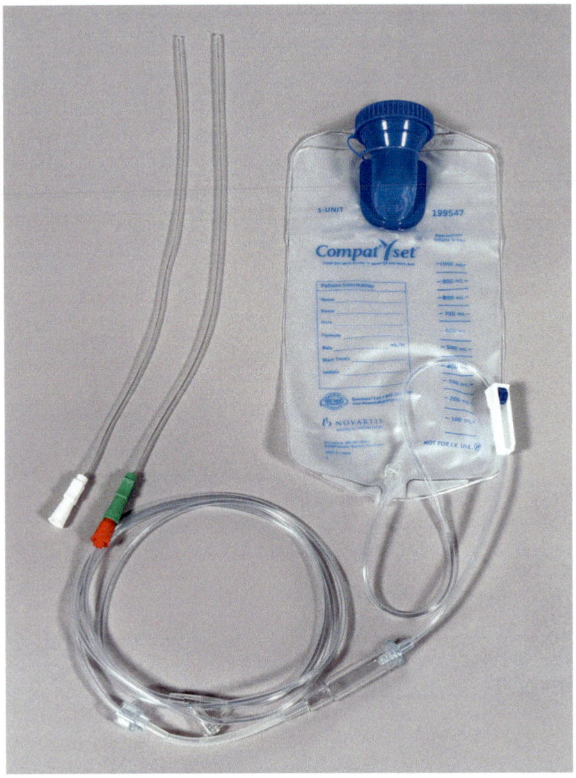

Fig. 17.2 A 12–14 Fr silastic catheter is used to intubate the stoma. A tube feeding bag with long tubing, to allow for adequate access, and a handheld control flow regulator is recommended

patients with constipation have shown decreased irrigation times and require less fluid compared to those patients with right colon access [18]. Percutaneous endoscopic placement of tubes into the left or right colon can provide minimally invasive access to the bowel for irrigation and decompression [19].

Indications/Patient Selection

Patients who have severe bowel dysfunction with fecal soiling or constipation who have failed medical or surgical treatments may be candidates for the ACE procedure. The ACE procedure does not preclude colectomy or stoma creation. Successful outcomes depend on patient expectations and motivations. Colonic irrigation is a life-long commitment and a rigid, time-consuming regimen. Bowel irrigation and evacuation takes approximately 45–60 min every day or every other day to adequately purge the bowel. Determining the correct volume of fluid irrigant and additives for optimal colonic wash out is achieved through trial and error. Nursing support to work with patients to determine the irrigation recipe is as important as the technical aspects of the procedure.

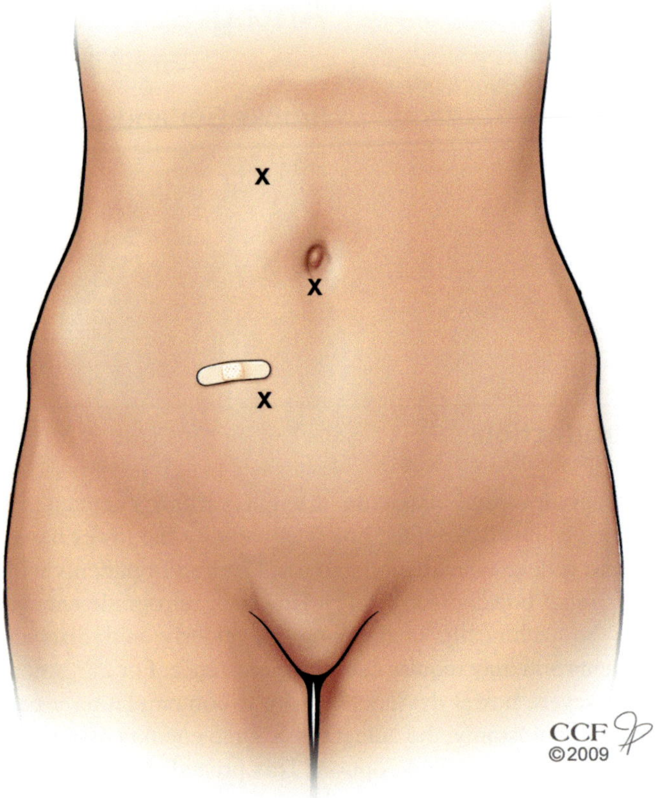

Fig. 17.3 The abdominal wall is marked preoperatively so that the conduit is not brought up into a fold in the abdominal wall and that access is easy in the sitting or lying position. Any of the three positions that are marked can be used depending on the patient body habitus. Illustration © CCF

Preoperative Preparation

Equipment: Patients are familiarized with the enema equipment preoperatively. A 12–14 Fr silastic catheter is used to intubate the stoma. A tube feeding bag with long tubing to allow for adequate access and a handheld control flow regulator is recommended (Fig. 17.2).

Stoma marking: The abdominal wall is marked preoperatively so that the conduit is not brought up into a fold in the abdominal wall and access is easy in the sitting or lying position. It is imperative that the site is visible to the patient. The conduit can be brought out through the umbilicus, right or left lower quadrant. Although the umbilicus may be cosmetically appealing the authors prefer the right lower quadrant in adults with a thick abdominal wall. For patients who are wheelchair bound it may be necessary to site the stoma on the upper abdomen for ease of access (Fig. 17.3).

Perioperative prophylactic antibiotics and bowel cleansing preparations are given to all patients.

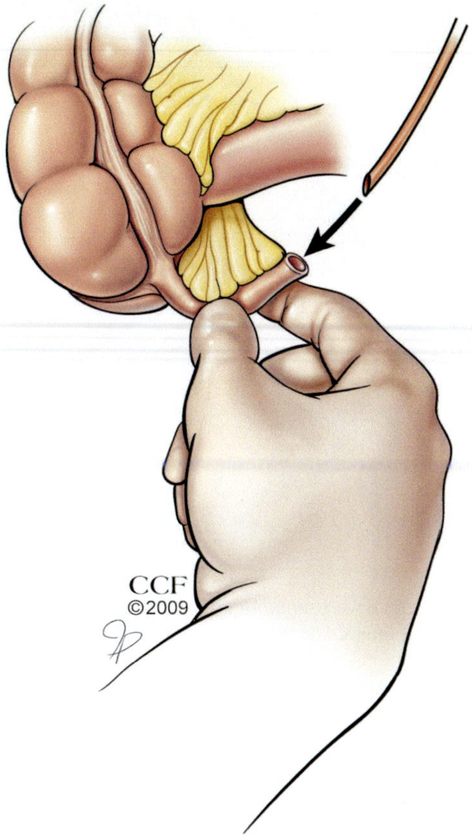

Fig. 17.4 The tip of the appendix is removed and a stay suture is inserted to stretch out the appendix to reveal the mesentery. A 12 Fr catheter is passed through the appendix to the cecum. Illustration © CCF

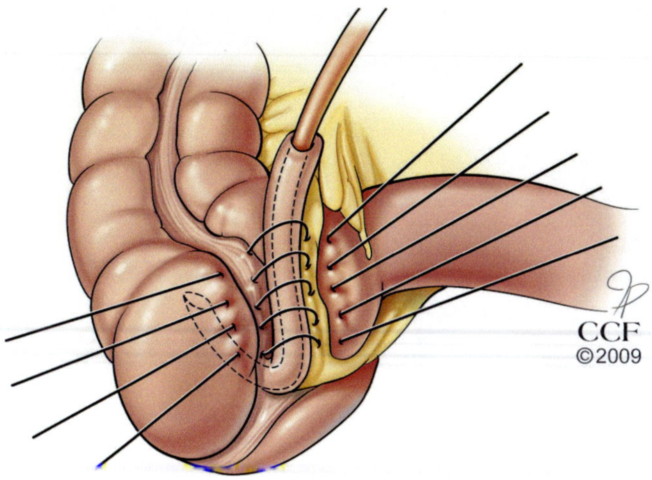

Fig. 17.5 A valve mechanism is created to avoid backflow of fecal material through the conduit. Illustration © CCF

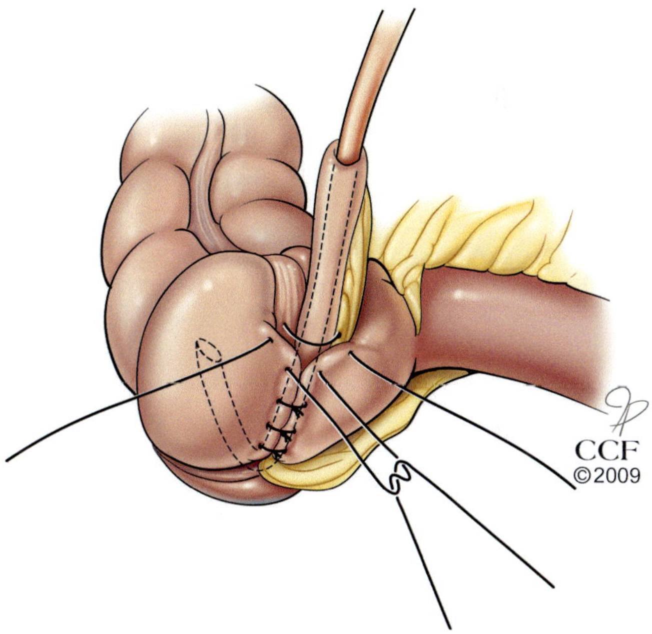

Fig. 17.6 The appendix is folded and the cecum is loosely wrapped around the appendix. Illustration © CCF

Operative Steps

1. The ACE can be performed via a laparoscopic or open technique with a midline, transverse, or right lower quadrant abdominal incision. The cecum is mobilized so that it easily reaches the abdominal wall. Malone initially described using the reversed appendix as the conduit with the amputated tip tunneled in the cecum, but this is no longer recommended and the appendix is left in situ.
2. The tip of the appendix is removed and a stay suture is inserted to stretch out the appendix to reveal the mesentery. A 12 Fr catheter is passed through the appendix to the cecum (Fig. 17.4).
3. A valve mechanism is created to avoid backflow of fecal material through the conduit. The appendix is folded and the cecum is loosely wrapped around the appendix (Figs. 17.5 and 17.6). The suture picks up the seromuscular layer on the cecum on each side of the appendix to anchor the tunnel. The cecum is anchored to the back of the anterior abdominal wall where the appendix emerges to prevent twisting and kinking of the conduit.
4. For patients without an appendix: A 5–10 cm segment of terminal ileum is isolated on its vascular pedicle (Fig. 17.7). A longer conduit is needed for a patient with a thicker abdominal wall. Bowel continuity is restored using a standard end-to-end anastomosis (Fig. 17.8). The isolated ileum is tubularized over a 12 Fr catheter by using a stapling device on the antimesenteric surface to narrow the lumen (Fig. 17.9). One end is then implanted into a submucosal tenial tunnel in the cecum and the other is brought to the skin as a stoma.
5. The colonic submucosal tunnel is created by incising the seromuscular layer of the tenia with a scalpel down to the

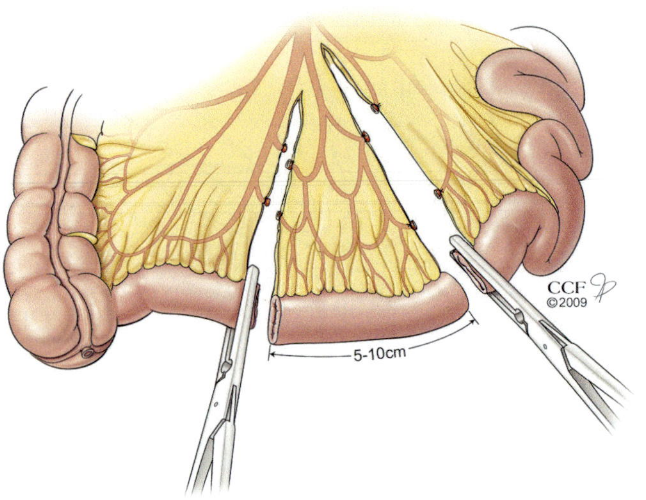

Fig. 17.7 For patients without an appendix, a 5–10 cm segment of terminal ileum is isolated on its vascular pedicle. Illustration © CCF

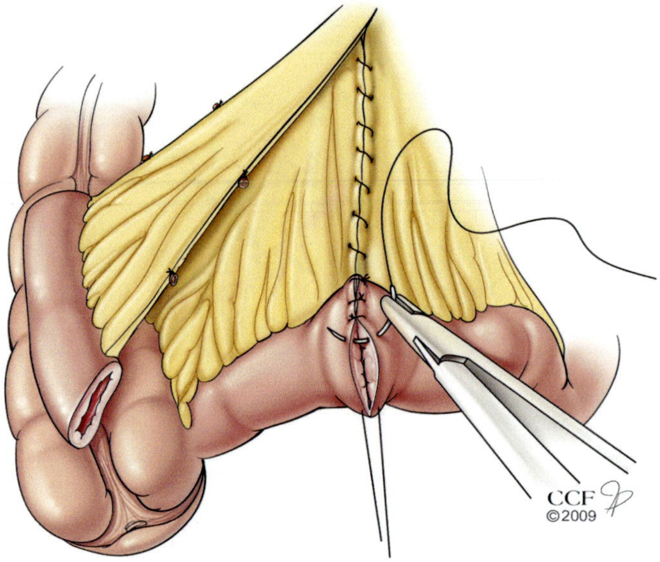

Fig. 17.8 Small bowel continuity is restored using a standard end-to-end anastomosis. Illustration © CCF

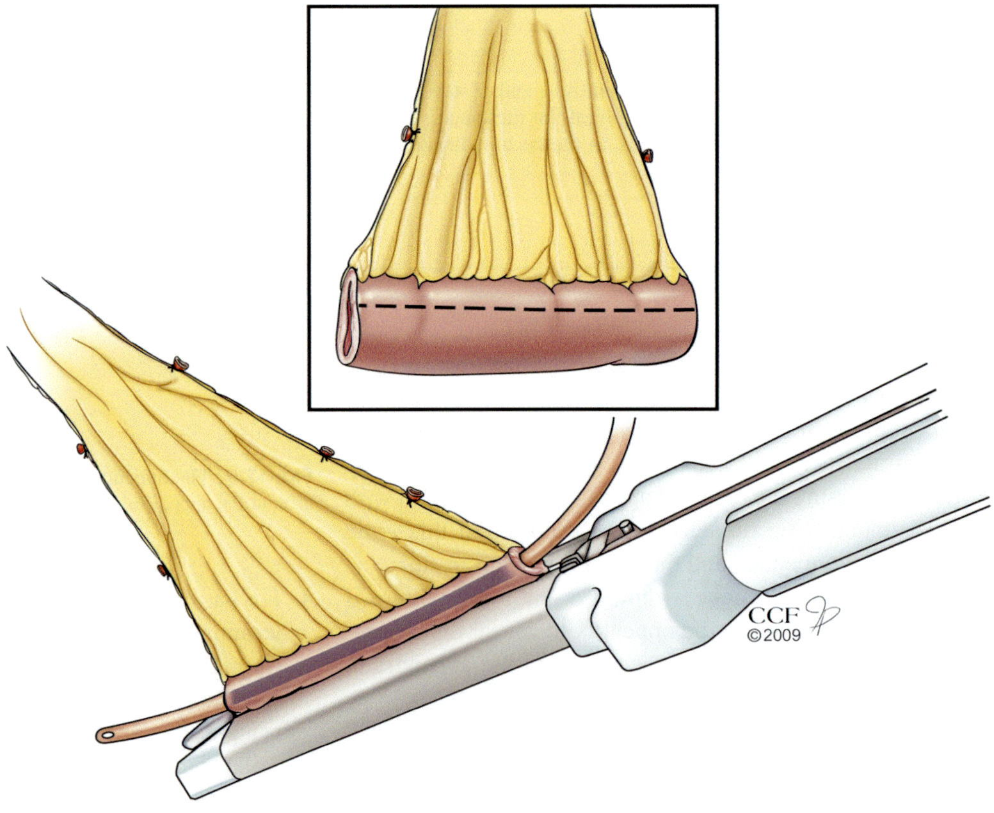

Fig. 17.9 The bowel is tubularized over a 12 Fr catheter by using a stapling device on the antimesenteric surface to narrow the lumen. Illustration © CCF

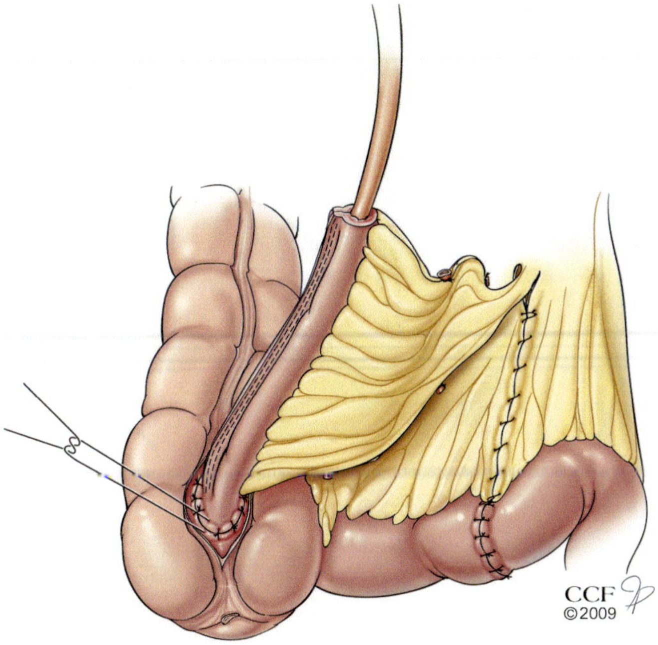

Fig. 17.10 An enterotomy is made at the distal end of the tunnel and the mucosa is sutured to the full thickness of the ileal conduit using absorbable sutures. Illustration © CCF

submucosa over a 7 cm length. An enterotomy is made at the distal end of the tunnel and the mucosa is sutured to the full thickness of the ileal conduit using 3.0 Vicryl sutures (Fig. 17.10). The seromuscular wall of the colon is closed over the conduit using 3.0 chromic sutures picking up partial thickness of the tunnel to prevent slippage (Fig. 17.11).

6. Stoma creation: A V-shape skin incision is made at the previously marked stoma location. An aperture is created through the abdominal wall that is sufficiently wide to allow the conduit to pass freely. The cecum is sutured to the anterior abdominal wall to prevent tension on the stoma or volvulus of the bowel on the conduit. If the conduit has a very small caliber, such as an appendix, it is spatulated and the apex of the V-flap is sutured into the defect using 4.0 chromic sutures with the knots outside the catheterizing channel (Figs. 17.12 and 17.13).

Postoperative Care

A 12 Fr silicone catheter remains in the conduit for a minimum of 21 days postoperatively. Irrigations start on postoperative day number 4, using 500–1000 cm^3 of normal saline as tolerated by patient.

The patient is started on a liquid diet on postoperative day number one and advanced to a GI soft diet as tolerated.

The patient is discharged with the indwelling catheter on day 5 and is expected to irrigate the indwelling daily with

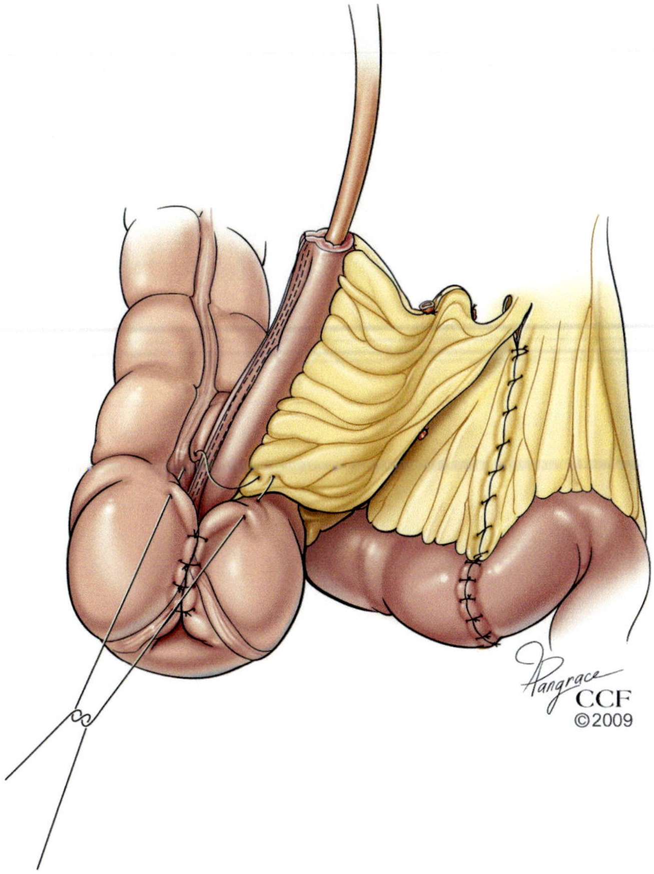

Fig. 17.11 The seromuscular wall of the colon is closed over the conduit, picking up partial thickness of the tunnel to prevent slippage. Illustration © CCF

500–1000 cm^3 of tap water. The patient returns 3 weeks later to learn intermittent catheterization.

The stoma should be catheterized daily whether or not an enema is being given to avoid stenosis.

Complications

Stoma stenosis and local wound infections are the most common complications reported.

Leakage of stool is an uncommon complication. If this occurs the valve mechanism can be revised.

Conclusion

The ACE procedure is an alternative for patients with refractory fecal incontinence or constipation who would like to avoid wearing a permanent stoma appliance. Colonic irrigation is a lifelong commitment and it requires a motivated patient and educated nursing staff for ongoing support. However, for the appropriate individual the ACE can be very gratifying.

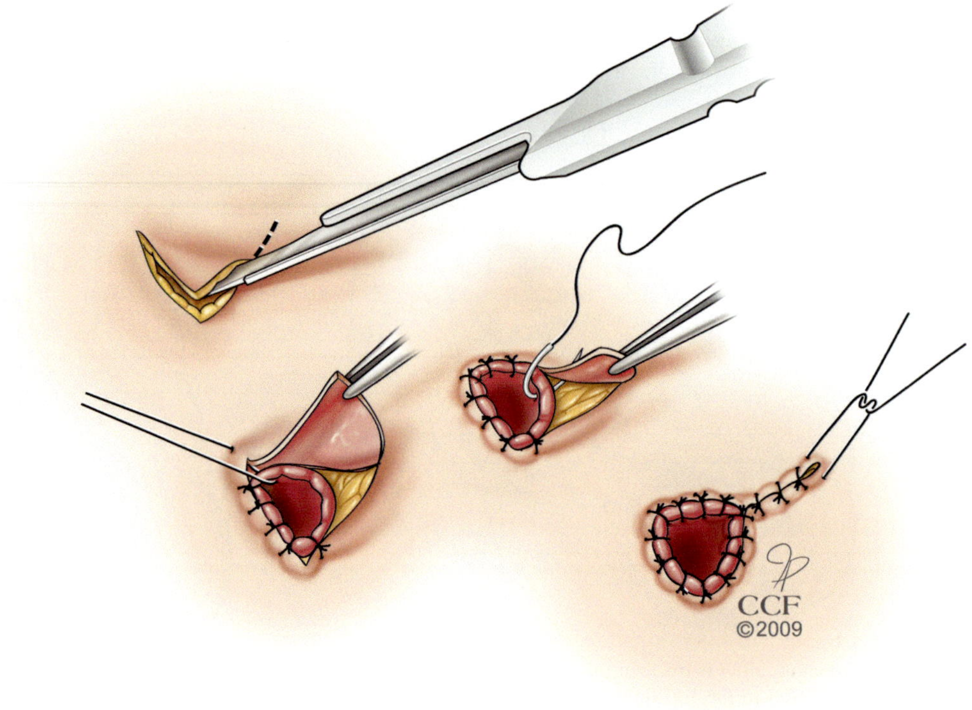

Fig. 17.12 A V-shape skin incision is made at the previously marked location and the stoma is created. Illustration © CCF

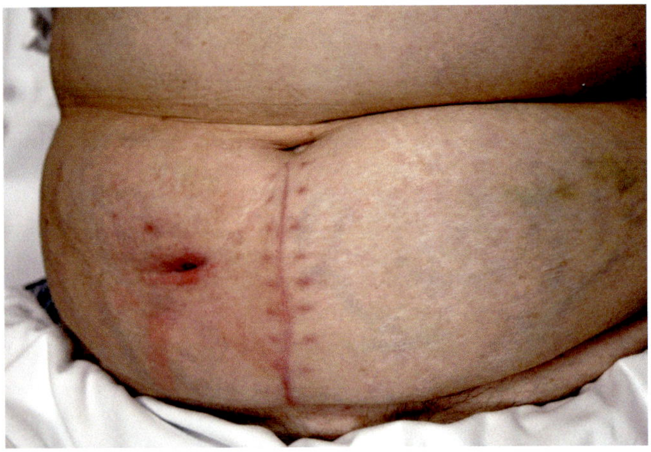

Fig. 17.13 The ACE orifice

References

1. Briel JW, Schouten WR, Vlot EA, Smits S, van Kessel I. Clinical value of colonic irrigation in patients with continence disturbances. Dis Colon Rectum. 1997;40(7):802–5.
2. Malone PS, Ransey PG, Kiely EM. Preliminary report: the antegrade continence mechanism. Lancet. 1990;336:1217–8.
3. Monti PR, Lara RC, Dutra MA, De Carvallo JR. New techniques for construction of efferent conduits based on the Mitranoff principle. Urology. 1997;49:112–5.
4. Willams NS, Hughes SF, Stuchfield B. Continent colonic conduit for rectal evacuation in severe constipation. Lancet. 1994;343(8909):1321–4.
5. Kiely EM, Ade-Ajayi N, Wheeler RA. Caecal flap conduit for antegrade continence enemas. Br J Surg. 1994;81(8):1215.
6. Mitrofanoff P. Cystostomie continenente trans-appendiculare dans le traitment des vessies neurologiques. Chir Pediatr. 1980;21:297–305.
7. Sinha CK, Grewal A, Ward HC. Antegrade continence mechanism (ACE): current practice. Pediatr Surg Int. 2008;24(6):658–8.
8. Worsoe J, Christensen P, Krogh K, Buntzen S, Laurberg S. Long-term results of antegrade colonic enema in adult patients: assessment of functional results. Dis Colon Rectum. 2008;51(10):1523–8.
9. Poirier M, Abcarian H, Nelson R. Malone antegrade continent enema: an alternative to resection in severe defecation disorders. Dis Colon Rectum. 2007;50(1):22–8.
10. Dick AC, McCallion WA, Brown S, Boston VE. Antegrade colonic enemas. Br J Surg. 1996;83:642–4.
11. Gerharz EW, Vik W, Webb G, Leaver R, Shah PJ, Woodhouse CR. The value of the MACE procedure in adult patients. JAM Coll Surg. 1997;185:544–7.
12. Teichman JM, Harris JM, Currie DM, Barber DB. Malone antegrade continence mechanism for adults with neurogenic bowel disease. J Urol. 1998;160:1278–81.
13. Hirst GR, Arumugam PJ, Watkins AJ, Mackey P, Morgan AR, Carr ND, et al. Antegrade continence enema in the treatment in the treatment of obstructed defecation with or without fecal incontinence. Tech Coloproctol. 2005;9:217–21.
14. Lees NP, Hodson P, Hill J, Pearson RC, MacLennan I. Long term results of the antergrade continent enema procedure for adults with constipation. Colorectal Dis. 2004;6(5):362–8.
15. Rongen MJ, van der Hoop Gerritsen, Baeten CG. Cecal access for antegrade colon enemas in medically refractory slow transit constipation. Dis Colon Rectum. 2001;44:1644–9.
16. Nanigian DK, Kurzrock EA. Intermediate – Term outcome of the simplified laparoscopic antegrade continence enema procedure: less is better. J Urol. 2008;179:299–303.
17. Webb HW, Barraza MA, Crump JM. Laparoscopic appendicostomy for management of fecal incontinence. J Pediatr Surg. 1997;32:457–8.
18. Sinha CK, Butler C, Haddad M. Left Antegrade Colonic Enema (LACE): review of the literature. Eur J Pediatr Surg. 2008;18(4):215–8.
19. Uno Y. Introducer method of percutaneous endoscopic cecostomy and antegrade continence enema by use of the Chait Trapdoor cecostomy catheter in patients with adult neurogenic bowel. Gastrointest Endosc. 2006;63:666–73.

Urinary Stomas

18

Amit R. Patel and Amr F. Fergany

Introduction

The formation of a urinary stoma may be indicated in the patient that requires urinary diversion. Patients with urologic/gynecologic malignancy such as bladder cancer or cervical cancer; benign conditions such as neuropathic bladder, extensive urethral stricture disease, complex urinary fistulas, or congenital malformations; and inflammatory disorders of the lower urinary tract with either irradiation or immunologic etiology are all indications for lower urinary tract diversion. The use of bowel has remained a constant for the last 150 years in diverting the genitourinary tract.

The first stomas were internal, such as ureterorectal ligations for bladder exstrophy by Sir John Simon in 1851, Boari's mechanical button in 1895 to avoid ureteral stenosis, and Madyl's intraperitoneal bladder trigone reimplantation into the sigmoid. Coffey developed the ureterosigmoidostomy in 1911, which remained the preferable alternative to noncontinent external drainage. Eventually urinary stomas evolved into cutaneous stomas. Verhoogen's continent catheterizable ileocecal pouch was introduced in 1909, later abandoned, brought back into favor by Gilchrist, and finally re-emerged as the Indiana pouch. Bricker's reintroduction of ileal conduit in 1950 as a diversion with fewer complications and greater technical feasibility [1] made it one of the most commonly used urinary stomas. Today, urologic surgeons can choose from an arsenal of urinary stomas from ileovesicostomies to noncontinent conduits to pouches with continent cutaneous catheterizable stomas.

A.R. Patel (✉)
Urologic Oncology, University of Chicago
Medical Center, Chicago, IL, USA
e-mail: amitpdoc@gmail.com

A.F. Fergany
Glickman Urological and Kidney Institute,
Cleveland Clinic Foundation, Cleveland, OH, USA

The scope of this chapter will cover urinary stomas, including the use of bowel to create urinary stomas. We will discuss the indications, operative techniques, and complications of cutaneous vesicostomies, conduits, and continent pouches with catheterizable cutaneous stomas.

Vesicostomy

Indications

The vesicostomy is the procedure of choice in patients requiring immediate, temporary urinary diversion. It is often used in children as a temporizing measure for acute renal failure, urinary sepsis, or bladder outlet obstruction from posterior urethral valves. The continent vesicostomy procedure can be performed for patients who have a large capacity bladder but do not have good bladder-emptying function. Patients with lower motor neuron lesion or prune belly syndrome may benefit from continent catheterizable vesicostomy made from the bladder itself.

Operative Technique: Noncontinent Vesicostomy

The noncontinent vesicostomy is usually placed between the pubic symphysis and the umbilicus. A 2–3-cm midline incision is made through the anterior rectus fascia. Using a Balfour or other self-retaining retractor, the rectus bellies are separated, and the space of Retzius is entered. The peritoneum is bluntly dissected off the bladder wall. The bladder is opened adjacent to the midline near the dome of the bladder. The bladder wall adjacent to the cystotomy is secured to the rectus fascia with interrupted 4-0 polydioxanone (PDS) suture. The mucosa is approximated to the skin edges using interrupted 4-0 chromic suture.

V.W. Fazio et al. (eds.), *Atlas of Intestinal Stomas*,
DOI 10.1007/978-0-387-78851-7_18, © Springer Science+Business Media, LLC 2012

Operative Technique: Continent Vesicostomy

The bladder is exposed through a midline or Pfannenstiel incision. The peritoneum is swept off of the dome and posterior aspect of the bladder. The bladder is filled with saline and distended through a urinary catheter. A bladder flap measuring approximately 7 cm in length and 2 cm in width is marked just lateral to the midline (Fig. 18.1a). The strip is rotated cephalad, and an additional 3 cm of mucosal flap is dissected free from the detrusor (Fig. 18.1b). The mucosal flap is tubularized over a 12 French catheter using a running 4-0 Vicryl suture (Fig. 18.1c, d). The full-thickness bladder flap is tubularized over the catheter using a running 3-0 Vicryl suture (Fig. 18.1e, f), ensuring full-thickness mucosa and serosa into the anastomosis. The tubularized bladder flap will serve as the continent catheterizable stoma.

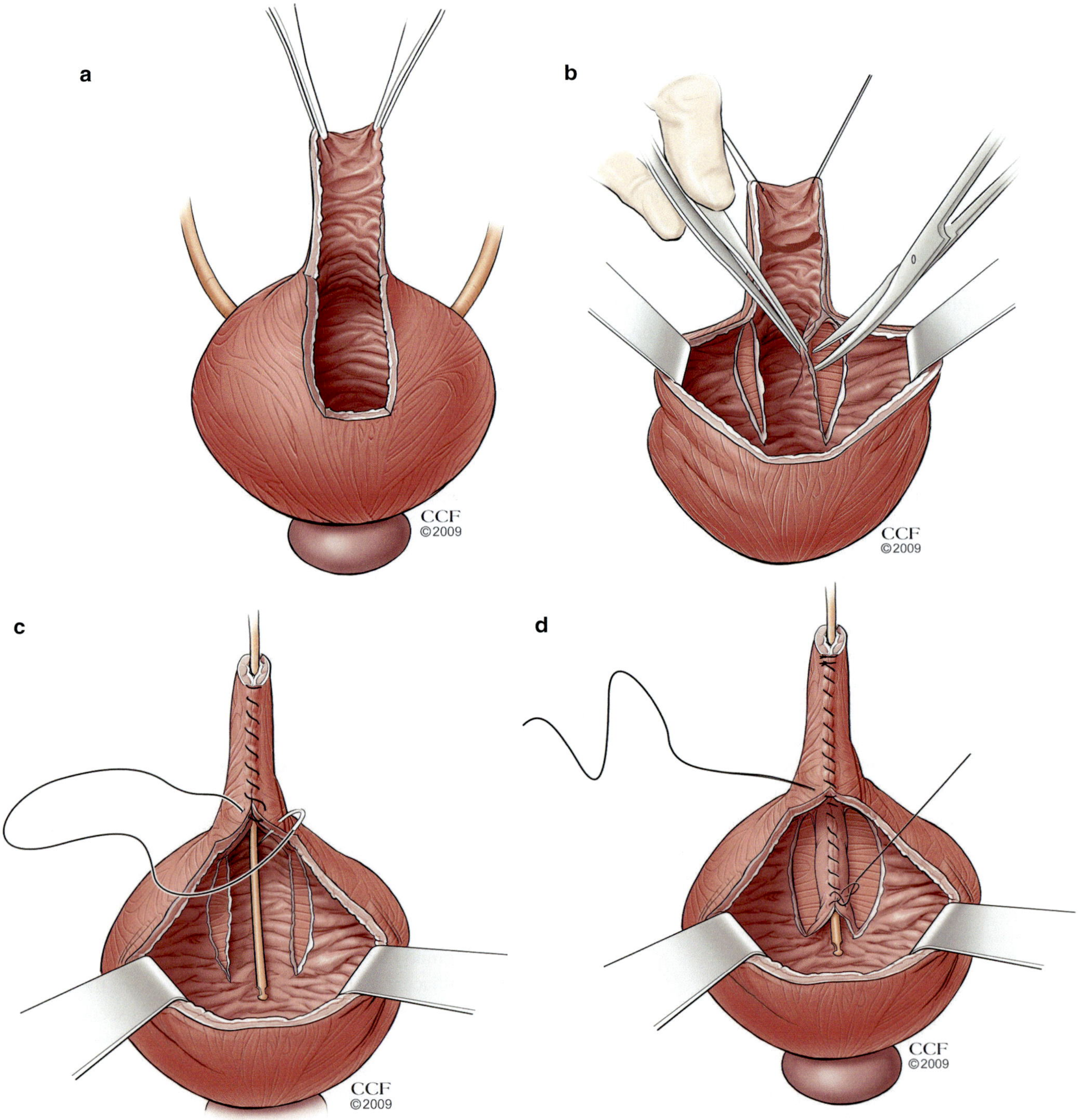

Fig. 18.1 Continent vesicostomy. (**a**) A flap is created from the mobilized bladder. (**b**, **c**) A submucosal flap is created and tubularized over a catheter. (**d**, **e**) The internal mucosal layers are closed over the catheter in two layers. (**f**) The bladder is closed with full-thickness sutures involving mucosa and serosa. Illustration © CCF

Fig. 18.1 (continued)

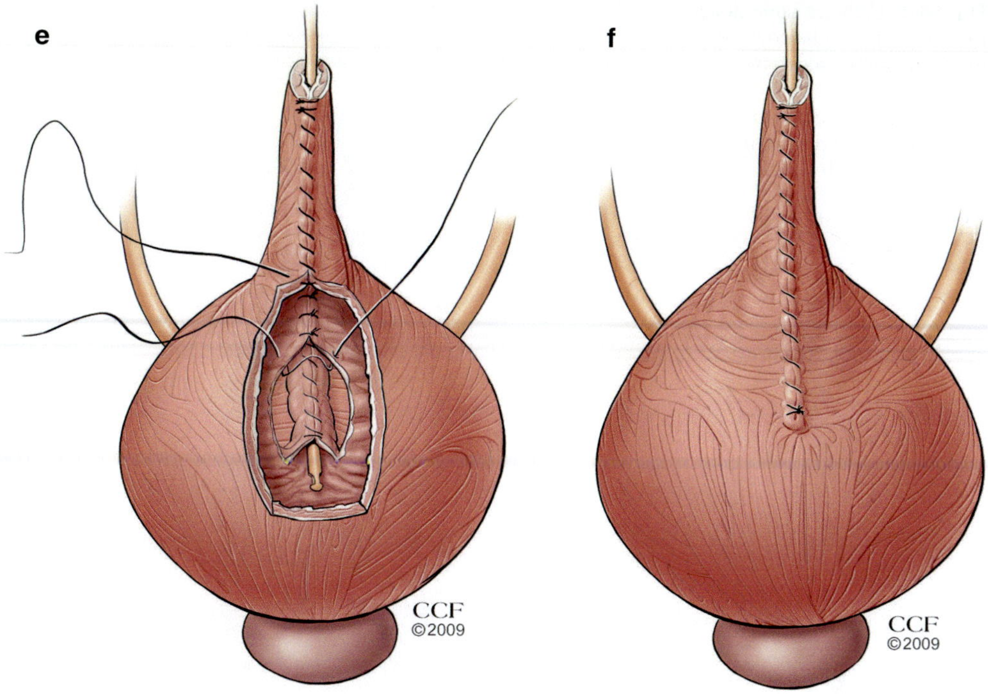

Catheterizable Stoma Formation (for Continent Vesicostomies and Pouches)

The stoma site should be selected to allow for a tension-free anastomosis. A V-shaped skin incision is made at the stomal site for interposition into the stoma. The flap is dissected through the subcutaneous fat to the fascia. A cruciate incision is made in the fascia and bluntly dilated to just beyond the caliber of the stoma. The stoma is brought out through the anterior abdominal wall to the skin and spatulated to allow for a cosmetic closure and to reduce stomal stenosis (Fig. 18.2a). The apex of the triangular skin flap is secured to the apex of the spatulated stoma using interrupted 4-0 Vicryl suture (Fig. 18.2b). The stomal anastomosis is completed using interrupted 4-0 Vicryl suture. The stoma should be catheterized several times to ensure ease of catheterization without kinking of the stoma. The stoma can also be secured with a single interrupted 3-0 Vicryl suture to the posterior abdominal wall to reduce kinking. The anterior bladder wall is secured to the posterior rectus sheath using 2-0 Vicryl suture.

Appendicovesicostomy and the Mitrofanoff Principle

Mitrofanoff reported the use of isolated appendix implanted into the bladder as a continent cystostomy [2]. The Mitrofanoff principle relies on a narrow conduit (appendix, ureter, or tapered bowel) connected between the skin and a large urinary reservoir (augmented bladder or urinary pouch) in an anti-refluxing manner. The conduit remains continent and is easy to catheterize to drain the reservoir.

Operative Technique

The right colon is mobilized beyond the hepatic flexure, and the appendix and its mesentery is carefully dissected off of the cecal attachments (Fig. 18.3a). Care is taken to preserve the appendiceal artery, a branch off of the ileocolic artery. Assessment of the mobilized appendix is necessary to ensure adequate reach to the bladder and chosen stoma site. The appendix is detached from the cecum sharply, and the cecal opening is closed using absorbable running suture, followed by Lembert sutures to over the closure line. An edge of cecum should be left on the appendix to provide a distal stoma that has reduced risk for stricture. The terminal end of the appendix is opened, and the lumen is dilated using serial metal sounds to ensure passage of a 12-Fr catheter.

A bladder hiatus is chosen for implantation of the appendix or Monti-Yang segment (see Yang-Monti Ileovesicostomy), ensuring adequate distance to reach the selected stoma site. The conduit is brought into the bladder through the hiatus (Fig. 18.3b). At least a 2–3-cm submucosal tunnel should be made and the conduit passed under the tunnel . Of note, the location of the hiatus and submucosal tunnel should be made away from the bladder neck and bladder trigone to avoid painful catheterization. The stoma is formed as discussed previously (see Catheterizable Stoma Formation). The catheter is usually secured in place for 3 weeks prior to initiating intermittent catheterization.

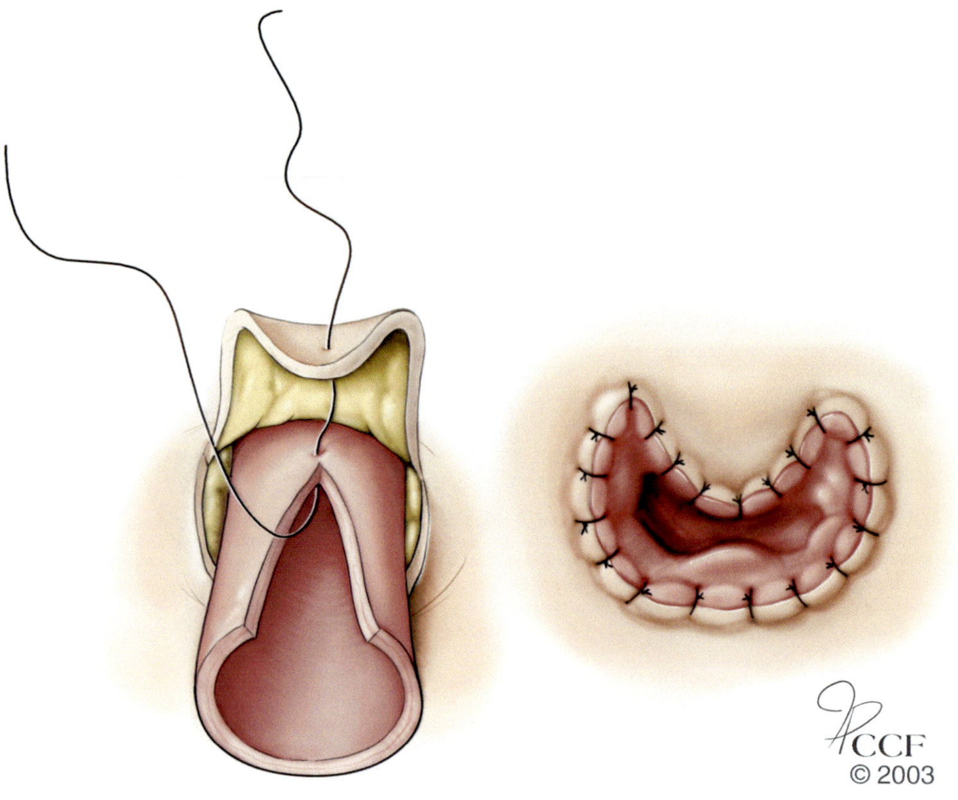

Fig. 18.2 Catheterizable stoma formation. The catheterizable tube is brought through the V-shaped skin incision, spatulated, and secured to the skin using interrupted sutures. Illustration © CCF

Yang-Monti Ileovesicostomy

The Mitrofanoff principle can be applied to a retubularized segment of ileum if the appendix has been removed or harvested for other purposes. A 2–3-cm segment of ileum is harvested with its mesentery demonstrating adequate vascular flow to the segment (Fig. 18.4). The segment is opened along its antimesenteric side. The opened segment is retubularized transversely in two layers over a 14 Fr catheter. The mucosa is approximated using running 5-0 Vicryl suture and the seromuscular layer is brought together using interrupted 4-0 Vicryl suture, leaving the stomal end spatulated for the stomal anastomosis. The tube is implanted into the bladder in similar fashion as the appendicovesicostomy. Stoma formation for this tube is described under Catheterizable Stoma Formation.

Complications

Difficulties with catheterization and/or stomal stenosis represent the most common complications in long-term studies, ranging from 20% to 60% for all types of catheterizable vesicostomies. Over 80% of patients remain continent after the initial surgery, with up to 96% achieving continence following a maximum of two revision procedures [3]. Most stomal complications are related to the technical placement of the stoma and may be avoidable [4]. Studies in pediatric populations demonstrate normal bladder function in a majority of patients with various congenital uropathies [5]. Urolithiasis complications can occur in up to 15% of patients [3]. The appendicovesicostomy, Yang-Monti ileovesicostomy, and continent vesicostomy, all provide adequate continent urinary stomas for patients when indicated.

Ileal Conduit

The uretero-ileal-cutaneous diversion was first described by Seiffert in 1935 [6]. Due to the technical difficulty to effectively collect and store urine, the procedure was abandoned. Bricker redescribed the procedure in 1950, and it has since gained widespread acceptance worldwide [1]. Advances in enterostomal treatment and therapy have increased the durability and tolerance of the ileal conduit. The ileal conduit is technically the fastest and simplest conduit to construct, and it is the simplest to take care of. The ileal conduit has one of the largest long-term outcomes, and therefore it is the urinary diversion procedure to compare to all other techniques. Any segment of ureter can be attached to the conduit from the renal pelvis to the trigone, making the ileal conduit construction a versatile method for diversion.

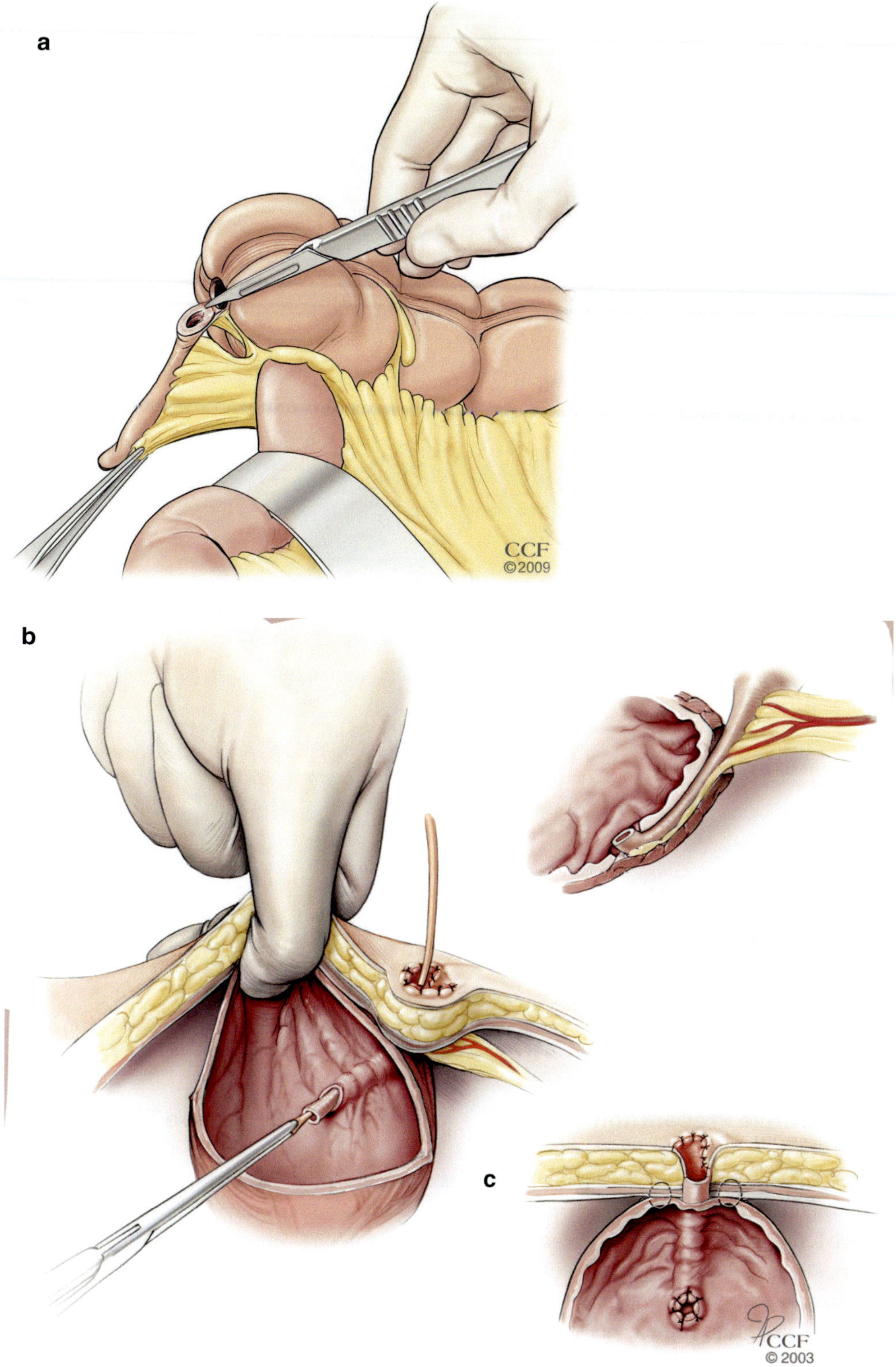

Fig. 18.3 Mitrofanoff catheterizable stoma. (**a**) The appendix is harvested with healthy mesoappendix. (**b**) It is traversed through a cystotomy and submucosal channel into the bladder. The proximal end is secured to the skin and a catheter is place through the stoma into the bladder. The appendiceal mucosa is secured to the bladder mucosa. (**c**) The bladder is secured to the anterior abdominal wall to prevent tension on the anastomosis. Illustrations © CCF

Indications

Any patient requiring urinary tract reconstruction following extirpative pelvic surgery may be considered for an ileal conduit. It can be used in cases where the bladder is left in-situ; for example, in neurogenic bladder, although modern management of neurogenic bladder has limited the role of supravesical diversion for this indication. The decision to choose the type of urinary diversion also relies heavily on the clinical condition of the patient, their comorbidities, body habitus, disability, and any other systemic illness that may preclude them from other types of urinary diversions.

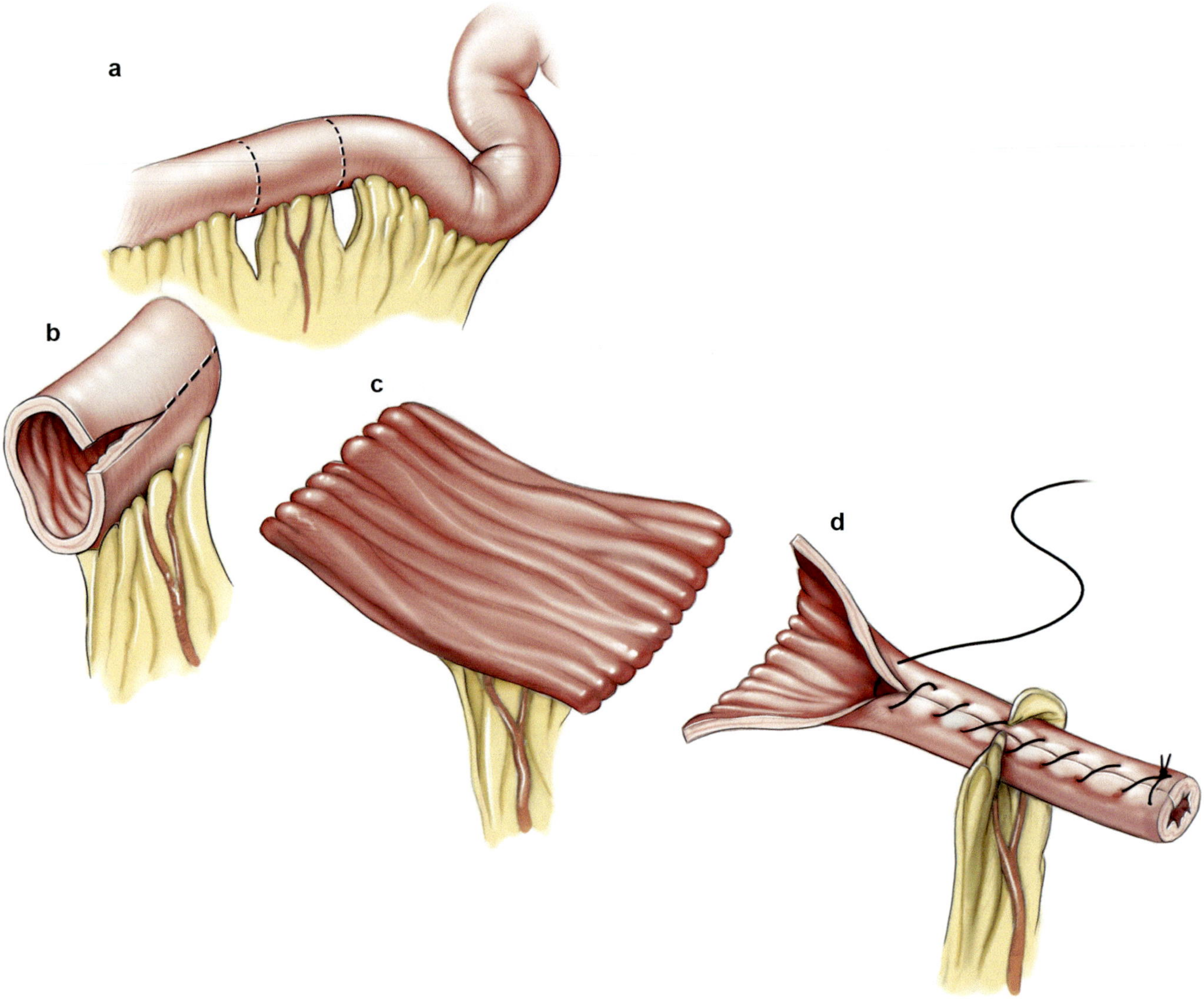

Fig. 18.4 Monti-Yang tube. (**a**) A 2–3-cm segment of well-vascularized ileum is harvested and (**b**, **c**) detubularized closer to the mesenteric edge. (**d**) The segment is retubularized transversely over a catheter, leaving one end spatulated for the stomal anastomosis. Illustration © CCF

Preoperative Preparation

Preoperative preparation of the patient includes a regimen of clear liquid diet starting 1–2 days prior to surgery, followed by a 4-L preparation of polyethylene glycol on the afternoon before surgery. Patients with indwelling urinary catheters or colonized urinary tracts are admitted the day prior to surgery for broad-spectrum intravenous antibiotics, which continue postoperatively for approximately 3–5 days.

The stoma site should be determined preoperatively in all patients by an enterostomal nurse or specialist. Patients are examined in the supine, sitting, and standing positions. The umbilicus, belt line, bony protuberances, prior surgical scars, and skin folds are noted and avoided when choosing the stoma site. The ideal stoma site is usually just medial to the linea semilunaris between the umbilicus and the anterior superior iliac spine.

Operative Technique

Following cystectomy or pelvic exenteration, the terminal ileum is identified and examined for length, and radiation enteritis, inflammatory bowel disease, or malignancy if applicable. The optimal length of conduit differs in each case due to patient body habitus and length of available ureter. The recommended length of conduit should not exceed the distance between the sacral promontory and the stoma site. Transillumination of the mesentery allows for inspection of the blood supply to the conduit. The ileocecal artery is spared to ensure vascular flow to the ileocecal junction. It is important to identify at least two vascular pedicles to the conduit to ensure adequate blood supply to the conduit. An incision is made in the peritoneum over the mesentery and the mesenteric vessels are clamped and tied (Fig. 18.5). The length and mobility of the segment that is

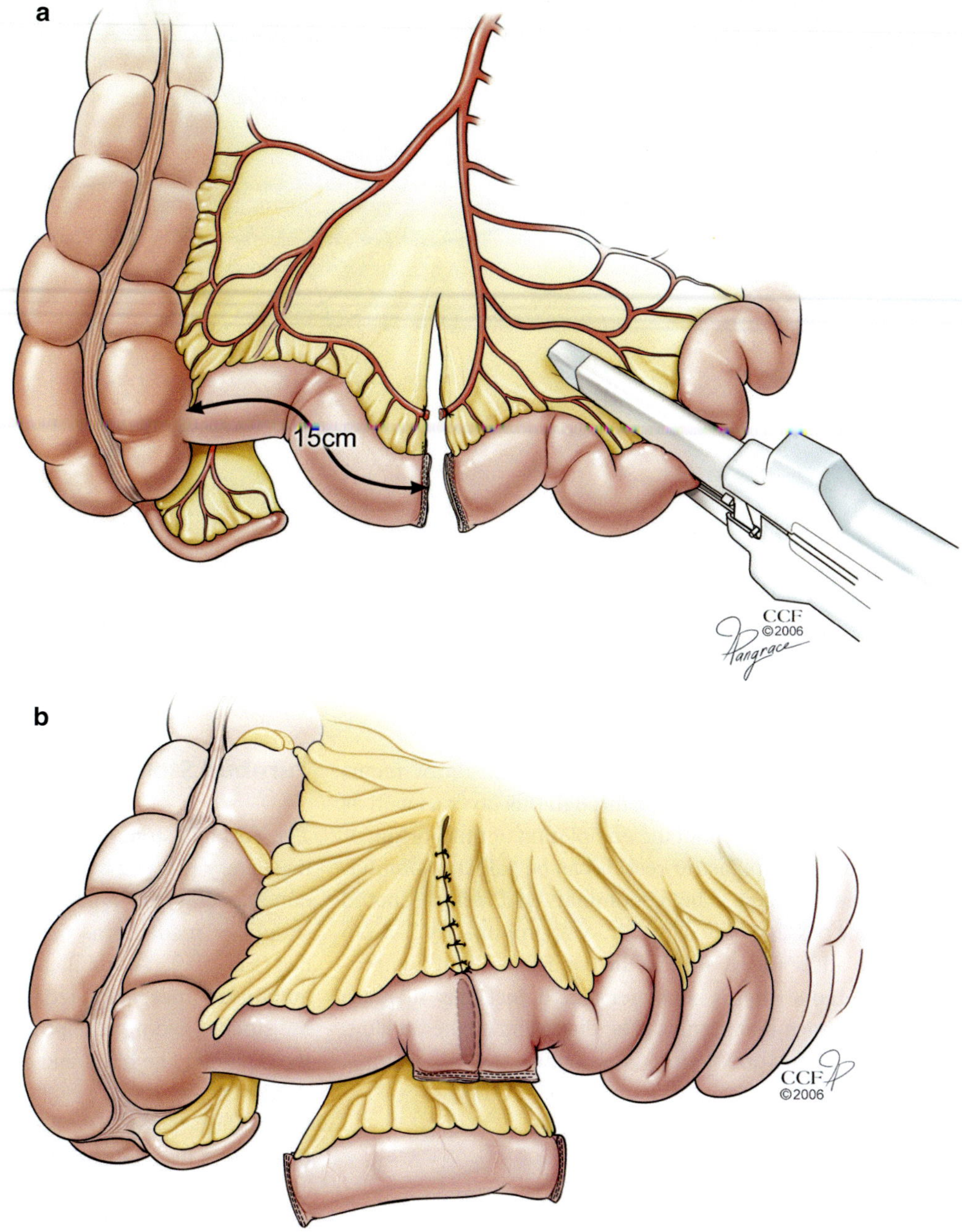

Fig. 18.5 Ileal conduit harvest. (**a**) An ileal segment 15 cm proximal to the ileocecal valve is isolated and (**b**) placed caudally to the anastomosis of the small bowel. Illustrations © CCF

to reach the skin is only dependent on the distal mesenteric division; thus, the proximal mesenteric division should be short, allowing for a broad vascular pedicle to the conduit. The bowel is divided using a bowel stapler, and the conduit segment is placed caudal to the remainder of bowel. The mesenteric window is closed using interrupted 3–0 silk suture to avoid mesenteric hernia, and bowel continuity is subsequently reestablished.

The staple line at the distal (efferent) end of the conduit is excised and the conduit lumen is opened. A small opening is made in the proximal end of the conduit and the conduit is irrigated free of enteric contents with normal saline irrigation. At this point, we prefer to prepare the stoma site to allow for more optimal localization of the ureteroileal anastomosis. The final maturation of the stoma in obese patients can be performed after the ureteroileal anastomosis is performed, to avoid difficulty in passing the stents through a large abdominal wall.

Stoma Formation

The skin edge, fascial layer, and peritoneal edge are brought into alignment using Kocher clamps. A circular plug of skin is excised from the predetermined stoma site. Dissection, using electrocautery, is carried through the subcutaneous fat to the anterior rectus fascia. A cruciate incision is made in the fascia, exposing the belly of the rectus muscle. The

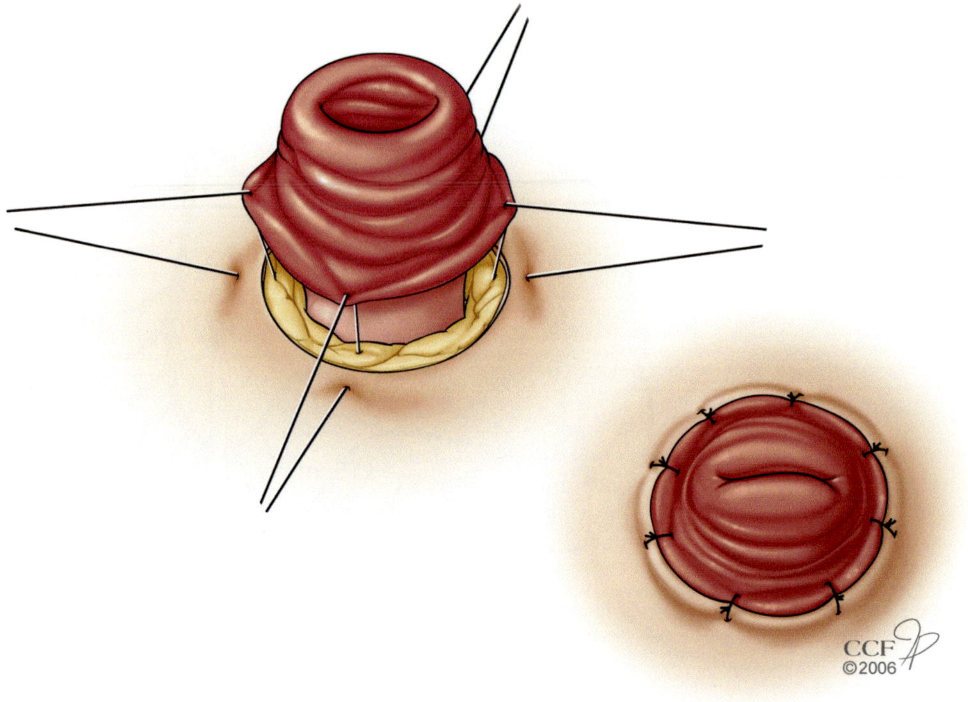

Fig. 18.6 End-loop stoma formation. The end-loop stoma is brought up 3 cm above the skin surface and sutured in an everting fashion in four quadrants. This is followed by supporting dermal sutures. Illustration © CCF

muscle is bluntly separated to expose the posterior rectus fascia. A linear incision is made through this layer as well as the peritoneum. Throughout the completion of this portion of the procedure, the epigastric vessels can be palpated simultaneously and avoided. The abdominal wall defect should allow for the passage of two fingers, or approximately 2–3-cm breadth, to allow for passage of the conduit without compromising the blood supply. A larger area defect may increase the risk of parastomal hernias. The distal end of the conduit, in an isoperistaltic orientation, is brought through the stoma site with care.

End-Loop Nipple Stoma

In the standard end-loop nipple stoma, the distal end of the conduit is brought through the previously prepared stoma opening using Babcock clamps to approximately 3 cm above the skin surface. Four quadrant sutures of 3-0 chromic are placed through the dermis edge, the serosa of the conduit well below the skin level, and through the full-thickness edge of the conduit (Fig. 18.6). Additional 3-0 chromic sutures are placed between the quadrant sutures to secure the conduit to the dermis. A securing suture of 2-0 Vicryl may be placed to secure the conduit to the inside of the abdominal wall. The proximal end of the conduit and the ureteroileal anastomosis can be covered with the posterior peritoneum to assist in minimizing leakage of urine and promote healing.

Turnbull Stoma

The Turnbull stoma may be used in obese patients with a short mesentery [7]. For this stoma, the distal (efferent) end of the conduit remains stapled closed. A small mesenteric opening should be made in the conduit segment 3 cm from the distal end (Fig. 18.7). A umbilical tape is placed through the opening and the antimesenteric side of the loop is brought out through the stoma opening at least 2–3 cm without tension or twisting the conduit. The blind end of the loop is positioned cephalad. A plastic rod replaces the umbilical tape and is secured in place (Fig. 18.8). The loop is opened transversely and is matured in the same everting manner as the end-loop stoma.

The Turnbull stoma provides an advantage to use over the end-loop nipple stoma when there is a short, bulky mesentery and thick abdominal wall commonly seen in obese patients. It has less of a tendency for retraction and stenosis; however, parastomal hernias are more commonly associated with the Turnbull stoma [8]. The end-loop nipple stoma provides for excellent appliance placement and less skin irritation, but stomal stenosis is more common with the end-loop nipple stoma.

Ureteroileal Anastomosis

The principles to consider during creation of the ureteroileal anastomosis include: maintenance of adequate distal ureteral blood supply, the maintenance of a tension-free anastomosis, absence of malignancy in the distal ureter (in cancer cases), and

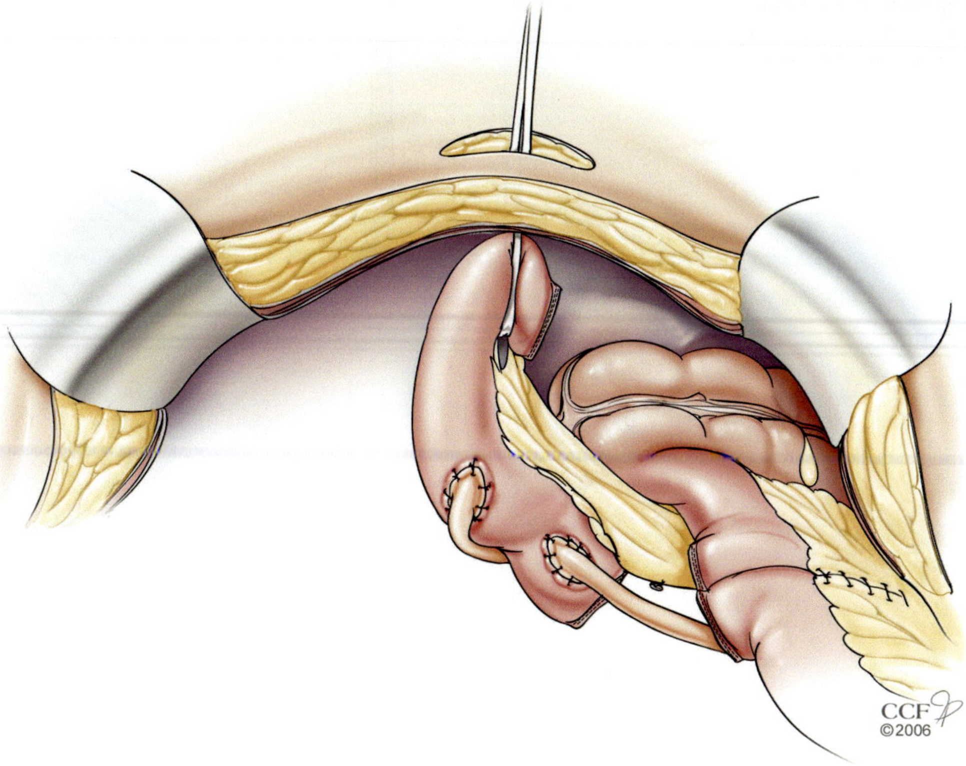

Fig. 18.7 Turnbull stoma formation. The Turnbull stoma is started by bringing up the distal loop of conduit by placing umbilical tape through the mesentery 3 cm from the distal end. Illustration © CCF

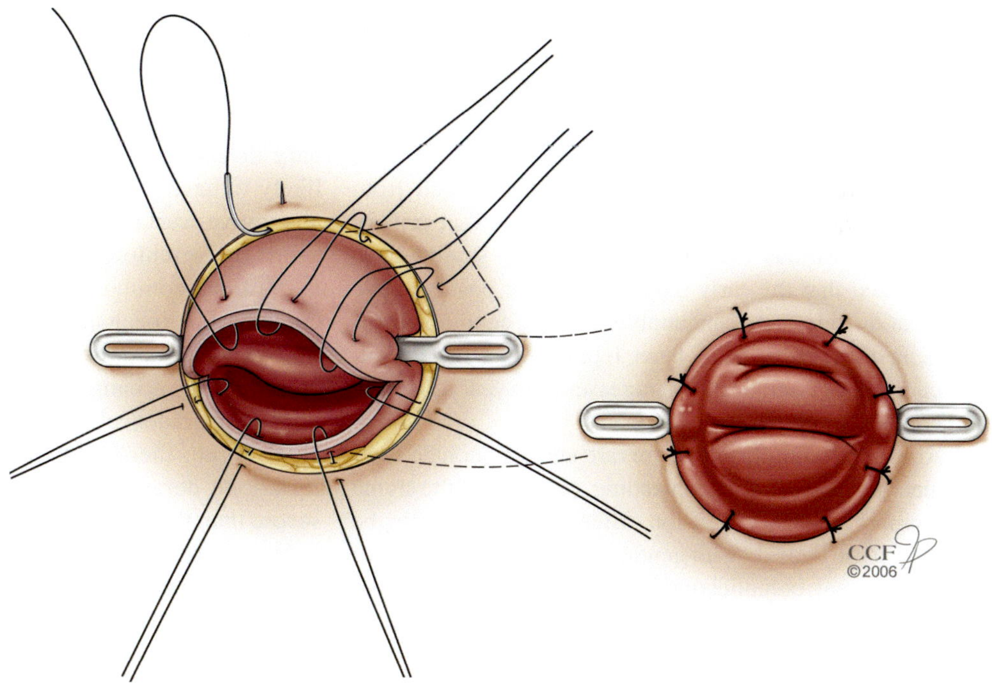

Fig. 18.8 Turnbull stoma completion. A plastic supporting rod replaces the umbilical tape. A myotomy is made transversely and the stoma is matured in an everting fashion. Illustration © CCF

the avoidance of ureteral kinking or twisting. If the stoma site is located on the right lower quadrant of the abdomen, the left ureter is passed under or through the sigmoid mesocolon to the right side. The hole in the sigmoid mesentery is usually made at the level of the sacral promontory; however, it may be more cephalad depending on the length of ureter and to avoid kinking the ureter. The ureteroileal anastomosis can be made using the Bricker, Wallace, or Lahey Clinic techniques and may be completed before or after the stoma maturation. The authors prefer securing the base of the conduit to the sacral promontory or to the retroperitoneal fibrous tissue after completing the ureteroileal anastomosis using 3-0 Vicryl suture (Fig. 18.9).

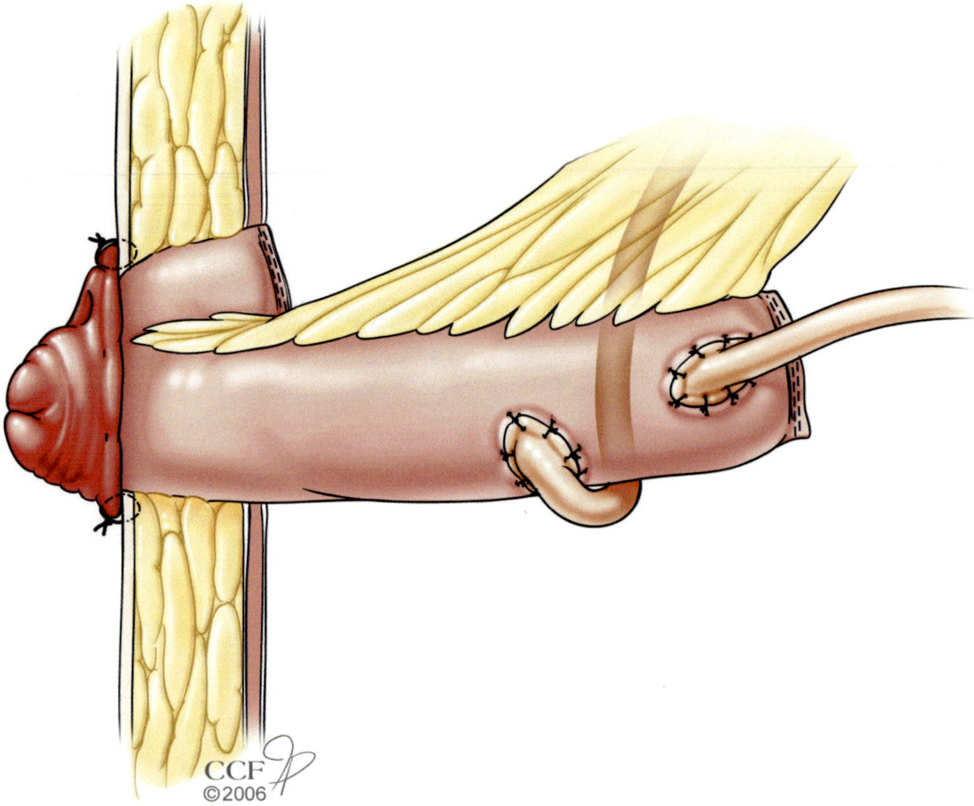

Fig. 18.9 Ileal conduit ureteral-ileal anastomosis and completion. The conduit as secured to the abdominal wall. The ureters are placed at the proximal end of the conduit. Illustration © CCF

Complications

The early mortality rates from early studies ranged from 0.3% to 13% for patients undergoing ileal conduit urinary diversion for various reasons. Contemporary studies have demonstrated that the early major and minor postoperative complication rates are comparable in ileal conduit versus continent diversions. It has been reported that the overall incidence of late complications increases each year following ileal conduit urinary diversion [9].

Early stomal complications are rare and can include ischemic necrosis and significant bleeding. Necrosis of the stoma site requires operative revision. Bleeding can usually be managed at the bedside with gentle pressure or placement of a stitch. Stomal complications include dermatitis, stomal stenosis, parastomal hernia, stomal prolapse, or retraction, which occurs in up to 31% of cases [10]. Parastomal hernias occur in 10–15% of cases [11].

Ureteroileal anastomotic complications can occur in the setting of urinary extravasation early postoperatively, with contemporary series reporting 0.3–1.3% incidence [9]. Late complications may include ureteral obstruction due to stricture at the ureteroileal anastomosis. Late and dense strictures usually do not respond to interventional treatment, and require open surgical repair.

Metabolic complications occur in all intestinal urinary diversions [12]. Patients with ileal conduits are less likely to have serious metabolic derangements due to less absorptive surface and minimal contact time with the urine. Hyperchloremic hypokalemic metabolic acidosis is the most common metabolic complication for the ileal conduit. The mechanism is increased ammonium absorption via the sodium receptors in addition to absorption of chloride in exchange for bicarbonate. Treatment of the metabolic acidosis lies in direct alkalinization. Oral potassium citrate therapy is effective and well-tolerated. The metabolic derangements of the jejunal conduit are more severe than the colonic or ileal conduits. Electrolyte imbalance is more common with the jejunal conduit, notably for hyponatremia, hypochloremia, hyperkalemia, azotemia, and acidosis. The jejunal conduit syndrome, which presents with nausea, emesis, anorexia, lethargy, and muscle weakness, is treated with salt and bicarbonate repletion and hydration [10].

Renal deterioration may occur long-term following ileal conduit urinary diversion. The etiology of this phenomenon is unknown as it can occur in the absence of obstruction and infections. Upper urinary tract deterioration can occur in 35% of patients at 5-year follow-up and up to 50% after 15-year follow-up [9].

Nephrolithiasis is a late complication of ileal conduit with increasing incidence at longer follow-up. The stones are usually located in the kidneys. Risk factors for stone formation include infection, hyperchloremic acidosis, and high conduit residual volumes. Struvite is the most common type of stone found in this cohort of patients.

Urinary tract infection is a common complication following urinary diversion and can occur either early or late in the postoperative course, and ranges from asymptomatic bacteriuria to pyelonephritis to urosepsis. All clinically significant infections should prompt evaluation of the urinary diversion anatomy to rule out obstruction from stomal stenosis or ureteroenteric stricture.

Sigmoid Colonic Conduit

Reports of deterioration of the upper urinary tracts in children due to the free reflux from ileal conduits led to redirecting attention to colonic conduits [13]. The use of sigmoid colon as a urinary conduit was first reported by Gross and Mogg in 1967 [14]. The colon, with its thicker musculature, is more amenable to the creation of submucosal tunnels and non-refluxing ureterocolonic anastomosis, allowing for adaptation of Coffey's ureteral anastomotic techniques. The sigmoid colon is usually redundant and mobile, allowing it to be a suitable urinary conduit.

Sigmoid urinary diversions can be used in the pediatric population where an anti-refluxing ureteroenteric anastomosis can reduce the potential for long-term renal scarring. Patients with Crohn's disease can be diverted using sigmoid colon. The sigmoid conduit should be avoided in patients with extensive pelvic radiation therapy. If the hypogastric arteries will be ligated during cystectomy, use of the sigmoid as a conduit might compromise the blood supply of the rectum. In contrast, the sigmoid colon is an ideal conduit following total pelvic exenteration as it eliminates the need for an intestinal anastomosis.

Operative Technique

The patient is positioned supine with the table flexed approximately 10°. The blood supply to the sigmoid colon from the inferior mesenteric artery is identified. The sigmoid colon is mobilized from its lateral and posterior attachments. A 15–20-cm segment of sigmoid colon is chosen for the conduit. A broad-based mesenteric blood supply is isolated for the sigmoid conduit. Division of the proximal mesentery is shorter than the distal mesentery to ensure adequate arterial blood supply to the isolated segment. The isolated sigmoid segment is placed lateral to the sigmoid colon (Fig. 18.10). The sigmoid colon is anastomosed using a two-layer end-to-end anastomosis and the mesenteric trap is closed. The isolated segment is irrigated free of colonic contents. The proximal end of the conduit is closed in two layers. The stoma is formed in the manner as an ileal conduit using the end-loop nipple stoma technique.

Ureterocolonic Anastomosis

The right ureter is brought through the sigmoid mesocolon to the left side. An incision is made using a #15 blade in the tenia libera. Dissection is carried through the muscularis to expose the mucosa. The submucosal layer is dissected approximately 1 cm on either side of the muscularis to create seromuscular flaps (Fig. 18.11a). The mucosa is incised for an approximately 3-mm opening (Fig. 18.11b). The ureter is spatulated and a stay suture is placed proximally attaching the ureter to the seromuscularis layer to minimize handling of the ureter during the anastomosis. An interrupted or running mucosal-to-mucosal anastomosis is completed. Prior to completion of the anastomosis, a ureteral stent is placed. The seromuscularis layer is closed loosely over the ureteral anastomosis in interrupted fashion (Fig. 18.11c, d). The closure should allow a right angle clamp to be passed easily into the tunnel.

Transverse Colonic Conduit

The transverse colonic conduit can be used in any patient requiring urinary diversion. It is ideal in children and adults who have received pelvic radiation; situations where the ileum and sigmoid colon are precluded from use. Patients with a history of recurrent retroperitoneal fibrosis, Crohn's disease, and unsuccessful primary urinary diversion (where the ureters are significantly shortened) can be managed with a transverse colonic urinary conduit. It offers non-refluxing ureteric anastomoses as well as the ability to position the stoma in the left or right upper quadrant. Contraindications for the transverse colonic conduit include ulcerative colitis, irradiation of the upper abdomen, and history of extensive colon resection.

Operative Technique

The patient is positioned supine and access is gained through a midline incision. The ureters are mobilized in standard fashion, inspected for areas of devascularization and irradiation damage, and brought through the retroperitoneum via mesenteric openings that are made bilaterally. These openings should be wide enough to accommodate the ureters and to avoid kinking or compression.

When selecting the transverse colon as the segment of conduit urinary diversion, the right colon and left colon must be mobilized to provide a tension-free colocolostomy.

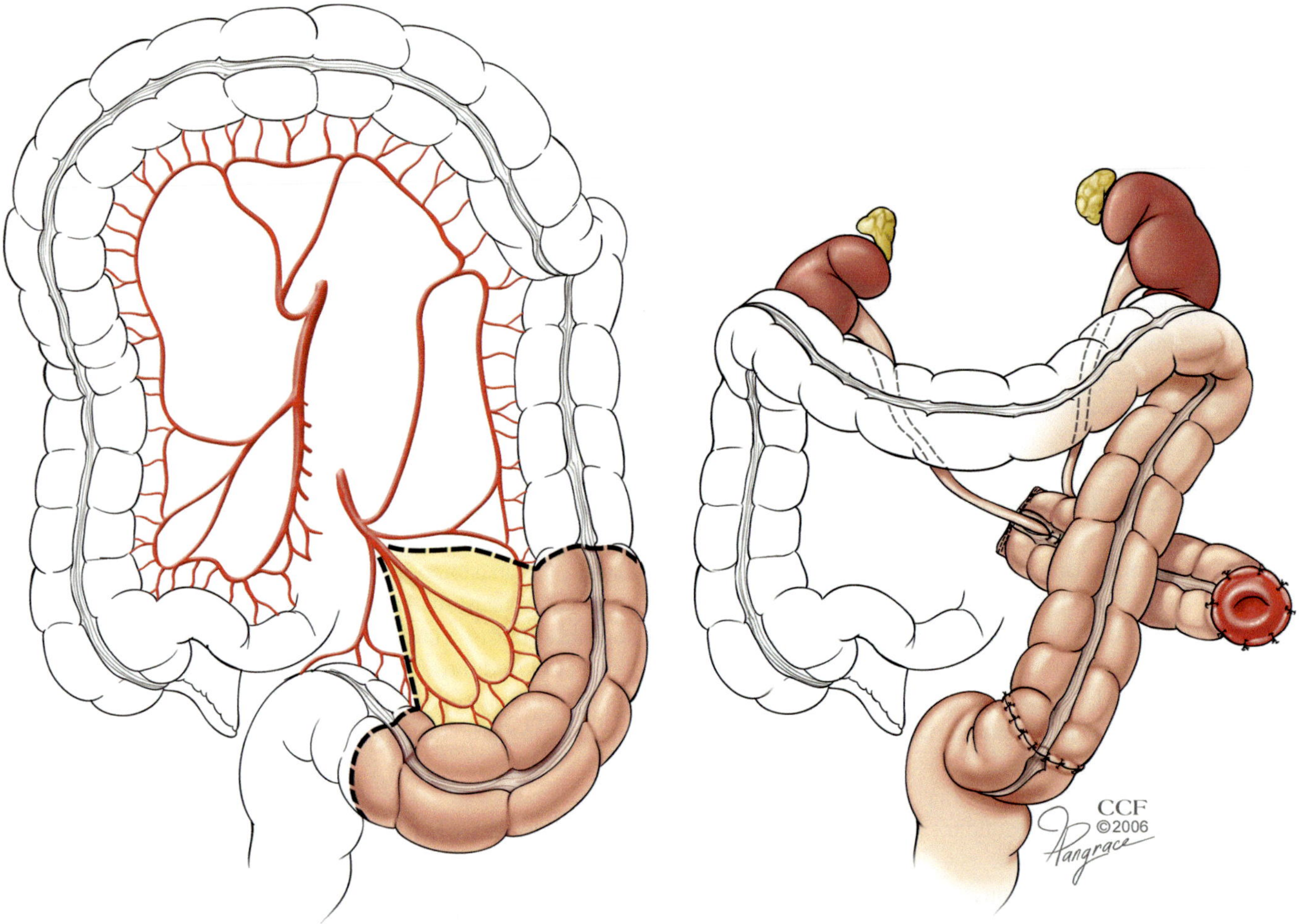

Fig. 18.10 Sigmoid conduit formation. The sigmoid conduit is isolated and placed laterally to the reconstituted bowel continuity. The ureters are anastomosed in a non-refluxing manner. The stoma is placed in the left lower quadrant. Illustration © CCF

A segment of transverse colon is selected approximately 15–20 cm in length (Fig. 18.12). The entire greater omentum is separated from the transverse colon. The mesentery is inspected and blood supply to the selected segment of conduit is identified. The mesenteric arcade of vessels is clamped and ligated. The selected colonic segment is divided proximally and distally with either a stapler or sharp division. Bowel continuity is established with either a stapled or a hand-sewn end-to-end colocolostomy. The mesenteric trap is closed in interrupted fashion. The segment is irrigated free of colonic contents. Depending on the type of ureterocolonic anastomosis, the proximal end of the transverse colonic conduit may be closed or left open (when using the Wallace technique).

Stoma Formation

The stoma for the transverse colonic conduit can be placed in either the right or left upper quadrant. The procedure for the formation of the conduit is technically similar to the sigmoid conduit stoma formation.

Complications

Due to the upper tract complications reported in children with ileal conduits, the colonic conduit was explored due to its viability as a non-refluxing conduit. Certain series on colonic conduit reported early complication rates up to 4.8% in the pediatric population (age <20). A majority of the complications were related to postoperative ileus [13].

Late complications include stomal stenosis rates of 15.5%, pyelonephritis rates of 7.6%. Renal calculi are reported to develop in 8.2% of renal units involved in urinary diversion. Ureterocolonic stenosis occurred in 6.9% of patients postoperatively after a mean of 5.8 months [13].

Dilatation and pyelonephritis changes in the upper tracts were tracked in 159 renal units in one study. In 77 renal units with no preoperative dilatation, 2 had mild/moderate postoperative dilatation and 2 required nephrectomy for nonfunctioning status [13].

Metabolic complications include hyperchloremic acidosis, a well-known complication in patients with continent ureterosigmoidostomies. However, in a contemporary

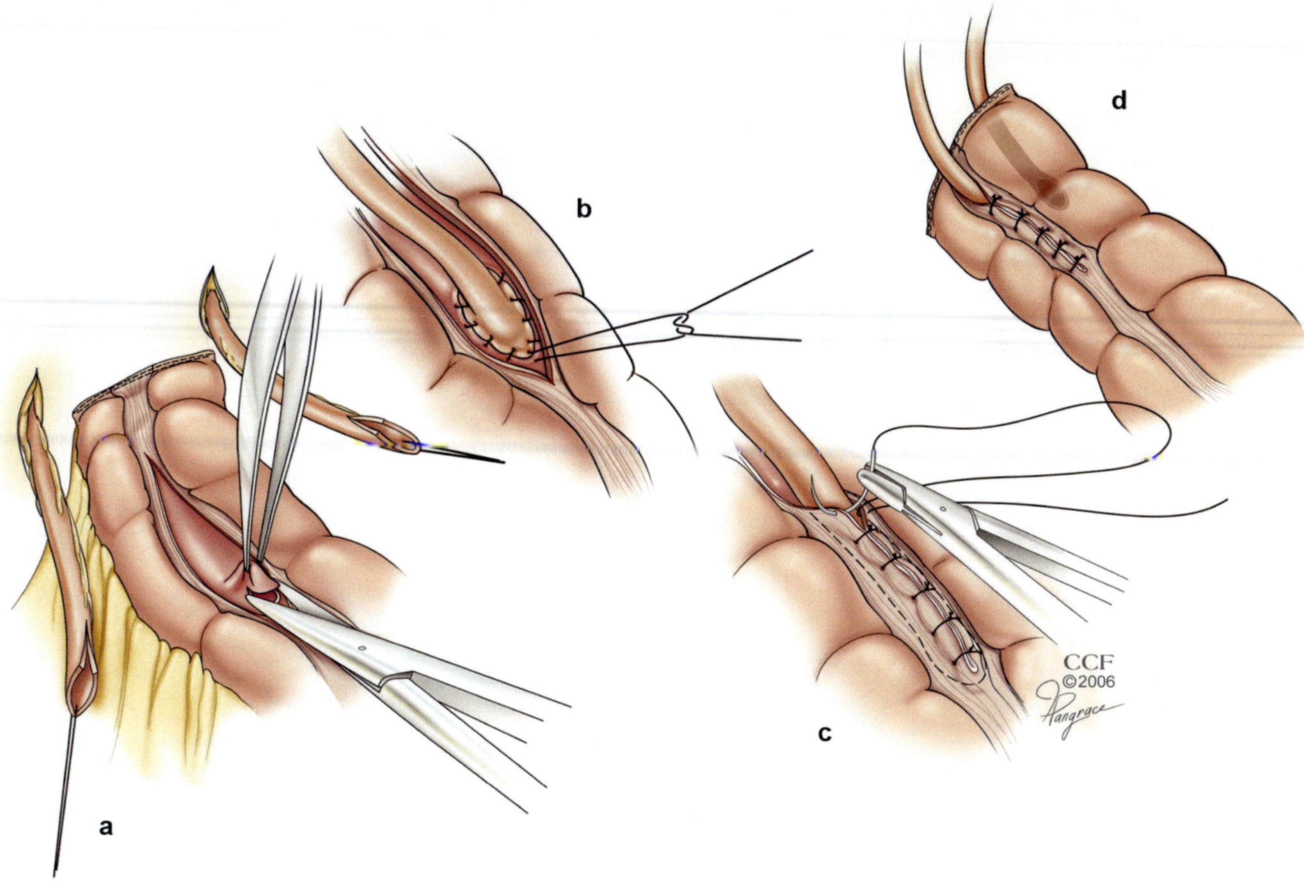

Fig. 18.11 Ureterocolonic anastomosis. The ureterocolonic anastomosis is placed along the tenia libera in a tunneled, anti-refluxing fashion. (**a**) The tenia is dissected free from the mucosa and flaps are formed. (**b**) The mucosa is incised and anastomosed to the ureter. (**c**, **d**) The tenia is closed loosely over the ureter completing the tunneled anastomosis. Illustration © CCF

series involving pediatric patients with minimum 5-year follow-up, <1% of patients were reported to have acidosis [13]. With stringent monitoring of acid–base level, osteomalacia can be avoided in patients in the long-term. Secondary malignancy in continent ureterosigmoidostomy is reported to be as high as 40% in patients observed long-term, with an average latency period of 26 years [15, 16]. However, cases of adenocarcinoma in the non-continent colonic conduit are extremely rare, with many long-term studies reporting no incidences of secondary malignancy [15].

Continent Catheterizable Pouches

General Principles

The construction of a continent cutaneous catheterizable urinary reservoir requires three main elements: (1) a low-pressure compliant reservoir, (2) an anti-refluxing ureterointestinal anastomosis, and (3) a continent stoma that allows easy catheterization. Various segments of bowel can be used to create a high-capacity, low-pressure reservoir, including: ileum, ileocolonic segment, ascending colon, transverse colon, and all of the above together. Attention to the blood supply of the bowel must be kept in mind when performing these procedures. Unlike the small bowel, the large bowel does not have straight arteries that give off longitudinal collateral circulation; thus, more of the vascular supply to the large bowel must be preserved.

Detubularized bowel segments provide a greater capacity at a lower pressure than intact segments of bowel. This is due to four factors:

1. The configuration takes advantage of the fact that the volume increases by the square of the radius; folding bowel once doubles the volume, and folding it twice will quadruple the capacity.
2. According to LaPlace's law, the greater the volume of the container, the greater the mural tension, which allows the pressure to remain low.
3. The compliance of detubularized bowel is greater than that of tubular bowel.
4. The contractile ability of detubularized bowel is blunted by lack of coordinated contraction [11].

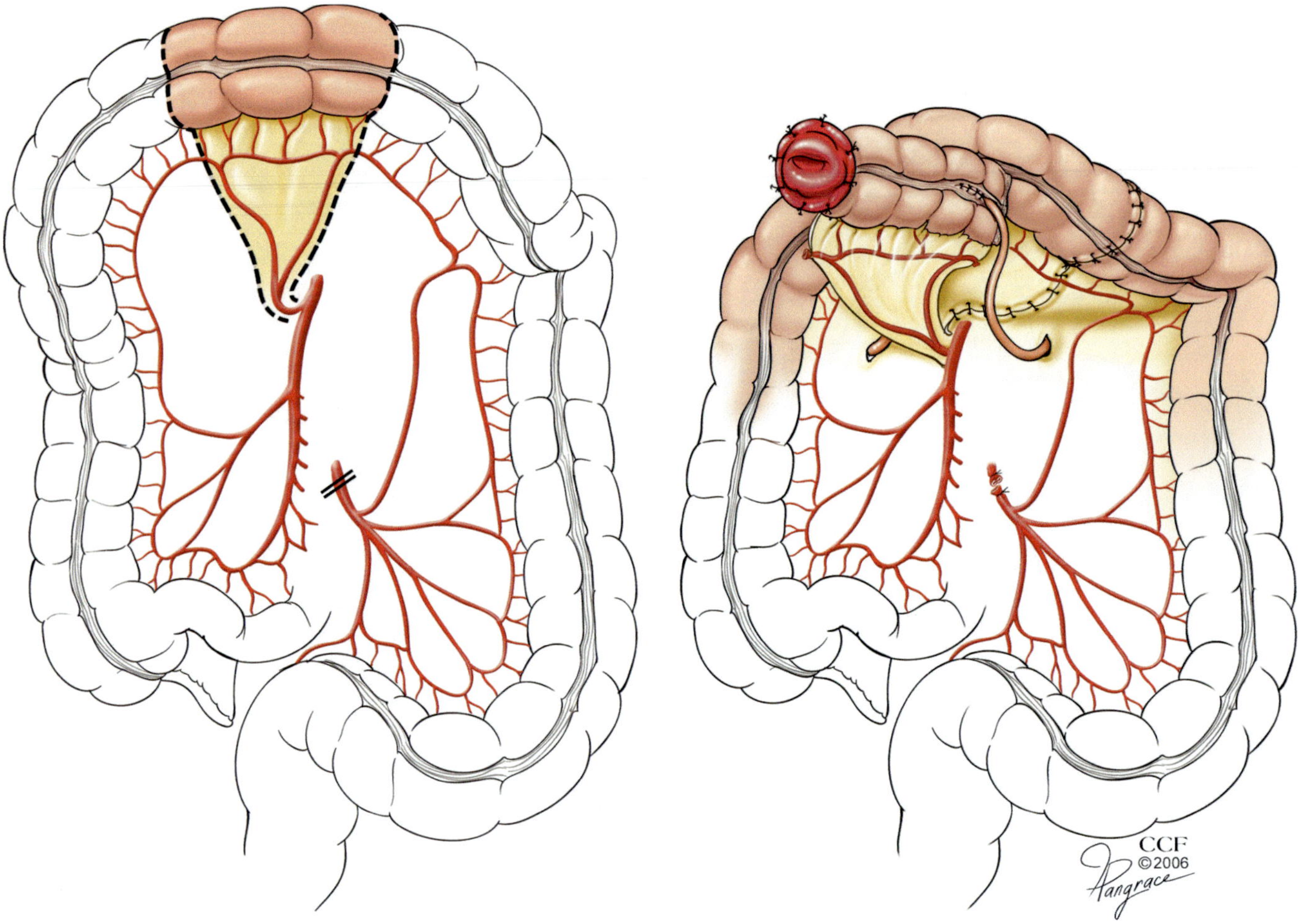

Fig. 18.12 Transverse colonic conduit formation. The isolated segment of transverse colon placed anterior to the colonic anastomosis. The ureters are brought out of the retroperitoneum through mesenteric windows. The stoma should be oriented in an isoperistaltic orientation. Illustration © CCF

Proof of concept arises from a study that examined cystometry findings on patients who underwent various types of enterocystoplasty. Clinically significant contractions (pressure >40 cmH_2O at volume <200 mL) occurred in 70% of tubular ileocystoplasty patients, 36% of tubular colonic cystoplasty patients, 10% for detubularized colon, and none of the detubularized ileocystoplasty patients [17].

History of the Continent Catheterizable Pouch

Verhoogen first reported the use of the ileocecal segment as a continent reservoir in 1908 for supravesical urinary diversion [15]. The cecum was used as the reservoir with the ileocecal valve serving as the anti-reflux mechanism; the appendix was brought out as a catheterizable stoma. The complications reported by Hinman and Weyrauch halted further attempts at continent catheterizable diversions until Gilchrist et al. reported the successful use of the ileocecal segment to achieve a continent urinary pouch via a catheterizable stoma [15, 18]. Rowland et al. first reported the use of the modified Gilchrist procedure in 29 patients in 1987 [19]. They reported that detubularizing the cecal segment increased compliance of the pouch and improved continence rates. The ileal limb was initially suture plicated to create a tapered, catheterizable stoma; subsequently, the stapler was used to plicate the limb. The initial reports were promising with short-term daytime continence rates >90%.

Indications

The indications include all of the previously cited indications for urinary diversion. Patients who do not qualify for orthotopic neobladders due to tumor involvement of the urethra may be eligible for a continent catheterizable pouch. Patient selection is important for postoperative care. Patients with poor manual dexterity may not be appropriate patients for this type of diversion as they will need to perform intermittent self-catheterization to empty the pouch several times daily. Patients with debilitating disorders, such as multiple sclerosis, or patients with quadriplegia who may have progressive debilitation may not be ideal patients. In addition, assessing the patient's motivation to take care of the pouch by emptying it regularly and irrigating the mucous out regularly is of paramount importance.

Preoperative Preparation

Preoperative bowel preparation can be achieved according to surgeon preference. At our institution, we employ a low-residue, clear liquid diet 72 h prior to surgery. This is followed by 4 L of oral polyethylene glycol with electrolytes solution 24 h prior to surgery. Antibiotic bowel regimen is generally not used in our practice as the mechanical bowel preparation has replaced it.

Operative Technique

Following cystectomy or other primary procedure, the right colon is mobilized from the ileocecal valve to the hepatic flexure (Fig. 18.13a). A measured length of right colon, approximating 25–30 cm from the ileocecal valve, is required. The ileum is taken 7–10 cm from the ileocecal valve. The mesentery is transilluminated to identify the mesenteric vessels; the blood supply to the ileocecal segment is derived from the ileocolic and right colic arteries. If the transverse colon is needed for length of the segment, the middle colic artery should be preserved for the segment. The colon and ileum are divided between clamps, and the ileocolostomy is performed with a stapled anastomosis. The ileocolic segment is irrigated with saline until clear of bowel content. The appendix is removed with a purse-string suture placed to invert the appendiceal stump.

The colonic segment is opened along its entire length between the anterior tenia (antimesenteric border) (Fig. 18.13a and b). The plication of the ileal continence limb is completed with the cecum open to visualize and digitally inspect the tapering of the ileum. A 12 French red rubber catheter is placed through the ileal limb into the cecum. Babcock clamps are placed on the antimesenteric edge of the ileum to allow for the gastrointestinal stapling device to taper the efferent limb. Care should be taken not to extend the stapling device through the ileocecal valve. The funnel-shaped proximal cecum is plicated over the ileocecal junction using 2-0 silk Lembert sutures. To ensure adequate placement for the sutures, the red rubber catheter is pinched against the mesenteric wall while the sutures are placed. This maneuver will tighten the ileocecal valve as well as cover the angled staple line at the ileocecal junction.

After completing the efferent ileal limb, the 12-French red rubber catheter should be removed and a 14-French or 16-French red rubber catheter should be used to test the limb for easy catheterization. The catheter should encounter mild resistance at the ileocecal valve.

The pouch is subsequently closed using 3-0 Vicryl suture in a Heineke-Mikulicz configuration by bringing the cephalad end of the detubularized pouch to the caudal end (Fig. 18.13c). Prior to completion of the closure, a 24-French Malecot catheter is placed as a cecostomy tube through the dependent portion of the cecum. At this point, the ureterointestinal anastomosis is completed. The ureters should be mobilized enough to reach the pouch without tension. The spatulated left ureter is passed under the sigmoid colon mesentery to the right side of the pelvis and through the pouch mesentery to be placed anteriorly. The spatulated right ureter is brought along the lateral edge of the pouch and placed anteriorly. The tenia is incised sharply and the mucosa is exposed. A 4-0 Vicryl holding suture is placed through the adventitia of the ureter and the tenia to decrease tension on the anastomosis. The mucosa-to-mucosa anastomosis is completed in running fashion using 4-0 Vicryl and the tenia is closed over the anastomosis using 4-0 Vicryl, incorporating the adventitia of the ureters at every other stitch (Fig. 18.13d). Ureteral stents are generally placed into the ureters and exit through the pouch in separate stab incisions. The stents and the Malecot catheter will be brought out of the abdomen through separate stab incisions. The pouch is subsequently closed and tested through the Malecot catheter for leaks and continence at the ileocecal valve with at least 500 mL of saline. The stoma is prepared as described earlier in this chapter (see Catheterizable Stoma Formation).

Complications

Early postoperative complications after the Indiana continent catheterizable pouch include pouch leak (4%) and inability to catheterize (2%) [20]. Bowel obstruction has been reported in up to 6% of patients and wound-related complications in 4%. Late complications include stomal stenosis (2%) which usually all requires revision surgery. Pyelonephritis occurs in up to 6% and may require operative intervention in up to 33% of patients. The overall late postoperative complication re-operation rate is 14%. Complication rates and re-operative rates are significantly higher in patients with prior abdomino-pelvic radiation therapy. Incontinence rates can approach 15% in radiated patients compared to nearly 0% in non-radiated patients [20]. These factors must be weighed when selecting patients for continent catheterizable pouch surgery.

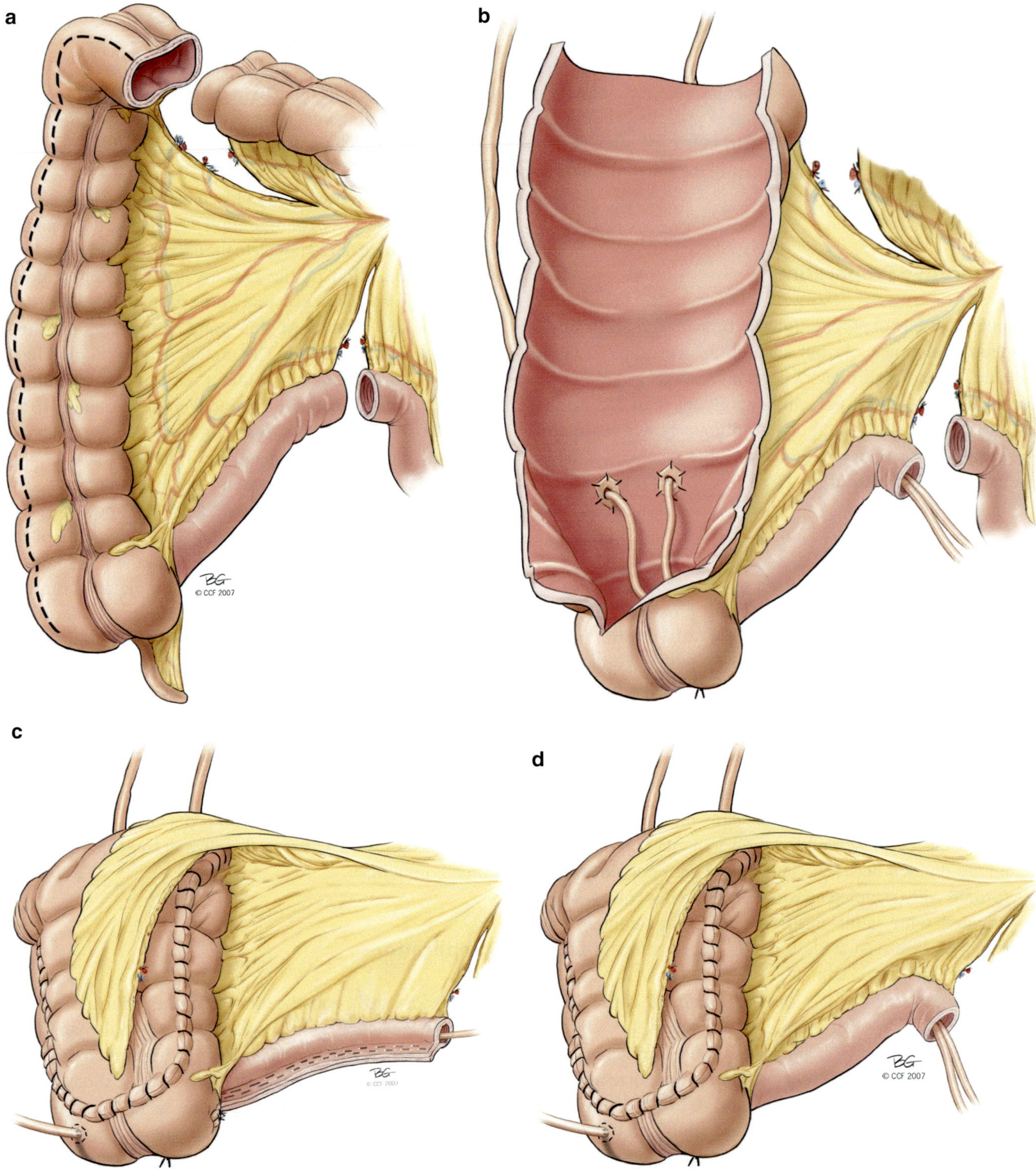

Fig. 18.13 Indiana pouch formation. (**a**) The ileal-colonic segment is isolated. (**b**) The segment is detubularized and the ureterocolonic anastomosis is completed. (**c**) The detubulized segment of colon is constructed into a pouch. (**d**) The efferent ileal limb is plicated and will function as the catheterizable stoma. Illustrations © CCF

Conclusion

Urinary stomas may be indicated for various reasons including malignant, infectious, neuropathic, or congenital disorders of the urinary tract. Although urothelium is the ideal tissue for use in urinary diversion, the use of bowel for urinary diversion has remained a durable alternative. Reconstructive techniques with bowel include formation of incontinent urinary stomas to bladder, incontinent urinary channels, as well as continent catheterizable stomas to reconstructed urinary pouches. Careful patient selection is paramount as the risks and complications are measureable when using bowel for urinary stomas. Thus, long-term follow-up is required in patients to follow renal function as well as metabolic derangements.

References

1. Bricker EM. Bladder substitution after pelvic evisceration. Surg Clin North Am. 1950;30:1511.
2. Mitrofanoff P. Trans-appendicular continent cystostomy in the management of the neurogenic bladder. Chir Pediatr. 1980;21:297.
3. Kaefer M, Tobin MS, Hendren WH, Bauer SB, Peters CA, Atala A, et al. Continent urinary diversion: the Children's Hospital experience. J Urol. 1997;157:1394.
4. Mollard P, Gauriau L, Bonnet JP, Mure PY. Continent cystostomy (Mitrofanoff's procedure) for neurogenic bladder in children and adolescent (56 cases: long-term results). Eur J Pediatr Surg. 1997; 7:34.
5. Jayanthi VR, McLorie GA, Khoury AE, Churchill BM. The effect of temporary cutaneous diversion on ultimate bladder function. J Urol. 1995;154:889.
6. Williams O, Vereb MJ, Libertino JA. Noncontinent urinary diversion. Urol Clin North Am. 1997;24:735.
7. Turnbull Jr RB, Hewitt CR. Loop-end myotomy ileostomy in the obese patient. Urol Clin North Am. 1978;5:423.
8. Bloom DA, Lieskovsky G, Rainwater G, Skinner DG. The Turnbull loop stoma. J Urol. 1983;129:715.
9. Madersbacher S, Schmidt J, Eberle JM, Thoeny HC, Burkhard F, Hochreiter W, et al. Long-term outcome of ileal conduit diversion. J Urol. 2003;169:985.
10. Hautmann RE, Abol-Enein H, Hafez K, Haro I, Mansson W, Mills RD, et al. Urinary diversion. Urology. 2007;69:17.
11. Hinman Jr F. Selection of intestinal segments for bladder substitution: physical and physiological characteristics. J Urol. 1988; 139:519.
12. McDougal WS. Metabolic complications of urinary intestinal diversion. J Urol. 1992;147:1199.
13. Stein R, Fisch M, Stockle M, Demirkesen O, Hohenfellner R. Colonic conduit in children: protection of the upper urinary tract 16 years later? J Urol. 1996;156:1146.
14. Mogg RA. The treatment of urinary incontinence using the colonic conduit. J Urol. 1967;97:684.
15. Thorne ID, Resnick MI. The use of bowel in urologic surgery. An historical perspective. Urol Clin North Am. 1986;13:179.
16. Gilchrist KW, Uehling DT, Starling JR. Cancer surveillance after ureterosigmoidostomy: colonic microscopic changes. J Surg Res. 1984;36:251.
17. Goldwasser B, Barrett DM, Webster GD, Kramer SA. Cystometric properties of ileum and right colon after bladder augmentation, substitution or replacement. J Urol. 1987;138:1007.
18. Merricks JW, Gilchrist RK. The ileocecal segment as a substitute bladder; a review of 18 cases. J Urol. 1954;71:591.
19. Rowland RG, Mitchell ME, Bihrle R, Kahnoski RJ, Piser JE. Indiana continent urinary reservoir. J Urol. 1987;137:1136.
20. Holmes DG, Thrasher JB, Park GY, Kueker DC, Weigel JW. Long-term complications related to the modified Indiana pouch. Urology. 2002;60:603.

19 Enterocutaneous Fistula

Hasan T. Kirat and Feza H. Remzi

Introduction

Enterocutaneous fistula (ECF) is an unusual communication between the bowel lumen and skin. It can occur spontaneously in patients with cancer, radiation enteritis, diverticular disease, inflammatory bowel disease, ischemic bowel, or perforated ulcer disease. However, most ECFs develop postoperatively when stool begins leaking from an anastomosis or unintended enterotomy.

The consequences of an ECF depend on the site of the fistula within the bowel, and the volume of stool that is leaking through it. High output fistulas (defined as more than 500 cm^3 per day) from the jejunum cause dangerous degrees of malnutrition, with loss of important electrolytes, minerals, trace metals, and vitamins. Therefore, appropriate nutritional and metabolic support is important. Low output, distal fistulas require less intensive care and are more likely to close spontaneously. Other factors influencing spontaneous closure rate include the health of the bowel from which the fistula originates, the presence of an abscess cavity between the bowel and the skin, the maturation of the fistula as bowel mucosa anastomoses itself to the dermis, and the presence of distal obstruction [1]. If spontaneous closure does not occur, surgery must be considered. Although management of all ECFs is usually based on the same principles regardless of the cause, this chapter focuses on management of postoperative ECFs.

H.T. Kirat (✉) • F.H. Remzi
Department of Colorectal Surgery, Digestive Disease Institute, Cleveland Clinic Foundation, Cleveland, OH, USA
e-mail: kirath@ccf.org

Management of ECF

Patient's Stabilization

Stool usually starts to leak from a defect in the bowel 5–10 days after an intra-abdominal operation, when peristalsis resumes after the postoperative ileus. Initial presentation is with pain and fever, a localized abscess or infection, that settles once the stool begins to drain. Patients may also develop peritonitis if the leak communicates with the peritoneal cavity (Fig. 19.1).

Treatment has three main goals: to correct or avoid nutritional deficits, achieve fistula closure, and maintain or restore

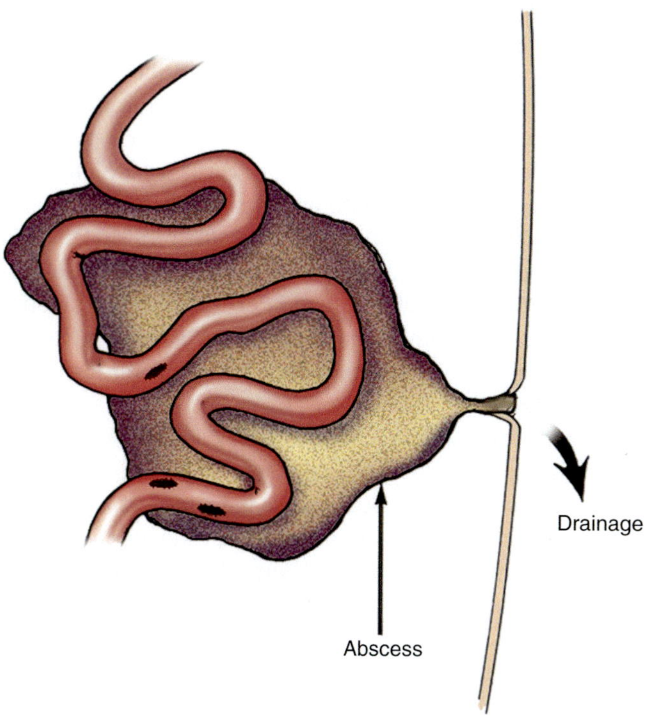

Fig. 19.1 Enterocutaneous fistula. Illustration © CCF

V.W. Fazio et al. (eds.), *Atlas of Intestinal Stomas*,
DOI 10.1007/978-0-387-78851-7_19, © Springer Science+Business Media, LLC 2012

bowel continuity. High output fistulas often lead to short bowel syndrome with malnutrition and electrolyte imbalances, which, if not treated properly, can lead to death [2, 3] (see also Chap. 8). Therefore, sick patients must be evaluated and resuscitated aggressively with crystalloids to reestablish intravascular volume. Infusion of albumin and transfusion of red blood cells restore plasma oncotic pressure and improve oxygen-carrying capacity, respectively. Electrolytes such as potassium, sodium, magnesium, phosphate, calcium, and zinc should be replaced, and levels should be monitored until they stabilize. In the meantime, the localized abscess should be drained and antibiotic therapy started.

Stool drainage through the fistula is controlled, and the surrounding skin is protected by the effective use of a pouching system (see also Chap. 19). Any undrained intra-abdominal collections are drained via computed tomography (CT) guidance [4]. The drain may be left in place to control further abscess formation.

After the initial resuscitation and control of sepsis, it usually becomes obvious whether the fistula output will spontaneously decrease or if the fistula is high output. When outputs rapidly dwindle, it may be possible for the patient to eat as the fistula closes. Normal bowel function is a good indicator that this will occur. For high output fistulas, or when there is extensive sepsis of disruption of the gastrointestinal (GI) tract, nutritional support should be initiated and continued until the ECF heals spontaneously or definitive repair is successful (see also Chap. 8).

Both enteral and parenteral nutrition via a single-lumen central catheter are generally provided until the patient can tolerate enteral feeding alone. Parenteral nutrition reduces morbidity and mortality by allowing the bowel to rest and the ECF to close. Enteral nutrition preserves gastrointestinal mucosa, supports the immunologic functions of the liver and the gut, and also avoids line sepsis. A total of 35–40 kcal/kg/day for men and 30–35 kcal/kg/day for women are required, unless there is continuing infection or underlying malnutrition. In patients with a proximal fistula and an adequate length of distal bowel with no obstruction, enteral feeds can be given through the fistula.

Patients with an ECF require at least 1.5 g/kg/day protein. Transferrin and prealbumin levels should be assessed weekly, since they are relatively acute phase indicators of a patient's nutritional status. Body surface area and estimation of existing deficits and losses can help determine the amount of fluid needed (see also Chap. 8).

Patients with a proximal fistula generally have a high output and are prone to dehydration. Such patients are generally receiving parenteral fluid, either with total parenteral nutrition (TPN) or as fluid alone. In patients with more variable fistula output who may not be receiving parenteral fluid, clinicians should be alert to the risk factors for and symptoms of dehydration. Such patients do best with a modified diet (e.g., avoid indigestible foods) and the use of liquid loperamide hydrochloride, diphenoxalate hydrochloride with atropine sulfate, liquid codeine, or tincture of opium to slow stool transit, increase absorption of water, and thereby thicken enteric output.

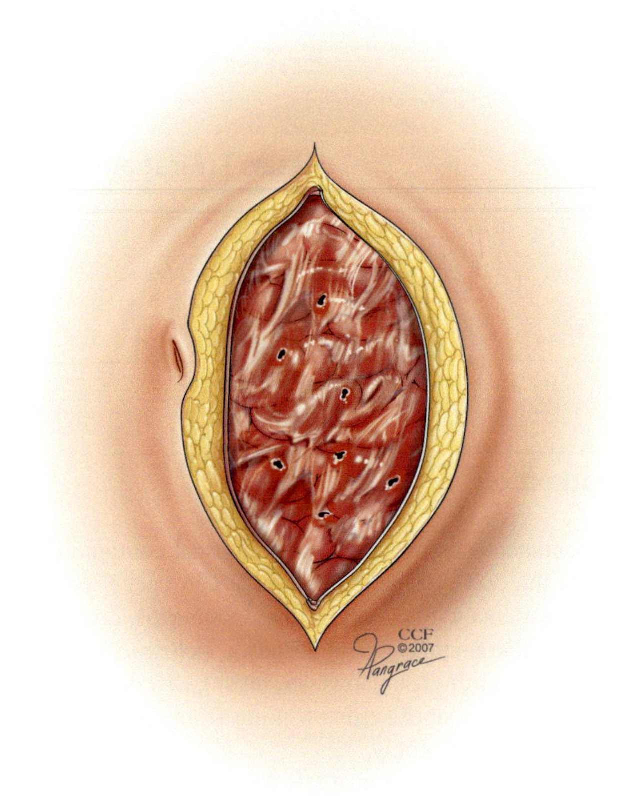

Fig. 19.2 Multiple fistulas and open abdomen. Illustration © CCF

Somatostatin (octreotide) inhibits the endocrine and exocrine secretions of many hormones in the gastrointestinal system. Although it may decrease fistula output and decrease time to healing, studies have failed to show a correlation with spontaneous closure rates [5]. Use of somatostatin is associated with hyperglycemia and increased risk of cholelithiasis. Hence, it is suggested that somatostatin and its analog octreotide be used only for high output ECFs (<500 mL/24 h).

Wound Care

An experienced enterostomal nurse is important in the control of the effluent from an ECF, especially in cases where there are multiple fistulas or an open abdominal wound (Fig. 19.2). Simple gauze dressing, skin barriers, pouches, and suction catheters can be used to manage fistula drainage. Although vacuum-assisted closure (VAC) systems or fibrin glue can promote ECF closure [6], the effectiveness of VAC on ECFs has not been proved. However, it may be used for large fistulas where control of the output is hard to maintain with a pouching system alone (see also Chap. 6).

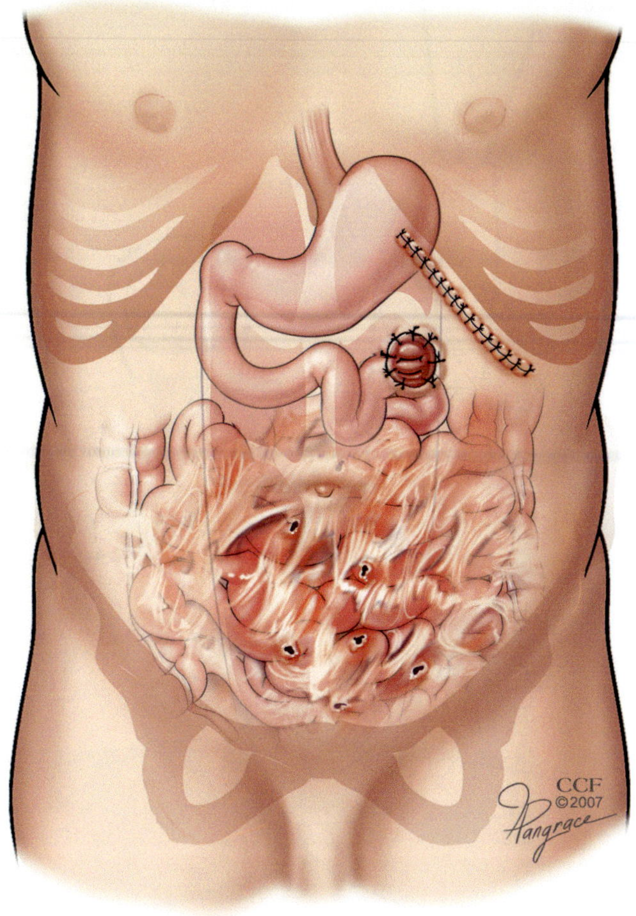

Fig. 19.3 A left subcostal incision for construction of a high jejunostomy for the management of chronic recurrent sepsis and fistula output. Illustration © CCF

Surgery

Early Repair

Early repair of an anastomotic leak or enterotomy is generally not a good idea as tissues are inflamed and weak. Under most circumstances, the leak should be diverted or exteriorized, so avoiding a fistula. If tissues are favorable, resection and reanastomosis can be done if accompanied by fecal diversion in the form of a proximal ileostomy or jejunostomy. This approach avoids the need for parenteral nutrition. In cases of severe peritonitis with difficult adhesiolysis, repeat laparotomy produces further enterotomies and small bowel injury, often requiring extensive resection, as well as new fistula formation. In patients with uncontrolled sepsis, multiple fistulas, and an open abdomen, a left subcostal incision can be made to construct a high jejunostomy (Fig. 19.3). The patient is maintained with TPN for a minimum of 6 months before reoperation and repair is contemplated. The other possibility is to make a high midline incision, avoiding

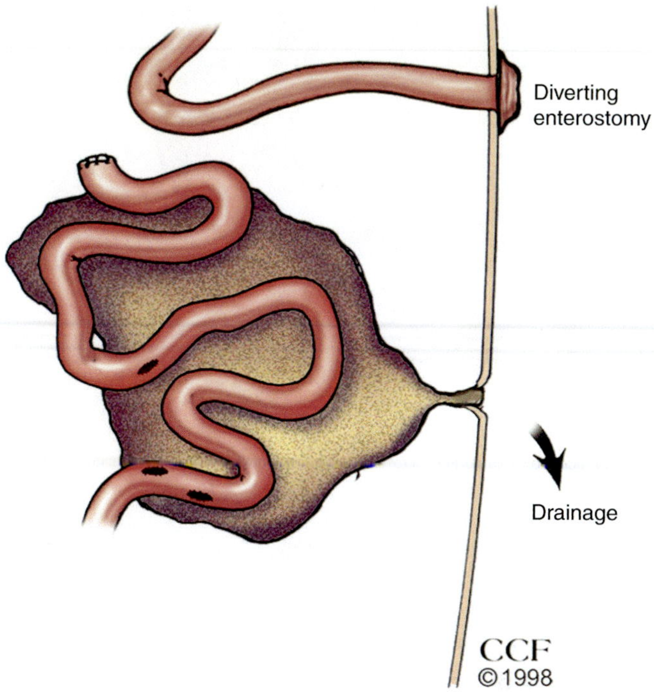

Fig. 19.4 A high jejunostomy. Illustration © CCF

the area of active sepsis/fistula, and create a high loop or end jejunostomy (Fig. 19.4).

Definitive Surgery

Timing

Reoperation during the first 2–10 weeks after the initial surgery doubles the mortality rate due to obliterative peritonitis and the problems that this causes when attempts are made to dissect the bowel. The more complex and complicated the initial surgery and its complications, the longer it takes for this obliterative peritonitis to settle. A judgment may be made about the status of intra-abdominal adhesions by palpating the abdomen and feeling how soft the contents are. Given the fact that many patients with an ECF have severe adhesions and intra-abdominal sepsis early after initial surgery (Fig. 19.5), delaying a definitive operation at least 6 months is wise.

Optimization

A multidisciplinary approach is necessary to manage the fistula until surgery can be performed. The surgeon integrates care from the stoma nurse, therapist, social worker, and sometimes psychiatrist to ensure the patient's health is optimal at the time of surgery (e.g., good nutritional status, absence of associated sepsis, etc.). Additionally, patients and their families should be aware of the prolonged recovery process, as well as possible postoperative complications and chances of fistula recurrence. Nutritional status should be adequately corrected and maintained before definitive surgery.

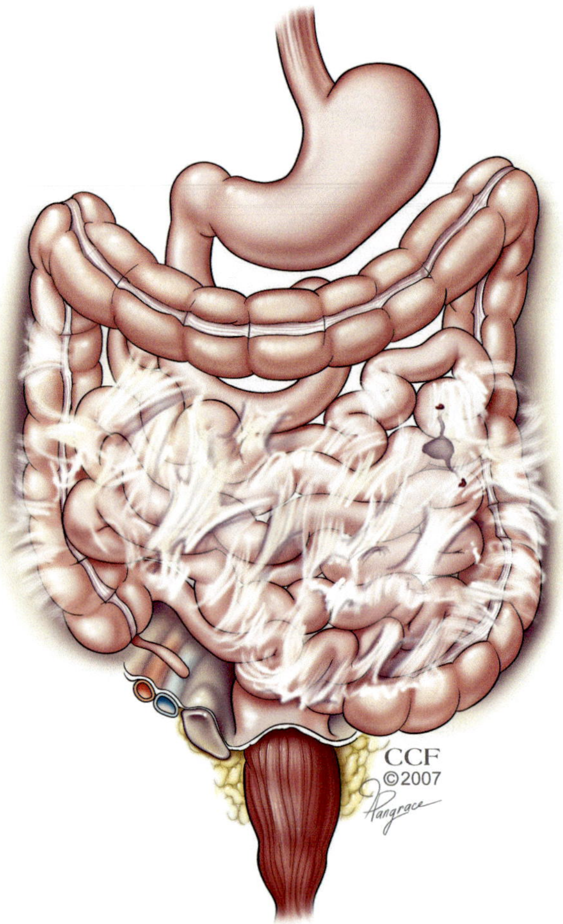

Fig. 19.5 Severe adhesions in the early period after initial surgery. Illustration © CCF

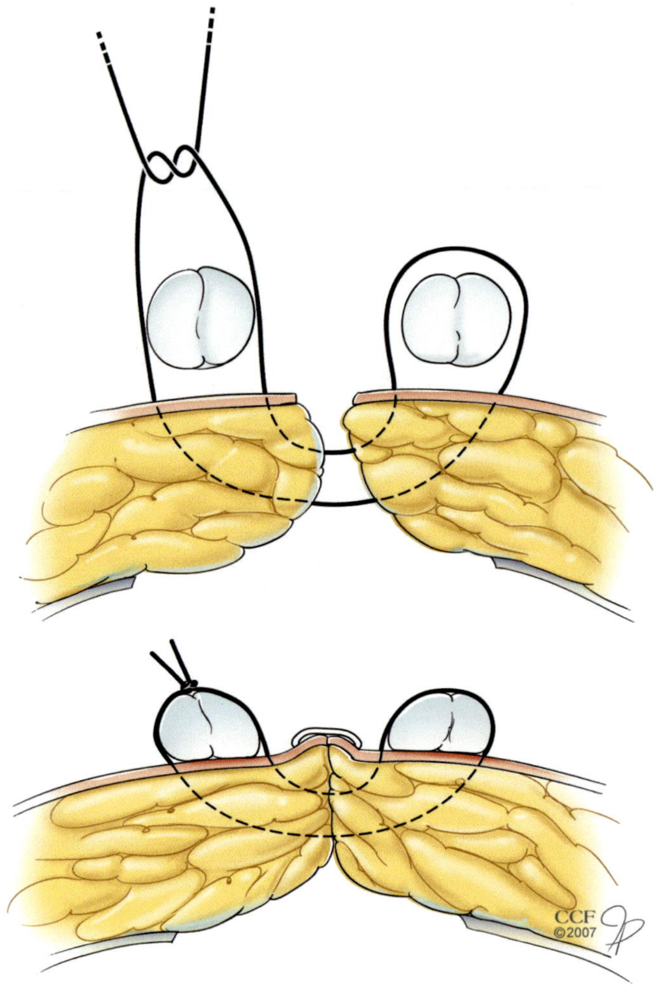

Fig. 19.6 Mobilization of full-thickness skin flaps to close the skin without tension using polypropylene suture over dental roles and staples. Illustration © CCF

Preoperative Preparation

Blood should be available, since these patients may require transfusion during this long procedure. Parenteral nutrition therapy should be discontinued on the date of operation and enteral feeding is stopped 48–72 h prior to surgery to allow for luminal antibiotic preparation. Fistulograms, gastrografin enemas, small bowel series, and stoma injection should be performed where appropriate to accurately map the anatomy of the gastrointestinal tract and the fistula.

The Procedure

At the time of surgery, the patient is placed in the Lloyd Davis position. Ureteral stents are placed when appropriate. The abdomen is opened, beginning just above the prior midline incision and skirting around the fistula opening if this is in the midline wound. It is wise to explore the upper part of the abdomen before incising the whole length of the incision, in case the operation has to be aborted because adhesions are inoperable. Once the abdominal cavity is opened, wound protectors can be placed to prevent wall contamination.

During the first stage of the operation, all adhesions to the small bowel are freed from the ligament of Treitz to the terminal ileum. Matted small bowel segments are released. An effective strategy is to dissect the most normal and least difficult areas first, leaving the segments of bowel involved in the fistula to last. During adhesiolysis, the use of sterile normal saline injection with hydro and extrafascial sharp dissection is recommended. If any serosal tears or enterotomies occur, they must be closed immediately.

Resection of the ECF and any other diseased segment of bowel is followed by a hand-sewn anastomosis. The anastomosis must be quarantined from any abscess cavity, often by interposing omentum. If the ECF is oversewn when a resection is not feasible due to the inability to adequately mobilize the bowel or concerns regarding possible short bowel syndrome, the fistula recurrence rate rises [7]. A temporary proximal jejunostomy is suggested in patients with oversewing of the ECF.

Before the abdominal cavity is closed, copious peritoneal irrigation with saline followed by inspection of the bowel surface is performed to ensure that there are no unrecognized injuries. Drains are not usually necessary unless there is a chronic abscess cavity lined by granulations. In this case, the granulations are curetted and the cavity either filled with omentum or protected by a large Penrose drain. Placement of a gastric tube can be considered if a prolonged postoperative ileus is anticipated.

In patients with bowel edema and distention, primary closure can be difficult. In these cases, lateral release of the external oblique aponeurosis or closure with absorbable mesh is helpful. If primary closure of the fascia is not possible, full-thickness skin flaps can be mobilized to close the skin without tension; polypropylene sutures are usually placed over dental rolls and staples (Fig. 19.6). When difficult primary closure is anticipated, a plastic surgery team is consulted. Permanent prosthetic material for closure should be avoided in order to prevent sepsis and further fistulization.

Conclusion

The management of an ECF includes control of fistula output with metabolic and nutritional support. Timing of definitive repair is key to its success. Early surgery should be avoided unless it is to control sepsis. Definitive repair involves resection of the fistula with the diseased segment of bowel and anastomosis and should not be attempted for at least 6 months after fistula onset. Multispecialty care in a tertiary institution results in good outcomes with low morbidity.

References

1. Evenson AR, Fischer JE. Current management of enterocutaneous fistula. J Gastrointest Surg. 2006;10:455–64.
2. Campos AC, Andrade DF, Campos GM, Matias JE, Coelho JC. A multivariate model to determine prognostic factors in gastrointestinal fistulas. J Am Coll Surg. 1999;188:483–90.
3. Remzi FH, Fazio VW. Enterocutaneous fistula. In: Bland KI, Sarr MG, Buchler MW, Csendes A, Garden OJ, Wong J, editors. General surgery: principles and international practice. 2nd ed. London: Springer; 2009. p. 649–59.
4. Fazio VW. Intestinal fistulas. In: Keighley MRB, Pemberton JH, Fazio VW, et al., editors. Atlas of colorectal surgery. New York: Churchill Livingstone; 1996. p. 363–77.
5. Lloyd DA, Gabe SM, Windsor AC. Nutrition and management of enterocutaneous fistula. Br J Surg. 2006;93:1045–55.
6. Becker HP, Willms A, Schwab R. Small bowel fistulas and the open abdomen. Scand J Surg. 2007;96:263–71.
7. Lynch CA, Delaney CP, Senagore AJ, Connor JT, Remzi FH, Fazio VW. Clinical outcome and factors predictive of recurrence after enterocutaneous fistula surgery. Ann Surg. 2004;240:825–31.

Parastomal Hernia

20

Matthew F. Kalady and Ian C. Lavery

Introduction

A parastomal hernia is defined as an incisional hernia at the site of a stomas. It is common with all types of stomas, and signs and symptoms are similar to those seen with any ventral hernia including a bulge, discomfort, or partial bowel obstruction. Factors specific to parastomal hernias include difficulty maintaining the stomas appliance or difficulty with irrigation or emptying the stomas. As corrective repair is often challenging and complex, surgery is reserved for symptomatic hernias. Various techniques, both open and laparoscopic, with and without mesh, have been described with myriad outcomes. This chapter describes the technical aspects of parastomal hernia repair.

Incidence

The overall incidence of parastomal hernia is widely variable in the literature due to differences in hernia definition, methods of diagnosis, and duration and types of follow-up. Physical examination is the cornerstone of diagnosis. Inspection and palpation of the stomal area with the appliance removed and with the patient straining allows for accurate examination. Often digitations of the stomas will reveal and define the hernia defect. Routine use of abdominal computed tomography increases the incidence of parastomal hernia detection and thus the reported incidence [1, 2]. However, the higher incidence of asymptomatic hernias does not equate to an increased need for repair. Overall, the likely incidence of parastomal hernia is between 30% and 50% [3]. Hernia rate varies by the type of stomas, and end colostomy has the highest incidence of 4–48.1%, followed by end ileostomy with an incidence of 1.8–28.3% [4]. Parastomal hernias are less common but still occur following creation of a loop ileostomy, loop colostomy, or urostomy.

A distinction should be made between a true parastomal hernia (Fig. 20.1) and a subcutaneous prolapse (Fig. 20.2). True hernias include a peritoneal sac that contains bowel or omentum. Subcutaneous prolapse, sometimes called a pseudohernia, results from slippage of the bowel through an intact fascial ring with accumulation of bowel in the subcutaneous space. It reproduces symptoms of a parastomal hernia, but because of the normal fascial opening, this problem can usually be managed by local revision.

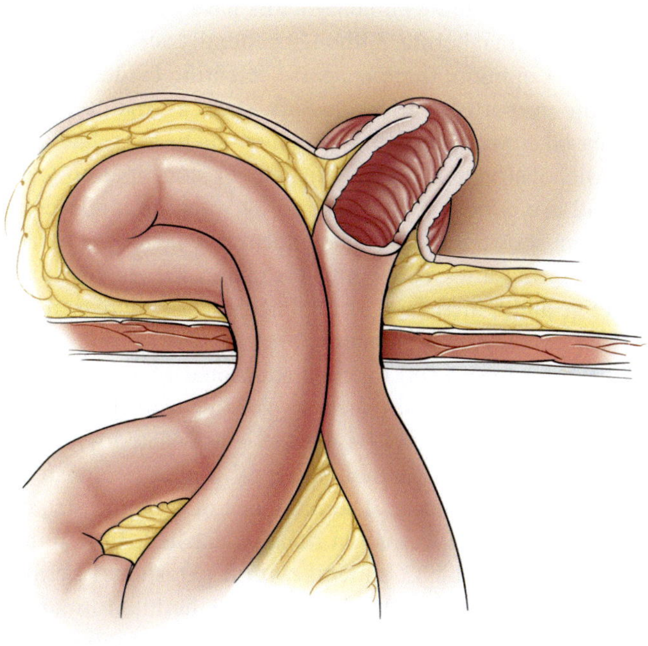

Fig. 20.1 Parastomal hernia. A true parastomal hernia includes protrusion of abdominal contents (bowel is shown here) through the stomal fascial defect. This may or may not be able to be reduced with gentle constant pressure on the herniated bowel back toward the fascial defect. Illustration © CCF

M.F. Kalady (✉) • I.C. Lavery
Assistant Professor of Surgery,
Department of Colorectal Surgery, Cleveland Clinic,
9500 Euclid Avenue, A30 Cleveland, Ohio 44195, USA
e-mail: kaladym@ccf.org

V.W. Fazio et al. (eds.), *Atlas of Intestinal Stomas*,
DOI 10.1007/978-0-387-78851-7_20, © Springer Science+Business Media, LLC 2012

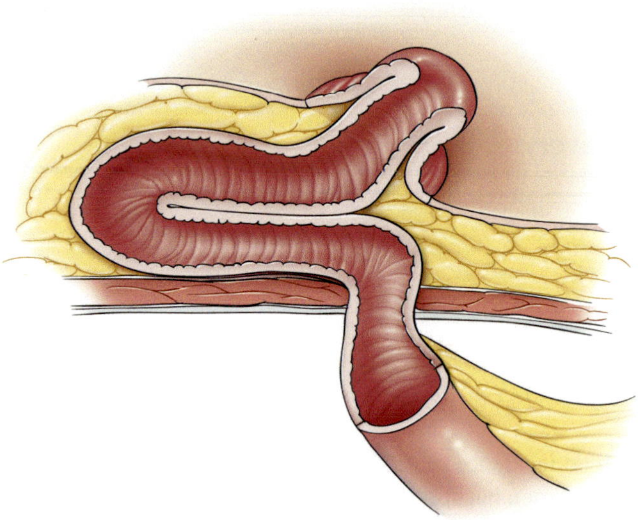

Fig. 20.2 Subcutaneous bowel prolapse. Occasionally, bowel will prolapse through the stoma aperture and fill the subcutaneous space, giving the appearance of a hernia. This is not reducible, but also usually not symptomatic other than creating a bulge. This does not create increased risk of strangulation and does not necessarily need to be fixed. Illustration © CCF

Predisposing Factors

Several patient and technical factors have been associated with parastomal hernia. Although generally accepted based on expert opinion, there is sparse scientific evidence supporting purported patient factors such as malnutrition, increased intra-abdominal pressure such as related to chronic obstructive airway disease or constipation, and steroid use. Obesity as measured by waist circumference has been shown to be an independent risk factor for parastomal hernia after colostomy formation [5]. In one prospective audit, increasing patient age slightly increased the risk of developing a parastomal hernia with an odds ratio of 1.04 (CI 1.00–1.08) for each additional year of age [6]. Technical consideration such as placement of the stomas aperture through the rectus muscle is associated with less hernia formation [7], although not all studies demonstrate a significant difference. The influence of trephine size on parastomal hernia formation remains debated. In a multivariate analysis of 33 patients with a parastomal hernia, aperture size independently predicted hernia formation with a 10% increase in risk for every millimeter increase in stomas aperture [6]. As a general rule, an aperture size that emits the bowel snugly without causing ischemia is best, although this varies for each patient and is difficult to quantify.

Primary Prevention

Due to the high incidence of parastomal hernia formation and difficulties with repair, primary prevention is favored. Some authors advocate a prophylactic approach to preventing parastomal hernias by using prosthetic mesh at the time of stomas creation [2, 8–11]. Earlier retrospective series using synthetic mesh for either prophylactic or therapeutic parastomal hernia repair has been associated with infection, seroma, and fistula formation [12–15]. However, two randomized prospective trials using lightweight mesh have demonstrated a reduced hernia formation in the underlay position during creation of an end colostomy [2, 11]. At a follow-up of 29 months, Serra-Aracil reported an incidence of 14.8% paracolostomy hernia with the use of mesh compared to 40.7% without mesh [2]. With a follow-up of 65 months, Janes reported showed a 7.5% parastomal hernia rate with mesh compared to 63% without mesh [11]. Both studies showed low rates of mesh-related complications.

Indications for Surgery

As with any hernia, incarceration, strangulation, obstruction, perforation, ischemia, and fistulization are absolute indications for surgical intervention. Relative indications include intermittent obstruction or incarceration, parastomal pain related to the hernia, difficulty with stomas care or appliance fit, and ulceration of skin overlying the hernia. There are some relative contraindications for stomas repair and these are mostly patient-related. In general, patients with severe comorbid disease, extreme morbid obesity, end-stage malignancy, or short life expectancy do not warrant repair of parastomal hernia, unless the current complication is life threatening.

Repair

The surgical management of parastomal hernia can be categorized into three main approaches: primary local fascial repair, relocation of the stomas to the contralateral side with repair of the hernia, and repair of the hernia with prosthetic mesh. There are no randomized trials directly comparing the efficacy of the various repairs. Most of the literature reports nonrandomized case series. One nonrandomized small series reported a higher recurrence rate after primary local tissue repair, but there was a higher incidence of surgical wound infection with the use of synthetic mesh [16].

Basic surgical principals should be followed regardless of the operative approach. A single dose of preoperative antibiotics is given within 1 h of the incision. The type of incision depends on the approach, but it should always be made

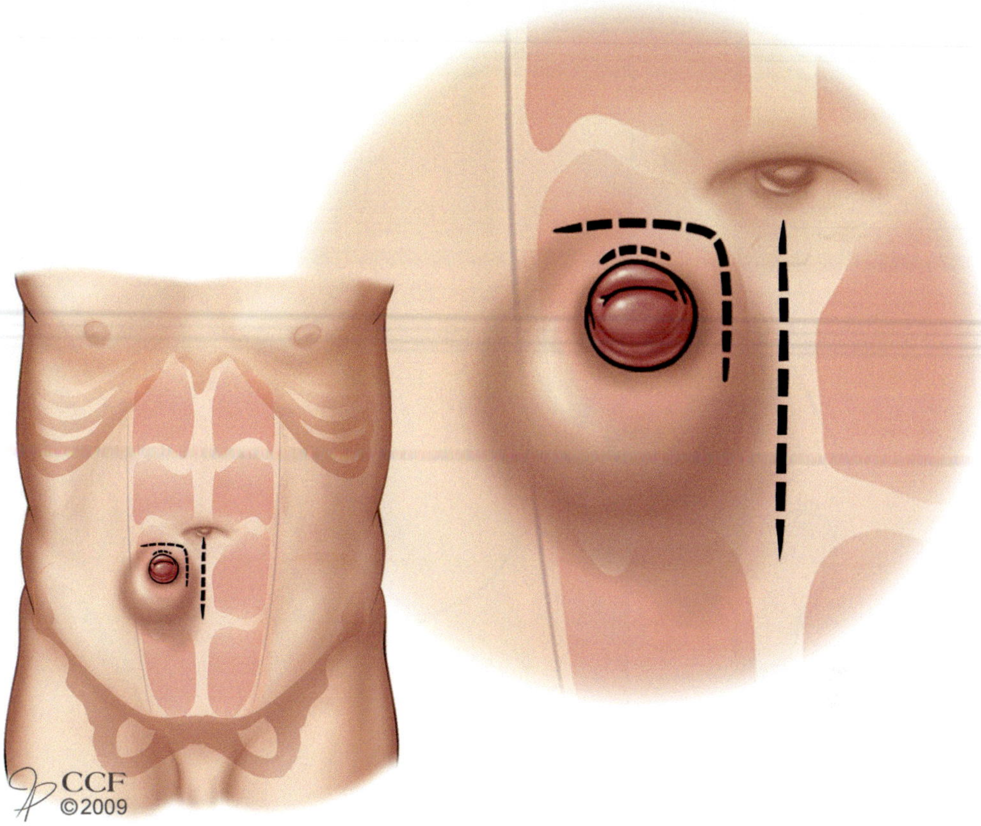

Fig. 20.3 Incision options for primary repair. If primary repair is going to be attempted, the skin incision should be made either just outside the mucocutaneous border or outside the plate of the stoma appliance. If the stoma needs to be revised, the near incision can be incorporated with the new stoma maturation site. If the stoma is not likely to be revised or rematured, the outer incision is an option as it will be outside the stoma appliance area and it will not interfere with forming a seal on the appliance nor will the wound be affected by stoma contents. A small midline incision is often preferred as it avoids creating additional skin creases in the peristomal area. Illustration © CCF

outside the area of the stomas appliance. The stomas itself is quarantined from the surgical field by covering with a clear occlusive dressing.

Local Repair

Local repair is associated with a high recurrence rate [16–18] and is not recommended as a long-term solution for durable repair. However, in certain circumstances when patients cannot tolerate a more extensive operation due to comorbidities and repair needs to be done, local repair may be utilized. The incision is either made at the mucocutaneous junction or outside the outline of the stomas template. A small midline incision is often preferred as it avoids creating additional skin creases in the peristomal area (Fig. 20.3). Dissection is carried down onto the fascia to identify the defect. The fascia is cleared circumferentially around the defect. The hernia sac is opened and excised and the contents reduced. The fascia is then reapproximated with non-absorbable sutures to create a snug stomas ring that admits the tip of a Kelly clamp. This technique is illustrated in Figs. 20.4 and 20.5. One other potential indication for utilizing local repair is the incidental finding of a small asymptomatic parastomal hernia identified at the time of surgery for another disease.

Relocation

Although there have been no randomized controlled trials, stomas relocation is associated with lower recurrence rates than primary repair [16]. Relocation of the stomas is usually to the contralateral side of the abdomen with repair of the hernia. Relocation may be done on the same side if the initial stomas was not brought through the rectus fascia and the remaining fascia on that side is still adequate. Stomas relocation normally requires a laparotomy, but some authors have described success without a laparotomy using a transperitoneal relocation [19]. This technique is hindered by the presence of adhesions. Relocation and hernia repair has been recommended as management of the first occurrence of a parastomal hernia. It is important to note that there is still a significant ventral hernia recurrence rate at the prior stomas site as high as 50% [20]. This is decreased with the use of mesh to repair that defect [21].

Repair with Mesh

Use of prosthetic mesh for hernia repair is becoming more common, particularly for recurrent hernias. The general approach involves reinforcing repair of the defect using

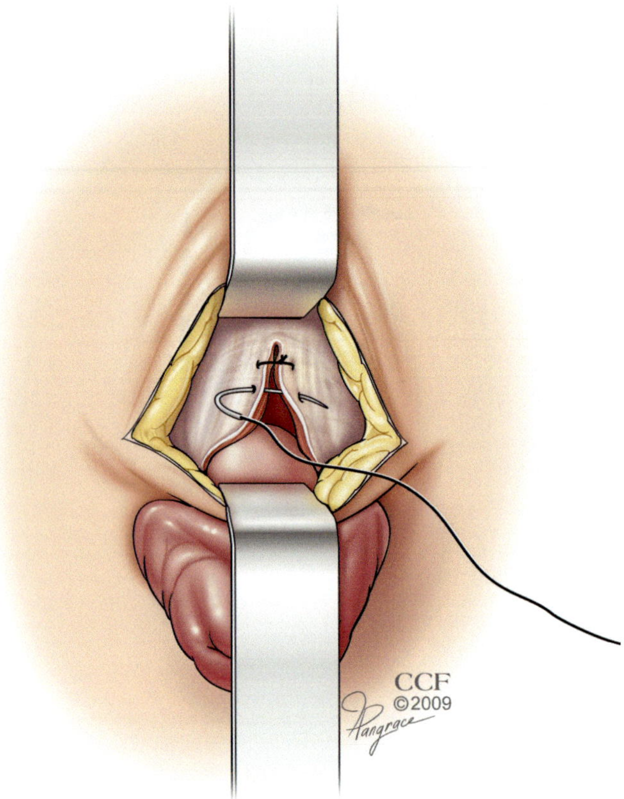

Fig. 20.4 Primary repair. Although primary repair is associated with a high rate of recurrence, it is still a feasible option in patients that cannot tolerate a more extensive procedure. With the hernia sac resected and the fascial edges cleared to healthy tissue, the fascial is closed primarily with simple interrupted or figure-eight #1 Prolene or PDS sutures. Illustration © CCF

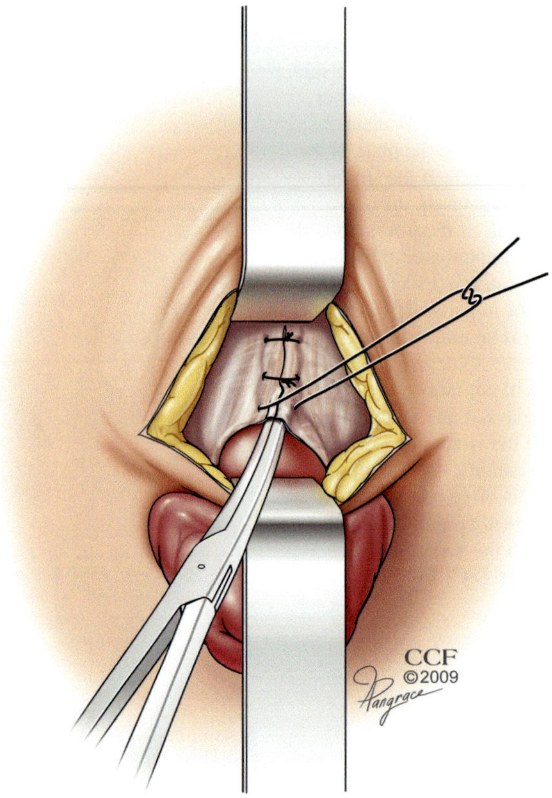

Fig. 20.5 Completed primary repair. The fascia is reapproximated so that the tip of a Kelly clamp can be inserted between the stoma and the repair. This prevents obstruction while making the repair tight enough to prevent recurrence. Illustration © CCF

prosthetic or biologic material with wide overlap of the fascia. Many different implants have been described [20, 22–26]. The insertion site of the prosthetic also varies in relation to the fascia: fascial onlay, fascia underlay (intraperitoneal), or fascia sublay (preperitoneal) placed dorsal to the rectus muscle and anterior to the posterior rectus sheath. No prospective studies have been performed to demonstrate the relative efficacy of one technique over another.

The least invasive approach entails inserting prosthetic mesh as an overlay on the anterior fascia. This has the advantage of not having to perform a laparotomy (Fig. 20.6). The hernia sac is opened and the bowel contents are reduced to identify the fascial defect. The anterior fascia is cleared for approximately 5 cm circumferentially around the stomas to create a sewing edge for the mesh. A slit is created in the mesh to allow the bowel to pass through and then the mesh is stitched to itself.

The authors prefer insertion of mesh with an underlay technique during a laparotomy. The previous midline incision is used to enter the peritoneal cavity and adhesions are lysed as necessary to clear the fascial edges. The fascial edge should be cleared for approximately 5–8 cm circumferentially to allow significant overlap of prosthetic and fascia. The appropriate mesh size is chosen and cut to fit as needed. In some circumstances, the mesh will overlap the midline incision and the underlay will cross over the midline. The mesh is secured with interrupted horizontal mattress sutures of #1 polydioxanone suture (PDS) or Prolene with 5 cm overlap on the posterior and anterior fascia.

Anchoring begins medially, superiorly, and inferiorly, with the lateral edge left for last. The lateral edge of the mesh may be handled using a keyhole approach or the Sugarbaker technique. In the keyhole approach, a slit is cut into the mesh as a keyhole through which the bowel passes. Once the mesh is secured around the bowel, the edges of the slit are sewn together to create a single sheet of mesh through which the bowel exits (Fig. 20.7). The snugness of the mesh can be adjusted by changing the degree of mesh overlap in closing the slit of the mesh. A second technique, described by Sugarbaker [27], involves lateralization of the bowel over a supportive mesh flap, essentially creating a lateral sling. The mesh is secured to the fascial ring with interrupted PDS horizontal mattress sutures circumferentially, except at the

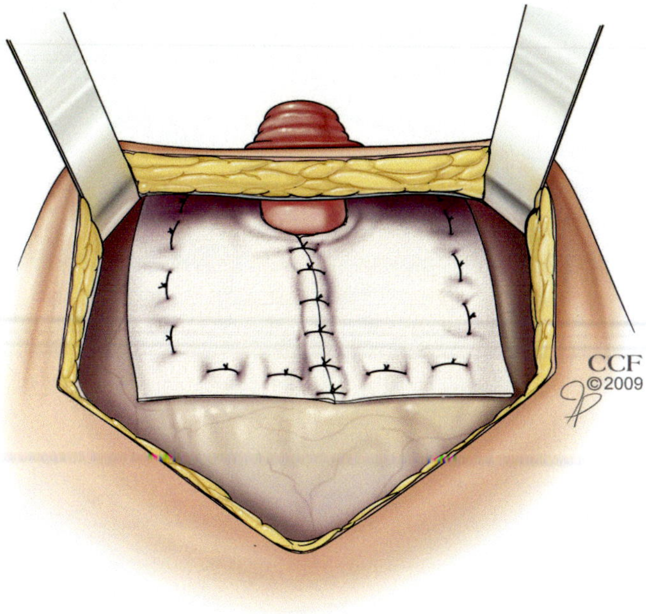

Fig. 20.6 Repair with prosthetic: overlay technique. After reducing the hernia, the anterior fascia is cleared of subcutaneous tissues for a 5-cm shelving edge and the mesh is secured with widely placed interrupted #1 PDS horizontal mattress sutures. Illustration © CCF

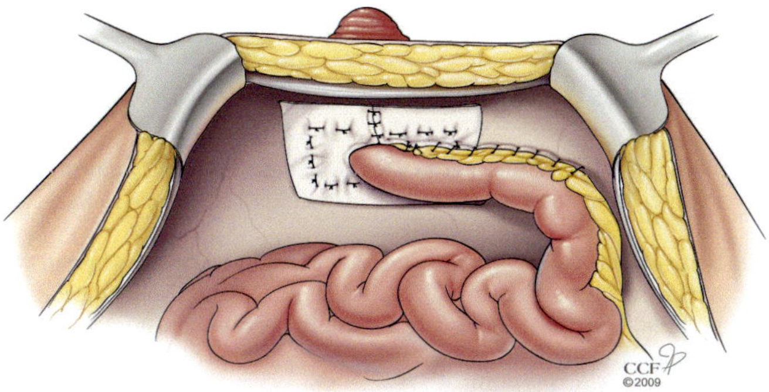

Fig. 20.7 Repair with prosthetic: underlay keyhole technique. A slit is cut into the mesh as a keyhole through which the bowel passes. Once the mesh is secured around the bowel, the edges of the slit are sewn together to create a single sheet of mesh through which the bowel exits. The snugness of the mesh can be adjusted by changing the degree of mesh overlap in closing the slit of the mesh. Illustration © CCF

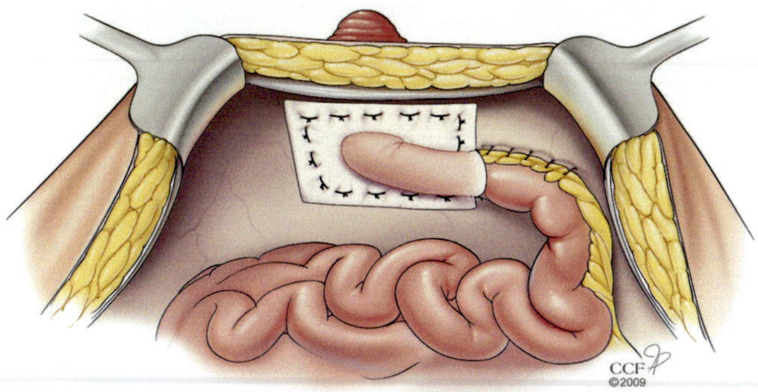

Fig. 20.8 Repair with prosthetic: underlay Sugarbaker technique. The mesh is secured to the fascial ring with interrupted PDS horizontal mattress sutures circumferentially, except at the lateral edge. Laterally, the mesh is secured to the posterior fascia on either side of the bowel as it exits laterally to create a type of flap. The mesenteric edge of the bowel is sewn to the peritoneum laterally. Illustration © CCF

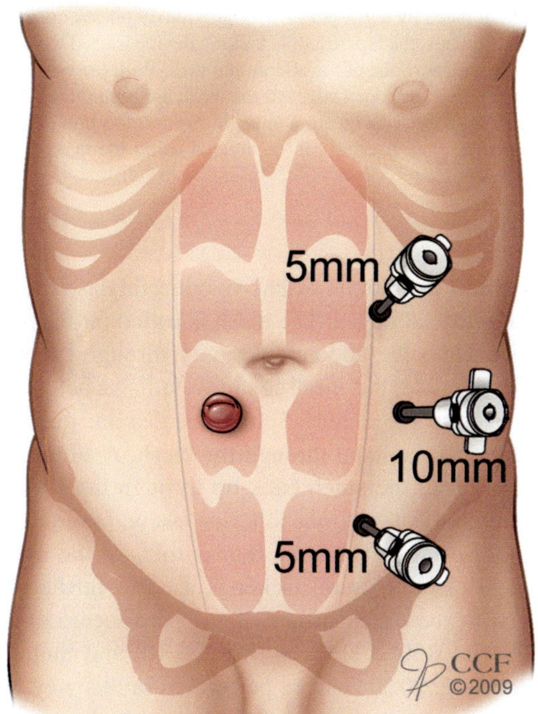

Fig. 20.9 Port placement for laparoscopic repair. The ports are placed on the contralateral side of the hernia so that the instruments can be triangulated to the pathology. A 10-mm or 5–12-mm port is placed at the level of the stoma for the camera and two 5-mm ports are placed laterally in the subcostal and lower quadrant, respectively. Ports may need to be adjusted depending on the extent of the hernia and location of adhesions. Additional 5-mm ports may be added as needed for retraction. Illustration © CCF

lateral edge. Laterally, the mesh is secured to the posterior fascia on either side of the bowel as it exits laterally to create a type of flap (Fig. 20.8). The mesenteric edge of the bowel is sewn to the peritoneum laterally. Theoretically, any increased abdominal pressure is absorbed by the mesh and decreases stress on the fascial opening.

Both the keyhole and Sugarbaker techniques have been employed using a laparoscopic approach [28–30]. Laparoscopic ports are placed to triangulate the working area. This involves placing a 10-mm or 5–12-mm port for the camera, and two additional 5-mm working ports. One example is shown in Fig. 20.9. If there is also a midline ventral hernia, the camera may need to be moved to the contralateral side of the stomas for better visualization.

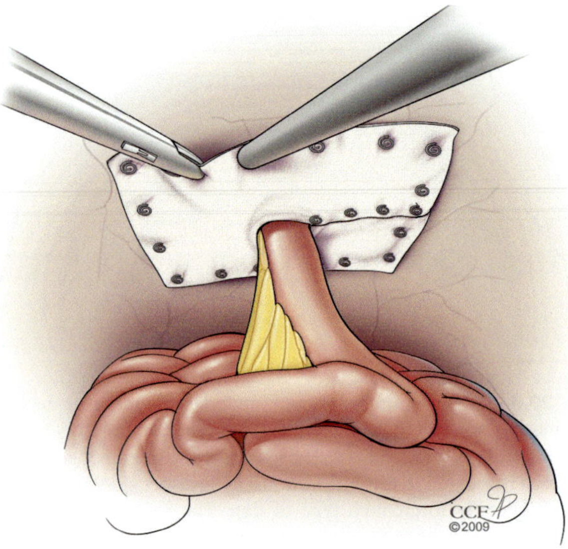

Fig. 20.10 Laparoscopic repair: underlay keyhole technique. With the mesh held in place by a grasper or with previously placed corner transabdominal stitches, the laparoscopic tacking device is used to secure the mesh to the undersurface of the abdominal wall. With the bowel mobile through the defect, the open edges of the mesh are brought together and overlapped as needed to create a snug fit around the bowel as in the open technique. The overlap can be created using the tacking device. Illustration © CCF

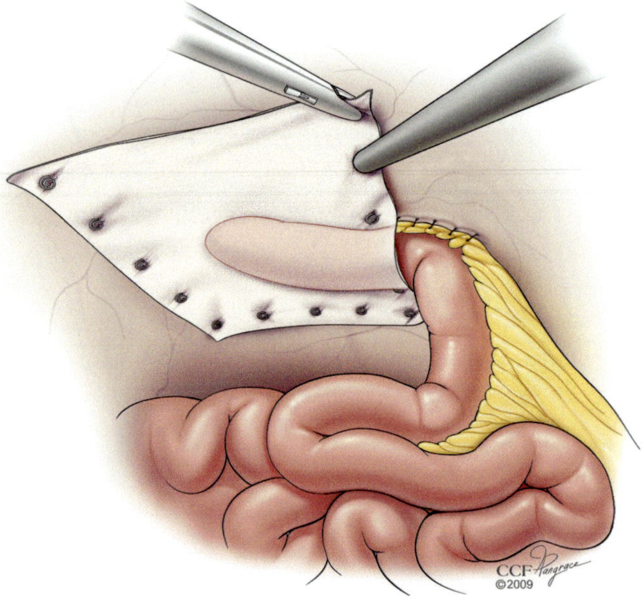

Fig. 20.11 Laparoscopic repair: underlay Sugarbaker technique. With the mesh held in place by a grasper or with previously placed corner transabdominal stitches, the laparoscopic tacking device is used to secure the mesh to the undersurface of the abdominal wall. As in the open Sugarbaker technique, the bowel exits laterally over a sling of mesh. A short segment of mesentery edge is stitched to the posterior fascia. Illustration © CCF

Just as with laparotomy, extensive adhesiolysis is required to free the fascial edges. The mesh is rolled into a cylinder and placed into the abdominal cavity through the 12-mm port. Once inside, the mesh is unraveled and held in position to overlap the defect. Spinal needles are passed into the abdominal wall and through the mesh. A suture passer is used to bring the stitch back up through the abdominal wall. The knot is tied to the anterior fascia, facilitated by a small skin incision. Once the four corners of the mesh are secured in place, a spiral tacker is used to further secure the mesh to the undersurface of the peritoneum and posterior fascia. Both a keyhole (Fig. 20.10) and Sugarbaker approach (Fig. 20.11) can be performed in this way. In one series, the laparoscopic keyhole technique had a recurrence rate of 37% at 36-month follow-up [29].

Conclusion

Despite improving techniques and technologies for prevention, parastomal hernias still remain a common problem with often difficult surgical solutions. Surgeons need to be aware of the advantages and outcomes of the various techniques and choose the best approach for the individual patient.

References

1. Williams JG, Etherington R, Hayward MW, Hughes LE. Paraileostomy hernia: a clinical and radiological study. Br J Surgery. 1990;77:1355–7.
2. Serra-Aracil X, Bombardo-Junca J, Moreno-Matias J, Darnell A, Mora-Lopez L, Alcantara-Moral M, et al. Randomized, controlled, prospective trial of the use of a mesh to prevent parastomal hernia. Ann Surg. 2009;249:583–7.
3. Israelsson LA. Parastomal hernias. Surg Clin North Am. 2008;88: 113–25.
4. Carne PW, Robertson GM, Frizelle FA, Carne PWG. Parastomal hernia. Br J Surg. 2003;90:784–93.
5. De Raet J, Delvaux G, Haentjens P, Van Nieuwenhove Y. Waist circumference is an independent risk factor for the development of parastomal hernia after permanent colostomy. Dis Colon Rectum. 2008;51:1806–9.
6. Pilgrim CHC, McIntyre R, Bailey M. Prospective audit of parastomal hernia: prevalence and associated comorbidities. Dis Colon Rectum. 2010;53:71–6.
7. Sjodahl R, Anderberg B, Bolin T. Parastomal hernia in relation to site of the abdominal stomas. Br J Surg. 1988;75:339–41.
8. Berger D. Prevention of parastomal hernias by prophylactic use of a specially designed intraperitoneal onlay mesh (Dynamesh IPST). Hernia. 2008;12:243–6.
9. Gogenur I, Mortensen J, Harvald T, Rosenberg J, Fischer A. Prevention of parastomal hernia by placement of a polypropylene mesh at the primary operation. Dis Colon Rectum. 2006;49: 1131–5.

10. Marimuthu K, Vijayasekar C, Ghosh D, Mathew G. Prevention of parastomal hernia using preperitoneal mesh: a prospective observational study. Colorectal Dis. 2006;8:672–5.
11. Janes A, Cengiz Y, Israelsson LA. Preventing parastomal hernia with a prosthetic mesh: a 5-year follow-up of a randomized study. World J Surg. 2009;33:118–21. discussion 22–3.
12. Aldridge AJ, Simson JN. Erosion and perforation of colon by synthetic mesh in a recurrent paracolostomy hernia. Hernia. 2001;5:110–2.
13. Geisler DJ, Reilly JC, Vaughan SG, Glennon EJ, Kondylis PD. Safety and outcome of use of nonabsorbable mesh for repair of fascial defects in the presence of open bowel. Dis Colon Rectum. 2003;46:1118–23.
14. Morris-Stiff G, Hughes LE. The continuing challenge of parastomal hernia: failure of a novel polypropylene mesh repair. Ann R Coll Surg Engl. 1998;80:184–7.
15. Steele SR, Lee P, Martin MJ, Mullenix PS, Sullivan ES. Is parastomal hernia repair with polypropylene mesh safe? Am J Surg. 2003;185:436–40.
16. Rubin MS, Schoetz Jr DJ, Matthews JB. Parastomal hernia. Is stoma relocation superior to fascial repair? Arch Surg. 1994;129:413–8. discussion 8–9.
17. Rieger N, Moore J, Hewett P, Lee S, Stephens J. Parastomal hernia repair. Colorectal Dis. 2004;6:203–5.
18. Horgan K, Hughes LE. Para-ileostomy hernia: failure of a local repair technique. Br J Surg. 1986;73:439–40.
19. Baig MK, Larach JA, Chang S, Long C, Weiss EG, Nogueras JJ, et al. Outcome of parastomal hernia repair with and without midline laparotomy. Tech Coloproctol. 2006;10:282–6.
20. Ellis CN. Short-term outcomes with the use of bioprosthetics for the management of parastomal hernias. Dis Colon Rectum. 2010;53:279–83.
21. Stephenson BM, Phillips RK. Parastomal hernia: local resiting and mesh repair. Br J Surg. 1995;82:1395–6.
22. Aycock J, Fichera A, Colwell JC, Song DH. Parastomal hernia repair with acellular dermal matrix. J Wound Ostomy Continence Nurs. 2007;34:521–3.
23. Ballas KD, Rafailidis SF, Marakis GN, Pavlidis TE, Sakadamis AK. Intraperitoneal ePTFE mesh repair of parastomal hernias. Hernia. 2006;10:350–3.
24. Franklin Jr ME, Trevino JM, Portillo G, Vela I, Glass JL, Gonzalez JJ. The use of porcine small intestinal submucosa as a prosthetic material for laparoscopic hernia repair in infected and potentially contaminated fields: long-term follow-up. Surg Endosc. 2008;22:1941–6.
25. Guzman-Valdivia G, Guerrero TS, Laurrabaquio HV. Parastomal hernia-repair using mesh and an open technique. World J Surg. 2008;32:465–70.
26. Kish KJ, Buinewicz BR, Morris JB. Acellular dermal matrix (AlloDerm): new material in the repair of stoma site hernias. Am Surg. 2005;71:1047–50.
27. Sugarbaker PH. Prosthetic mesh repair of large hernias at the site of colonic stomas. Surg Gynecol Obstet. 1980;150:576–8.
28. Berger D, Bientzle M. Laparoscopic repair of parastomal hernias: a single surgeon's experience in 66 patients. Dis Colon Rectum. 2007;50:1668–73.
29. Hansson BM, de Hingh IH, Bleichrodt RP. Laparoscopic parastomal hernia repair is feasible and safe: early results of a prospective clinical study including 55 consecutive patients. Surg Endosc. 2007;21:989–93.
30. Muysoms F. Laparoscopic repair of parastomal hernias with a modified Sugarbaker technique. Acta Chir Belg. 2007;107:476–80.

21 Surgical Treatment of Peristomal Skin Conditions

Eoghan Condon and David Dietz

Introduction

In the United States, 250,000 ostomies are created every year; 23% of which will, at some time, require revision. The majority of surgical revisions are for early complications of stoma formation, while up to 20% of revisions are performed for late ostomy complications relating to peristomal skin conditions. At least two-thirds of ostomates experience skin problems that interfere with the normal use of their stoma appliance, and peristomal skin problems are the most common reasons for a visit to outpatient stoma services. Most peristomal skin conditions are secondary to the effects of the stoma on what would otherwise be healthy skin. Primary diseases of the skin around the stoma, such as dermatitis, eczema, cancer, or manifestations of inflammatory bowel disease, are relatively rare. This discussion will relate mainly to the secondary conditions.

Prevention is obviously the key to minimizing the impact of peristomal skin disorders. This is accomplished by making a good stoma with correct location and proper eversion, by using properly fitting stoma appliances and with hygienic management of the peristomal skin. If prevention fails and the skin around the stoma becomes abnormal, medical management resolves many of the issues. Only a small proportion of patients need surgery. This chapter will identify peristomal skin conditions that may require surgery and discuss the indications and various surgical techniques for their treatment.

E. Condon (✉)
Department of Surgery, Limerick University Hospital, Limerick, Ireland
e-mail: eoghancondon@mac.com

D. Dietz
Department of Colorectal Surgery, Digestive Disease Institute, Cleveland Clinic Foundation, Cleveland, OH, USA

Dermatitis

Chronic Irritation and Wetness

Chronic stool leakage secondary to an ill-fitting device most commonly causes dermatitis of the peristomal skin. The most common causes of leakage are the changes that occur in the abdominal wall after surgery, usually related to weight gain or surgical scarring. Skin that is chronically wet and irritated will become hyperkeratinized and acanthotic. It will be whitish, heaped up, and tender, and may even ulcerate (see Fig. 14.32 in Chap. 14). A properly fitting, appropriately applied appliance can solve most cases. Sucralfate powder applied to erosions and roll-on antiperspirant may also be of benefit. However, some severe cases may require a short course of topical corticosteroid. In some cases, tender, hyperkeratinized skin may need to be excised under local anesthetic in the office. If the stoma is an ileostomy and does not have an adequate spout, revision to create a spout may help by minimizing the tendency of stool to leak under the faceplate.

Allergic Dermatitis

Allergic dermatitis can be identified clinically by its distribution and timing. It occurs at the onset of use of a new appliance and only areas in direct contact with the appliance are affected. Changing the type or brand of appliance and application of a topical steroid agent usually results in complete resolution. Testing the reactivity of various types of skin barriers before stoma construction minimizes the chance of allergic dermatitis.

Peristomal Pyoderma Gangrenosum (PG)

Pyoderma gangrenosum (PG) is an inflammatory skin disease characterized by rapidly growing, painful ulcers with purple edges, developing around the stoma (Fig. 21.1). PG is associated with inflammatory bowel disease, particularly

V.W. Fazio et al. (eds.), *Atlas of Intestinal Stomas*,
DOI 10.1007/978-0-387-78851-7_21, © Springer Science+Business Media, LLC 2012

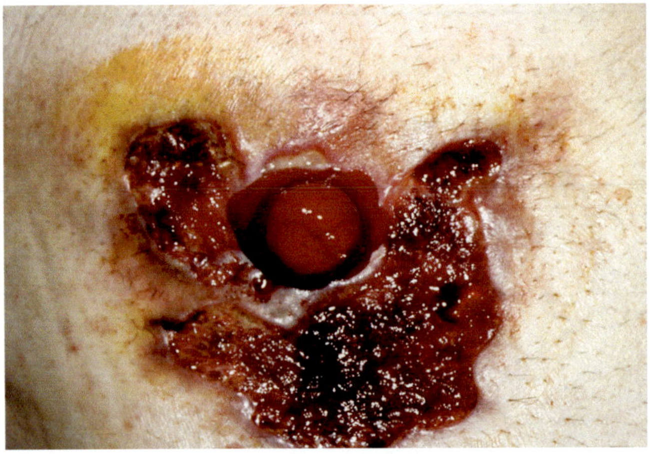

Fig. 21.1 Characteristic PG ulcers, which are deep, punched vertical edges in varying distributions away from the stoma site. With a normal ileostomy, we usually deroof the necrotic areas of these ulcers and inject them with long-acting steroids. This technique mainly involves injecting the edges of the ulcers

ulcerative colitis. Its immediate cause remains unknown, but it is most common after resiting or refashioning of a stoma. We recommend unroofing the ulcer, trimming overhanging edges, and giving intralesional corticosteroid. In a study of this approach, we demonstrated a 40% complete response rate and 40% partial response rate [1]. A sustained response rate of 80% was achievable with infliximab for patients who fail first-line therapy. Ultimately, patients may require resiting of the stoma, which is successful in 87% of patients.

Peristomal Ulceration: Traumatic or Due to Leakage

Nonspecific peristomal ulceration may be difficult to distinguish from pyoderma, but in general does not have the purplish edges. It may be due to pressure from an ill-fitting stoma device, or leakage of alkaline stool resulting in maceration. Maceration of the skin subsequently leads to skin breakdown and ulceration, forming superficial ulcers with sloping edges. Successful management depends on correcting pouching and treating the ulcer with a silicone-based film or hydrocolloid powder (Fig. 21.2).

Granulomas

Small granulomas can develop at the mucocutaneous junction, usually from excessive friction around the stoma. This can be unsightly for the patient and sometimes can cause small amounts of bleeding. The primary treatment is repeated applications of silver nitrate until the lesion has disappeared. Rarely, surgical excision is required in the office under local anesthetic (Fig. 21.3).

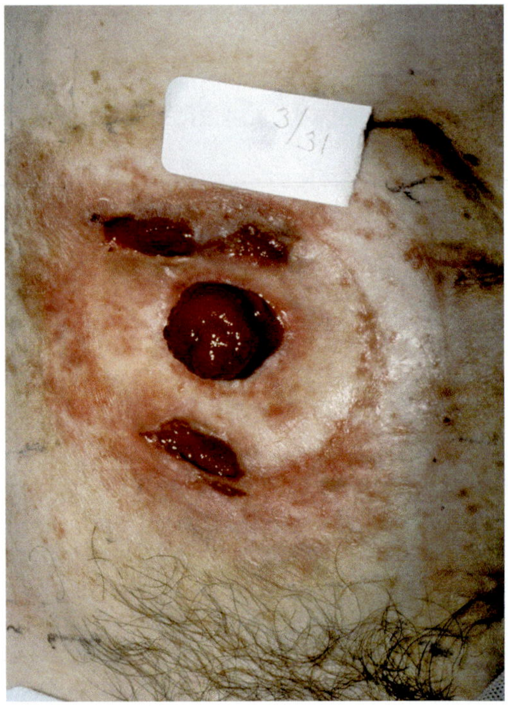

Fig. 21.2 This is an example of a traumatic pressure ulcer secondary to a change in the patient's body habitus without altering their stoma appliance. Application of hydrocolloid-based powder and a change to a concave appliance resulted in complete resolution of the ulcer

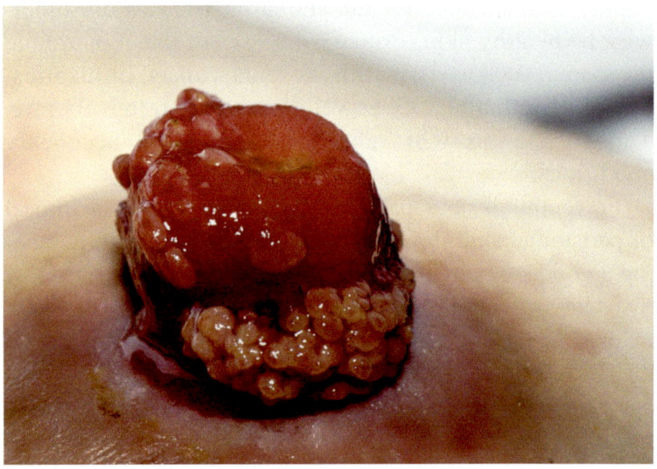

Fig. 21.3 This is an example of multiple granuloma at the mucocutaneous junction from an ill-fitting stoma device. This responded to repeated silver nitrate applications. In patients with familial adenomatous polyposis, it is advisable to send any stomal growth or polyp for histological examination as it may be an adenomatous polyp

Portal-Systemic Venous Communication at the Stoma (Vascular Proliferation)

Patients with portal hypertension develop portal-systemic venous communications around a stoma. This gives rise to the so-called *caput medusa* appearance of dilated veins around the stoma site. These veins can present with intractable stoma

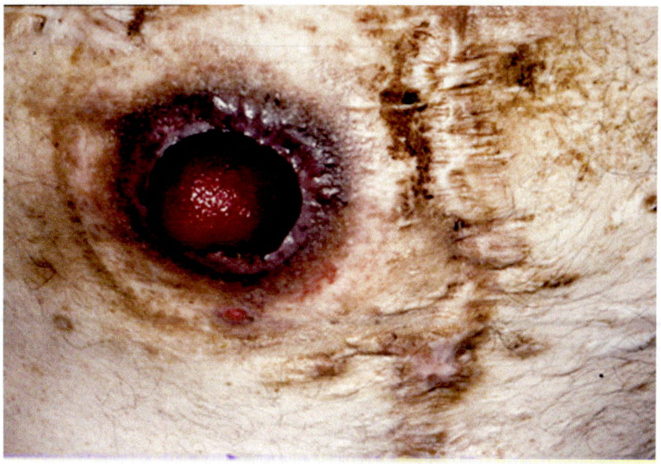

Fig. 21.4 This is an example of caput medusa. Note the circumferential dilation of veins around the stoma site. The ileostomy itself is unaffected

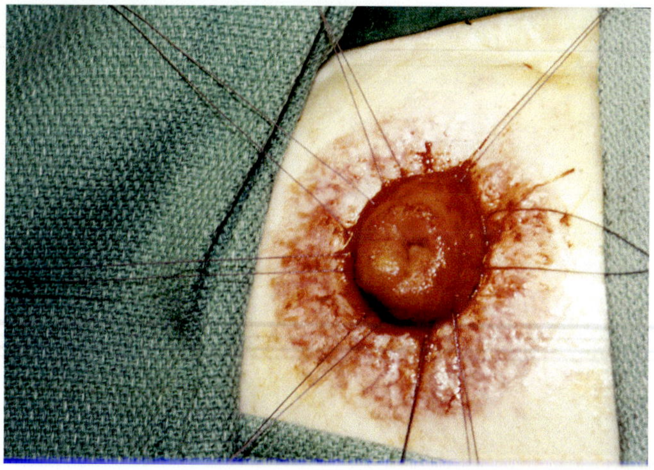

Fig. 21.5 This is an ileostomy with caput medusa. It demonstrates the first part of the surgical procedure. The mucocutaneous junction has been divided circumferentially around the ileostomy. Stay sutures have been placed with 3/0 braided absorbable sutures at 8 points equidistance apart. These sutures prevent rotation of the stoma and allow for identification of the adherent everted edge. A 3/0 braided absorbable suture can be used to ligate dilated veins between the subcuticular layer and the fascial layer in a sequential manner. We recommend this to be done in an interrupted fashion, as continuous blind suturing may result in an uneven skin surface around the ileostomy. They are full thickness at the everted edge and can be used to reapproximate the stoma by a subcuticular technique at the mucocutaneous junction after the dilated veins have been approximated

hemorrhage from even minor trauma such as removing or inserting the stoma bag. Initial management should be to stabilize the patient and correct any coagulation deficiencies. The application of pressure and injection of adrenaline may temporize the situation but rarely results in a complete stoppage of hemorrhage. A well-placed suture at the exact point of hemorrhage may help. Some authors advocate local surgery where the stoma is mobilized at the mucocutaneous junction and the varices identified and ligated. This stomal disconnection can be very bloody and is more difficult than it seems, and the venous connections re-establish themselves quite quickly (Figs. 21.4 and 21.5). A more permanent solution is to treat the underlying cause of increased venous portal pressure.

Infections

Folliculitis

Folliculitis is an inflammation of cutaneous hair follicles, which appear as red, raised spots in the skin around the stoma (see Fig. 14.42 in Chap. 14). Folliculitis may be due to the trauma of removing the stoma appliance or the trauma of shaving or clipping hair.

Folliculitis is rarely infectious but may require antibiotics if an infection supervenes. Mild folliculitis clears up on its own after 7–10 days, with gentle pouching technique.

Abscess

A peristomal abscess may herald an underlying fistula tract opening. Gentle ileoscopy may demonstrate active Crohn's disease and so will guide the management. Basic principles of treatment include control of sepsis and treatment of underlying bowel disease (Fig. 21.6). Sometimes there is an associated stricture, which nearly always ultimately requires revision. Local revision is not feasible as the involved segment is usually longer than 6 cm and the chronic sepsis around the stoma precludes safe local mobilization.

The development of a fistula early in the postoperative period is likely to be related to a missed serosal tear or enterotomy. In immunocompromised or diabetic patients, peristomal sepsis can quickly get out of control, leading to severe cellulitis and ultimately necrotizing fasciitis.

Early ileostomy fistulae by their nature are high fistulae and will not heal with conservative treatment. It is best to do a local revision of ileostomy. Colostomy fistula can be treated conservatively; a fistulotomy can be performed in the office under local anesthetic and the tract allowed to heal by secondary intention. An unmotivated patient or failure to heal within 2 weeks is an indication to revise the colostomy in the operating room.

Conclusion

Peristomal skin complications rarely require surgical intervention and the vast majority respond to either conservative or medical management (Figs. 21.7 and 21.8). The mainstay of surgical management is revision. The decision to do a local or open revision relates to the timing since a complication and associated disease.

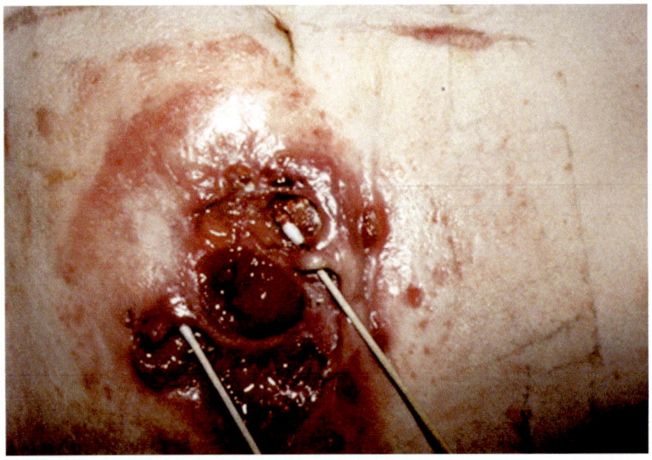

Fig. 21.6 This is an example of a Crohn's ileostomy with multiple abscesses and fistulae. Initially, the sepsis was treated locally with antibiotics and drainage. The patient's Crohn's ileostomy was then medically treated, but ultimately laparotomy was required with resection of 20 cm of strictured ileum and resiting of the ileostomy

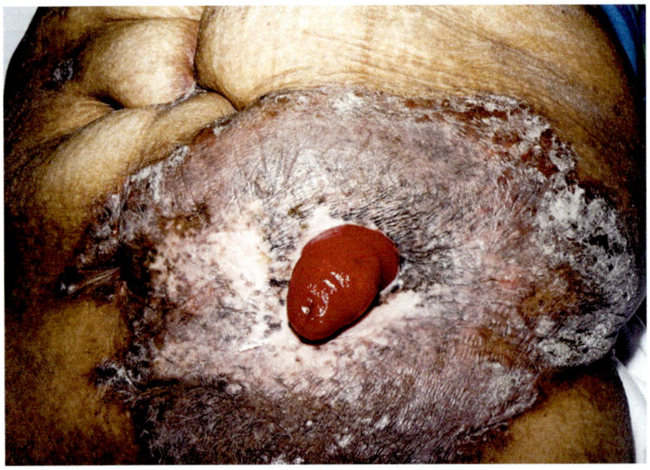

Fig. 21.7 This is primary psoriasis around a normal healthy ileostomy. Note the mucocutaneous junction is intact. The site of psoriasis rarely arises de novo; previous history of sites of abdominal wall psoriasis should be taken into account when considering stoma sites

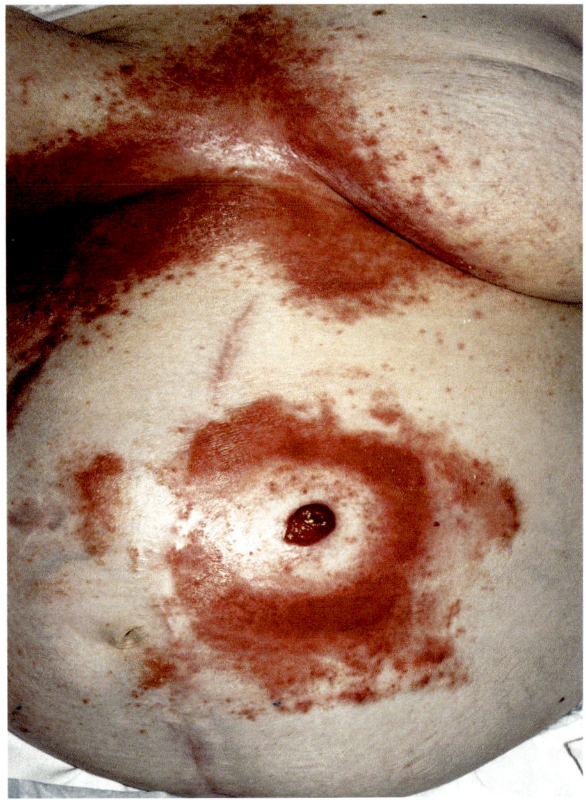

Fig. 21.8 Typical fungal rash surrounding an ileostomy. Invariably brought on by the moist environment around the adhesive stoma bag. There may also be concomitant infection with *Staphylococcus aureus*. This case responded to antibacterial and antifungal powder application over the course of 5 weeks

Reference

1. Kiran RP, O'Brien-Ermlich B, Achkar JP, Fazio VW, Delaney CP. Management of peristomal pyoderma gangrenosum. Dis Colon Rectum. 2005;48(7):1397–403.

Stoma Prolapse

22

Ursula M. Szmulowicz and Tracy A. Hull

Introduction

Stomas are frequently constructed both on elective and emergent bases. The indications for a stoma range from cancer and inflammatory bowel disease to trauma and fecal incontinence. Stomas are often beset by complications such as stenosis, retraction, and prolapse. Prolapse represents one of the most common late complications involving stomas. Indeed, the second documented colostomy – a loop sigmoid colostomy performed in 1793 on a child with imperforate anus – was complicated by prolapse [1]. Prolapse may affect all types of stoma, including colostomy, ileostomy, urostomy, and Koch pouch. Additionally, both loop and end stomas may develop prolapse (Figs. 22.1 and 22.2).

This chapter reviews the etiology, incidence, and symptoms of stoma prolapse. Also, the methods to prevent and treat stoma prolapse are discussed.

Etiology

Stoma prolapse is categorized as either fixed or sliding. A fixed prolapse results from suboptimal construction of the stoma: The stoma bud extends too far above the abdominal wall, with the length of the prolapse stable [2, 3]. In the case of a fixed ileostomy prolapse, the stoma protrudes more than 5 cm beyond the skin level [2]. Primarily, the fixed prolapsed stoma poses difficulties with fitting the stoma appliance, giving rise to bleeding from trauma to the stoma or to peristomal skin irritation due to leakage of the effluent [4]. Patients may also be distressed by poor cosmesis secondary to the protruding bowel [4].

A sliding stoma prolapse, similar to a fixed prolapse, involves the protrusion of everted intestine, either small bowel or colon, via the stoma site itself [3] (Fig. 22.3).

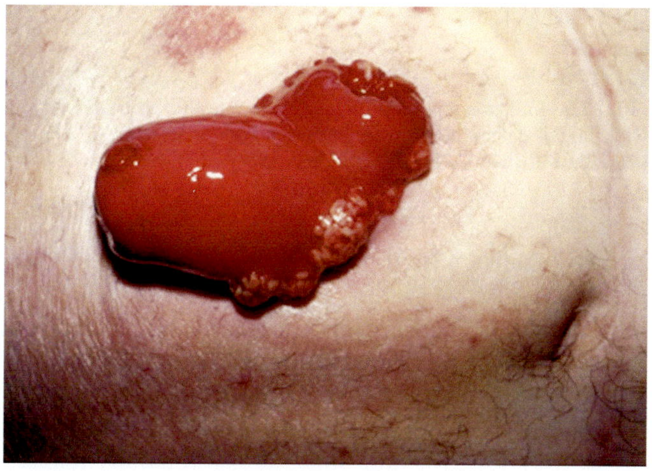

Fig. 22.1 Loop ileostomy prolapse

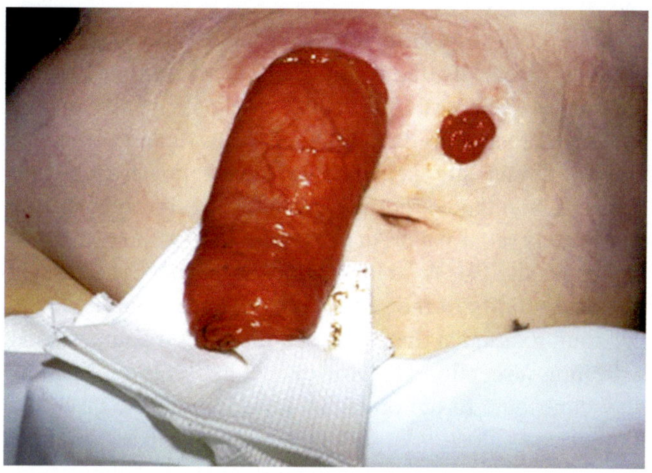

Fig. 22.2 A prolapsed end ileostomy adjacent to a mucous fistula

U.M. Szmulowicz (✉)
Department of Colorectal Surgery,
Cleveland Clinic Foundation, Cleveland, OH, USA
e-mail: szmulou@ccf.org

T.A. Hull
Department of Colon and Rectal Surgery, Digestive Disease Institute,
Cleveland Clinic Foundation, Cleveland, OH, USA

V.W. Fazio et al. (eds.), *Atlas of Intestinal Stomas*,
DOI 10.1007/978-0-387-78851-7_22, © Springer Science+Business Media, LLC 2012

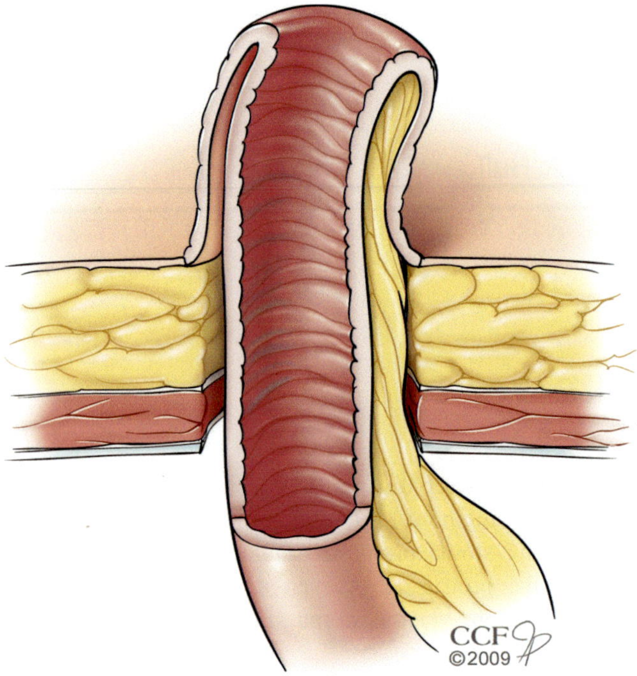

Fig. 22.3 End stoma prolapse. The mobile intestine protrudes via the wide fascial defect, along with its mesentery (Adapted from Abrams [51]. Illustration © CCF)

However, unlike a fixed prolapse, the length of the sliding prolapsed intestine varies according to the degree of intra-abdominal pressure [5]. Earlier authors divided end colostomy prolapse into three stages, each determined by the size of the prolapsed bowel: 3 cm, several inches, and up to several feet for first-, second-, and third-degree prolapses, respectively [6]. A sliding stoma prolapse usually reduces spontaneously. However, in contrast to a fixed stoma prolapse, sliding stoma prolapse carries a risk of incarceration and strangulation [3].

The etiology of a sliding stoma prolapse is a source of controversy. Generally, the condition is ascribed to an unfixed mesentery, which allows the full-thickness of the mobile intestine, along with its mesentery, to protrude excessively via the stoma site [2]. The prolapsed bowel emanates from an untethered portion of intestine located several centimeters proximal or, in the case of loop stomas, distal to the stoma site [4]. As such, Chandler and Evans suggested that the mobility of the prolapsing intestine combined with the point fixation at the stoma site indicates a commonality with intussusception [1]. However, a large fascial opening may contribute to the prolapse, especially in the case of a loop or end colostomy [1]. Turnbull and Weakley reported that, while stoma prolapse is a consequence of the herniation of the bowel through a large fascial aperture, repair of the opening does not necessarily obviate the problem [7]. Additionally, Stevenson and Volwiler noted that stoma prolapse may ensue if the opposing serosal surfaces of the stoma bud fail to become fixed or do so in an improper position [8].

Incidence

Prolapse is among the most common complications affecting stomas. The overall incidence ranges from 1% to 16% [3]. Park et al. reported a 2% rate of stoma prolapse among 1,616 stomas performed at Cook County Hospital over a 20-year period [9]. The frequency of prolapse depends upon the site of the stoma – colostomy or ileostomy – as well as the type of stoma – loop or end (Table 22.1). A shorter duration of follow-up may underestimate the extent of stoma prolapse [21].

Prolapse occurs in 2.6–26% of end ileostomies and in 0–12.5% of loop ileostomies [1, 22]. Leong and colleagues identified 12 (8%) cases of prolapse among 150 patients with a permanent end ileostomy over an average of 9.2 years of follow-up; the calculated probability of a stoma prolapse in this group was 11% at 20 years [18]. The series from Cheung found that none of the ileostomies – eight end ileostomies and two loop ileostomies – experienced a prolapse during the 38-month observation period [10]. In the case of loop ileostomies, their often temporary duration limits the opportunity for the development of prolapse [21].

The incidence of end colostomy prolapse varies from 1% to 13% [22]. An audit from Porter and colleagues described four cases of prolapse (3.2%) among 126 end colostomies over the 35-month observation period [19]. Of the 203 permanent end colostomies in the series from Londono-Schimmer et al., 11 (5.4%) stomas developed prolapse during a mean of 5.5 years of follow-up, while the actuarial rate of colostomy prolapse at 13 years was calculated to be 11.8% [11].

Loop transverse colostomies are accorded the highest frequency of stoma prolapse, ranging from 7% to 25% (Fig. 22.4) [23]. However, Cheung reported a rate of 47% in a series of 19 loop transverse colostomies; in contrast, only one of the six "bridged" transverse colostomies, in which the proximal and distal limbs were drawn through separate fascial incisions, were affected by this complication [10]. A lower incidence of 17.4% was recorded by Harris et al. in an audit of 345 stomas [16]. Edwards and colleagues compared loop transverse colostomies and loop ileostomies, demonstrating that prolapse is more common in the former group – 5.6% versus 0%, respectively (no p value) [12].

In children, colostomies – frequently performed for anorectal malformations and Hirschsprung's disease – have a frequency of prolapse that ranges from 8.1% to 58%

Table 22.1 The incidence of stoma prolapse in adult patients

	Patients	Median follow-up[a]	Loop ileostomy	Loop colostomy	End ileostomy	End colostomy
Chandler and Evans [1]	448	Unspecified		26% (52/200)		2.4% (6/248)
Cheung [10]	199	38 months	0% (0/2)	30.3% (10/33) (47% for transverse alone)	0% (0/8)	4.5% (7/156)
Londono-Schimmer et al. [11]	203	5.5 years				5.4% (11/203)
Edwards et al. [12]	34	62 days[a]	0% (0/34)			
	36	73 days[a]		5.6% (2/36)		
García-Botello et al. [13]	127	9.13 months[a]	3.1% (4/127)			
Gooszen et al. [14]	70	3 months[a]	3.1% (1/32)	2.6% (10/38)		
Hoffman et al. [15]	111	10.4 months[a]		5.3% (2/38)		1.4% (1/73)
		22 months				
Harris et al. [16]	345	Unspecified	2% (1/44)	13% (6/47) (17.4% for transverse alone)	0% (0/44)	1.4% (3/210)
Law et al. [17]	77	183 days[a]	0% (0/39)			
		180 days[a]		7.9% (3/38)		
Leong et al. [18]	150	9.2 years			8% (12/150)	
Porter et al. [19]	126	35 months				3.2% (4/126)
Wexner et al. [20]	83	10 weeks[a]	0% (0/83)			

[a]Or time to stoma closure

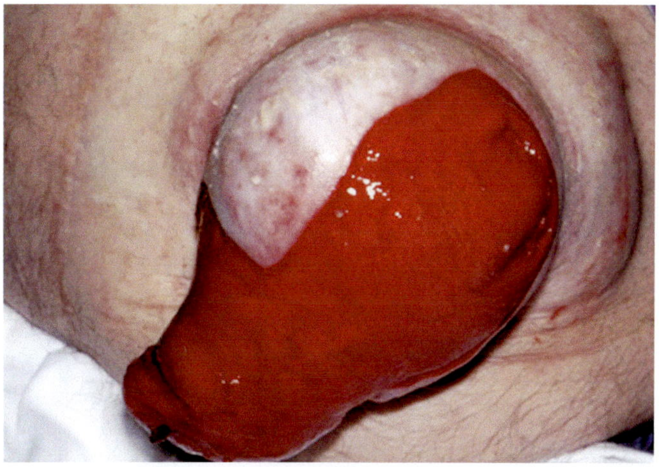

Fig. 22.4 Loop colostomy prolapse

Table 22.2 The incidence of stoma prolapse in pediatric patients

	Total patients	Time to colostomy closure	Colostomy prolapse
Al-Salam et al. [24]	74	Unspecified	18.90%
Chandler and Evans [1]	43 (19 between 1 and 13 years old)	Unspecified	25.6% (58% in 1–13 year olds)
Çiğdem et al. [25]	473	6.7 months (ARM) 6.9 months (HD) 3.6 months (other)	20.50%
Lister et al. [26]	189	Unspecified	12%
Mollitt et al. [27]	146	6–15 months	12%
Nour et al. [28]	138	10.7 months (HD) 12.4 months (ARM)	18.8% (73% for loop transverse)
Pena et al. [29]	1470	Unspecified	8.10%

ARM anorectal malformation, *HD* Hirschsprung's Disease

(Table 22.2). This high rate for colostomy prolapse belies the often temporary nature of these stomas, which are generally reversed once the underlying pathology is addressed. Çiğdem and colleagues retrospectively reviewed their experience with 473 children who underwent a colostomy, observing a 20.5% incidence of stoma prolapse, the second most common complication in the series following skin excoriation, over the up to 6.7-month follow-up [25]. A similar study from Pena et al. demonstrated that colostomy prolapse developed in 119 (8.1%) of the 1,470 children who had a colostomy, primarily the Hartmann's procedure (16.1%) and loop colostomy (15.6%) [29]. The transverse loop colostomy specifically was most impacted by stoma prolapse in a retrospective analysis of pediatric colostomies from Nour and colleagues, accounting for 73% of the 26 cases of colostomy prolapse among 138 children [28].

Prolapse is a frequently encountered complication of the myriad stoma types. Although prolapse most commonly involves loop transverse colostomies, all stomas are at risk. The colostomies created for childhood disease are especially prone to prolapse [1]. The variation in the rates of prolapse among series may rest upon differences in follow-up, with the incidence increasing over time.

Onset

Turnbull and Weakley categorized stoma prolapse as acute or chronic in onset [7]. The less frequently encountered acute prolapse follows a sudden increase in intra-abdominal pressure, or a "sudden expulsive effort" [7]. Due to the associated edema of the prolapsed bowel, manual reduction often fails, resulting in gangrene or strangulation [4]. In contrast, chronic prolapse progressively develops over a long time [7].

Prolapse is considered a late complication of stoma creation, occurring at least 1 month following surgery, with the majority developing within a year of the procedure [1]. Allen-Mersh and Thomson determined that 8 (50%) of their 16 patients experienced prolapse of an end colostomy within this time frame [30]. In contrast, in a series from Duchesne and colleagues, 2 (22.2%) of the nine cases of stoma prolapse took place within 1 month of surgery, as an early complication [31]. Additionally, Allen-Mersh and Thomson further noted that stomas are perpetually at risk for prolapse: The remaining 8 (50%) patients were found to have end colostomy prolapse between 1 and 20 years after stoma construction [30].

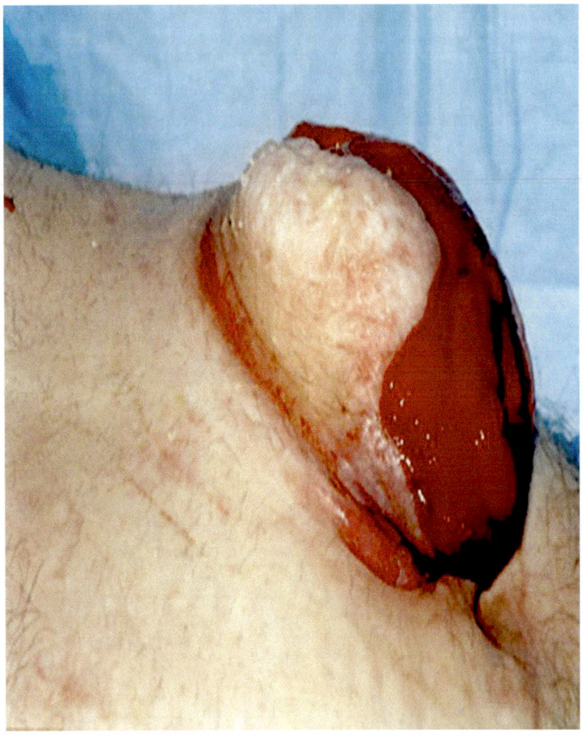

Fig. 22.5 A traumatized prolapsing end colostomy with active bleeding

Symptoms and Signs

The presentation of stoma prolapse ranges from asymptomatic to incarceration and strangulation. Robertson et al. reported that 50% of their cases of ileostomy prolapse were considered "minor" [21]. Cosmesis is the principal complaint in most patients, with the prolapsed stoma appearing as a prominent and unattractive bulge, not easily hidden by clothing [3]. Stoma prolapse also poses difficulties related to pouching. The prolapsed intestine may force the appliance from the flange, resulting in the leakage of enteric contents and subsequent peristomal skin irritation [8]. Additionally, the presence of a concomitant parastomal hernia may further exacerbate the management of the appliance [8]. The tip of the prolapsed stoma easily becomes traumatized, developing pressure necrosis and ulceration with bleeding [8, 32] (Fig. 22.5). Weaver and colleagues noted that three (37.5%) of their eight patients with ileostomy prolapse experienced accidental injury to the stoma, causing bleeding and necrosis [33]. Abdominal discomfort may arise in association with the prolapsed stoma [32]. Moreover, stoma prolapse has a negative impact upon the quality of life of the patients (Fig. 22.6). A review of Dutch stoma patients from Gooszen and colleagues found that stoma prolapse resulted in category III social restriction (38%) – "complete isolation" – significantly more often than in category I (6%) – "social restriction less than once per week" ($p<0.05$) [14]. Despite these difficulties, an uncomplicated stoma prolapse does not impinge upon bowel function. However, prolapse of a loop stoma potentially leads to incomplete fecal diversion [3].

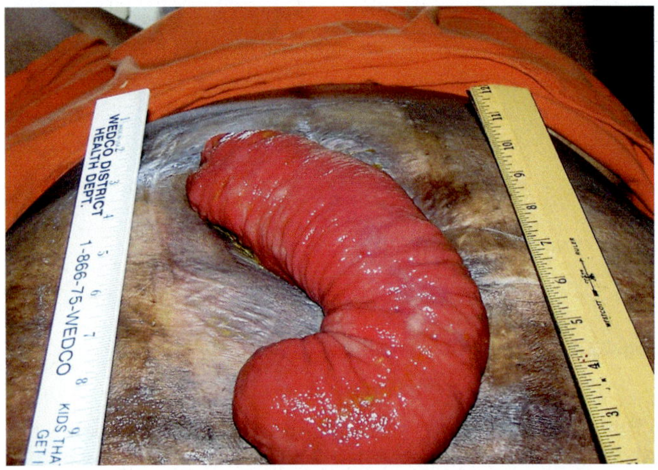

Fig. 22.6 A markedly prolapsed loop colostomy (Courtesy of Dr. Luca Stocchi)

An incarcerated, or irreducible, prolapsed stoma is a rare occurrence. An incarceration presents with abdominal pain and compromised bowel function due to the associated edema [7, 8]. Moreover, its progression to strangulation may be accompanied by peritonitis and, ultimately, systemic signs of sepsis [8].

Risk Factors

A variety of factors, both patient-related and technical, predispose to stoma prolapse.

An increase in intra-abdominal pressure is strongly associated with stoma prolapse. Pomeranz first proposed this relation, noting that persistent outward pressure upon the stoma, in conjunction with periodic straining efforts and peristalsis, allows for the intussusception of bowel via the stoma [5]. In their series of 58 adults with colostomy prolapse, Chandler and Evans determined that 11 (18.9%) had a known reason for elevated intra-abdominal pressure: two with chronic obstructive pulmonary disease and nine with malignant ascites [1]. Constipation and chronic coughing have also been identified in patients with stoma prolapse [34]. Ng and colleagues commented that the high incidence of stoma prolapse in infants and children may stem from the higher intra-abdominal pressures from frequent crying [35].

Obesity has also been charged with a greater propensity for stoma prolapse, in addition to other stoma complications [3]. This association is also ascribed to an increased intra-abdominal pressure [34]. Yet, Park and colleagues discerned no correlation between obesity and late stoma complications in the series of 1,616 stomas from Cook County Hospital [9]. Arumugam and colleagues concluded that obesity was only independently linked to stoma retraction and early skin excoriation, not to stoma prolapse [36]. In contrast, Duchesne et al. reported that obesity (BMI > 30) was significantly related to an increase in overall stoma complications (OR = 2.66, 95% CI = 1.15–6.16); although stoma prolapse was not considered separately, three (33%) of the nine cases of stoma prolapse occurred in this population [31]. Similarly, in a retrospective review of 345 stomas, Leenen and Kuypers recorded an overall complication rate of 47% in those with a BMI of 30–40 and of 36% in patients with a normal weight; yet, only stoma necrosis was significantly more common in the obese as compared to patients of normal weight ($p < 0.003$) [37].

Pregnancy has also been correlated with stoma prolapse [38]. Yet, Scudamore et al. observed that only 1 (8.3%) of the 12 women with stomas who underwent a total of 18 pregnancies developed a stoma prolapse [39]. Daly and Brooke found no stoma complications among the eight pregnancies in their series of end ileostomies performed in association with a total proctocolectomy [40]. Furthermore, a report from Gopal and colleagues, based upon questionnaires sent to members of the American Society of Colon and Rectal Surgeons in 1985, revealed that 5 (7.5%) cases of stoma prolapse occurred in a group of 66 ostomates who underwent 82 pregnancies: four in end ileostomies and one in an end colostomy [41]. The authors opined that stoma prolapse during pregnancy results from the outward force of the enlarging uterus upon the stoma [41]. Additionally, stoma prolapse is promoted by the increased intra-abdominal pressures caused by hyperemesis gravidarum [42]. However, Wu and Fazio stated that an increased protrusion of the stoma, by as much as 2–3 cm, is common during pregnancy, especially in the third trimester; the pseudoprolapse generally resolves following delivery and should not be surgically corrected unless persistent [39, 43]. A large fascial defect and a lack of mesenteric fixation contribute to this finding [43].

Children are considered to be at a greater risk for stoma prolapse [1]. In a series from Chandler and Evans, 58% of the 19 children from the ages of 1–13 years old experienced a colostomy prolapse – a significant difference when compared to the 13% of the 448 adults (>13 years old) with the same complication ($p < 0.001$) [1]. Among the children and adults, the proportion of end and loop colostomies involved in stoma prolapse was similar [1].

Advanced age purportedly results in a greater proclivity to stoma prolapse [34]. Yet, Chandler and Evans did not note a significant difference in the incidence of loop colostomy prolapse in those younger (27%) as compared to older (25%) than 60 years old [1]. Similarly, Harris et al. did not encounter more instances of stoma prolapse in the elderly, despite the greater number of stomas in that age group [16]. Also, Park and colleagues reported no correlation between late stoma complications and older age; however, the authors did associate aging with a significant increase in overall and early complications ($p = 0.0097$ and 0.009, respectively) [9].

Gender has not been shown to influence the risk of stoma prolapse. Chandler and Evans observed a non-significant difference between men and women with regard to colostomy prolapse, 16% and 11%, respectively [1]. Overall complication rates were unaffected by the gender of the patient in the series of 1,616 stomas from Cook County Hospital [9]. A similar lack of correlation between gender and overall stoma complications was demonstrated by a review of the Charity Hospital experience with 164 patients with stomas [34].

Patients with a spinal cord injury are more susceptible to stoma prolapse. Arun and colleagues reviewed their experience with stomas in an Acute Spinal Cord Injury Unit, finding a rate of prolapse of 54.5% [44]. Moreover, in three patients, the prolapse recurred up to three times despite surgical intervention [44]. Of the six patients with stoma prolapse, all had injuries at T-10 or higher; only 2 (18.8%) of the 11 patients without prolapse had a spinal cord injury above this level [44]. The authors concluded that stoma prolapse is more frequent in patients with a spinal cord injury above T-10, due to the associated denervation of the lower quadrants of the abdomen [44]. Similarly, Goldsmith and colleagues contended that abdominal wall atony in general acts as a predisposing factor for stoma prolapse [6].

Emergency stoma procedures reportedly increase the rate of complications such as prolapse, when compared to elective cases [10]. Yet, in a review of the experience of the Harborview Medical Center with 51 stomas created under emergency conditions, only one proximal colostomy (1.9%) developed a prolapse, attributed to poor technique [45]. Leenen and Kuypers also demonstrated no significant difference in overall stoma complications, including prolapse, between the emergent (36%) and elective groups (36%), with the exception of necrosis and high output in the former situation ($p<0.01$) [37]. The incidence of prolapse was similar in the emergency and elective stomas, as detailed by Robertson et al. (4% versus 6%) [21]. Although Harris and colleagues established that stoma prolapse was more common in the emergency (4%) rather than the elective (2.6%) setting in a series of 345 stomas, this disparity did not reach statistical significance [16].

A failure to perform preoperative stoma marking, especially in the emergent setting, has been cited as a risk factor for stoma prolapse [22]. In a series of 49 patients with stomas secondary to inflammatory bowel disease from Weaver et al., four (50%) of the eight stomas developed prolapse in conjunction with a malpositioned stoma [33]. Yet, although Park and colleagues observed a reduction in the overall rate of stoma complications after preoperative stoma marking ($p=0.0089$), this finding did not apply to either early or late complications alone [9]. Additionally, in a series of 127 loop ileostomies, García-Botello et al. did not identify an increase in the incidence of complications, including stoma prolapse, in stomas created without preoperative stoma marking [13]. A study from Bass and colleagues revealed that preoperative stoma marking significantly improved outcomes for early ($p<0.03$) but not late complications such as stoma prolapse ($p<0.34$) [46]. The authors remarked that such late complications as prolapse depend more upon errors in technique than in stoma position [46]. In particular, Leong and colleagues concluded that constructing an end ileostomy or colostomy via the oblique muscles instead of the rectus abdominus muscles did not influence the probability of stoma prolapse [18]. Also, Chandler and Evans did not encounter a greater frequency of prolapse in those stomas placed through the incision [1].

An absence of mesenteric immobilization proximal to the stoma has been implicated in the etiology of prolapse [6]. The resulting redundant, unfixed intestine is thus capable of prolapsing via the stoma site [6]. In a retrospective review of children with colostomy complications, Pena et al. noted that the prolapse consistently included the mobile segment of the colon [29]. A fluoroscopic evaluation of seven right transverse loop colostomies with prolapse of the distal limb revealed that the involved segment was redundant in each case, with a length of 30–45 cm [47]. Yet, Turnbull and Weakley proffered that mesenteric fixation by any method does not preclude stoma prolapse [7]. Leong et al., in an audit of 150 patients with an end ileostomy, found that mesenteric fixation did not result in a significant reduction in the incidence of prolapse [18]. This assertion was also reflected by the experience of the St. Mark's group with permanent end colostomies and prolapse [11]. In addition, Warren and McKittrick recorded a 13.3% rate of stoma prolapse among 210 patients despite their standard practice of mesenteric fixation [48].

A large fascial aperture is a common finding in stomas that develop prolapse. Turnbull and Weakly suggested that stoma prolapse is defined by the herniation of bowel through an overly large fascial defect [7]. Allen-Mersch and Thomson established that 50% of the prolapsed colostomies, primarily end colostomies, in their series had an associated parastomal hernia [30]. In a review of their experience with trephine stomas, Kini et al. observed that, among 25 patients, 3 (12%) cases of prolapse occurred, attributed to the larger fascial defect necessitated by this technique [49]. A large fascial opening is similarly implicated as the cause of prolapse in stomas performed for distal obstruction [50]. In order to accommodate the dilated, obstructed bowel, a sizeable fascial defect is created at the time of the procedure; however, as the obstruction is relieved, the bowel returns to its normal proportions, leaving a commodious opening [50]. The audit from Chandler and Evans demonstrated a 38% rate of prolapse in those colostomies constructed to relieve a distal obstruction, a significantly greater incidence than the 7% rate for colostomies not performed for distal obstruction ($p<0.001$) [1]. The authors also ascribed the higher frequency of stoma prolapse in infants to the large fascial defect required in the setting of distal obstruction, as with Hirschsprung's disease [1]. Additionally, a defect created by excision – as opposed to incision – of the fascia weakens the abdominal wall and predisposes to stoma prolapse [34, 51].

Loop stomas, especially transverse loop colostomies, are more prone to prolapse [35]. Chandler and Evans encountered prolapse in their loop colostomies 10 times more frequently than in their end colostomies: 26% versus 2.4% ($p<0.001$) [1]. The distal limb of loop stomas is particularly given to prolapse [7, 35] (Fig. 22.7). However, in their series of colostomies, Chandler and Evans observed that both limbs of the loop colostomies prolapsed in 79% of the 63 cases, although the prolapsed distal limb was significantly longer [1]. In ten patients (15.8%), only the distal limb of the loop colostomy prolapsed, as compared to three cases (4.4%) in which the proximal limb alone protruded [1]. Edwards et al. found 2 (5.5%) stoma prolapses among the 36 patients with temporary loop transverse colostomies but none in the 34 patients in the loop ileostomy group following low anterior resection [12]. The authors attributed this difference in stoma prolapse to the larger fascial opening of the loop transverse colostomy (no p value) [12]. Similarly, loop colostomies are more likely to prolapse with a more proximal location, where the greater diameter of the bowel dictates a larger fascial defect for exteriorization [1]. Chandler and Evans determined that loop cecostomies, as compared to right or distal transverse colostomies, have a greater incidence of prolapse, at 100%, 39.5%, and 12.2%, respectively [1].

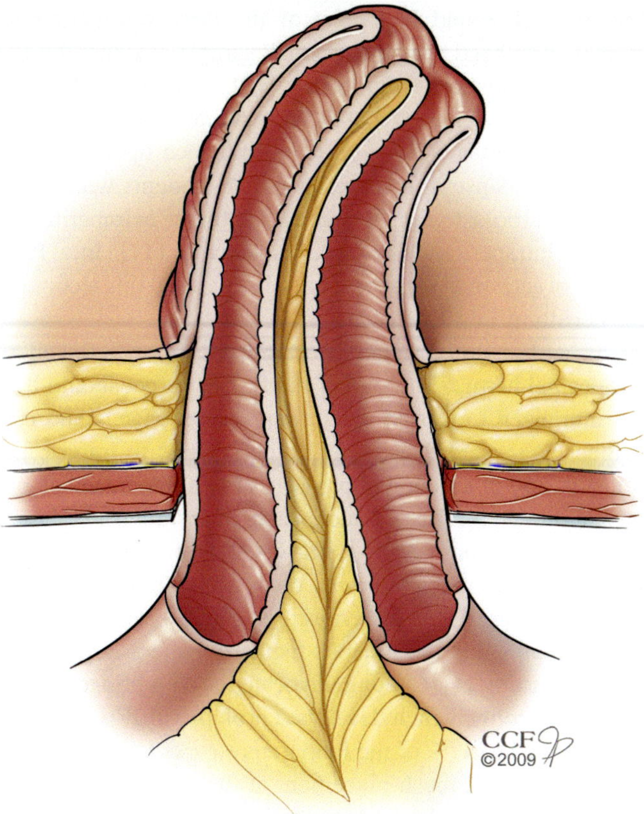

Fig. 22.7 Loop stoma prolapse. Prolapse usually originates with the distal limb of the loop stoma, which is pictured as longer than the proximal limb. The mesentery is included with the prolapsing intestine (Adapted from Abrams [51]. Illustration © CCF)

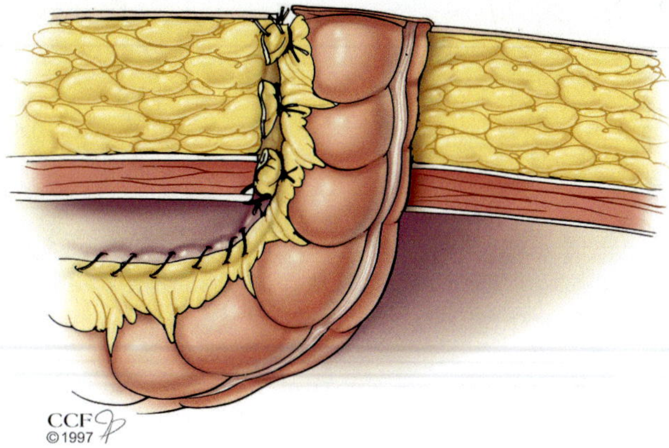

Fig. 22.8 Mesenteric fixation. The mesentery of an end stoma is secured to the peritoneum, in addition to the fascia and subcutaneous fat (Adapted from Wu and Fazio [43]) Illustration © CCF)

Numerous factors, both patient-related and technical, have been linked to the development of stoma prolapse. Various series support the connection between stoma prolapse and an increase in intra-abdominal pressure, young age, and spinal cord injury. Although both pregnancy and obesity result in an elevation in intra-abdominal pressure, neither definitively leads to a greater incidence of stoma prolapse. Stomas performed in an emergency setting without the benefit of preoperative stoma marking also have not been shown to be more susceptible to prolapse. The importance of mesenteric fixation remains controversial. However, a large fascial opening – often in association with a loop stoma, a proximal stoma location, or distal obstruction – does predispose to stoma prolapse.

Prevention

Kim and Kumar noted that avoidance of a stoma is the best measure to prevent stoma complications [3]. However, stoma creation often is inescapable. Thus, technical excellence in constructing a stoma is the primary deterrent against stoma prolapse. This begins with preoperative marking of an appropriate stoma site, ideally through the rectus abdominus muscle. Nevertheless, even a well-made stoma does not entirely eliminate the risk of prolapse [52]. As such, the technique of stoma creation has undergone various modifications over time. In an early example, in 1841, Schinzinger divided the standard loop colostomy, leaving the distal limb in the abdomen, thus obviating the even by-then well-recognized complication of prolapse [53].

As previously discussed, controversy surrounds the efficacy of fixing the mesentery to the anterior abdominal wall to prevent prolapse (Fig. 22.8). Pena et al. suggested that colostomy prolapse in children may be averted if the mesentery is secured approximately 6–7 cm from the fascial defect [29]. Todd recommended a nonabsorbable suture for this purpose [54]. Chandler and Evans also advocated mesenteric fixation, although their data did not indicate a statistically significant improvement in the rate of colostomy prolapse with this technique: 12% versus 31% without suture fixation [1]. Pearl emphasized that the mesentery, not the intestine, be attached to the anterior abdominal wall, pointing to the finding that the prolapsing intestine emanates from a site several centimeters proximal to the stoma; thus, fixation of the bowel alone still allows for prolapse from a point located still more proximally [55]. Conversely, according to Maeda and colleagues, since prolapse begins at the mucocutaneous suture line, mesenteric fixation would not eliminate stoma prolapse [47].

Ng and colleagues proposed that the intestine itself, not the mesentery, be secured to the abdominal wall [35] (Fig. 22.9). The authors performed a prospective trial in which 27 infants were randomized to undergo a traditional loop colostomy constructed over a fascial bridge and 28 infants to a loop colostomy with tethering of the distal limb of intestine to the parietal peritoneum using catgut suture [35]. Prolapse of the distal limb developed in 7 (25.9%)

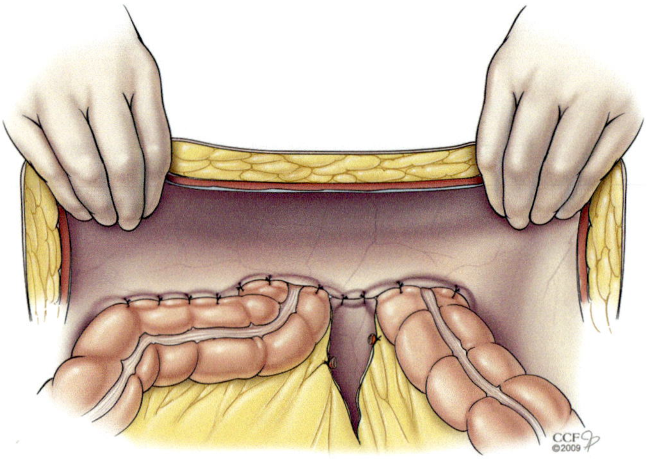

Fig. 22.9 Tethering of the distal limb of a loop stoma to the anterior abdominal wall (Adapted from Ng et al. [35]. Illustration © CCF)

infants in the former group and in 2 (7%) infants in the latter group, a difference that did not reach statistical significance ($p=0.078$) [35]. At the time of colostomy closure, one of the two infants with stoma prolapse despite tethering sutures was found to have a near-complete disruption of the sutures while, in the other infant, only the most distal sutures were partially rent [35]. Notably, those infants with intact tethering sutures did not experience a stoma prolapse [35]. The authors attributed the two cases of prolapse in the tethered group to the catgut suture, recommending instead a long-term absorbable suture [35]. Similarly, Pomeranz suggested that, in patients with an end ileostomy, the terminal ileum be attached with catgut to the peritoneum along the right lateral abdominal wall; the author obtained good results in ten patients, with no prolapse occurring during a follow-up of 2 months to 4 years [5]. Yet, Abcarian and Pearl maintained that prolapse is not proscribed by securing the bowel around the fascial defect to the peritoneum [56]. Additionally, other authors noted that suture fixation to the bowel may be complicated by fistula formation [5].

Alternatively, Goligher and Sames recommended passing an end ileostomy through a retroperitoneal tunnel, created between the cut edge of the white line of Toldt and the anterior abdominal wall fascial defect [8] (Fig. 22.10a–c). A series from Whittaker and Goligher comparing the complications of intraperitoneal and extraperitoneal end colostomies demonstrated an overall significantly higher incidence of pericolostomy hernia, prolapse, and recession in the former group ($p<0.1$); yet, in the intraperitoneal group, 28 (72%) of these 39 complications were comprised solely of parastomal hernias [57]. Although a difference in the rate of stoma prolapse alone was not assessed in the review, this particular complication only took place in 6.7% of the intraperitoneal and 2.2% of the extraperitoneal group [57]. Also, in their series of 150 patients with an end ileostomy, Leong et al. found that none of the three retroperitoneal stomas developed prolapse, a small sample size that did not allow for statistical significance [18]. Londono-Schimmer and colleagues reported that the extraperitoneal approach did not have a statistically significant influence upon the incidence of prolapse in their series of 203 patients with a permanent end colostomy: 7.1% and 5.3% for the extraperitoneal and the intraperitoneal routes, respectively [11]. In a 1985 survey of intestinal surgeons, only 12.5% used this technique for ileostomy construction [55].

As earlier noted, stoma prolapse is strongly linked to parastomal hernia. The size of the fascial defect should thus be minimized to proscribe stoma prolapse. Maeda and colleagues suggested that a smaller defect acts to impede the transmission of abdominal pressure around the mucocutaneous suture [47]. Also, Chandler and Evans advised that the colostomy be constructed as far distally as possible, recognizing that the more proximal colostomies require a larger fascial opening [1]. Furthermore, separate fascial incisions for the stoma and the mucous fistula obviate a large single fascial opening [1]. Cheung advocated such a bridged transverse colostomy, which developed prolapse in 17% of cases, as compared to 47% of the loop transverse colostomies [10].

The utility of mesh placement at the time of stoma creation has not been studied as a means to prevent stoma prolapse. However, a randomized clinical trial from Jänes et al. indicated that the incorporation of mesh around the fascial defect of a permanent colostomy reduces the incidence of paracolostomy hernia when compared to the traditional technique after a 12-month follow-up: 3.7% versus 48.1%, respectively ($p=0.00$) [58]. The authors emphasized that the mesh – a synthetic large-pore lightweight material with a high absorption – was placed as a sublay between the rectus abdominus muscles and the posterior rectus sheath [59]. No patient experienced infection, fistula, or pain secondary to the mesh [58]. As stoma prolapse is often associated with parastomal hernia, the addition of mesh at the time of permanent stoma creation may reduce both complications. This was suggested by an audit by Voitk of four patients with a paracolostomy hernia along with a colostomy prolapse, treated with mesh [60]. These four patients underwent laparoscopic repair using a nonabsorbable synthetic mesh that was applied over the hernia defect, the distal colon, and the colostomy without reducing the hernia contents or repairing the defect; the mesh was secured to the abdominal wall as well as to the colon [60]. The author reported no recurrence of the paracolostomy hernia or the prolapse over a follow-up of 2–12 months, as well as no complications due to the mesh such as erosion into the bowel, infection, or bowel obstruction [60].

The Cook County Hospital group developed the rodless end-loop stoma in order to avoid the management issues and complications associated with the traditional loop stoma.

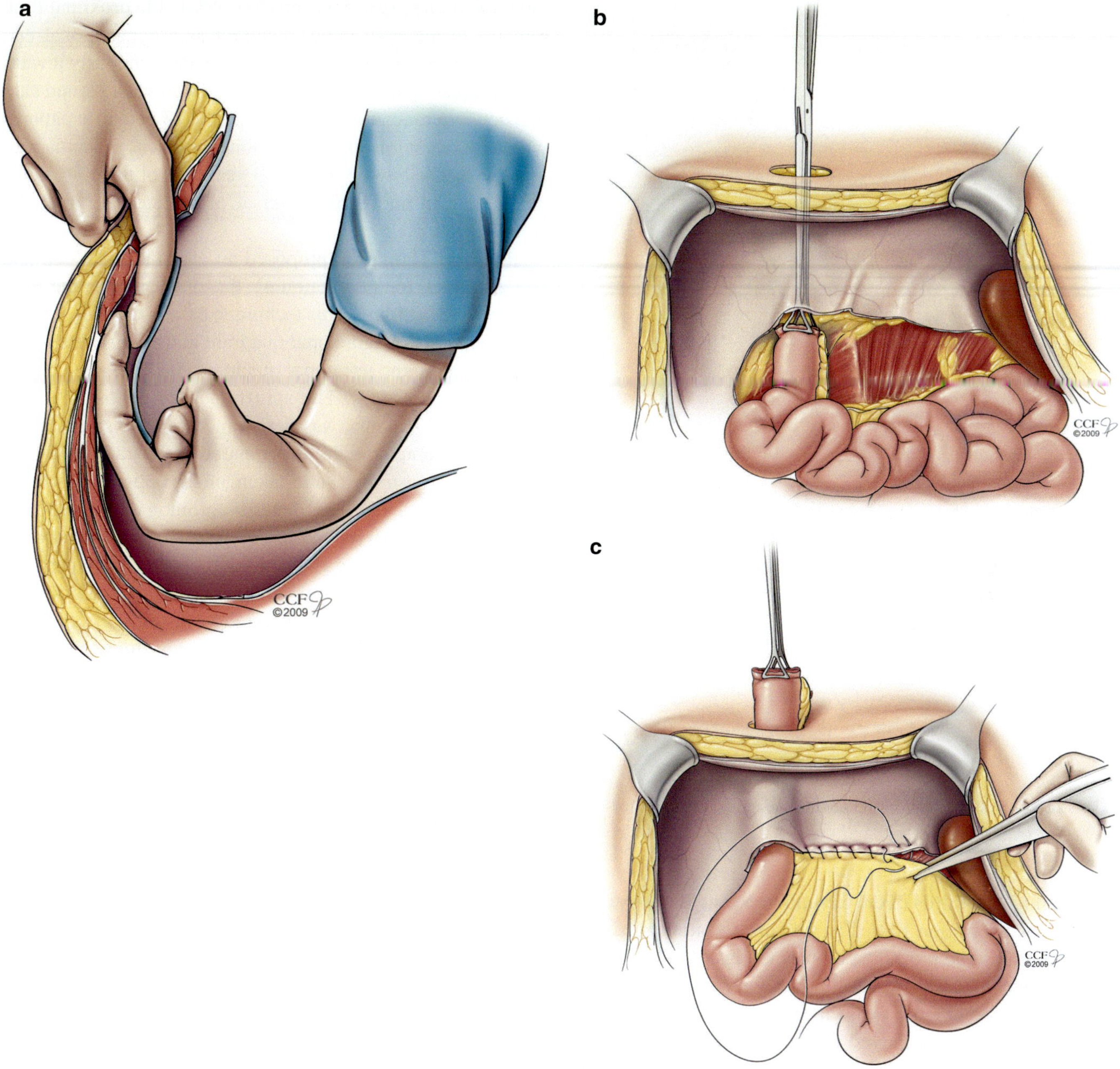

Fig. 22.10 Retroperitoneal end ileostomy. (**a**) The tunnel is bluntly created between the cut edge of the white line of Toldt and the anterior abdominal wall fascial defect. (**b**) The ileostomy is passed through the tunnel to the fascial defect. (**c**) The small bowel mesentery is secured to the cut edge of the peritoneum (Adapted from Stevenson and Volwiler [8]. Illustrations © CCF)

After exteriorizing the stapled loop of intestine through a single fascial defect, the proximal limb is matured as an end stoma, along with a small segment of the antimesenteric aspect of the distal limb [56] (Fig. 22.11). No external supporting device is required. A total of 229 stomas were created in this fashion – 135 colostomies, 70 ileocolostomies, and 24 ileostomies – only 1 (0.4%) of which prolapsed [61]. The group attributed this one instance of prolapse to an overly large fascial opening in conjunction with breakdown of the staple line of the distal limb [61]. In general, the authors noted that the design of this stoma precludes prolapse of the distal limb of the traditional loop stoma [61].

A method for stabilizing an end ileostomy with a stapling device was introduced by Ecker and colleagues. By examining histologic cross-sections of conventional ileostomies, the authors determined that the fixity of an ileostomy depends upon a small segment of adhered serosal surface, located contramesenterically, within the stoma bud [62]. The tendency to ileostomy prolapse, they concluded, resulted from the interference of the mesenteric fat, which occupies

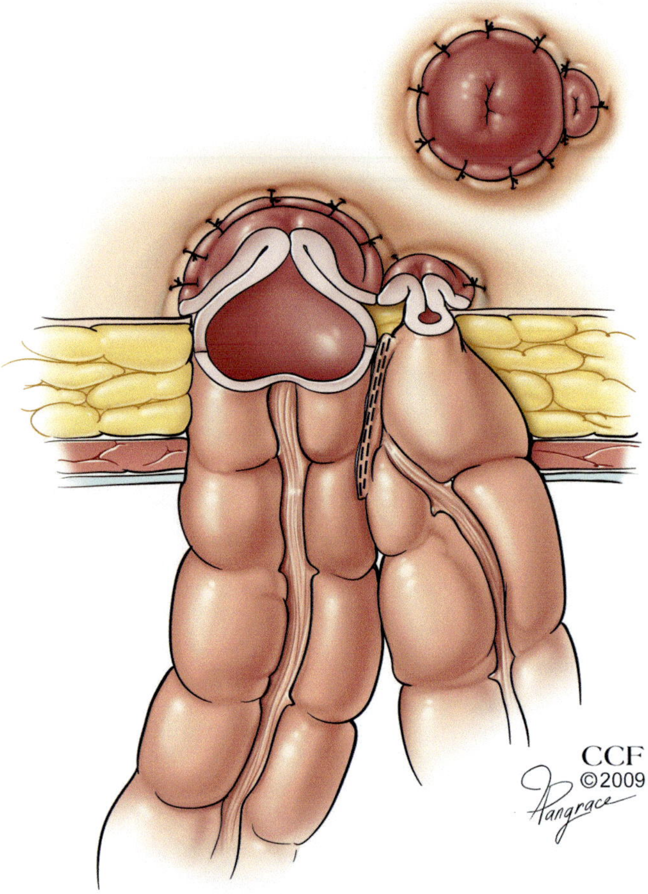

Fig. 22.11 Rodless end-loop stoma (Adapted from Rosen and Nogueras [34]. Illustration © CCF)

one-half to two-thirds of the circumference of the ileostomy, in serosal apposition [62]. The authors recommended that stoma prolapse be prevented by promoting serosal adhesion of the stoma bud at its weakest points with a stapling device [62]. In this technique, with the laparotomy incision open, the small bowel is prolapsed through a plane-sutured ileostomy, created flush to the abdominal skin, with a Babcock clamp for a distance of 3 cm; this intussuscepted ileum is secured by firing a linear stapler on the mesenteric and contramesenteric aspects of the ileostomy [62]. The resulting perforations from the guide post are repaired in several layers [62]. The authors reported that, after an average observation of 2.6 years, no stoma prolapses arose among the 11 patients thus treated, nor did ischemia complicate the procedures [62].

As the distal limb of a loop stoma is particularly at risk for prolapse, Ein suggested a divided loop colostomy for fecal diversion in infants and children [53]. In this technique, a right upper quadrant transverse colostomy is constructed through a small transverse incision [53]. Once exteriorized, the loop of transverse colon is divided, keeping the distal longer than the proximal limb [53]. While the proximal limb remains in the right upper quadrant as a conventional end colostomy, the distal limb is tunneled subcutaneously toward the left upper quadrant, where it is matured via a second skin incision as a mucous fistula [53]. Of the 13 pediatric patients who underwent this procedure, none experienced stoma prolapse over a follow-up of up to 3 years; 10 of the 13 patients underwent an uneventful reversal of the stoma during the study period [53].

Riaz and Thompson proposed an alternative to loop and end ostomies for defunctioning the distal colon: the split transverse colostomy. This technique entails creating a proximal stoma in the right upper quadrant and a separate smaller distal stoma in the left upper quadrant via a 5–7-cm vertical midline incision [63]. The split transverse colostomy, performed in 24 patients, was determined to have significantly fewer total complications as compared to the traditional loop transverse colostomy, undertaken in 25 patients ($p < 0.05$) [63]. Stoma prolapse was the most common complication in both groups, observed in 2 (8%) in the split transverse colostomy group and in 10 (40%) of those treated with a loop transverse colostomy (no p value reported) [63]. Of note, in this non-randomized trial, the split colostomy group had a markedly shorter survival than the loop colostomy group due to their underlying disease [63]. A disadvantage is that reversal of the split transverse colostomy requires a formal laparotomy [63].

In the pediatric population, a purse-string technique has been advanced by Golladay and colleagues to avoid colostomy prolapse (Fig. 22.12). After an end colostomy is fashioned, with either an oversewn distal limb or a mucous fistula as appropriate, separate purse-string sutures of an absorbable material are placed between the seromuscular layer of the bowel and both the fascial layers [64]. By tightening these sutures, the fascial opening is minimized [64]. The colostomy is matured using a similar purse-string suture, securing the exteriorized colon to the subcutaneous tissue and skin [64]. The authors reported that none of the 85 colostomies produced in this fashion developed a prolapse, although the average follow-up was not specified [64].

Laparoscopic stoma formation is a relatively recent addition to the surgical armamentarium. With the laparoscopic technique, mobilization of the bowel to be exteriorized is facilitated, not requiring enlargement of the fascial defect, as with the trephine method [65]. Yet, the impact of the relative lack of adhesions upon stoma prolapse is unclear. Fuhrman and Ota retrospectively reviewed their experience with 17 patients in whom a colostomy had been successfully created laparoscopically [65]. During the 24.3-week average follow-up, one patient (5.8%) developed a prolapse, which did not require operative intervention as the patient shortly died of her disease [65]. An audit from Kini and colleagues established that stoma prolapse did not complicate the six colostomies

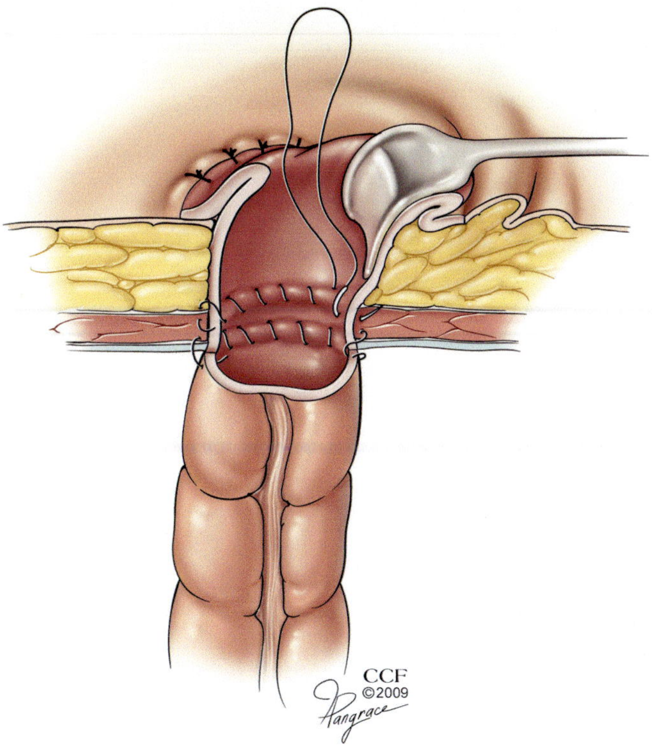

Fig. 22.12 Colostomy purse-string technique (Adapted from Rosen and Nogueras [34]. Illustration © CCF)

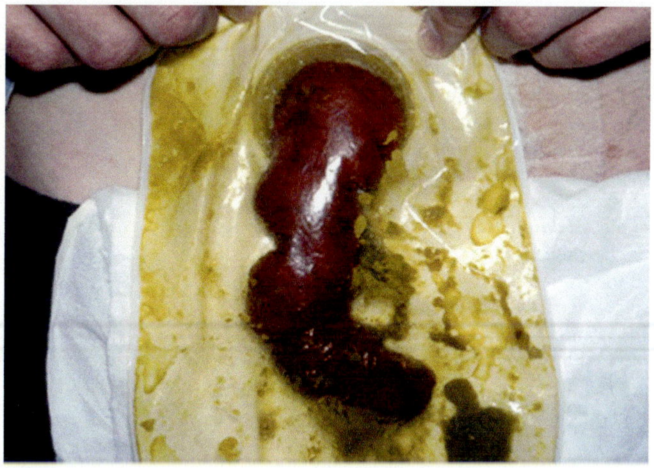

Fig. 22.13 The prolapsing end ileostomy is clearly visualized through the clear plastic appliance

and one ileostomy performed via the laparoscopic technique over the 6- to 18-month observation period [49].

The risk of stoma prolapse is best, albeit not entirely, addressed by a well-constructed stoma. Various modifications to the procedure have been proposed to reduce the proclivity to stoma prolapse. The efficacy of mesenteric or intestinal fixation has not been definitively proven. Nor has the retroperitoneal tunneling of stomas, a little-used technique, significantly affected the incidence of stoma prolapse. As a large fascial defect is a known predisposing factor for stoma prolapse, it is essential to minimize the size of the aperture to avoid this complication. Of the modified techniques of stoma construction, the rodless end-loop stoma has shown the most promise in preventing stoma prolapse in a large series. The role of mesh placement has yet to be examined specifically for stoma prolapse. Also, the impact of laparoscopic stoma creation on stoma prolapse remains to be determined.

Management

The majority of cases of stoma prolapse are either asymptomatic or minimally symptomatic. In such cases, the prolapse can be initially addressed by modifying or changing the stoma appliance as well as with reassurance [8]. McErlain et al. suggested the use of a clear appliance for better assessment of the stoma, a stoma shield or abdominal support, and a wider adhesive area to secure the pouch [32] (Fig. 22.13). An external fixation device, secured to the appliance, was proposed for the nonoperative reduction of stoma prolapse by Fucini as well as by Hsieh et al. [66, 67] (Fig. 22.14). In five patients with colostomy prolapse – three with temporary and two with permanent loop colostomies – Fucini obtained good control of the prolapse, although one patient ultimately required surgical correction due to a coexisting parastomal hernia; none of the patients developed complications due to the device [66]. Nonsurgical management is also advised in patients with significant comorbidities who are unable to tolerate surgery.

A more significant or symptomatic stoma prolapse mandates surgical intervention. Common complaints prompting surgical management include peristomal skin irritation, difficulties with the appliance, as well as pressure necrosis and bleeding from the traumatized stoma [43]. Additionally, repair is warranted based upon issues with cosmesis [43]. Stoma prolapse leads to surgery in 2.9–100% of cases, depending upon the series (Table 22.3). When surgery is required, it primarily is performed on an elective basis, with only incarceration and strangulation compelling emergent intervention. Porter and colleagues indicated that one (25%) of their four cases of end colostomy prolapse underwent surgery [19]. Furthermore, Leong et al. revised 4 (33%) of their 12 prolapsed permanent end ileostomies [18]. When examining their experience with prolapsed permanent end colostomies, the same group found that a procedure was necessary in 2 (18.1%) of the 11 affected patients: a local approach in one patient and a laparotomy with stoma re-siting in the other [11]. Allen-Mersh and Thomson noted that neither age nor obesity negatively impacted the surgical management of colostomy prolapse [30].

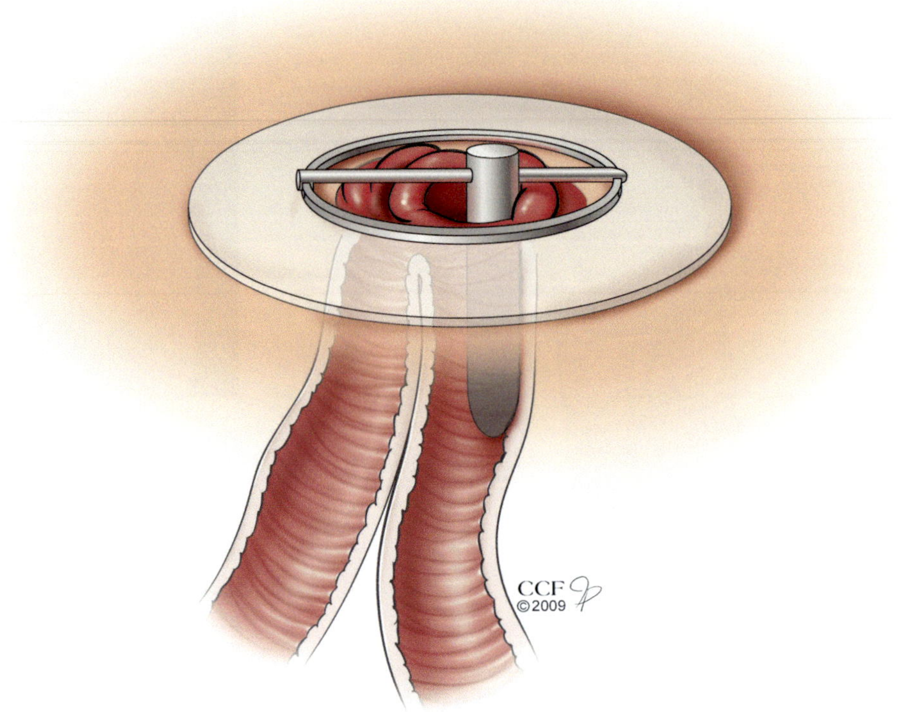

Fig. 22.14 A device for preventing recurrent loop colostomy prolapse. The device is comprised of a 6.8-cm flexible plastic rod and a 5–6-cm rubber tube, oriented perpendicularly as depicted. After reducing the prolapsing bowel, the rubber tube is placed within the stoma. The device is secured by the application of the stoma bag, fixing the plastic rod (Adapted from Fucini [66]. Illustration © CCF)

A higher proportion of children with colostomy prolapse require surgical correction [28]. The series from Çiğdem et al. demonstrated that only 12% of the children who developed colostomy prolapse had a surgical revision [25]. In contrast, 14 (53.8%) of the 26 children with colostomy prolapse underwent surgery – primarily abdominal wall plication – in the review from Nour and colleagues [28]. Additionally, Pena et al. observed that repair of the colostomy prolapse was needed in 91 (76.4%) of the 119 children with a colostomy [29].

In general, stoma prolapse may be approached via a local parastomal revision or laparotomy. A local repair is usually tolerated even by high-risk patients. However, Abrams stated that a local procedure is doomed if the prolapsing intestine had been progressively lengthening prior to surgery [51]. In the case of a temporary stoma, prolapse is best treated by its reversal. Ultimately, re-siting of the stoma may become necessary if local revision is unsuccessful, especially if a parastomal hernia is an associated finding [7]. Unlike other stoma complications, stoma prolapse is linked to an increased risk of recurrence following surgical management [30]. Allen-Mersh and Thomson determined that colostomy prolapse (50%) required more than one surgical repair in a greater proportion of patients than colostomy stenosis (18%) or paracolostomy hernia (19%) [30].

An ileostomy prolapse is usually first addressed by a local approach. Stevenson and Volwiler described a procedure in which the ileostomy, once incised at the mucocutaneous junction, is mobilized from the subcutaneous tissue, after which an appropriate length of excess small bowel is resected [8]. Opinions vary regarding whether a rim of mucosa should be left behind on the peristomal skin or a small amount of skin be removed with the ileostomy [22]. Kim and Kumar emphasized that a limited length of small bowel be excised to avoid metabolic and nutritional derangements [3]. An ileostomy is then recreated in the usual fashion, taking care to fix the stoma to the fascia [8]. Fixation of the new ileostomy to prevent recurrent prolapse is encouraged with the placement of suture, bidirectional seromyotomies, or a serosal strip [38]. According to Sohn et al., the bidirectional seromyotomies – vertical and horizontal scoring of the seromuscular surface of the stoma with the electrocautery – promote fixation by reducing the peristaltic activity of the stoma [68] (Fig. 22.15). Todd similarly advocated incising the seromuscular surface in addition to securing the serosa of the stoma to the peritoneum, Scarpa's fascia, and the skin [54]. The previously described stapling technique from Ecker and colleagues also enhances the stability of a prolapsed end ileostomy when performed at the time of stoma formation, with no recurrences among the nine patients over the 2.6-year follow-up [62]. Weaver et al. reported good results in 7 (88%) of 8 patients with inflammatory bowel disease who underwent local revision of an ileostomy prolapse; the remaining patient developed stenosis secondary to Crohn's disease [33]. The authors nevertheless remarked

Table 22.3 The reoperation rate for stoma prolapse among adult and pediatric patients

	Patients with stoma prolapse	Rate of reoperation (%)	Type of procedure
Allen-Mersh and Thomson [30]	16	>100	Local revision 20 Stoma resiting 6 Colectomy with ileostomy 3
Al-Salem et al. [24][a]	14	14.3	
Chandler and Evans [1]	69	8.7	Button colopexy 3 Abdominal wall plication 1 Local revision 2
Cheung [10]	17	11.80	Local revision 2
Çiğdem et al. [25][a]	97	12.4	
García-Botello et al. [13]	4	25	
Hoffman et al. [15]	3	100	
Leong et al. [18]	12	33.30	
Lister et al. [26][a]	23	17.4	
Londono-Schimmer et al. [11]	11	18.10	Local revision 1 Stoma resiting 1
Mollitt et al. [27][a]	17	2.9	
Nour et al. [28][a]	26	53.80	Purse-string suture 2 Abdominal wall plication 12
Pena et al. [29][a]	119	76.40	
Porter et al. [19]	4	25	Local revision 1

[a]Pediatric

that a sliding stoma prolapse may not be amenable to a local procedure [33]. Failure of a local intervention is followed by a laparotomy for revision or re-siting of the stoma. Turnbull and Weakley stressed that relocation of a prolapsed ileostomy is the best method of treatment [7]. Also, a loop ileostomy may be converted to an end ileostomy, which is less prone to prolapse [7].

Prior to the widespread use of the Brooke ileostomy, a split-thickness skin graft was commonly used in the construction of end ileostomies [68]. The resulting rigid stoma was immune from prolapse, leading to a recommendation from Turnbull and Weakley that stoma prolapse be treated with skin grafting [7]. In this technique, after a circumstomal incision is created, the stoma is mobilized and the prolapsed bowel excised in the usual fashion [7]. Once the redundant mesentery is removed from the terminal portion of the ileum, a 3-cm wide unmeshed split-thickness skin graft is secured to the unmatured stoma and the peristomal skin with a zero nonabsorbable suture material [7] (Fig. 22.16a, b). Although, in the series from Dragstedt et al., recurrent stoma prolapse was rare following this approach, stenosis was inevitable due to contraction of the skin graft, starting on the tenth postoperative day [7, 34]. Turnbull and Weakley noted that such stenosis is easily addressed by incising the skin graft, a maneuver that does not compromise its efficacy in preventing prolapse [7]. Sohn and colleagues later modified this procedure, adding bidirectional myotomies over the last 2 in. of the ileum, upon which a meshed split-thickness skin graft (0.012 in., expanded 1–3) is sutured to the serosa and to the peristomal skin [68] (Fig. 22.17). The single patient who underwent this technique experienced no recurrence of the ileostomy prolapse as well as no stoma stenosis after a 3-year follow-up [68].

As with ileostomy prolapse, colostomy prolapse, especially in the case of a permanent stoma, is usually initially approached locally. The method is similar to that previously recounted for ileostomy prolapse, wherein the stoma is mobilized and the excess intestine excised. In contrast, there is no constraint upon the resection of redundant colon. Allen-Mersh and Thomson performed 20 local revisions for end colostomy prolapse, accounting for 69% of the surgical procedures for prolapse [30]. In the majority of these local revisions – 55% – the result was judged "poor," with only 35% and 10% experiencing a "good" or "moderate" outcome, respectively [30]. Conversely, Chandler and Evans achieved good results in two patients after local procedures for loop colostomy prolapse, although the two limbs of the stoma were separated by a fascial bridge [1]. A modification of the local revision for a prolapsed loop transverse colostomy was described by Agrez, in which only the prolapsed distal limb is mobilized, leaving the mucocutaneous junction of the proximal limb intact [69]. After stapling closed the prolapsed distal limb, a small portion of its antimesenteric aspect is matured as a "blowhole" [69]. No results were reported. Goldsmith and colleagues detailed the "amputation" technique for colostomy prolapse, wherein the prolapsed colostomy is excised, leaving a small stomal cuff behind, to which the colon is then re-anastomosed [6] (Fig. 22.18a, b). The authors, not advocates of the technique, cautioned against a larger cuff, which hazards gangrene, and the possibility of an interceding enterocele [6].

In a majority of cases, prolapse of the loop colostomy involves the defunctionalized distal limb [35]. Turnbull and Weakley suggested that a prolapsed loop colostomy be refashioned into an end colostomy to treat this complication [7]. In most cases, this procedure may be performed by a local technique, with resection of the redundant colon followed by creation of an end colostomy (Fig. 22.19a–d). The distal limb is then left as a mucous fistula in the case of distal obstruction, either at the same or at a separate site, or as a long stump in its absence [3, 7]. Abrams reported that, in the case of a proximal loop transverse colostomy, the prolapse will recur in 33% of cases despite conversion to an end transverse colostomy, due to the persistence of redundant colon [51].

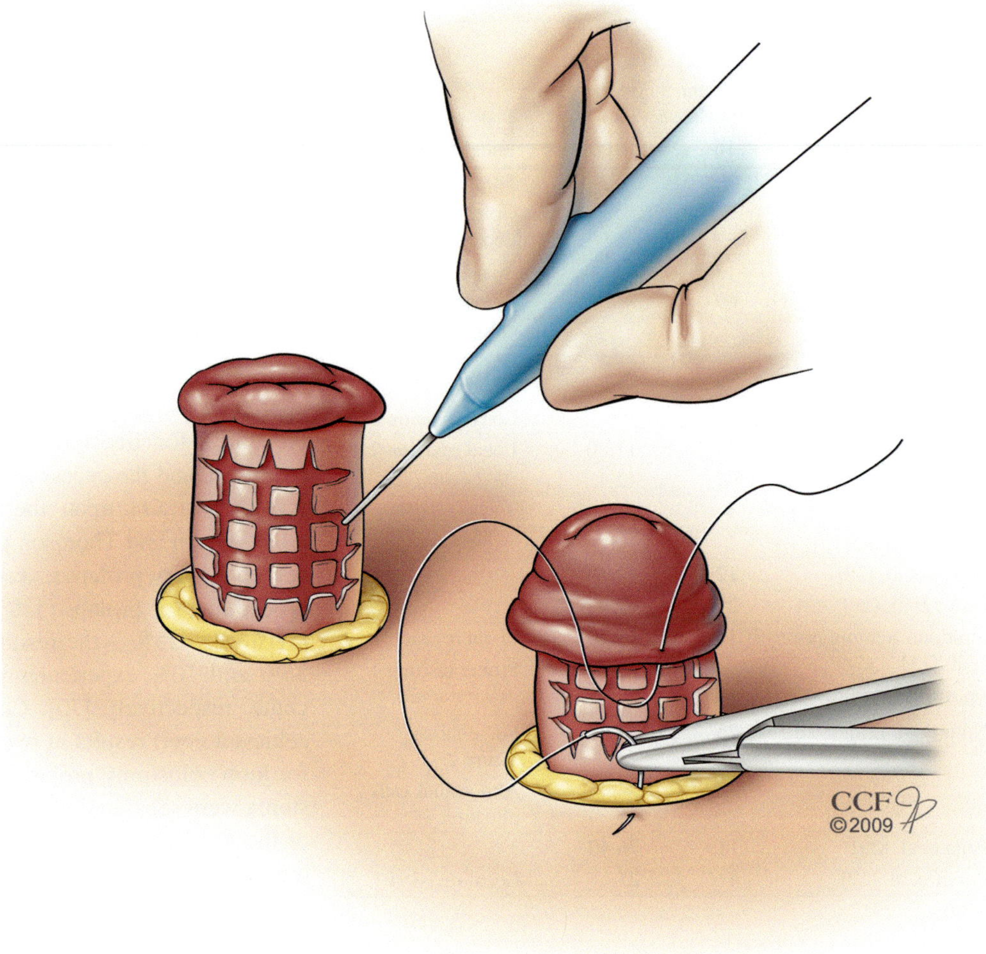

Fig. 22.15 Bidirectional seromyotomies (Adapted from Steele and Wu [38]. Illustration © CCF)

In the event of the failure of a local approach, colostomy prolapse is approached by a laparotomy. However, Chandler and Evans unsuccessfully treated one patient with an unspecified colostomy prolapse via laparotomy, by securing the redundant intestine to the parietal peritoneum [1]. If feasible, intestinal continuity should be re-established to eliminate the prolapse. A recurrence of an end colostomy prolapse may, in select cases, require a completion colectomy with end ileostomy [3]. Allen-Mersh and Thomson applied this method following unsuccessful local revisions for three separate prolapsed end colostomies, obtaining good results in two cases (67%) and a "moderate" outcome in 1 (33%) [30]. The authors observed that the results of a completion colectomy with end ileostomy were superior to those yielded by resiting the colostomy: "good" in 2 (33%) patients but "moderate" and "poor" in 1 (17%) and 3 (50%) patients, respectively [30]. For prolapsed colostomies associated with a parastomal hernia, the ideal method of repair is that which best addresses the hernia, either a local approach or a laparotomy with revision or resiting of the stoma [3].

A number of other minimally invasive techniques have been introduced as an alternative remedy for stoma prolapse: a modified Délorme procedure, post-reduction bowel fixation, and stapling procedures.

A modified Délorme procedure was applied by Abulafi and colleagues for colostomy prolapse (Fig. 22.20a, b). With this method, the mucosa of the prolapsed stoma is incised circumferentially 1–1.5 cm from the mucocutaneous junction [70]. As with the Délorme procedure for rectal prolapse, the mucosa is stripped until the apex of the prolapse is attained [70]. Approximately 6–8 absorbable sutures are then placed to plicate the muscular layer of the denuded stoma, after which the bowel is reduced [70]. The mucosal sleeve is then resected and a mucosa-to-mucosa anastomosis completed [70]. Two patients experienced no recurrence of the prolapse after 3 years of follow-up [70].

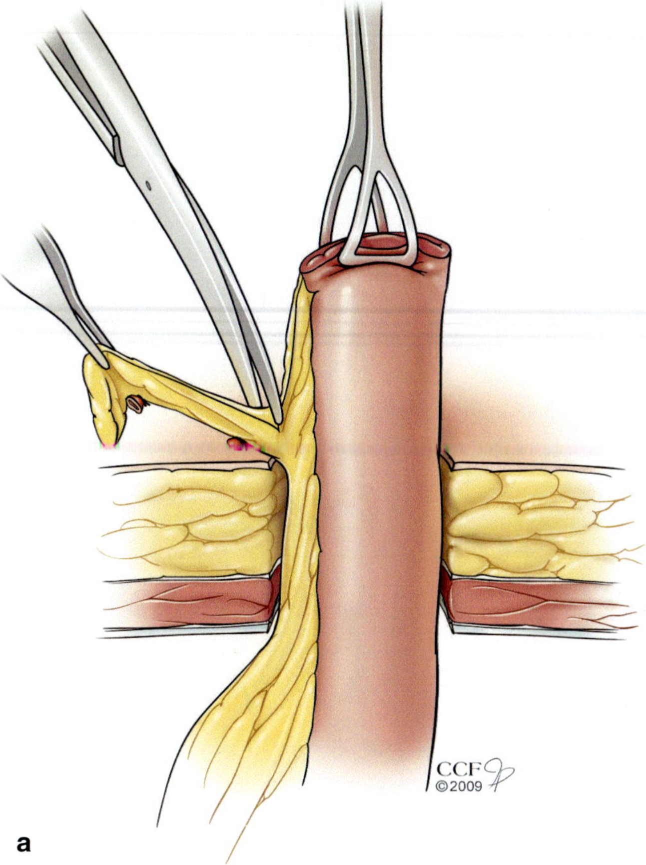

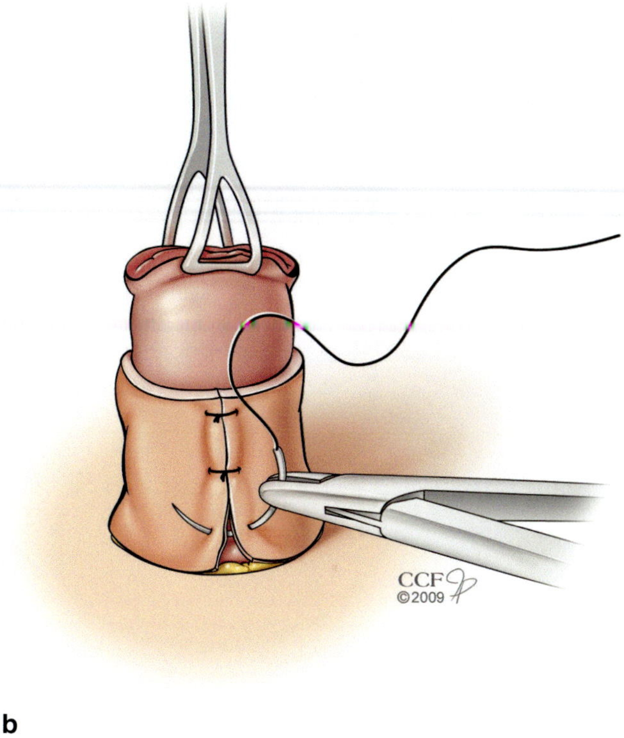

Fig. 22.16 Unmeshed split-thickness skin graft. (**a**) The redundant mesentery is removed from the exteriorized stoma, in preparation for placement of the unmeshed split-thickness skin graft. (**b**) The skin graft is placed, securing it to the unmatured stoma and the peristomal skin (Adapted from Turnbull and Weakley [7]. Illustrations © CCF)

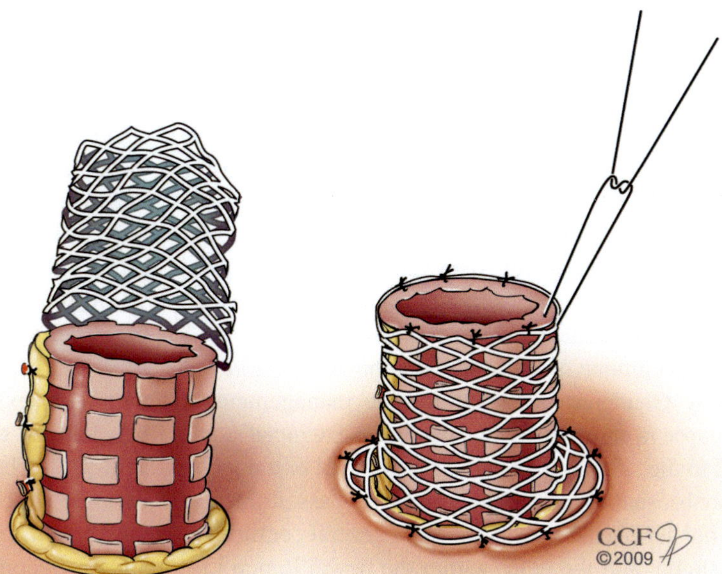

Fig. 22.17 Meshed split-thickness skin graft with bilateral seromyotomies (Adapted from Sohn et al. [68]. Illustration © CCF)

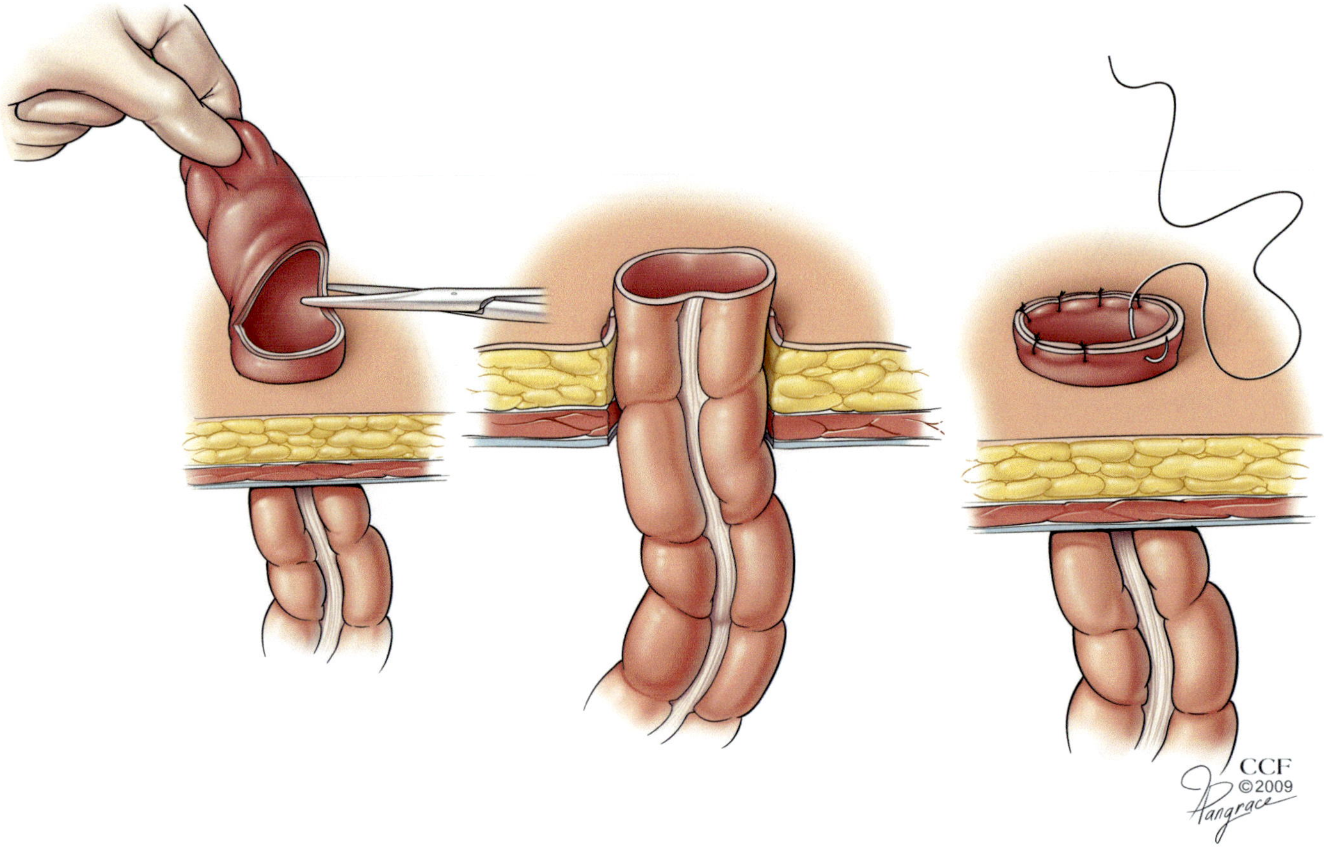

Fig. 22.18 Local "amputation" repair for end colostomy prolapse. The prolapsed colon is excised, leaving behind a cuff of stoma. An anastomosis is completed between the colon and the remaining cuff (Adapted from Goldsmith et al. [6]. Illustration © CCF)

Mogilner et al. detailed a minimally invasive method to treat colostomy prolapse in children: a modified latex tube colopexy. This technique involves placing two 2-0 nylon sutures through a latex tube and a 4×5 cm Stomahesive wafer, both lying over the skin adjacent to the stoma, and then through the walls of the abdomen and reduced stoma [50]. By tying the two sutures, the colon is secured to the abdominal wall [50]. The authors advocated leaving the sutures in place until the colostomy is reversed [50]. However, in two patients, the sutures were removed 3 weeks subsequent to the procedures due to necrosis of the skin and bowel wall, resulting in an immediate recurrent prolapse [50].

A similar technique of post-reduction bowel fixation was proposed by Gauderer and Izant for the management of stoma prolapse in children. In this method, the reduced stoma is secured to the skin with a U-stitch comprised of a double-armed nonabsorbable monofilament suture, passed through one latex bolster placed against the skin, several centimeters from the stoma, and the other within the bowel lumen [52] (Fig. 22.21a–c). The suture and bolsters are removed 2 weeks following the procedure, once adhesions have formed [52]. In their series of four infants – two with loop colostomies, one with a loop colostomy with a skin bridge, and one with two separate stomas – the prolapse was successfully reduced in three infants (75%) until the planned stoma reversal [52]. However, in the infant with the separate stomas, the prolapse partially recurred 8 months after unfastening the suture and bolsters but was again addressed using this modality without a repeat prolapse until the death of the child 2 weeks later [52]. The authors noted that injury to an adjacent loop of intestine potentially could occur while placing the suture [52]. Yet, the procedure is advantageous in that intestine is preserved while avoiding a major operation [52].

Originally described by Mayo in 1939, button-pexy of a prolapsed stoma is another example of post-reduction bowel fixation [71]. The technique applies the same principle of temporary external fixation, allowing for adhesions to form between the redundant intestine and the anterior abdominal wall [71]. The latex bolsters, however, are replaced by two buttons, which better distribute pressure upon the skin and bowel wall, preventing necrosis [71] (Fig. 22.22). Also, the authors recommended 0 silk suture to promote the foreign body reaction and, thus, scarring [71]. These sutures are left in place for 3–4 weeks. In their experience of six children with stoma prolapse, five were successfully managed with the button-pexy method [71]. Erosion of the button into the

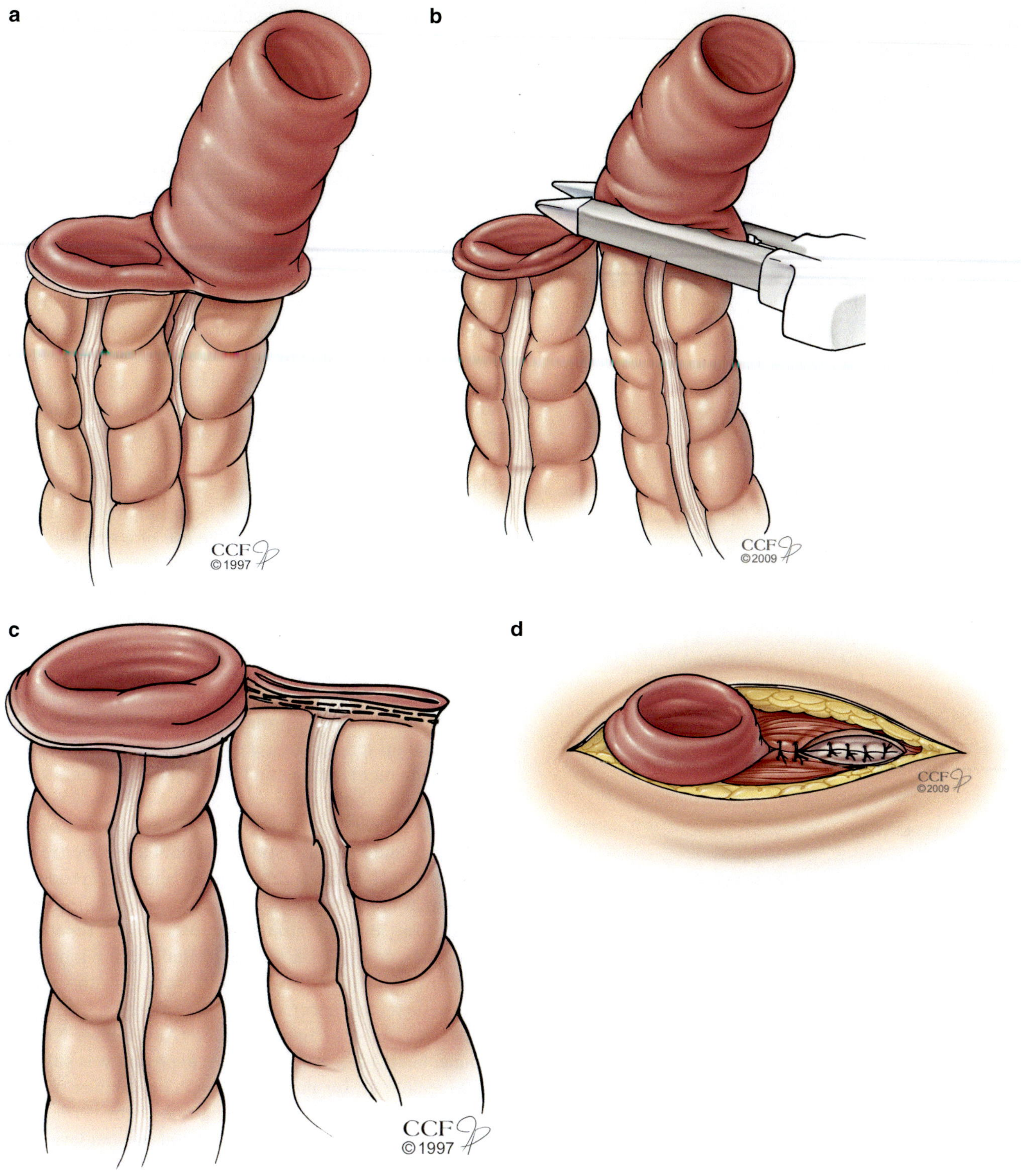

Fig. 22.19 Conversion of a prolapsed loop colostomy to an end stoma via a local technique. (**a**) Both limbs of the loop colostomy are fully mobilized. (**b**, **c**) The prolapsed distal limb is divided and closed with a stapling device. (**d**) The stoma is refashioned as an end colostomy, leaving the stapled distal limb within the peritoneal cavity (Adapted from Wu and Fazio [43]. Illustrations © CCF)

skin in one case led to its removal after 1 week; the prolapse recurred 1 month later, after which button-pexy was again used with good results [71]. Chandler and Evans treated two patients with the button-pexy technique; while the prolapse recurred twice in the child, the adult was able to undergo an uneventful colostomy closure [1].

a

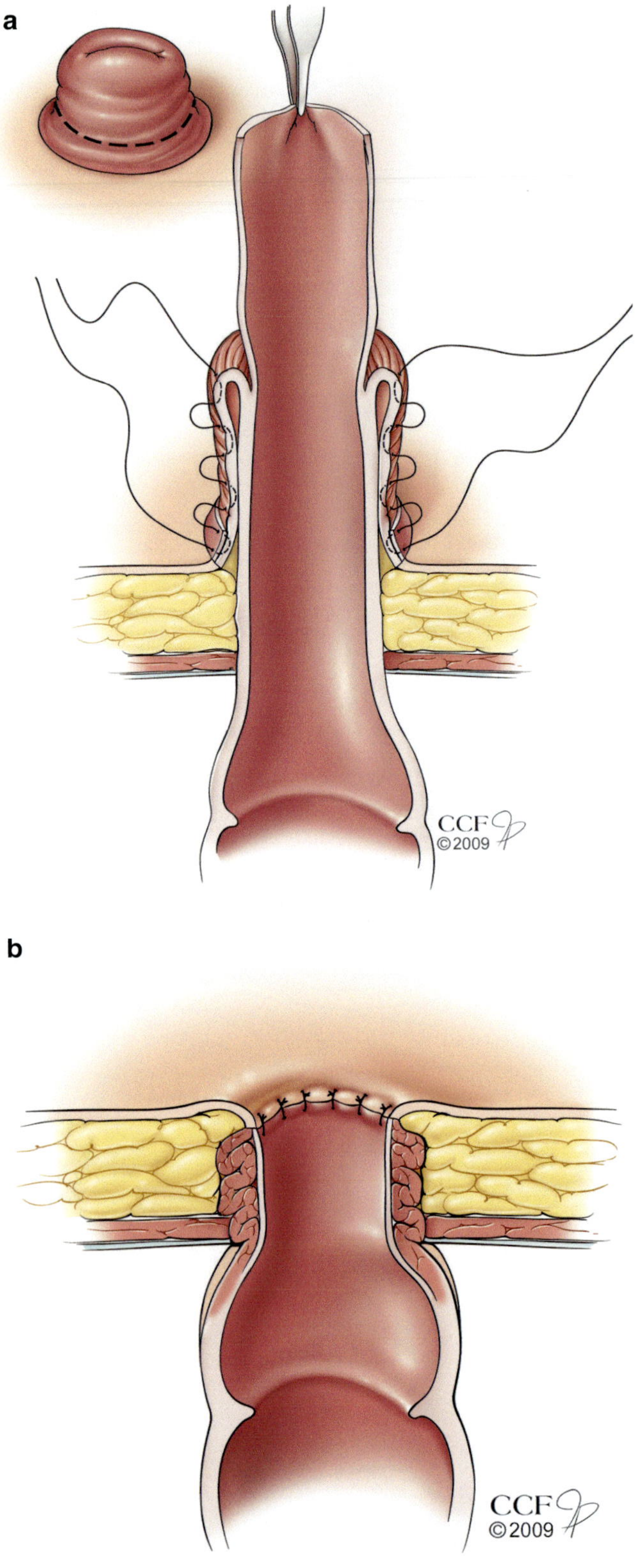

b

Fig. 22.20 Modified Délorme procedure for colostomy prolapse. (a) After the mucosa is stripped from the prolapsed colon, 6–8 plicating sutures are placed. (b) The plicated colon is reduced and a mucosa-to-mucosa anastomosis performed (Adapted from Abulafi et al. [70]. Illustrations © CCF)

An analogue to the Thiersch procedure was advocated by Corry for prolapse of end and loop colostomies. Two small transverse incisions are created at the 3 and 9 o'clock positions adjacent to the colostomy, through which #1 monofilament suture is then passed within the deep subcutaneous fat, encircling the stoma [72]. While tying the suture, an index finger is left in the stoma to prevent obstruction [72]. Four patients treated with this procedure remained free of prolapse after 1 year [72]. Krasna developed a similar procedure for colostomy prolapse in children, in which a 1-0 nylon suture is placed as a circumstomal purse-string within the subcutaneous fat [73]. The author reported no recurrence of the prolapse in an unspecified number of patients prior to closure of the colostomy [73]. In one case, the suture was removed as it had eroded through the mucous membrane of the stoma but immediately replaced [73]. It was noted that the technique is not applicable to pediatric colostomies intended for longer than a year, as the suture will not adapt to the growth of the child [73].

Intestinal staplers have also been employed for stoma prolapse. Hata et al. promoted the use of a stapling device for the treatment of end colostomy prolapse. With the prolapsed intestine exteriorized, one limb of a PROXIMATE™ 100 mm Linear Cutter (Ethicon Endo-Surgery, Cincinnati, OH) is inserted into the stoma lumen in a vertical orientation and then fired [74] (Fig. 22.23a, b). A second firing of the stapling device is applied in the opposite location, producing two flaps of prolapsed stoma [74]. Each flap of tissue is transversely transected with the stapler, leaving a small remnant of stoma as a bud [74]. Five patients with an incarcerated stoma were successfully managed with this method – four with an end colostomy and one with an end ileostomy and mucous fistula – without a recurrence of the prolapse [74]. The authors noted that the procedures, performed under conscious sedation, resulted in minimal blood loss and no stoma necrosis [74]. Tepetes and colleagues described a similar technique for loop colostomy prolapse in an 85-year-old woman with extensive metastatic rectal cancer, using a gastrointestinal anastomosis (GIA™) 60-mm linear stapler (Autosuture, Norwalk, Connecticut) [75]. An alternative approach was suggested by Maeda et al. for prolapsed loop colostomies. With the patient under general anesthesia, a 2–3-cm vertical incision is made approximately 1–2 cm above the level of the skin through the lateral aspect of the full-thickness of the prolapsed intestine [76] (Fig. 22.24a–c). A GIA 60-mm stapler (Tyco Healthcare, Tokyo, Japan), inserted horizontally through this defect, is then fired repeatedly until the prolapsed segment is completely resected [76]. The remainder of the initial incision is then repaired with sutures [76]. The authors reported no recurrence of the prolapse in the two treated patients until their deaths from metastatic colon cancer [76].

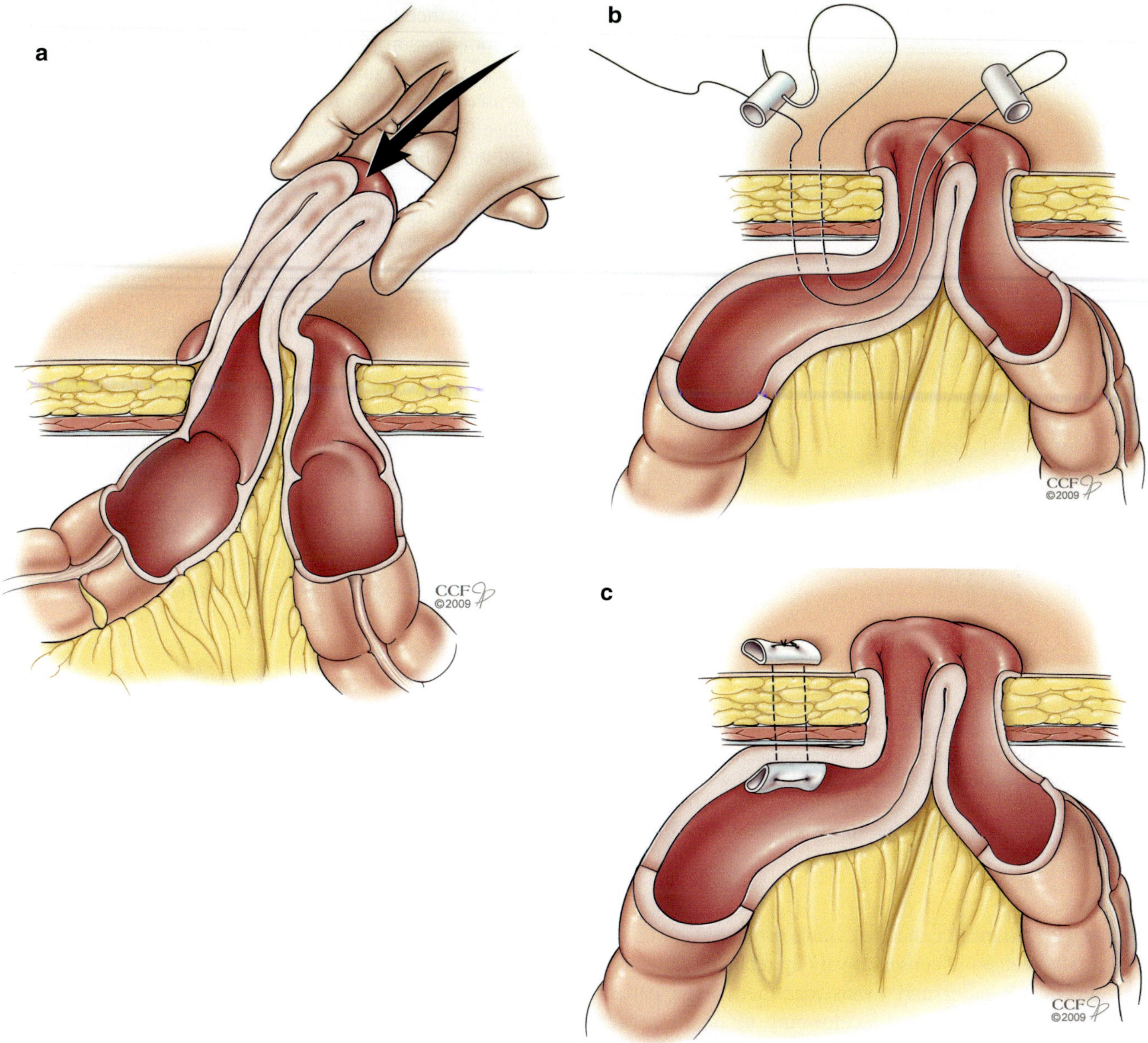

Fig. 22.21 Post-reduction bowel fixation for stoma prolapse using latex bolsters. (**a**) The prolapsed stoma is first reduced. (**b**) A double-armed suture is placed through two latex bolsters, one on the skin and the other within the lumen of the prolapsed limb. (**c**) In tying the suture, the intestine is secured to the anterior abdominal wall (Adapted from Gauderer and Izant [52]. Illustrations © CCF)

In conclusion, prolapse is a significant complication following stoma creation. Primarily, its management rests on alteration of the stoma appliance and reassurance. A more symptomatic prolapse, however, necessitates surgical intervention. In the majority of cases, a local revision initially is pursued. However, failure of a parastomal procedure is followed by a laparotomy with relocation of the stoma, especially in the case of a concurrent parastomal hernia. Ideally, when feasible, intestinal continuity is re-established. Methods such as the modified Délorme procedure, post-reduction bowel fixation, and stapler repair remain unproven in large studies.

Incarceration

Incarceration and strangulation are uncommon sequelae of stoma prolapse (Fig. 22.25). The sliding type of stoma prolapse is primarily prone to this complication [3]. Moreover, an acute prolapse is more often associated with strangulation than the chronic, recurrent form [4]. A stoma prolapse becomes incarcerated when the exteriorized prolapsed bowel grows increasingly edematous, preventing spontaneous reduction. Manual decompression of the incarcerated prolapsed stoma is generally futile due to the edema and patient

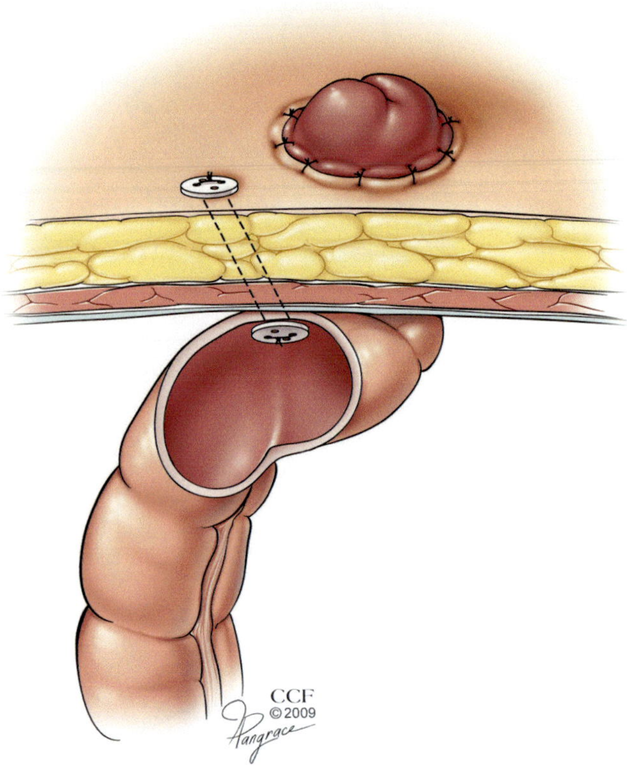

Fig. 22.22 Button colopexy. A double-armed 0 silk suture is threaded via the two holes of a coat button. Both sutures are then passed through the lateral wall of the reduced stoma, approximately 2–4 cm proximal to the opening, and through the anterior abdominal wall, securing the button inside the bowel to the peritoneum. The suture is then tied over a second button on the abdominal wall (Adapted from Rosen and Nogueras [34]. Illustration © CCF)

anxiety [3]. An incarcerated but viable prolapsed stoma may be initially addressed conservatively by reducing the intestinal edema. Chandler and Evans identified seven patients (10%) with incarceration of a colostomy, all of whom were treated with sedation and the application of sugar and ice [1]. Table sugar is a desiccating agent that, when placed on the incarcerated prolapsed stoma, rapidly decreases the edema; the bowel is then reducible, either spontaneously or by manual decompression [77]. Myers and Rothenberger reported two cases in which table sugar was profitably used to reduce an incarcerated rectal prolapse as well as an end ileostomy prolapse [78]. As an alternative, Chaudhuri and Prasai promoted the submucosal injection of hyaluronidase (3,000 units in 20 mL of water) into the incarcerated prolapsed stoma, a technique that they successfully employed in a case of rectal prolapse [79].

Prolonged incarceration of a stoma may result in compromise of the blood supply as the edema develops, leading to strangulation and bowel ischemia [8]. The appearance of gangrene necessitates emergent surgical intervention. Chandler and Evans remarked that such emergency surgery is rare, with none in their series of 491 patients [1]. Attempts at reduction of gangrenous intestine should be avoided to avoid peritoneal contamination. In the absence of sepsis and peritonitis, a local approach may be selected, in which the strangulated, prolapsed segment is resected and a new stoma created [34]. However, peritonitis mandates an exploratory laparotomy with excision of the ischemic bowel and reconstruction of an ostomy at a new site [34].

Summary

Stoma prolapse is a common late complication, occurring in 1–16% of stomas. Primarily, stoma prolapse presents a challenge for ostomy care, although cosmesis is also a concern. In rare cases, a prolapsed stoma may develop incarceration and strangulation. The risk factors for stoma prolapse include both patient-related and technical factors. Prevention of stoma prolapse is facilitated by good technique in constructing the stoma. The initial management of stoma prolapse involves reassurance of the patient and adjustments to the stoma appliance. However, symptomatic or progressive stoma prolapse requires surgical repair, either via a local approach or a laparotomy. Incarceration and strangulation mandate immediate intervention.

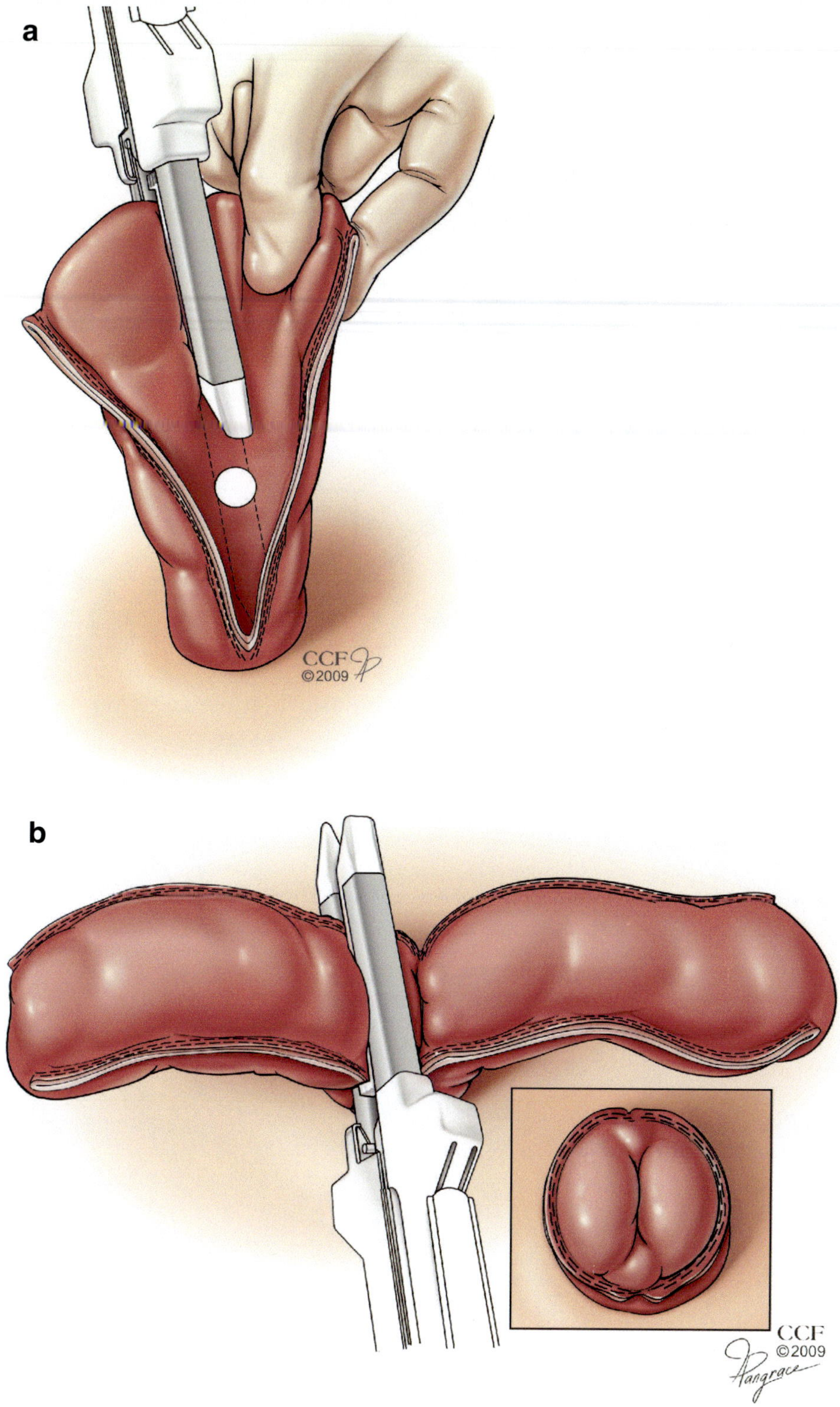

Fig. 22.23 (**a**, **b**) Repair of a prolapsed end colostomy using a stapling device (Adapted from Hata et al. [74]. Illustration © CCF)

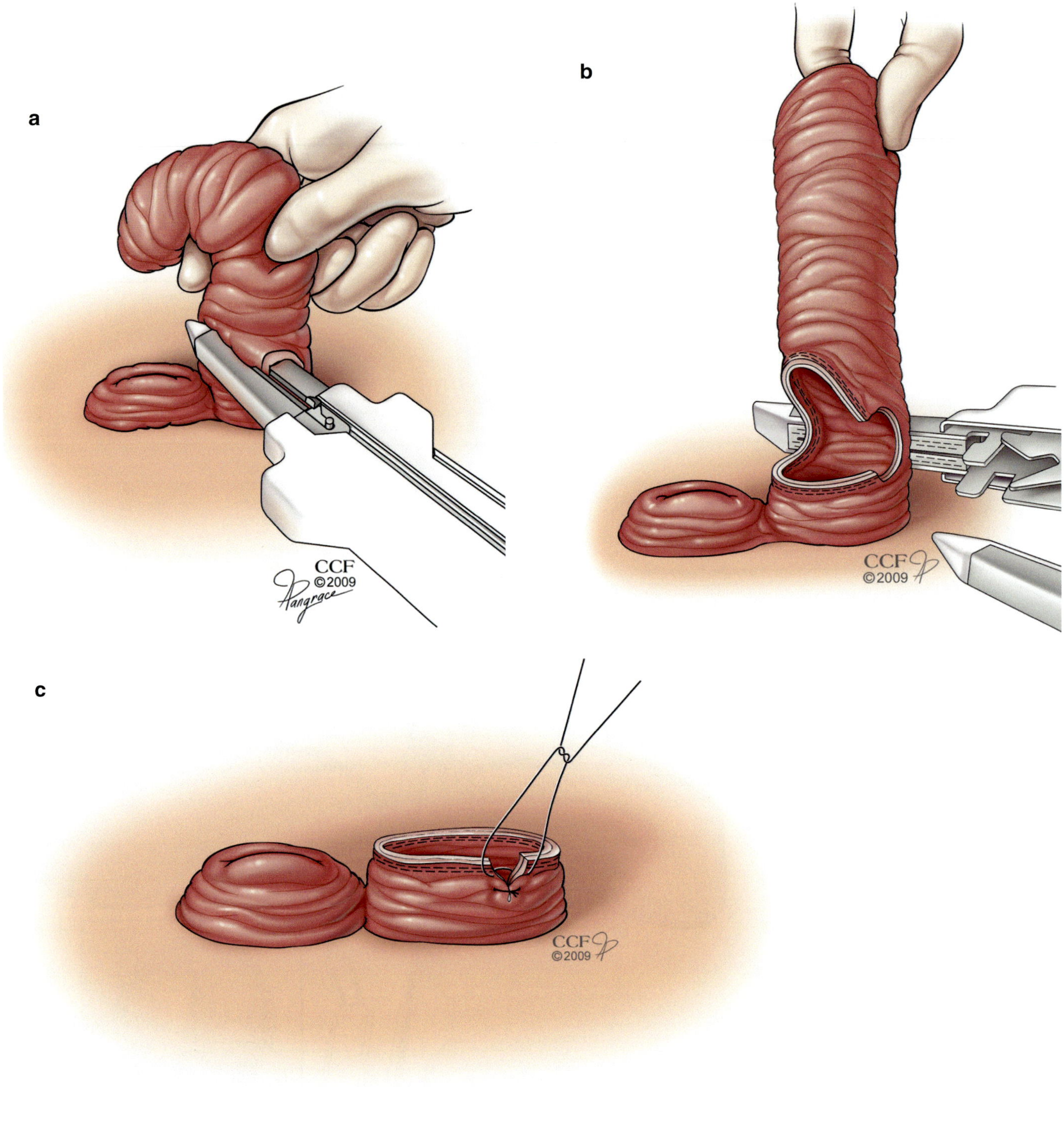

Fig. 22.24 (**a–c**) Repair of a prolapsed loop colostomy with a stapler (Adapted from Maeda et al. [76]. Illustration © CCF)

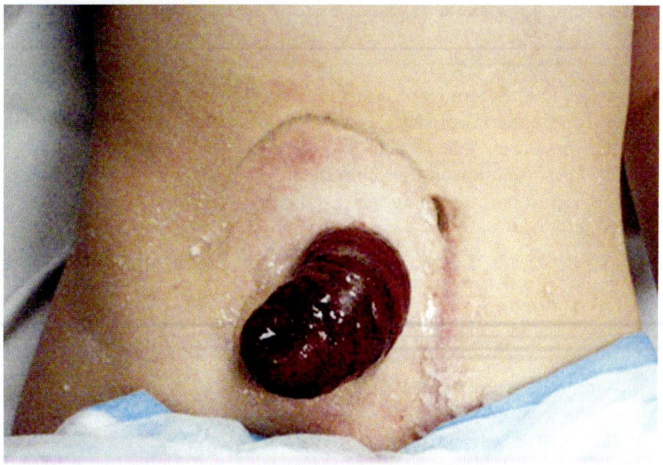

Fig. 22.25 A strangulated end ileostomy prolapse

References

1. Chandler JG, Evans BP. Colostomy prolapse. Surgery. 1978; 84:577–82.
2. Gordon PH, Rolstad BS, Bubrick MP. Intestinal stomas. In: Nivatvongs S, Gordon PH, editors. Principles and practices of surgery for the colon, rectum, and anus. 2nd ed. St. Louis: Quality Medical Publishing; 1999. p. 1117–80.
3. Kim JT, Kumar RR. Reoperation for stoma-related complications. Clin Colon Rectal Surg. 2006;19:207–12.
4. Pearl RK. Complications of ileostomy. In: Nelson RL, Nyhus LM, editors. Surgery of the small intestine. Norwalk: Appleton & Lange; 1987. p. 499–509.
5. Pomeranz AA. An operation for prevention of ileostomy prolapse. Dis Colon Rectum. 1963;6:381–4.
6. Goldsmith HS, Tignor S, Byrne JJ. Terminal colostomy prolapse. Am J Surg. 1964;108:105–6.
7. Turnbull RB, Weakley FL. Atlas of intestinal stomas. St. Louis: C.V Mosby Company; 1967.
8. Stevenson JK, Volwiler W. Ileostomy stoma complications—prevention and correction. In: Cooper P, Nyhus LM, editors. Surgery annual, vol. 3. New York: Meredith Corporation; 1971. p. 305–22.
9. Park JJ, Del Pino A, Orsay CP, Nelson RL, Pearl RK, Cintron JR, et al. Stoma complications: the Cook County Hospital experience. Dis Colon Rectum. 1999;42:1575–80.
10. Cheung MT. Complications of an abdominal stoma: an analysis of 322 stomas. Aust N Z J Surg. 1995;65:808–11.
11. Londono-Schimmer EE, Leong APK, Phillips RKS. Life table analysis of stomal complications following colostomy. Dis Colon Rectum. 1994;37:916–20.
12. Edwards DP, Leppington-Clarke A, Sexton R, Heald RJ, Moran BJ. Stoma-related complications are more frequent after transverse colostomy than loop ileostomy: a prospective randomized clinical trial. Br J Surg. 2001;88:360–3.
13. García-Botello SA, García-Armengol J, García-Granero E, Espí A, Juan C, López-Mozos F, et al. A prospective audit of the complications of loop ileostomy construction and takedown. Dig Surg. 2004;21:440–6.
14. Gooszen AW, Geelkerken RH, Hermans J, Lagaay MB, Gooszen HG. Quality of life with a temporary stoma: ileostomy vs colostomy. Dis Colon Rectum. 2000;43:650–5.
15. Hoffman MS, Barton DPJ, Gates J, Roberts WS, Fiorica JV, Finan MA, et al. Complications of colostomy performed on gynecologic cancer patients. Gynecol Oncol. 1992;44:231–4.
16. Harris DA, Egbeare D, Jones S, Benjamin H, Woodward A, Foster ME. Complications and mortality following stoma formation. Ann R Coll Surg Engl. 2005;87:427–31.
17. Law WL, Chu KW, Choi HK. Randomized clinical trial comparing loop ileostomy and loop transverse colostomy for faecal diversion following total mesorectal excision. Br J Surg. 2002;89:704–8.
18. Leong APK, Londono-Schimmer EE, Phillips RKS. Life-table analysis of stomal complications following ileostomy. Br J Surg. 1994;81:727–9.
19. Porter JA, Salvati EP, Rubin RJ, Eisenstat TE. Complications of colostomies. Dis Colon Rectum. 1989;32:299–303.
20. Wexner SD, Taranow DA, Johansen OB, Itzkowitz F, Daniel N, Nogueras JJ, et al. Loop ileostomy is a safe option for fecal diversion. Dis Colon Rectum. 1993;36:349–54.
21. Robertson I, Leung E, Hughes D, Spiers M, Donnelly L, Mackenzie I, et al. Prospective analysis of stoma-related complications. Colorectal Dis. 2005;7:279–85.
22. Nogueras JJ, Wexner SD. Stoma prolapse. In: MacKeigan JM, Cataldo PA, editors. Intestinal stomas: principles, techniques, and management. St. Louis: Quality Medical Publishing, Inc.; 1993. p. 268–77.
23. Shellito PC. Complications of abdominal stoma surgery. Dis Colon Rectum. 1998;41:1562–72.
24. Al-Salam AH, Grant C, Khawaja S. Colostomy complications in infants and children. Int Surg. 1983;77:164–6.
25. Çiğdem MK, Onen A, Duran H, Öztürk H, Otçu S. The mechanical complications of colostomy in infants and children: analysis of 473 cases of a single center. Pediatr Surg Int. 2006;22:671–6.
26. Lister J, Webster PJ, Mirza S. Colostomy complications in children. Practitioner. 1983;227:229–37.
27. Mollitt DL, Malangoni MA, Ballantine TV, Grosfeld JL. Colostomy complications in children. An analysis of 146 cases. Arch Surg. 1980;115:455–8.
28. Nour S, Beck J, Stringer MD. Colostomy complications in infants and children. Ann R Coll Surg Engl. 1996;78:526–30.
29. Pena A, Migotto-Krieger M, Levitt MA. Colostomy in anorectal malformations: a procedure with serious but preventable complications. J Pediatr Surg. 2006;41:748–56.
30. Allen-Mersh TG, Thomson JPS. Surgical treatment of colostomy complications. Br J Surg. 1988;75:416–8.
31. Duchesne JC, Wang Y-Z, Weintraub SL, Boyle M, Hunt JP. Stoma complications: a multivariate analysis. Am Surg. 2002;68:961–6.
32. McErlain D, Kane M, McGrogan M. Prolapsed stoma. Nurs Stand. 2004;18:41–2.
33. Weaver RM, Alexander-Williams J, Keighley MRB. Indications and outcome of reoperation for ileostomy complications in inflammatory bowel disease. Int J Colorectal Dis. 1988;3:38–42.
34. Rosen S, Nogueras JJ. Stomal prolapse. In: Cataldo PA, MacKeigan JM, editors. Intestinal stomas: principles, techniques, and management. 2nd ed. New York: Marcel Dekker, Inc.; 2004. p. 307–22.
35. Ng WT, Book KS, Wong MK, Cheng PW, Cheung CH. Prevention of colostomy prolapse by peritoneal tethering. J Am Coll Surg. 1997;184:313–5.
36. Arumugam PJ, Bevan L, Macdonald L, Watkins AJ, Morgan AR, Beynon J, et al. A prospective audit of stomas—analysis of risk factors and complications and their management. Colorectal Dis. 2003;5:49–52.
37. Leenen LPH, Kuypers JHC. Some factors influencing the outcome of stoma surgery. Dis Colon Rectum. 1989;32:500–4.
38. Steele MCA, Wu JS. Late stomal complications. Clin Colon Rectal Surg. 2002;15:199–207.
39. Scudamore HH, Rogers AG, Bargen JA, Banner EA. Pregnancy after ileostomy for chronic ulcerative colitis. Gastroenterology. 1957;32:295–303.
40. Daly DW, Brooke BN. Ileostomy and excision of the large intestine for ulcerative colitis. Lancet. 1967;2:62–4.

41. Gopal KA, Amshel AL, Shonberg IL, Levinson BA, VanWert M, VanWert J. Ostomy and pregnancy. Dis Colon Rectum. 1985;28: 912–6.
42. Nicholl MC, Thompson JM, Cocks PS. Stomas and pregnancy. Aust N Z J Obstet Gynaecol. 1993;33:322–4.
43. Wu JS, Fazio VW. Difficult stomas. In: Schrock TR, editor. Perspectives in colon and rectal surgery. St. Louis: Quality Medical Publishing, Inc.; 1998. p. 33–60.
44. Arun H, Ledgerwood A, Lucas CE. Ostomy prolapse in paraplegic patients: etiology, prevention, and treatment. J Am Paraplegia Soc. 1990;13:7–9.
45. Stothert JC, Brubacher L, Simonowitz DA. Complications of emergency stoma formation. Arch Surg. 1982;117:307–9.
46. Bass EM, Del Pino A, Tan A, Pearl RK, Orsay CP, Abcarian H. Does preoperative stoma marking and education by the enterostomal therapist affect outcome? Dis Colon Rectum. 1997;40: 440–2.
47. Maeda K, Maruta M, Utsumi T, Sato H, Masumori K, Aoyama H. Pathophysiology and prevention of loop stomal prolapse in the transverse colon. Tech Coloproctol. 2003;7:108–11.
48. Warren R, McKittrick LS. Ileostomy for ulcerative colitis: technique, complications and management. Surg Gynecol Obstet. 1951; 93:555.
49. Kini SU, Perston Y, Radcliffe AG. Laparoscopically assisted trephine stoma formation. Surg Laparosc Endosc. 1996;6:371–4.
50. Mogilner JG, Rode H, Siplovich L, Cywes S. Bedside modified latex tube colopexy for the treatment of colostomy prolapse in children. Isr J Med Sci. 1990;26:410–1.
51. Abrams JS. Abdominal stomas: indications, operative techniques, and patient care. Boston: John Wright; 1984.
52. Gauderer MWL, Izant RJ. A technique for temporary control of colostomy prolapse in children. J Pediatr Surg. 1985;20:653–5.
53. Ein SH. Divided loop colostomy that does not prolapse. Am J Surg. 1984;147:250–2.
54. Todd IP. Mechanical complications of ileostomy. Clin Gastroenterol. 1982;11:268–73.
55. Pearl RK, Prasad L, Orsay CP, Abcarian H, Tan AB. A survey of technical considerations in the construction of intestinal stomas. Am Surg. 1985;51:462–5.
56. Abcarian H, Pearl RK. Stomas. Surg Clin N Am. 1988;68: 1295–305.
57. Whittaker M, Goligher JC. A comparison of the results of extraperitoneal and intraperitoneal techniques for construction of terminal iliac colostomies. Dis Colon Rectum. 1976;19:342–4.
58. Jänes A, Cengiz Y, Israelsson A. Preventing parastomal hernia with a prosthetic mesh: a randomized study. Arch Surg. 2004;139:1356–8.
59. Israelsson LA. Preventing and treating parastomal hernia. World J Surg. 2005;29:1086–9.
60. Voitk A. Simple technique for laparoscopic paracolostomy hernia repair. Dis Colon Rectum. 2000;43:1451–3.
61. Unti JA, Abcarian H, Pearl RK, Orsay CP, Nelson RL, Prasad L, et al. Rodless end-loop stomas: seven-year experience. Dis Colon Rectum. 1991;34:999–1004.
62. Ecker KW, Schmid T, Xu HS, Feifel G. Improved stabilization of conventional (Brooke) ileostomies with the stapler technique. World J Surg. 1992;16:525–9.
63. Riaz AA, Thompson HH. Split transverse colostomy: an alternative method of defunctioning the distal colon. Tech Coloproctol. 2006; 10:57–60.
64. Golladay ES, Bernay F, Wagner CW. Prevention of prolapse in pediatric enterostomas with purse string technique. J Pediatr Surg. 1990;25:990–1.
65. Fuhrman GM, Ota DM. Laparoscopic intestinal stomas. Dis Colon Rectum. 1994;37:444–9.
66. Fucini C. A simple device for prolapsing loop colostomies. Dis Colon Rectum. 1989;32:534–5.
67. Hsieh M-Y, Liu C, Ho S-H, Wung S-H, Chin T, Wei C. Simple device for treating prolapsing loop colostomy. J Chin Med Assoc. 2006;69:138–9.
68. Sohn N, Schulman N, Weinstein MA, Robbins RD. Ileostomy prolapse repair utilizing bidirectional myotomy and a meshed split-thickness skin graft. Am J Surg. 1983;145:807–8.
69. Agrez MV. Revision of transverse colostomy prolapse without stoma resiting. Ann R Coll Surg Engl. 1997;79:383–4.
70. Abulafi AM, Sherman IW, Fiddian RV. Délorme operation for prolapsed colostomy. Br J Surg. 1989;76:1321–2.
71. Canil K, Fitzgerald P, Lau G, Cameron G, Walton M. Button-pexy fixation for repair of ileostomy and colostomy prolapse. J Pediatr Surg. 1995;30:1148–9.
72. Corry M. Colostomy prolapse [letter]. Br J Surg. 1984;71:81.
73. Krasna IH. A simple purse string suture technique for treatment of colostomy prolapse and intussusception. J Pediatr Surg. 1979;14: 801–2.
74. Hata F, Kitagawa S, Nishimori H, Furuhata T, Tsuruma T, Ezoe E, et al. A novel, easy, and safe technique to repair a stoma prolapse using a surgical stapling device. Dig Surg. 2005;22:306–10.
75. Tepetes K, Spyridakis M, Hatzitheofilou C. Local treatment of a loop colostomy prolapse with a linear stapler. Tech Coloproctol. 2005;9:156–8.
76. Maeda K, Maruta M, Utsumi T, Sato H, Aoyama H, Katsuno H, et al. Local correction of a transverse loop colostomy prolapse by means of a stapler device. Tech Coloproctol. 2004;8:45–6.
77. Fligelstone LJ, Wanendeya N, Palmer BV. Surgical workshop: osmotic therapy for acute irreducible stoma prolapse. Br J Surg. 1997;84:390.
78. Myers JO, Rothenberger DA. Sugar in the reduction of incarcerated prolapsed bowel: report of two cases. Dis Colon Rectum. 1991;34: 416–8.
79. Chaudhuri A, Prasai A. Hyaluronidase in the reduction of prolapsed colostomy. Ann R Coll Surg Engl. 2003;85:209.

23 Challenging Stomas

Ryan S. Williams and Victor W. Fazio

Introduction

Intestinal stomas play an important role in surgical care as they are used to divert the intestinal stream from its normal course – relieving an obstruction, protecting an anastomosis, or as the outlet for intestinal contents. Stomas can be considered an intestinal anastomosis, and constructed with the same care as any other anastomosis. Despite our best efforts, problems and difficulties do occur. Ostomy complications occur in more than 30% of patients, with some studies showing long-term rates greater than 50% [1–5]. Many of these complications impact patients' daily routines and decrease their quality of life [6–8]. These may be minor problems ranging from pseudoepitheliomatous hyperplasia and irritation of the peristomal skin to major problems such as peristomal hernia or complete ischemic necrosis. A significant number of patients with these complications will require reoperation [1, 4, 9–11]. This chapter will present techniques to diminish the possibility of complications when a difficult ostomy formation is present.

Preoperative Considerations

Counseling and Marking

Elective surgery provides the opportunity for proper preparation and evaluation of patients who need a stoma. It is the Joint Position Statement and recommendation of The American Society of Colon and Rectal Surgeons (ASCRS) and the Wound Ostomy Continence Nurse Society (WOCN) that all patients scheduled for ostomy surgery, even urgent surgery if possible, undergo preoperative ostomy site marking (ASCRS and WOCN) [12]. This provides the opportunity for counseling and education of a patient soon to be confronted with the need for ostomy care. Patients undergoing ostomy creation have been found to have a lower quality of life based upon observational questionnaire studies [8, 13, 14]. There are many emotional, psychological, and physiologic implications associated with ostomy placement; and preparing patients for this major life change can aid in their adjustment [15]. It also provides an opportunity to identify patients where ostomy formation might be unusually difficult.

Temporary Stomas

Ideally, surface marking should be done with the patient sitting, standing, and lying down. Ideally, the mark is placed below the umbilicus, through the rectus abdominus, at a fat mound away from scars, incisions, and bony protuberances (Fig. 23.1). Most importantly, it should be in a visible location, which in patients with a prominent abdomen, may be above the umbilicus. The ostomy traditionally is centered at the rectus abdominus, but selecting a location approximately 2 cm slightly lateral to this can diminish the problems with medial leakage and proximity to a complicated midline wound. The ostomy is at times the only evidence that an operation has occurred for the patient and "pride" should be taken in the construction of their ostomy. With the possibility that at least 20% of "temporary" stomas are never closed, temporary ostomies should be constructed with this possibility in mind [16–19]. Additionally, temporary ostomies are constructed to permit closure locally, without the need for a laparotomy. If the bowel is divided to construct the temporary ostomy, the efferent limb of ostomy is placed in a location easily accessible from the afferent limb location. To facilitate closure, adhesive barriers, such as Seprafilm® (Genzyme Corporation, Cambridge, MA), can be used to decrease adhesion formation and thereby decrease ostomy closure operative times (Fig. 23.2) [20–22]. With the decreased adhesion formation, ostomies may be closed as early as 3 weeks after formation, which is significantly earlier than the conventional 6–12 weeks [21].

R.S. Williams (✉) • V.W. Fazio
Department of Colorectal Surgery, Digestive Diseases Institute, Cleveland Clinic Lerner College of Medicine of Case Western Reserve University, Cleveland Clinic Foundation, Cleveland, OH, USA
e-mail: williar4@ccf.org; faziov@ccf.org

V.W. Fazio et al. (eds.), *Atlas of Intestinal Stomas*,
DOI 10.1007/978-0-387-78851-7_23, © Springer Science+Business Media, LLC 2012

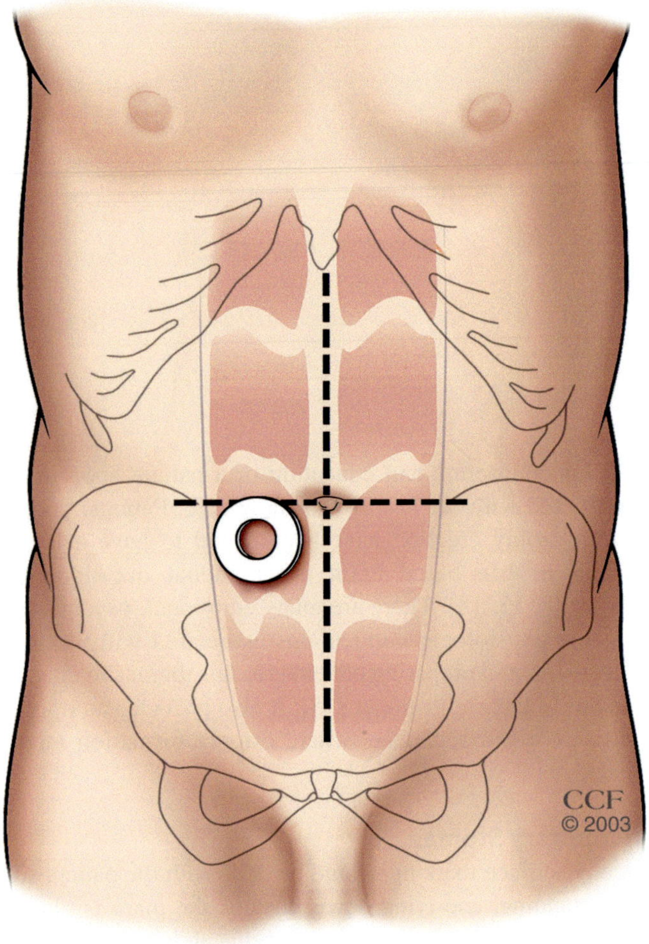

Fig. 23.1 Traditional placement for an ostomy, below the umbilicus on the rectus abdominus. Illustration © CCF

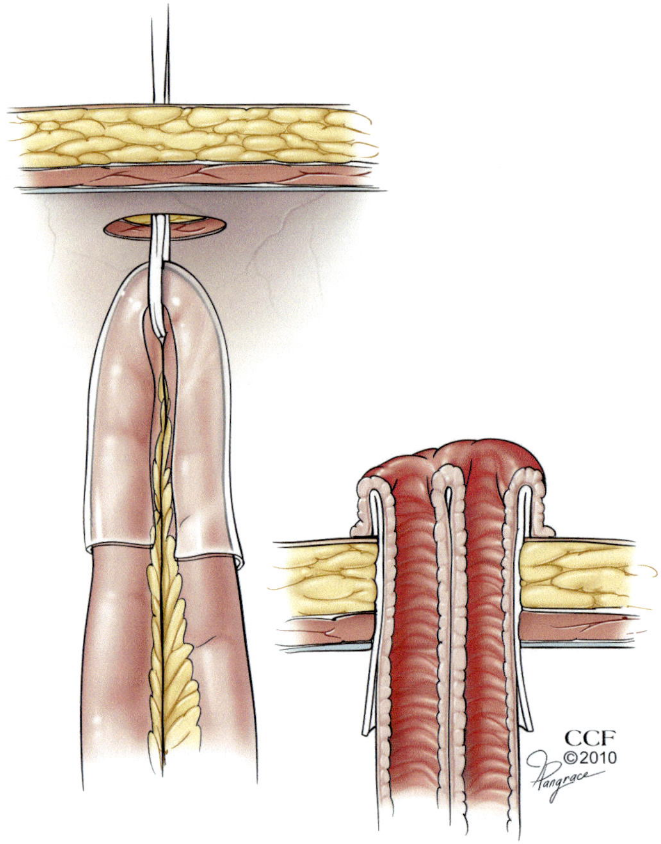

Fig. 23.2 Loop-end ileostomy with adhesive barriers. Illustration © CCF

Risk Factors for a Difficult Stoma

Preoperative

Some preoperative patient variables are uncontrollable and these are associated with difficult ostomy placement. These include a high body mass index (BMI), age, emergency surgery, and inflammatory bowel disease (IBD) [3, 23–25]. Other preoperative factors that can make placement more difficult include previous abdominal scars or incisions, abdominal wall hernias, and skin problems. These should be avoided or corrected at the time of operation.

One variable that is often overlooked is the need for an ostomy. Does the patient really need a stoma or is it possible to avoid placing an ostomy without increasing the risk of a complication? The idea of avoiding ostomy placement has been most obviously seen in relation to trauma and the early dogma of required intestinal diversion. It has been shown that intestinal ostomies are not always necessary in penetrating traumatic injuries to the colon or small intestine as well as in selected cases of low rectal reconstruction and with ileal pouch anal anastomosis (IPAA) [7, 26, 27]. The ostomy carries added risks when compared to patients who do not have an ostomy (discussed later) [3, 5, 10, 11, 28–30]. Similarly, ostomy closure itself carries a complication rate [11, 31–33].

Just as enterostomal nurses play a key role in the preoperative preparation of the stoma patient, they also provide valuable input in the postoperative care. They can help determine if a problem can be handled nonoperatively or if the problem may require surgery (see Chap. 6).

Operative

Operative variables that make ostomy construction difficult revolve around having adequate length of bowel and mesentery to allow for a tension-free stoma, and adequate blood supply or perfusion. Obesity, large pannus, a foreshortened or thickened mesentery secondary to inflammation, mesenteric fibrosis, short bowel syndrome (SBS), and IBD, all may create length issues, and subsequent tension on the stoma, with the potential for an ischemic ostomy segment. Intraperitoneal fibrosis from previous extensive abdominal surgery, carcinomatosis, and desmoid tumors make for difficult exteriorization of the ostomy. Some of these same

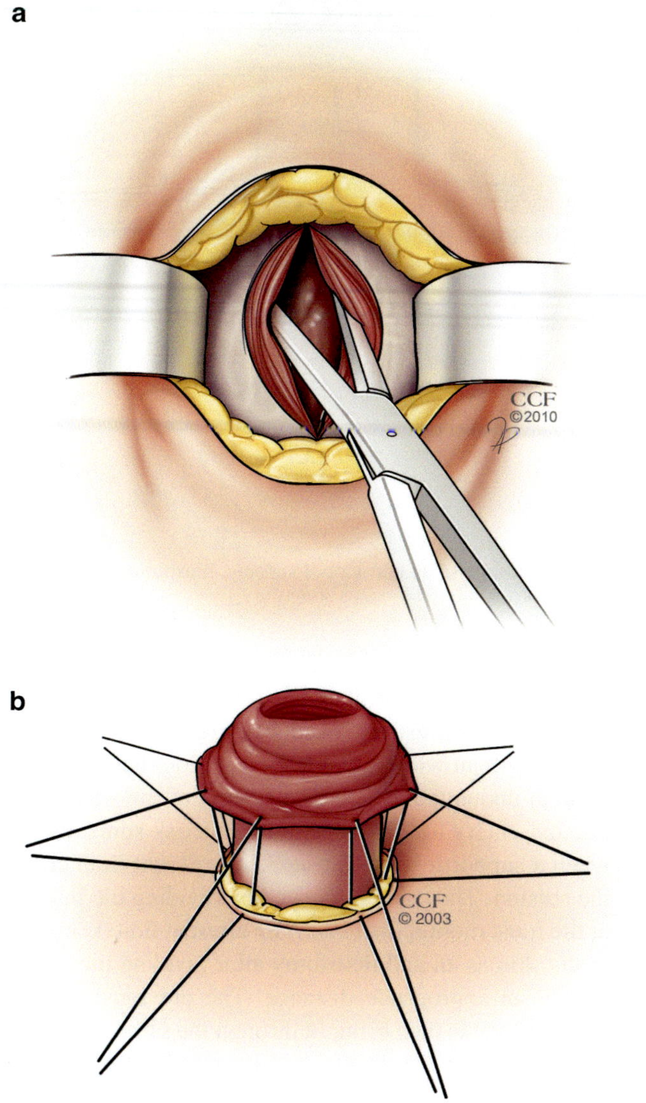

Fig. 23.3 (**a**) A rectus abdominus muscle-splitting incision approximately 3 cm (a two-finger aperture). (**b**) The cut edge of the ileum is sutured to the dermis. Illustration © CCF

variables predispose to an increased complication rate. The goal in elective as well as emergency surgery is to lessen their impact on ostomy construction.

Ileostomy Construction

After siting, ileostomy construction is usually not difficult owing to the highly vascularized, intraperitoneal nature of the small bowel. An ileostomy should be constructed with a rectus abdominus muscle-splitting incision, with an aperture large enough to allow the bowel to pass through without any additional intestine, approximately 3 cm, equaling a two-finger aperture (Fig. 23.3a). The cut edge of the ileum is

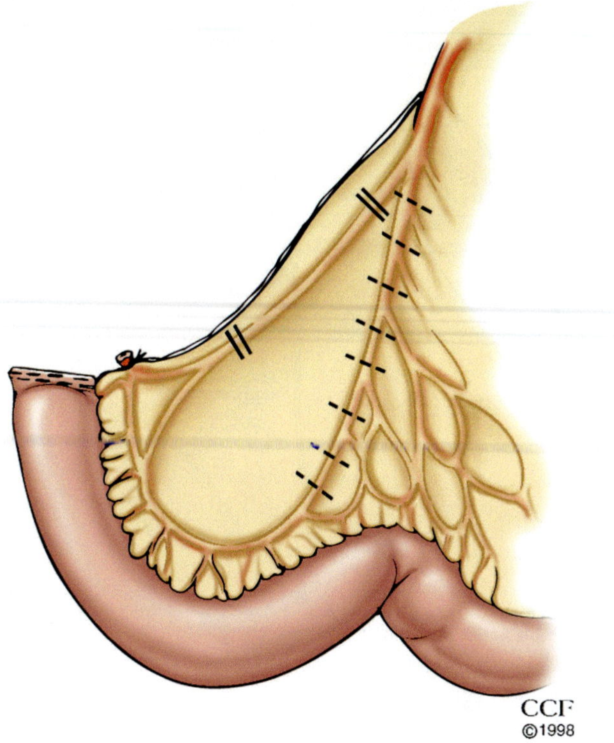

Fig. 23.4 Ligation of the ileocolic artery at its origin. Illustration © CCF

sutured to the dermis and not the epidermis, to prevent mucosal implants (Fig. 23.3b). A 2.5-cm spout allows easy pouching.

Difficulty with the bowel reaching the skin without tension most often arises with obese patients or patients with inflammatory bowel disease, who have had previous extensive resection of the small intestine. If an ostomy can be deferred in an obese patient, weight-loss surgery can aid in the formation of the ostomy. This can decrease the distance the ostomy needs to travel through the abdominal wall as the patient loses weight. Other patients with reach issues include those with a previous history of intestinal ischemia, necrotizing enterocolitis, desmoid tumor, omphalacele, or gastroschisis where a small bowel resection was performed.

Techniques for maximizing length include complete release of tethering structures:

- Division of the terminal ileum as close to the cecum as possible.
- Ligation of the ileocolic artery at its origin (Fig. 23.4).
- Dissection of the base of the small bowel mesentery to the third portion of the duodenum.
- Creation of windows in the small bowel mesentery overlying the superior mesenteric artery after injecting the mesentery with saline, thus lessening the chance of injuring the main feeding vessel (Fig. 23.5).

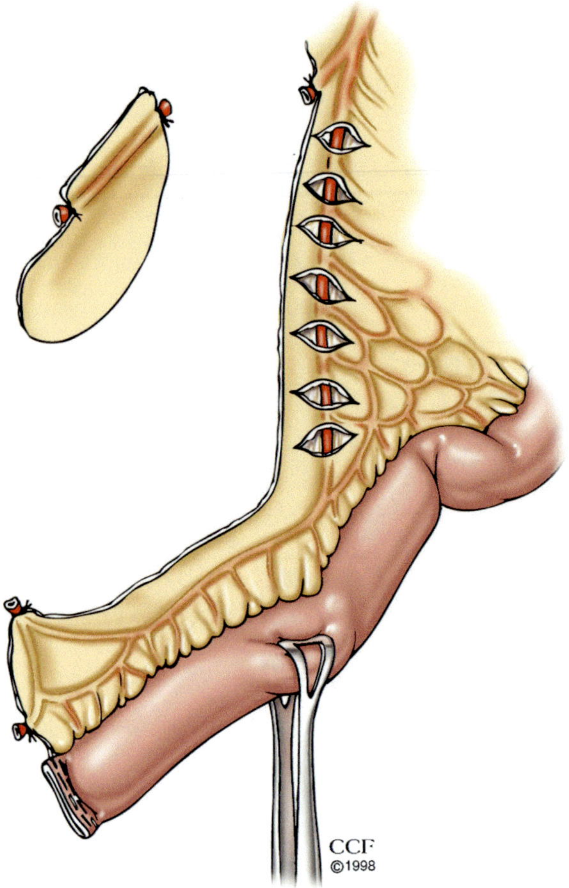

Fig. 23.5 Creation of windows in the small bowel mesentery overlying the superior mesenteric artery. Illustration © CCF

- Creation of a pedicalized ostomy, by incompletely skeletonizing the arcade and potentially the vasa recta from which they branch from the superior mesenteric artery. Additional maneuvers that can be used include:
- Division of the peristomal mesentery for 5 cm or less. This can be done as long as there is adequate submucosal collateral blood supply or the marginal artery is not ligated. This can provide up to an additional 5 cm of length.
- Supraumbilical placement of the stoma in obese patients with large and thick abdominal walls. Superior visualization and subsequent care is provided compared to a hidden lower abdominal ostomy.
- Creation of an end-loop ileostomy. Occasionally, the intestinal segment providing the greatest length is proximal to the proposed end ostomy. In this situation, the tethering structure is an important feeding artery. Its division would devascularize distal bowel, making ileostomy construction more difficult as an ischemic distal end may need to be resected. In this situation, using a more proximal intestinal segment with the greatest length to create an end-loop ileostomy may be beneficial (Fig. 23.6).

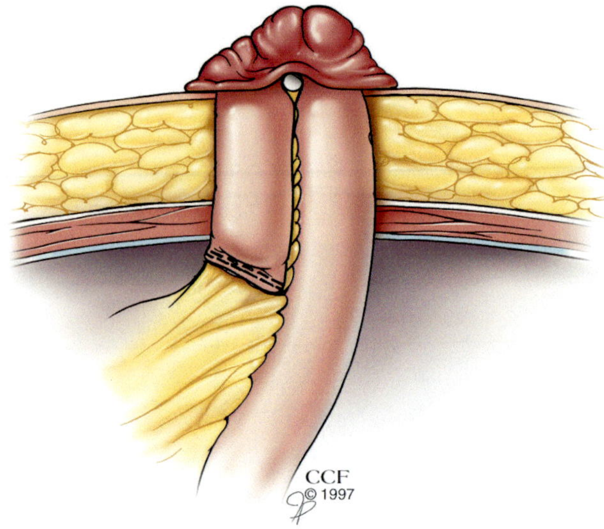

Fig. 23.6 Creation of an end-loop ileostomy. Illustration © CCF

- Creation of a loop-end ileostomy. This situation may occur with obese patients when a loop ostomy is needed. An everted loop ostomy cannot be created when the proposed segment will not reach the anterior abdominal wall without undue tension despite freeing of the small intestine mesentery to the duodenum. This risk spurs division when a supporting rod is used. The efferent limb creates the tension. This can be relieved by dividing the intestine at the most mobile ileal site. The afferent limb is brought to the skin as an end ileostomy after dividing the mesentery at an appropriate distance. The previously stapled efferent limb is then brought through the same trephine as the ileostomy (Fig. 23.7a, b). Panniculectomy may be done to excise the abdominal fat. This shortens the abdominal wall traverse. Elliptical skin excision is usually required with subcutaneous sump drainage.
- Division of the anterior and posterior rectus fascia and muscle to minimize the possibility of vascular compression. An 8–10-cm incision is placed through the peritoneum and posterior fascia. This incision is then approximated with interrupted sutures, left untied, until after bringing the ostomy through its aperture (Fig. 23.8). After suture tying, if an element of ischemia is present during the closure of the long division, fascial sutures are removed as needed.
  - Alternatively, to decrease the risk of potential trauma to an ostomy and its blood supply as it is delivered through its aperture, an Alexis® wound retractor (Applied Medical, Rancho Santa Margarita, CA 92688) can be used as a delivery device, facilitating passage.
- Insertion of a long mesenteric support rod may be used in near-desperate situations. This can be seen in cases of severe obesity, carcinomatosis, dense adhesions that prevent adequate mobilization, or in cases of extensive bowel

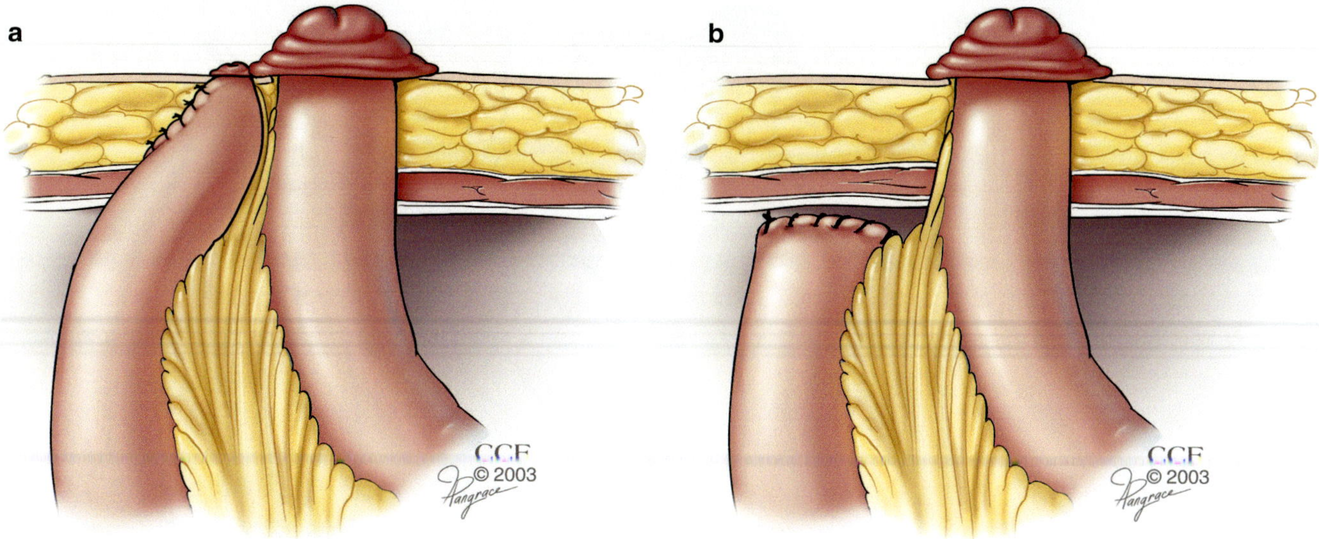

Fig. 23.7 (**a**, **b**) Creation of a loop-end ileostomy. The afferent limb is brought to the skin as an end ileostomy after dividing the mesentery at an appropriate distance. Illustration © CCF

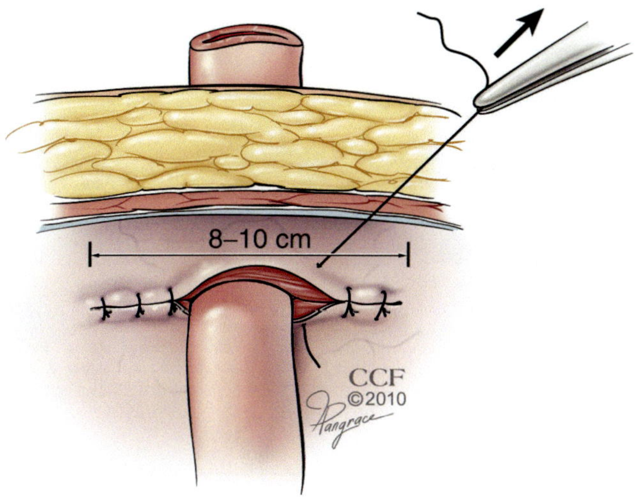

Fig. 23.8 An 8–10-cm incision is placed through the peritoneum and posterior fascia. Illustration © CCF

resection. In these situations, the inability to adequately mobilize the bowel can lead to spur division and ostomy necrosis. To help prevent this, the support rod, which can be attached to a ureteric filiform catheter, is inserted through the skin away from the ostomy, passing through the subcutaneous tissues as well as the mesentery and again back to the skin (Fig. 23.9a–c). The rod can also be placed so as to have the ostomy at the posterior fascia.

Colostomy Construction

Placement of a colostomy can have some similar difficulties; and similar construction techniques are used for a colostomy as for an ileostomy. However, for a sigmoid/descending colostomy, the ostomy site is located on the left of the abdomen, through the rectus abdominus, and the ostomy is everted less. Additionally, the epidermal mucosal implants are not seen with colostomies.

As much of the colon is a retroperitoneal structure, it is tethered to the posterior abdominal wall. These attachments along with inflammation and a large pannus in an obese patient can make constructing a colostomy difficult.

Again, techniques that can be used to gain length for a colostomy revolve around release of all tethering structures with vascular presentation. The steps then are:

- Takedown of lateral peritoneal attachments.
- Splenic flexure mobilization.
- Release of omental attachments.
- Early ligation of inferior mesenteric artery when needed for descending colon length. This allows evaluation of the adequacy of blood flow from the middle colic artery.
- High ligation of inferior mesenteric vein.
- Creation of windows in the colon mesentery.

Additional maneuvers that can be used include:

- Division of the peristomal mesentery for 2 cm or less. This can be done as long as there is adequate submucosal collateral blood supply or the marginal artery is not ligated. This can provide an additional 2 cm of length.
- Supraumbilical placement for obese patients with large and thick abdominal walls. The colostomy is easier to see compared to a hidden lower abdominal ostomy.
- Creation of an end-loop colostomy similar to its small intestine counterpart.
- Panniculectomy can be done to excise the substantially thick abdominal wall and its large amount of the intervening adipose tissue. This shortens the distance the ostomy must be positioned.

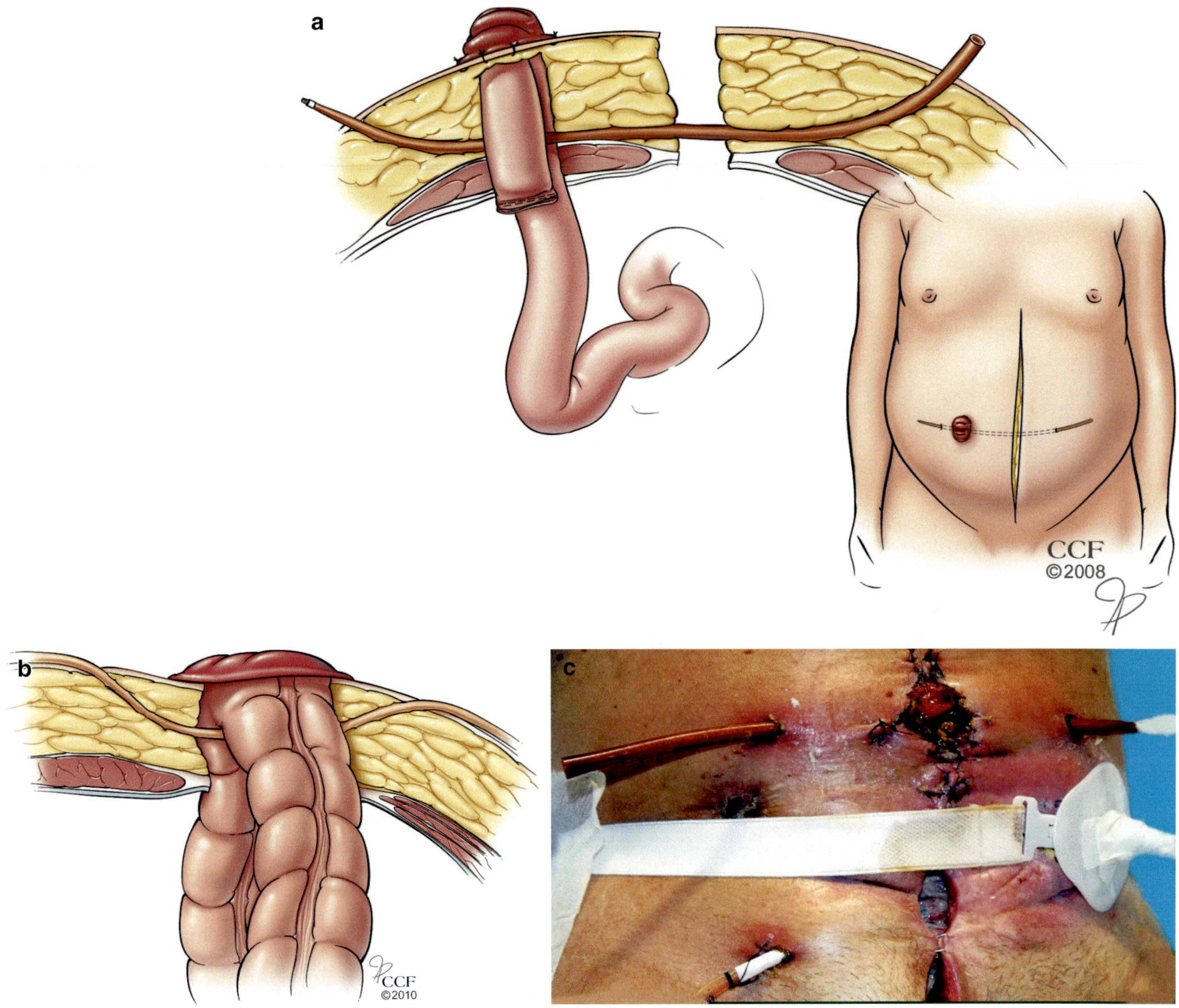

Fig. 23.9 (**a**) A long mesenteric support rod is inserted through the skin away from the ostomy, (**b**, **c**) passing through the subcutaneous tissues as well as the mesentery and again back to the skin. Illustration © CCF

Another factor possibly making colostomy construction difficult is insufficient collateral blood flow from the middle colic artery when the inferior mesenteric artery (IMA) is ligated at its origin. The adequacy of collateral flow can be tested prior to IMA ligation by placing a small vascular clamp on the IMA origin and assessing the viability of the intended ostomy segment. If the segment remains perfused, an ostomy can be constructed with the intended segment of colon. If ischemia is present, then a more proximal segment of viable colon will need to be used.

A difficult situation that may arise is with a friable inflammatory process involving the distal colon. In this situation, excision of all inflamed bowel may involve removal of an excessive amount of intestine. The alternative is to leave a very inflamed rectosigmoid junction. The inflammatory process creates a situation where the bowel is thickened, friable, and edematous and not easily accepting of suture. What can be done is a delayed maturation of an ostomy. After all grossly inflamed and involved intestine is resected, the rectosigmoid stump is brought through the abdominal wall, but not matured. It is covered with a gauze dressing and is left for maturation in the following days when inflammation has resolved and the bowel can be matured without the sutures tearing through the wall. This is done in the technique of a Turnbull-Cutait procedure. Alternatively, a non-sutured ostomy has been reported in the literature as being comparable to a sutured ostomy [34]. To perform both of the techniques described, sufficient length of an ostomy segment is obviously needed.

Early Postoperative Ostomy Complications

High Output

High ileostomy output is an expected sequelae when an ostomy is constructed using jejunum or proximal ileum. Patients undergoing IPAA are susceptible to this. When the stoma is temporary, the high output is temporary and resolves after stoma closure. Treatment of high ileostomy output revolves around providing adequate hydration, with appropriate electrolyte components as these patients tend to become hyponatremic. Additional measures to increase transit time and decrease output include administration of codeine elixir, tincture of opium, diphenoxylate/atropine, loperamide, as well as bile-binding agents like cholestyramine [35–39].

Obstruction

Ostomy obstruction falls into two categories – obstruction secondary to mechanical issues or secondary to functional problems. Obviously a mechanical obstruction in the early postoperative period may be adhesion-related or due to a tight aperture in the abdominal wall, or may be technical (a mesenteric twist or misplaced suture). Aid in the diagnosis can come from administering a gentle water-soluble contrast enema through the stoma or by endoscopy of the stoma.

In the early postoperative period, a functional obstruction is an ileus. There may be stoma effluent in the presence of an ileus, but this is usually pale green or yellow, watery, without gas, and without odor. It is often referred to as "bowel sweat" and does not mean that bowel function has returned. The patient may be nauseated or may vomit. The initial treatment in this situation is intestinal decompression with fluid and electrolyte replacement. The presence of bowel function is heralded by symptom resolution, ostomy flatus, and the presence of a thicker more feculent ostomy effluent.

Ischemia

Early postoperative ostomy ischemia and necrosis is a very serious and potentially life-threatening complication. The incidence of necrosis ranges from 1% to 21% [3, 4, 24, 25, 40]. Its degree can be mild and transient from minor trauma during ostomy construction to full-thickness necrosis. Its causes range from inadequate arterial blood supply to venous congestion. The initial step in dealing with ostomy ischemia is recognizing patients who are at risk – obese and those with foreshortened, tethered mesenteries. Prevention of this complication involves an uncompromising attitude to the blood supply of the stoma. At time of construction, there should be "nuisance" bleeding or bleeding requiring deliberate efforts to stop this bleeding at the bowel edge.

The most common cause of an ischemic stoma is devascularization of a segment's mesenteric blood supply. In general, dividing the mesentery at the bowel edge can be performed without ischemia for 2–5 cm from the cut end of the bowel [9, 41]. If a stoma looks ischemic when pulled through the aperture, the possibilities of fascial tension, mesenteric venous obstruction, vascular kinking from the trephine opening, or a mesenteric twisting should be considered. These problems should be corrected as discovered. Mesenteric venous obstruction or congestion should be suspected when a seemingly well-vascularized ileostomy begins to appear ischemic once passed through its abdominal aperture. This can be alleviated by "de-fatting" the areas between the vasa recta, allowing the veins to dilate further and relieve the congestion or obstruction.

Colonic ostomy ischemia can also occur if a segment's arterial supply is inadequate. This can be from its main blood supply; i.e., inferior mesenteric artery or collateral supply from the middle colic artery. It can also occur if the marginal artery, pericolonic fat, or epiploic appendices are divided. At the time of colon resection, if brisk bleeding is not seen from the marginal artery, an inadequate blood supply may be present. The procedure from here requires further colonic resection until brisk bleeding from the marginal vessels is seen.

Postoperatively, a darkening, grayish ostomy should prompt evaluation for ischemia. This can be determined by examining the ostomy mucosa with a glass test tube and light or gently scoring the mucosa with a needle, looking for adequate perfusion. If a demarcated segment is superficial to the fascia, a delayed revision can be performed. If the necrotic involvement extends below the fascia, immediate revision is performed as this segment can retract and lead to peritonitis and intra-abdominal sepsis [42]. Ostomy discoloration alone does not mandate immediate revision [40]. Mildly ischemic, but viable ostomies will often develop inflammatory exudates on their surface, which if wiped off will reveal underlying pink regenerating mucosa. A "Bishop's collar" stricture may develop as a late complication of no or delayed maturation of the ostomy. Almost always, an end ileostomy with mucosal ischemia results in a fibrotic ring of the muco-cutaneous junction, which may require revision later (Fig. 23.10; see also Chap. 14 Figs. 14.25, 14.26a, b and 14.27).

Peristomal Sepsis

A peristomal abscess is heralded by surrounding erythema, fluctuance, warmth, and tenderness. The source is commonly from an infected fluid collection or contamination at the time of ostomy creation. Another source is fistula formation. With any of these cases whether associated with an ileostomy or

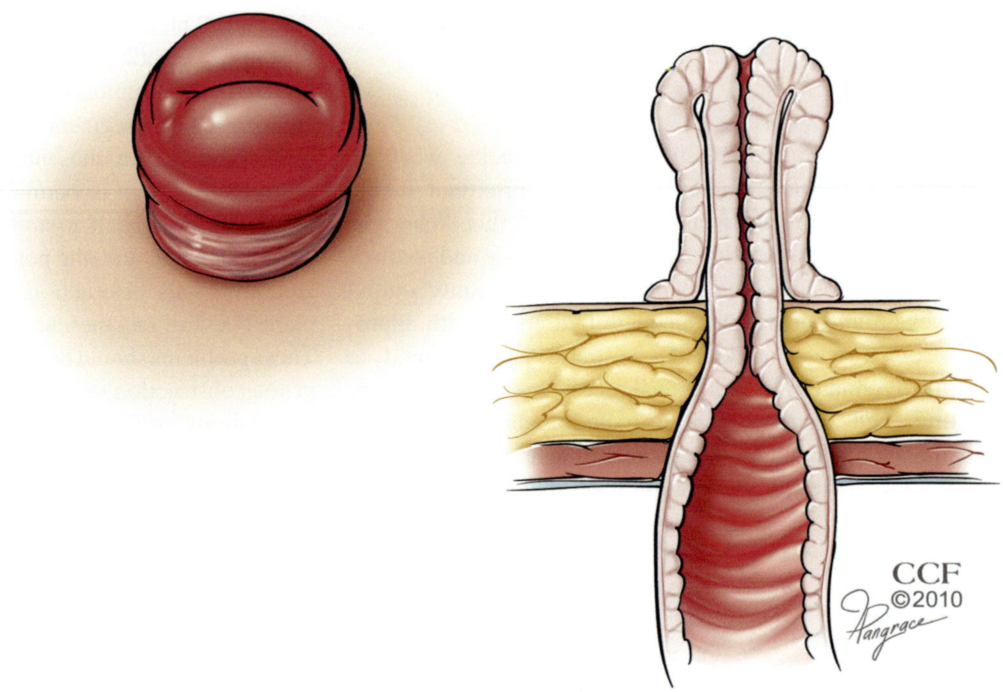

Fig. 23.10 A "Bishop's collar" stricture may develop as a late complication of the ostomy. Illustration © CCF

colostomy, the abscess should be drained. The drainage site should be either away from the pouching system or at the muco-cutaneous junction (Fig. 23.11). Both sites allow continued pouching without difficulty.

The usual cause for peristomal fistula is some form of trauma. This can be associated with disease exacerbation in patients with Crohn's Disease (CD). Seromuscular suturing of diseased or inflamed bowel, unknown enterotomy, and ostomy irrigation systems can be common sources of trauma. If the fistula is thought to be from local trauma and not an intra-abdominal process, with its external opening at the muco-cutaneous junction, a conservative approach can be taken. It can be pouched with the ostomy. Suspicion of an intra-abdominal source should prompt investigation and immediate correction with ostomy revision.

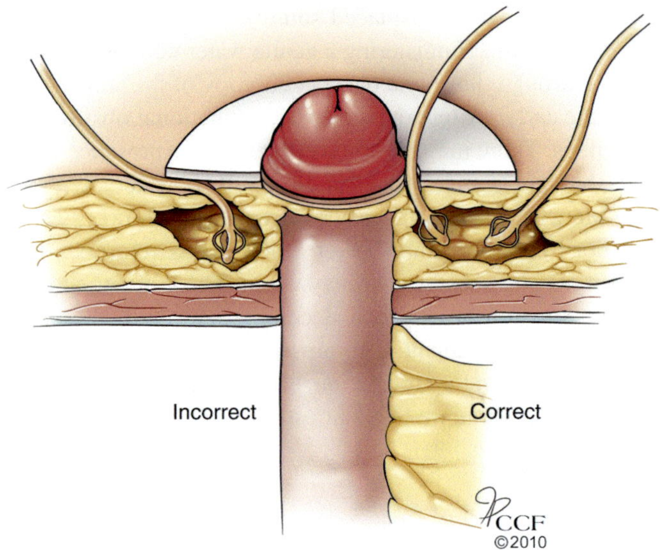

Fig. 23.11 Correct and incorrect drainage systems. Illustration © CCF

Late Ostomy Problems

Peristomal Hernia

Peristomal herniation occurs as bowel traverses a large ostomy aperture (see Chap. 20). It is an incisional hernia, and thought to occur more often with colostomies than with ileostomies [3, 16, 43–46]. Factors contributing to its development include those for the development of any hernia – obesity, a large fascial aperture, weakened abdominal wall from previous incisions, placement of an ostomy outside of the rectus muscle [3, 47, 48].

In the acute postoperative period, the development of a hernia is obviously a technical problem, the fascial trephine being made too large. This should be repaired immediately, usually reopening of the midline incision for adequate exposure for bowel reduction.

Not all peristomal hernias need repair. Patients who are asymptomatic or who cannot tolerate reoperation may be best served with an abdominal binder. Peristomal hernias that are symptomatic in patients who are surgical candidates may be repaired. Indications include:

1. Entrapment/irreduciblity
2. Obstructive symptoms
3. Enlarging hernia
4. Overlying skin stretching
5. Cosmetic countenance in some cases

The repair will be with or without relocation and with or without the use of prosthetic material. The incision used for repair must take into account the surrounding area normally used for pouching. If possible, it should be left undisturbed. This can be accomplished by using a semi-circular incision outside of the pouching stoma plate [49]. A radial incision can also be placed outside of the stoma plate, preventing interference with pouching. The hernia sac can be addressed through a racket incision also. Ideally, the fascial should be closed primarily. This is most possible when adequate fascia is present in a thin patient, not prone to placing detrimental pressure and tension on the repair. If the defect cannot be closed primarily, a mesh material should be used, with the ostomy site lateral to the repair. Newer biological acellular dermal mesh materials may help prevent infectious complications associated with surgery in contaminated fields [50, 51]. The same biologic meshes can be used prophylactically in patients with increased risk for development of herniation – obese, malnourished, immunosuppressed, chronic cough (chronic obstructive pulmonary disease [COPD]) (see Chap. 20).

For patients with recurrent peristomal hernias and those in whom a good appliance seal cannot be maintained, relocating the ostomy site with closure of the hernia defect is the best option. This can be accomplished with placement of the new ostomy on the contralateral side or through a new rectus abdominus site on the ipsilateral side. The choice of relocation site should be the best possible site even though it is on the same side.

Stoma Prolapse

A similar condition to peristomal hernia is stomal prolapse, as a large fascial trephine predisposes patients to this. Mesenteric fixation sutures can help prevent this from occurring. As with hernias, an asymptomatic patient need not have a repair. Those patients who are symptomatic may be candidates for surgery. This most often occurs with colostomies and the first decision revolves around the need for the ostomy. If continuity can be restored, it should. If the ostomy cannot be closed, then local repair can be performed. With an end ostomy, this will involve an ostomy revision with or without a resection and placement of mesenteric fixation sutures to prevent recurrent prolapse. Additionally two-directional myotomy can be made. This is done by making serial incisions through the bowel serosa. This will allow fixating adhesions to form when the bowel edge is reflected upon itself, thus decreasing the possibility of prolapse.

Temporary loop ostomies may be closed. Loop ostomies that cannot be closed, such as those proximal to complete bowel obstruction, can be revised locally by dividing the bowel and creating an end ostomy with adjacent mucous fistula or loop-end ostomy. This will allow decompression proximally and distally. At times, ostomy relocation may be needed, especially if the fascial aperture is very large and repair cannot be accomplished easily or the original ostomy is in a suboptimal site.

Retraction

Ostomy retraction can occur due to inadequate mobilization of a bowel segment, poor location or fixation, steroid dependence, and obesity. Occasionally, this can still be pouched with minimal problems using concave stoma plates and belts and with weight reduction [52]. When pouching becomes an issue, surgical correction by revision is warranted. Fixation sutures are placed at the mesentery-fascial interface and the mesentery-subcutaneous fat. The ostomy is then matured to the dermis. Other techniques include creation of a loop-end ostomy, placement of longitudinal staples paramesenterically, and two-directional myotomy.

Stricture

Ostomy stricture is an uncommon problem that usually is the result of ischemia of the ostomy. In the case of CD patients, recurrent disease is the likely cause. Other causes include previous radiation therapy, or external compression (e.g., constricting skin or fascial opening) [9]. When this complication does occur, symptomatic patients should undergo local revision of the ostomy with relocation reserved for patients with local skin problems precluding the use of current ostomy site. Dilatation of the stricture rarely provides lasting improvement.

In patients who are poor surgical candidates in need of ostomy revision, ostomy resiting using a "railroading" or "tunneling" technique can be used. This is done by making a circumferential ostomy incision, delivering it outside the abdomen. An umbilical tape is placed around the end. After making the re-sited ostomy incision, a large Kelly clamp or similar is passed through the new aperture, grasping the umbilical tape and delivering the ostomy through the new aperture. This technique is best used in patients without dense anterior abdominal wall adhesions [53].

Conclusions

As with any surgery, ostomy creation is a life-changing event and deserves careful attention. Its construction influences a person's quality of life. It should be constructed with the utmost care to lessen the problems associated with an ostomy. In the best situations, problems will still occur and this is more so when a difficult ostomy creation is encountered. By minimizing complications, a viable, well-perfused, tension-free ostomy can be created in difficult situations. This is facilitated by preoperative marking, meticulous construction technique, and the application of the maneuvers discussed in this chapter.

References

1. Londono-Schimmer EE, Leong APK, Phillips RKS. Life table analysis of stomal complications following colostomy. Dis Colon Rectum. 1994;37(9):916–20.
2. Makela JT, Niskasaari M. Stoma care problems after stoma surgery in Northern Finland. Scand J Surg. 2006;95:23–7.
3. Park JJ, Del Pino A, Orsay CP, Nelson RL, Pearl K, Cintron JR, et al. Stoma complications: the cook county hospital experience. Dis Colon Rectum. 1999;42(12):1575–80.
4. Leong APK, Londono-Schimmer EE, Phillips RKS. Life-table analysis of stomal complications following ileostomy. Br J Surg. 1994;81:727–9.
5. O'Toole GC, Hyland JM, Grant DC, Barry MK. Defunctioning Loo ileostomy: a prospective audit. J Am Coll Surg. 1999;188:6–9.
6. Gooszen AW, Geelkerken RH, Hermans J, Lagaay MB, Gooszen HG. Quality of life with a temporary stoma: ileostomy vs. colostomy. Dis Colon Retum. 2000;43:650–5.
7. Tsunoda A, Tsunoda Y, Narita K, Watanabe M, Nakao K, Kusano M. Quality of life after low anterior resection and temporary loop ileostomy. Dis Colon Rectum. 2008;51:218–22.
8. O'Leary DP, Fide CJ, Foy C, Lucarotti ME. Quality of life after low anterior resection with total mesorectal excision and temporary loop ileostomy for rectal carcinoma. Br J Surg. 2001;88:1216–20.
9. Wu JS, Fazio VW. Difficult stomas. Persp Colon Rectal Surg. 1998;10:33–60.
10. Gooszen AW, Geelkerken RH, Hermans J, Lagaay MB, Gooszen HG. Temporary decompression after colorectal surgery: randomized comparison of loop ileostomy and loop colostomy. Br J Surg. 1998;85:76–9.
11. Winslet MC, Barsoum G, Pringle W, Fox K, Keighley MRB. Loop ileostomy after ileal pouch-anal anastomosis—Is it necessary? Dis Colon Rectum. 1991;34:267–70.
12. American Society of Colon and Rectal Surgeons and the Wound Ostomy Continence Nurse Society. Joint position statement on the value of preoperative stoma marking for patients undergoing ostomy surgery. J Wound Ostomy Continence Nurs. 2007;34:627–8.
13. Engel J, Kerr J, Schlesinger-Raab A, Eckel R, Sauer H, Holzel D. Quality of life in rectal cancer patients. Ann Surg. 2003;238:203–13.
14. Nugent KP, Daniels P, Stewart B, Patankar R, Johnson C. Quality of life in stoma patients. Dis Colon Rectum. 1999;42:1569–74.
15. Rozen BL. The value of a well-placed stoma. Cancer Pract. 1997;5(6):347–52.
16. Rullier E, Le Toux N, Laurent C, Garrelon J, Parneix M, Saric J. Loop ileostomy versus loop colostomy for defunctioning low anastomoses during rectal cancer surgery. World J Surg. 2001;25: 274–8.
17. den Dulk M, Smit M, Peeters K, Kranenbarg E, Rutten H, Wiggers T, et al. A multivariate analysis of limiting factors for stoma reversal in patients with rectal cancer entered into the total mesorectal excision (TME) trial: a retrospective study. Lancet Oncol. 2007;8: 297–303.
18. Peeters KC, Tollenaar RA, Marijnen CA, Klein KE, Steup WH, Wiggers T, et al. Risk factors for anastomotic failure after total mesorectal excision of rectal cancer. Br J Surg. 2005;92:211–6.
19. Tilney HS, Sains PS, Lovegrove RE, Reese GE, Heriot AG, Tekkis PP. Comparison of outcomes following ileostomy versus colostomy for defunctioning colorectal anastomoses. World J Surg. 2007;31: 1142–51.
20. Tjandra JJ, Chan MK. A sprayable hydrogel adhesion barrier facilitates closure of defunctioning loop ileostomy: a randomized trial. Dis Colon Rectum. 2008;51:956–60.
21. Tang CL, Seow-Chen F, Fook-Chong S, Eu KW. Bioresorbable adhesion barrier facilitates early closure of the defunctioning ileostomy after rectal excision: a prospective, randomized trial. Dis Colon Rectum. 2003;46:1200–7.
22. Salum M, Wexner SD, Nogueras JJ, Weiss E, Koruda M, Behrens K, et al. Does sodium hyaluronate- and carboxymethylcellulose-based bioresorbable membrane (seprafilm) decrease operative time for loop ileostomy closure? Tech Coloproctol. 2006;10:187–90; discussion 190–1.
23. Harris DA, Egbeare D, Jones S, Benjamin H, Woodward A, Foster ME. Complications and mortality following stoma formation. Ann R Coll Surg Engl. 2005;87(6):427–31.
24. Arumugam PJ, Bevan L, Macdonald L, Watkins AJ, Morgan AR, Beynon J, et al. A prospective audit of stomas—analysis of risk factors and complications and their management. Colorectal Dis. 2003;5(1):49–52.
25. Duchesne JC, Wang Y, Weintraub SL, Boyle M, Hunt JP. Stoma complications: a multivariate analysis. Am Surg. 2002;68(11):961–6; discussion 966.
26. Demetrios D, Murray J, Chan L, Ordonez C, Bowley D, Nagy KK, et al. Penetrating colon injuries requiring resection: diversion or primary anastomosis? An AAST prospective multicenter study. J Trauma. 2001;50:765–75.
27. Remzi FH, Fazio VW, Gorgun E, Ooi BS, Hammel J, Preen M, et al. The outcome after restorative proctocolectomy with or without defunctioning ileostomy. Dis Colon Rectum. 2006;49:470–7.
28. Wexner SD, Taranow DA, Johansen OB, Itzkowitz F, Daniel N, Nogueras JJ, et al. Loop ileostomy is a safe option for fecal diversion. Dis Colon Rectum. 1993;36:349–54.
29. Senapati A, Nicholls RK, Ritchie JK, Tibbs CJ, Hawley PR. Temporary loop ileostomy for restorative proctocolectomy. Br J Surg. 1993;80:628–30.
30. Carlsen E, Bergan AB. Loop ileostomy: technical aspects and complications. Eur J Surg. 1999;165:140–3.
31. Pokorny H, Herkner H, Jakesz R, Herbst F. Predictors for complications after loop stoma closure in patients with rectal cancer. World J Surg. 2006;30:1488–93.
32. Pokorny H, Herkner H, Jakesz R, Herbst F. Mortality and complications after stoma closure. Arch Surg. 2005;140:956–60.
33. Mansfiel SD, Jensen C, Phair AS, Kelly OT, Kelly SB. Complications of loop ileostomy closure: a retrospective cohort analysis of 123 patients. World J Surg. 2008;32(9):2101–6.
34. Mackay G, Goldberg J. Self-everting ileostomy. Colorectal Dis. 2007;9:763–4.
35. King RF, Norton T, Hill GL. A double-blind cross-over study of the effect of loperamide hydrochloride and codeine phosphate on ileostomy output. Aust N Z J Surg. 1982;52:121–4.
36. Newton CR. Effect of codeine phosphate, lomotil and isogel on ileostomy function. Gut. 1978;19:377–83.
37. Modlin M. Urinary calculi and ulcerative colitis. Br Med J. 1972;3(821):292.

38. Fukushima T, Sugita A, Masuzawa S, Yamazaki Y, Takemura H, Tsuchiya S. Prevention of uric acid stone formation by sodium bicarbonate in an ileostomy patient: a case report. Jpn J Surg. 1988;18:465–8.
39. Christl SU, Scheppach W. Metabolic consequences of total colectomy. Scand J Gastroenterol Suppl. 1997;222:20–4.
40. Carlsen E, Bergan AB. Technical aspects and complications of end-ileostomies. World J Surg. 1995;19:632–6.
41. Fleshman Jr JW. Ostomies. In: Hicks TC, Beck DE, Opelka FG, Timmcke AE, editors. Complications of colon and rectal surgery. Baltimore: Williams and Wilkins; 1996. p. 357–81.
42. Kann BR, Cataldo TE. Early stomal complications. Clin Colon Rectal Surg. 2002;15:191–8.
43. Pearl RK. Parastomal hernias. World J Surg. 1989;13:569–72.
44. Martin L, Foster G. Parastomal hernia. Ann R Coll Surg Engl. 1996;78:81–4.
45. Williams JG, Etherington R, Hayward MWJ, Hughes LE. Paraileostomy hernia: a clinical and radiological study. Br J Surg. 1990;77:1355–7.
46. Steel MCA, Wu JS. Late stomal complications. Clin Colon Rectal Surg. 2002;15:199–207.
47. Turnbull Jr RB, Weakley FL. Atlas of intestinal stomas. St. Louis: Mosby; 1967.
48. Sjodahl R, Anderberg B, Bolin T. Parastomal hernia in relation to the site of the abdominal stoma. Br J Surg. 1988;75:339–41.
49. Thorlakson RH. Technique of repair of herniations associated with colonic stomas. Surg Gynecol Obstet. 1965;120:347–50.
50. Kim H, Bruen K, Vargo D. Acellular dermal matrix in the management of high-risk abdominal wall defects. Am J Surg. 2006; 192:705–9.
51. Patton Jr JH, Berry S, Kralovich KA. Use of human acellular dermal matrix in complex and contaminated abdominal wall reconstructions. Am J Surg. 2007;193:360–3.
52. Young MJ. Convexity in the management of problem stomas. Ostomy Wound Manage. 1992;38:53–60.
53. Taylor Jr RL, Rombeau JL, Turnbull Jr RB. Transperitoneal relocation of the ileal stoma without formal laparotomy. Surg Gynecol Obstet. 1978;146(6):953–8.

Index

V.W. Fazio et al. (eds.), *Atlas of Intestinal Stomas*,
DOI 10.1007/978-0-387-78851-7, © Springer Science+Business Media, LLC 2012

Q

R

S

MIX
Papier aus verantwortungsvollen Quellen
Paper from responsible sources
FSC® C105338

If you have any concerns about our products,
you can contact us on
ProductSafety@springernature.com

In case Publisher is established outside the EU,
the EU authorized representative is:
Springer Nature Customer Service Center GmbH
Europaplatz 3, 69115 Heidelberg, Germany

Printed by Libri Plureos GmbH
in Hamburg, Germany